AIRWAY MANAGEMENT

AIRWAY MANAGEMENT

EDITORS

Leland H. Hanowell, M.D.
Associate Professor
Director, Post Anesthesia Care Unit
Attending Physician, Surgical Intensive Care Unit
Department of Anesthesiology
University of California, Davis School of Medicine and Medical Center
Sacramento, California

Richard J. Waldron, M.B.B.S., F.A.N.Z.C.A.
Staff Specialist Anaesthetist
Department of Anaesthetic Services
Royal Hobart Hospital
Honorary Senior Clinical Lecturer
University of Tasmania
Hobart, Tasmania, Australia

ASSOCIATE EDITOR

Judith C.F. Hwang, M.D.
Assistant Professor
Department of Anesthesiology
University of California, Davis School of Medicine and Medical Center
Sacramento, California

Lippincott - Raven
PUBLISHERS
Philadelphia • New York

Printed in the United States of America

9 8 7 6 5 4 3 2 1

Library of Congress Cataloging-in-Publication Data

Airway management / editors, Leland H. Hanowell, Richard J. Waldron; associate editor, Judith C. F. Hwang.
p. cm.
Includes bibliographical references and index.
ISBN 0-397-51520-0
1. Airway (Medicine) 2. Trachea—Intubation. 3. Respiratory intensive care. 4. Anesthesiology. I. Hanowell, Leland H. II. Waldron, Richard J. III. Hwang, Judith C. F.
[DNLM: 1. Airway Obstruction—therapy. 2. Intubation. 3. Drug Therapy. 4. Emergencies. WF 140 A2978 1996]
RC732.S37 1996
616.2—dc20
DNLM/DLC 96-14755
for Library of Congress CIP

Care has been taken to confirm the accuracy of the information presented and to describe generally accepted practices. However, the authors, editors, and publisher are not responsible for errors or omissions or for any consequences from application of the information in this book and make no warranty, express or implied, with respect to the contents of the publication.

The authors, editors, and publisher have exerted every effort to ensure that drug selection and dosage set forth in this text are in accordance with current recommendations and practice at the time of publication. However, in view of ongoing research, changes in government regulations, and the constant flow of information relating to drug therapy and drug reactions, the reader is urged to check the package insert for each drug for any change in indications and dosage and for added warnings and precautions. This is particularly important when the recommended agent is a new or infrequently employed drug.

Some drugs and medical devices presented in this publication have Food and Drug Administration (FDA) clearance for limited use in restricted research settings. It is the responsibility of the health care provider to ascertain the FDA status of each drug or device planned for use in their clinical practice.

Contents

Contributing Authors

Roblee P. Allen, M.D., F.A.C.C.P.
Associate Professor
Division of Pulmonary/Critical Care Medicine
Department of Internal Medicine
University of California
Davis School of Medicine and Medical Center
2315 Stockton Boulevard
Sacramento, California 95817

Malcolm B. Anderson, M.B.B.S, F.A.N.Z.C.A.
Senior Lecturer in Anaesthetics
University of Tasmania
Staff Anaesthetist
Department of Anaesthetic Services
Royal Hobart Hospital
Liverpool Street
Hobart, Tasmania
Australia 7001

Felix D. Battistella, M.D.
Assistant Professor of Surgery
Department of Surgery
University of California
Davis School of Medicine and Medical Center
4301 X Street
Sacramento, California 95817

Anthony J. Bell, M.B., B.S., M.D., F.R.A.C.P.
Associate Professor and Director
Department of Critical Care Medicine
Royal Hobart Hospital
Liverpool Street
Hobart, Tasmania
Australia 7001

Alison M. Berry, M.B., Ch.B., F.R.C.A.
Staff Anaesthetist
Nambour Hospital
Nambour, Queensland
Australia

Joseph R. Brimacombe, M.B., Ch.B., F.R.C.A.
Clinical Associate Professor
Department of Anaesthesia and Intensive Care
Queensland University
Cairns Base Hospital
Cairns, Queensland
Australia 4870

Christopher S. Butler, M.B.B.S., F.A.N.Z.C.A.
Staff Anaesthetist
Department of Anaesthesia and Intensive Care
Townsville General Hospital
Eyre Street
Townsville, Queensland
Australia 4810

Sheila D. Cooper, M.D.
Assistant Clinical Professor of Anesthesiology
Department of Anesthesia
University of California,
San Diego Medical Center
200 West Arbor Drive # 8770
San Diego, California 92103

Suanne M. Daves, M.D.
Assistant Clinical Professor of Anesthesiology
Department of Anesthesiology
University of California
Irvine Medical Center
101 City Drive South
Orange, California 92668

Jan M. Davies, M.Sc., M.D., F.R.C.P.C.
Professor of Anaesthesia
Department of Anaesthesia
Foothills Hospital and
University of Calgary
1403 Twenty-Ninth Street Northwest
Calgary, Alberta
Canada T2N 2T9

Christopher J. Eagle, B.Sc., M.D., F.R.C.P.C.
Associate Professor of Anaesthesia
Department of Anaesthesia
Foothills Hospital and
University of Calgary
1403 Twenty-Ninth Street Northwest
Calgary, Alberta
Canada T2N 2T9

Mark R. Ezekiel, M.D., M.S.
Assistant Clinical Professor and
Director of Cardiothoracic Anesthesia
Department of Anesthesiology
University of California
Irvine Medical Center
101 City Drive South
Orange, California 92668

Wendy J. Falloon, M.B.B.S., D.A.(U.K.), F.A.N.Z.C.A.
Specialist Anaesthetist
303 Macquarie Street
Hobart, Tasmania
Australia 7000

Dennis L. Fung, M.D.
Professor of Anesthesiology
Department of Anesthesiology
University of California
Davis School of Medicine
4150 V Street
Sacramento, California 95817

Ahmed Ghouri, M.D.
Anesthesia Resident
Department of Anesthesiology
University of California
Irvine Medical Center
101 City Drive South
Orange, California 92668

Adolph H. Giesecke, M.D.
Jenkins Professor of Anesthesiology
Department of Anesthesiology
University of Texas
Southwestern Medical School
5323 Harry Hines Boulevard
Dallas, Texas 75235-9068

Thomas J. Gilman, M.D.
Assistant Professor
Department of Anesthesiology
University of California
Davis School of Medicine and Medical Center
2315 Stockton Boulevard
Sacramento, California 95817

Jennifer Hall, M.B., B.S., F.A.N.Z.C.A.
Assistant Professor
Department of Anesthesiology
University of California
Davis School of Medicine and Medical Center
2315 Stockton Boulevard
Sacramento, California 95817

Leland H. Hanowell, M.D.
Associate Professor
Director, Post Anesthesia Care Unit
Attending Physician, Surgical Intensive Care Unit
Department of Anesthesiology
University of California
Davis School of Medicine and Medical Center
2315 Stockton Boulevard
Sacramento, California 95817

Jonathan L. Howes, M.B.B.S., D.A., F.R.C.A.
Senior Anaesthetic Registrar
Sir Humphry Davy Department of Anaesthesia
Bristol Royal Infirmary
Bristol, United Kingdom
BS2 8HW

Judith C.F. Hwang, M.D.
Assistant Professor
Department of Anesthesiology
University of California
Davis School of Medicine and Medical Center
4150 V Street, Suite 1200
Sacramento, California 95817

Richard S. Isaacs, M.D.
Department of Otolaryngology–Head and Neck Surgery
University of California
Davis School of Medicine and Medical Center
2315 Stockton Boulevard
Sacramento, California 95817
Attending Head and Neck Surgeon
Kaiser-Permanente, Northern California Region
Sacramento, California 95823

Ronald L. Katz, M.D.
Chairman, Department of Anesthesiology
University of Southern California
School of Medicine, and
Los Angeles County/University of Southern California Medical Center
Los Angeles, California 90033

Charles P. Kingsley, M.D.
Associate Professor of Anesthesiology
Department of Anesthesiology
The Pennsylvania State University School of Medicine
Hershey, Pennsylvania 17033

Robert G. Loeb, M.D.
Associate Professor of Anesthesiology
Department of Anesthesiology
University of California
Davis Medical Center
4150 V Street, Suite 1200
Sacramento, California 95817

Douglas R. Mest, M.D.
Staff Anesthesiologist
Long Beach Community Medical Center; and
Assistant Clinical Professor
Department of Anesthesiology
University of California
Irvine Medical Center
101 City Drive South
Orange, California 92668

Peter G. Moore, M.D., Ph.D.
Professor of Clinical Anesthesiology
Department of Anesthesiology
University of California
Davis Medical Center
4150 V Street, Suite 1200
Sacramento, California 95817

Debra E. Morrison, M.D.
Assistant Clinical Professor
Department of Anesthesiology
University of California
Irvine Medical Center
101 City Drive South
Orange, California 92668

James E. Morrison, M.D.
Department of Surgery
University of California
Davis School of Medicine and Medical Center
4301 X Street, Room 2310
Sacramento, California 95817

John M. Mott, M.D.
Department of Anesthesiology
University of California
Davis School of Medicine and Medical Center
2315 Stockton Boulevard
Sacramento, California 95817

Mark T. Murphy, M.D.
Department of Anesthesia
University of Texas
Southwestern Medical School
5323 Harry Hines Boulevard
Dallas, Texas 75235-9068

Michael J. Paech, M.B.B.S., D.R.C.O.G., F.R.C.A., F.A.N.Z.C.A.
Head, Department of Anaesthesia
King Edward Memorial Hospital for Women
374 Bagot Road
Subiaco
Perth, Western Australia
Australia 6008

Rajesh V. Patel, M.D.
Assistant Professor of Anesthesiology
Department of Anesthesiology
University of Southern California
School of Medicine, and
Los Angeles County/University of Southern California Medical Center
Los Angeles, California 90033

Russell T. Reid, R.C.P., R.R.T., C.P.F.T.
Adult Intensive Care Unit Coordinator
Department of Respiratory Care
University of California
Davis Medical Center
2315 Stockton Boulevard
Sacramento, California 95817

Jalil Riazi, M.D.
Associate Clinical Professor and Vice Chairman
Department of Anesthesiology, and
Director of Pediatric Anesthesia
University of California
Irvine Medical Center
101 City Drive South
Orange, California 92668

Antonio Sanchez, M.D.
Associate Clinical Professor of Anesthesia
Department of Anesthesiology
University of California
Irvine Medical Center
101 City Drive South
Orange, California 92668

William C. Santos, M.D.
Assistant Clinical Professor of Anesthesia
Department of Anesthesiology
University of California
Davis Medical Center
4150 V Street, Suite 1200
Sacramento, California 95817; and
Staff Physician
Central Anesthesia Service Exhange
3315 Watt Avenue
Sacramento, California 95821

Vance E. Shearer, M.D.
Assistant Professor of Anesthesiology
Department of Anesthesiology
University of Texas
Southwestern Medical Center
5323 Harry Hines Boulevard
Dallas, Texas 75235-9068

Marcus W. Skinner, M.Sc., B.Med.Sc., M.B.B.S.
Senior Anaesthetic Registrar
Department of Anaesthetic Services
Fremantle Hospital
Alma Street
Perth,
Western Australia 6160

Jonathan M. Sykes, M.D.
Associate Professor, Facial Plastic and Reconstructive Surgery
Department of Otolaryngology–Head and Neck Surgery
University of California
Davis School of Medicine and Medical Center
2315 Stockton Boulevard
Sacramento, California 95817

Richard J. Waldron, M.B.B.S., F.A.N.Z.C.A.
Staff Specialist Anaesthetist
Department of Anaesthetic Services
Royal Hobart Hospital; and
Honorary Senior Clinical Lecturer
University of Tasmania
GPO Box 1061L
Hobart, Tasmania
Australia 7001

David A. White, M.D.
Associate Professor of Anesthesiology
Department of Anesthesiology
University of California
Davis School of Medicine and Medical Center
2315 Stockton Boulevard
Sacramento, California 95817

William C. Wilson, M.D.
Assistant Clinical Professor
Department of Critical Care Medicine and Cardiothoracic Anesthesiology
University of California
San Diego Medical Center
200 West Arbor Drive #8770
San Diego, California 92103

Preface

Airway Management presents the fundamental principles in assessing, managing, and treating various airway problems encountered in the prehospital period, emergency room, operating room, and intensive care unit. This book is intended for practicing physicians, residents in the medical and surgical specialties, medical students, paramedics, and emergency and critical care nurses. It will also be of value in the training of respiratory therapists. It provides a detailed review of the anatomy of the airway, pharmacology of the various drugs used for urgent airway access, and descriptions of equipment used for maintaining and intubating the airway, as well as discussions of prehospital strategies. Clinical circumstances addressed include trauma, pediatrics, cardiac arrests, and other case scenarios. This book is designed to be an on-hand reference with drawings and photographic illustrations of various techniques, in addition to tables and drug dosages to aid the practicing physician. The five appendices give detailed information regarding difficulties in intubation, indications for intubation, appropriate tube sizes, and drug dosages. Specific chapters are devoted to paramedic issues, and there is a detailed review of transport ventilators and the clinical issues pertinent to patient transport and rescue.

Airway Management will be an essential reference for any physician or other key medical care provider interested in airway assessment and instrumentation, surgery, or special techniques in the management of the airway.

Acknowledgments

The editors wish to acknowledge the International Trauma Anesthesia and Critical Care Society (ITAACS) for its efforts to improve both the level of prevention and clinical management of trauma on a global basis. The efforts of the Society to advance airway management and other modalities of trauma management will improve patient care worldwide.

PART I

Airway Basics

Airway Management, edited by
L.H. Hanowell, M.D. and R.J. Waldron, M.D.,
Lippincott-Raven Publishers, Philadelphia © 1996.

CHAPTER 1

Applied Anatomic Considerations in Airway Management

Jonathan M. Sykes and Richard S. Isaacs

INTRODUCTION

Normal respiration involves a highly detailed neurophysiologic process that results in the exchange of inspired and expired air through various anatomic structures. An understanding of these structures is important before mastering the techniques of maintaining or re-establishing the normal airway. The following anatomic discussion focuses on the features crucial for the establishment and maintenance of a tracheal airway.

THE NOSE

The external nose is formed by the nasal bones, the upper and lower lateral cartilages, the cartilaginous portion of the nasal septum, and skin. The surface anatomy and associated infrastructure of the nose are depicted in Figs. 1 and 2. The paired elliptical nostrils are separated by the pliable portion of the nasal septum and columella. The nose has a bony framework in its upper portion comprised of the two nasal bones and the bones that form the posterior septum: the vomer (inferiorly) and the perpendicular plate of the ethmoid (superiorly). The lower and anterior portions of the nose are supported mainly by cartilage.

Nasal Cavity

The nasal cavity is divided into two passages or fossae by the nasal septum. The nasal septum is a rigid partition formed by the perpendicular plate of the ethmoid, the vomer, and the septal cartilage (Fig. 3). The nasal septum, contained within its mucoperichondrial and mucoperiosteal envelope, is normally a midline structure but is frequently deviated to one side.

Each nasal fossa is described as having a roof, a floor, a medial wall (nasal septum) and a lateral wall. The pas-

R.S. Isaacs: Department of Otolaryngology–Head and Neck Surgery, University of California, Davis School of Medicine and Medical Center, Sacramento, California 95817; and Kaiser-Permanente, Northern California Region, Sacramento, California 95823.
J.M. Sykes: Department of Otolaryngology–Head and Neck Surgery, University of California, Davis School of Medicine and Medical Center, Sacramento, California 95817.

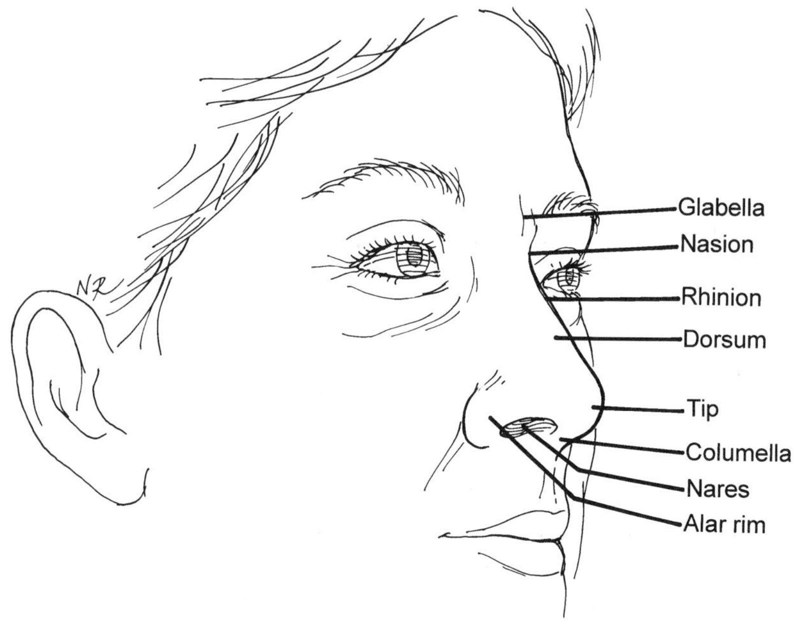

FIG. 1. Surface anatomy of the nose.

sages open anteriorly by way of the anterior naris, or nostril. The nasal passages open posteriorly by way of the posterior naris, or choana, into the nasopharynx. The anterior nares are located at the base of the nose and open inferiorly. Directly above each naris is the anterior aspect of the nasal cavity, which is termed the "nasal vestibule." The nares and vestibule are bounded by the medial and lateral crura of the alar cartilage and surrounding fibrofatty tissue. The skin of the vestibule is thin and tightly adherent to the underlying lower lateral cartilages. The medial wall of the nasal vestibule contains the supporting structure of the anterior part of the cartilaginous septum and the connective tissue septum (i.e., the columella). In the lateral portion of the vestibule, the skin contains course hairs (vibrissae) that guard the nasal entrance and assist in air filtration.

Lateral Walls

The lateral walls of the nasal passages are composed of irregular bony projections covered by soft tissue and

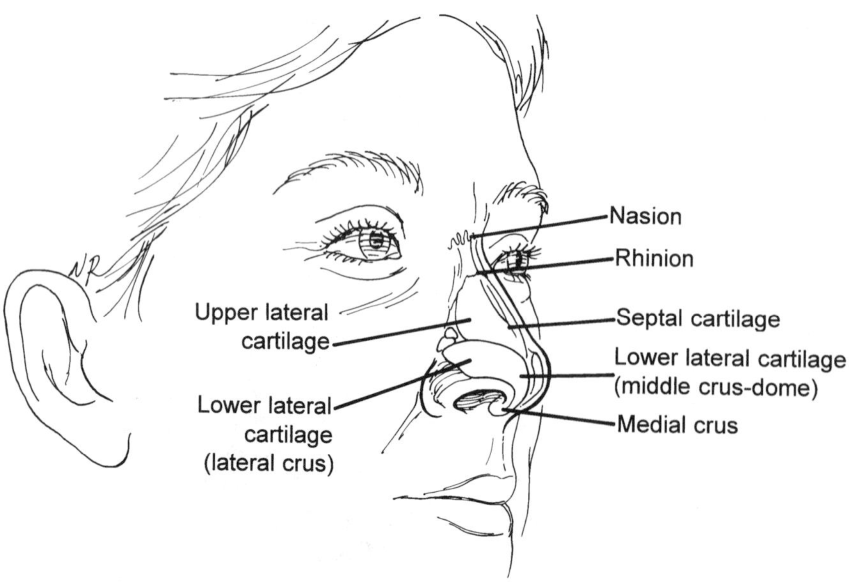

FIG. 2. Infrastructure of the nose.

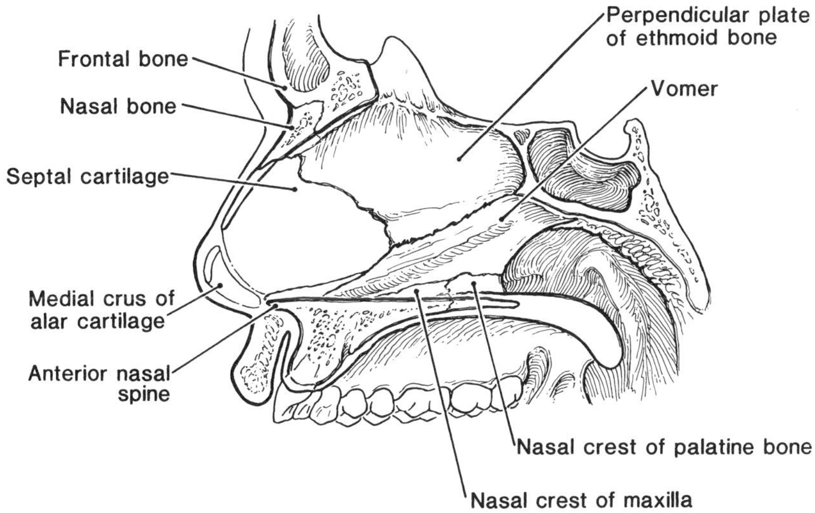

FIG. 3. Schematic diagram of the nasal septum. Note that the septum is made up of the anterior nasal septal cartilage and the perpendicular plate of the ethmoid bone and the vomer. Other contributions include portions of the palatine bone and the maxilla.

mucous membrane (Fig. 4). These elevations, whose course is roughly parallel to the nasal floor, are the inferior, middle, superior, and supreme nasal conchae or turbinates. The space beneath each turbinate is called a "meatus"; its nomenclature corresponds to that of the adjacent turbinate (e.g., the middle meatus is located directly beneath the middle turbinate). The ethmoid bone contributes to the structure of the supreme, superior, and middle turbinates. The inferior turbinate, however, derives its structure from a separate bone. The lateral nasal wall also contains the ostia or openings of the paranasal sinuses and the nasolacrimal duct (Fig. 4). The inferior meatus lies between the floor of the nose and the insertion of the inferior turbinate. The inferior meatus does not contain a sinus ostium, but the opening of the nasolacrimal duct is located approximately 3 cm posterior to the external nasal opening. The middle meatus is located between the inferior and middle turbinates and contains the ostia of the nasofrontal duct, the anterior ethmoid cells, and the maxillary sinus. The superior meatus is located superior to the middle turbinate and contains the opening for the posterior ethmoid cells. The sphenoid ostium lies on the anterior wall of the sphenoid sinus in the area of the sphenoethmoidal recess.

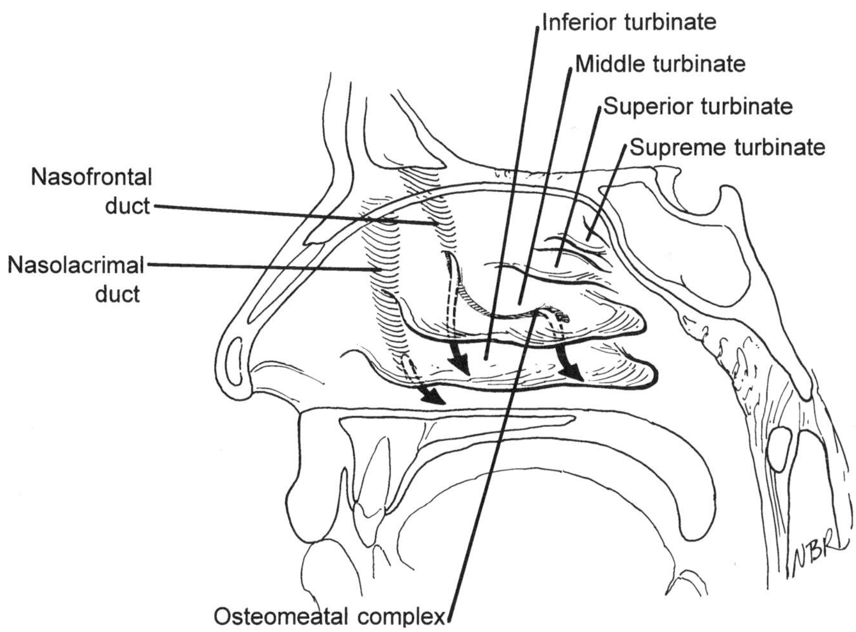

FIG. 4. Schematic diagram of the right lateral wall of the nose (the left side of the nose and nasal septum have been removed). The *arrows* depict the course of the nasolacrimal duct, the nasofrontal duct, and the opening to the maxillary sinus through their corresponding bones.

Posterior Nares (Choana)

Each posterior naris or choana is oval in shape and measures approximately 2.5 cm vertically and 1.5 cm horizontally. The posterior naris is completely bounded by bone covered by mucoperiosteum. The posterior nares are usually symmetric as the posterior portion of the septum is consistent and does not usually deviate in this region. There are, however, occasional cases of congenital choanal atresia and posttraumatic bony septal deviations. In these instances, posterior obstruction of the septum may occur.

Functions of the Nose

The nose has several very important functions in addition to its role as a conduit to the lower respiratory tract. Inspired air is warmed, humidified, and cleansed during its turbulent flow over the membranous lining of the nasal passages. The rich vascular supply of the turbinates allows the nasal airway to expand or contract according to the degree of vascular engorgement. Trauma to the nasal passages may result in profuse hemorrhage because of their rich blood supply. Other nasal functions include olfaction and phonation (the nose acts as an additional resonating chamber for certain consonants).

THE PHARYNX

The pharynx is a musculofascial tube that connects the nasal and oral cavities with the larynx and esophagus. The pharyngeal tube is composed of a thin outer fascial layer that thickens posteriorly to become the buccopharyngeal fascia. Inferiorly, this fascia becomes continuous with the adventitia of the esophagus, while superiorly it attaches to the skull base.

Constrictor Muscles

The middle muscular layer is composed of the three pharyngeal constrictor muscles: The superior constrictor inserts at the base of the skull, the middle constrictor muscle inserts into the hyoid bone, and the inferior constrictor muscle inserts into the cricoid cartilage (Fig. 5). The inferior constrictor contributes to a muscular band, the cricopharyngeus, which forms the upper esophageal sphincter. Each muscular segment is overlapped at its lower border by the adjacent inferior muscle segment. All muscle segments are inserted posteriorly into a tendinous median raphe (Fig. 5).

Divisions of the Pharynx

The pharynx is divided into three sections: the nasopharynx, the oropharynx, and the hypopharynx (Fig. 6).

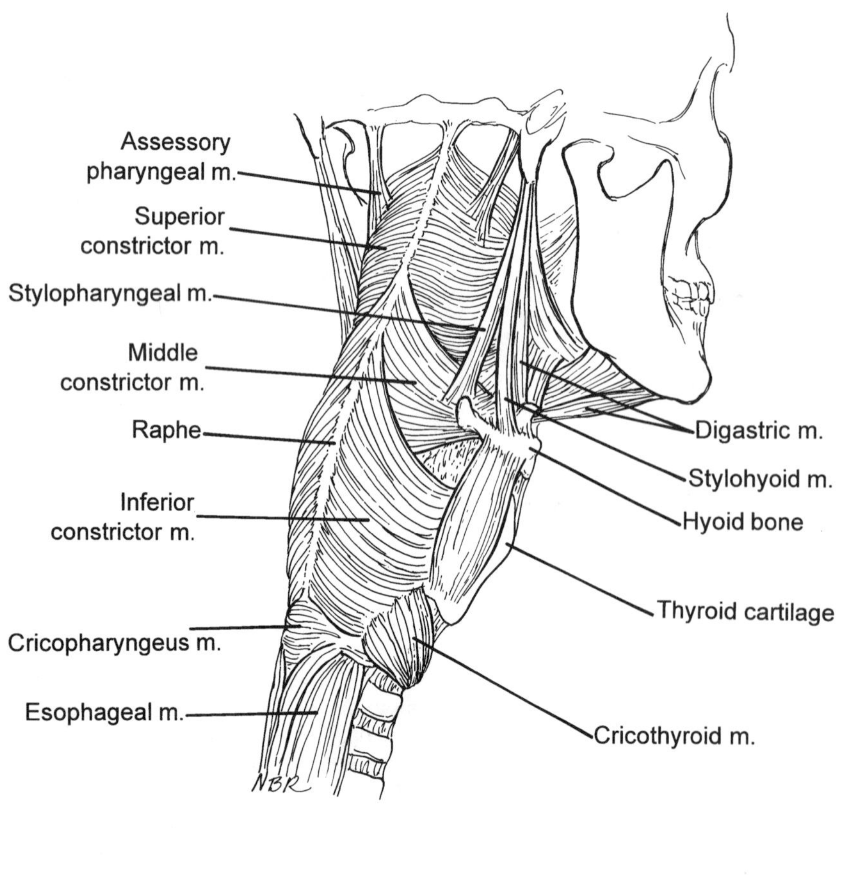

FIG. 5. Right posterior oblique view of the pharynx depicting the pharyngeal musculature. Note the overlapping of the pharyngeal constrictors and their insertion into the posterior midline as a tendinous raphe.

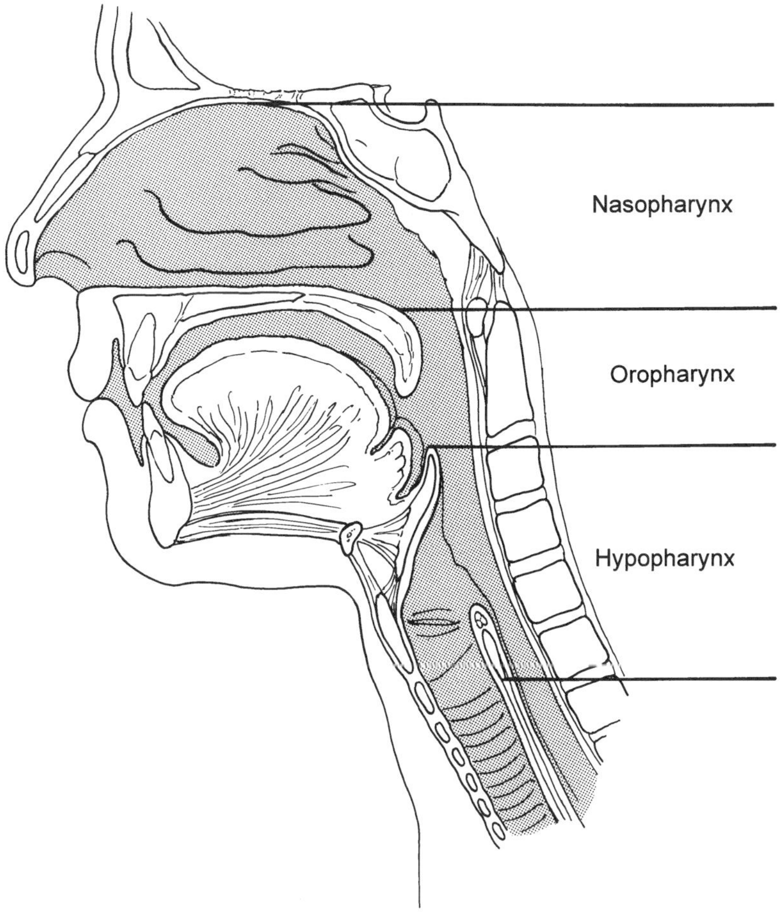

FIG. 6. Parasagittal view of the upper aerodigestive tract depicting the delineation of the nasopharynx, oropharynx, and hypopharynx.

The very delicate muscular framework of the pharynx makes this structure prone to lacerations, retropharyngeal dissection, and the iatrogenic creation of false passages. Therefore, a knowledge of these structures is critical for the practitioner before attempting tracheal intubation.

Nasopharynx

The nasopharynx is situated directly behind the nasal cavity. Its inferior boundary is a line drawn transversely at the level of the soft palate. Five passages communicate with the nasopharynx: the two nasal choanae, the orifices of the two eustachian tubes, and the inferior outlet to the oropharynx. The roof of the nasopharynx is formed by the sphenoid and occipital bones of the skull base. The roof slopes gradually posteriorly and is continuous with the posterior nasopharyngeal wall. The posterior wall of the nasopharynx is separated from the spinal column by the tough prevertebral fascia, which covers the longus capitis muscle, the deep prevertebral musculature, and the arch of the first cervical vertebra.

Each eustachian tube orifice is located medial to the lateral cartilaginous prominence called the "torus tubarius." Above and behind the torus is a recess called the "fossa of Rosenmüller." The eustachian tube functions to equalize middle ear and atmospheric pressure when pulled open by the specialized action of the palatal muscles.

The mucous membrane of the roof and posterior walls of the nasopharynx contains lymphoid tissue termed the "single pharyngeal or adenoid tonsil." Massive hypertrophy of the adenoid can result in chronic nasal airway obstruction. This condition may create difficulty in establishing a nasotracheal airway, or it may contribute to sleep apnea/altered arterial CO_2 levels. The adenoid tonsil, however, typically involutes during puberty.

Oropharynx

The oropharynx lies directly posterior to the oral cavity and extends from the soft palate superiorly to the tip of the epiglottis inferiorly. The posterior wall consists of the prevertebral fascia and the bodies of the second and third cervical vertebrae. The lateral walls of the oropharynx contain the paired tonsillar fossae (Fig. 7). These fossae are formed by the palatoglossal (anterior pillar) and palatopharyngeal (posterior pillar) folds and contain the palatine tonsils.

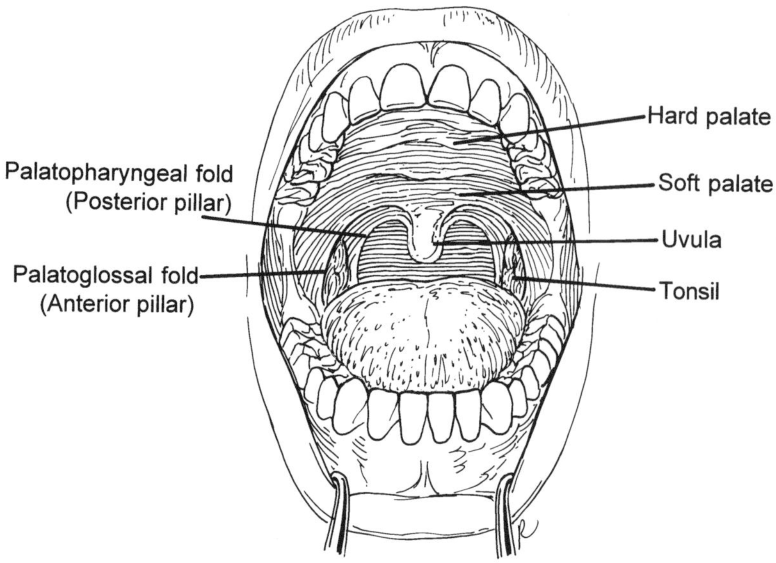

FIG. 7. Intraoral view of the open mouth depicting the tonsillar fossae and the corresponding tonsillar pillars.

Directly medial to the tonsillar fauces lies the posterior aspect, or base, of the tongue. The tongue base is anterior to the laryngeal inlet and attaches to the epiglottis by the paired lateral glossoepiglottic folds and by the single median glossoepiglottic fold. The glossoepiglottic folds bound two spaces, called the "epiglottic valleculae." The posterior dorsal tongue surface is irregular in contour because of the lingual tonsils.

In some children, the palatine tonsils may reach considerable size and actually obstruct exposure of the larynx during intubation. As is commonly seen with the adenoid tonsil, the palatine tonsils usually involute after puberty.

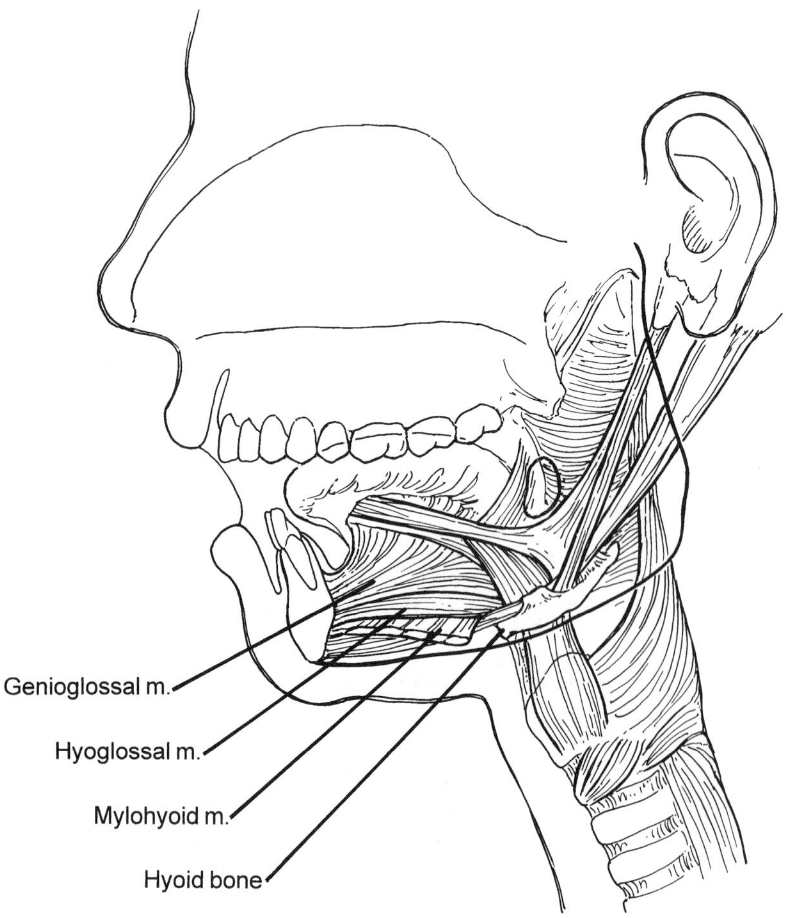

FIG. 8. Parasagittal view of the muscles of the floor of the mouth with their corresponding insertions into the tongue, mandible, and hyoid bone.

Figure 8 demonstrates the parasagittal view of the oropharynx with emphasis on the musculature of the tongue and the floor of the mouth. The tongue is comprised of a specialized group of paired muscles that provide it with extreme mobility. The tongue musculature is divided into two groups: those muscles that are attached to fixed points (the styloglossus, the genioglossus, the hyoglossus, and the palatoglossus muscles), and those muscles that run freely in the body of the tongue (the transverse, superior, and inferior longitudinal muscles, and the vertical muscles). The floor of the mouth is supported mainly by the paired mylohyoid muscles, which arise from the mandible and insert into the hyoid bone.

Cellulitis of the submandibular and submental spaces can involve the floor of the mouth, located superior to the mylohyoid muscle. This process, known as "Ludwig's angina," usually follows a dental extraction or infection. The tongue muscles are usually involved and become edematous and displaced posteriorly. Rapid progression of the infection can produce airway obstruction. A tracheotomy is commonly required to secure the airway before incision and wide drainage of the floor of the mouth is performed.

Hypopharynx

The hypopharynx extends inferiorly from the upper edge of the epiglottis to the inferior edge of the cricoid cartilage and communicates with three structures: the oropharynx, the laryngeal inlet, and the esophagus. On each side of the larynx are the funnel-shaped piriform recesses. These recesses are bounded superiorly by the lateral glossoepiglottic folds and lie between the aryepiglottic folds and the internal lining of the thyroid cartilage (Fig. 9). The piriform recesses function to divert the food bolus laterally and away from the larynx in transit to the esophagus. The posterior border of the hypopharynx comprises the buccopharyngeal and prevertebral fascia and deep prevertebral musculature. The hypopharynx is located approximately at the level of the fourth through sixth cervical vertebrae.

THE LARYNX

Functions of the Larynx

The larynx is continuous with the trachea and has a specialized constrictor-dilator mechanism in the airway. The sphincteric, protective function is the oldest phylogenetic function of the larynx, having developed from aquatic amphibian predecessors. The constrictor mechanism of the larynx results in an effective and rapid closure that prevents food, liquid, and other foreign material from entering the lower airway. In addition, the vocal cords have a vibratory effect on the expiratory air column and produce the sound used in voice production.

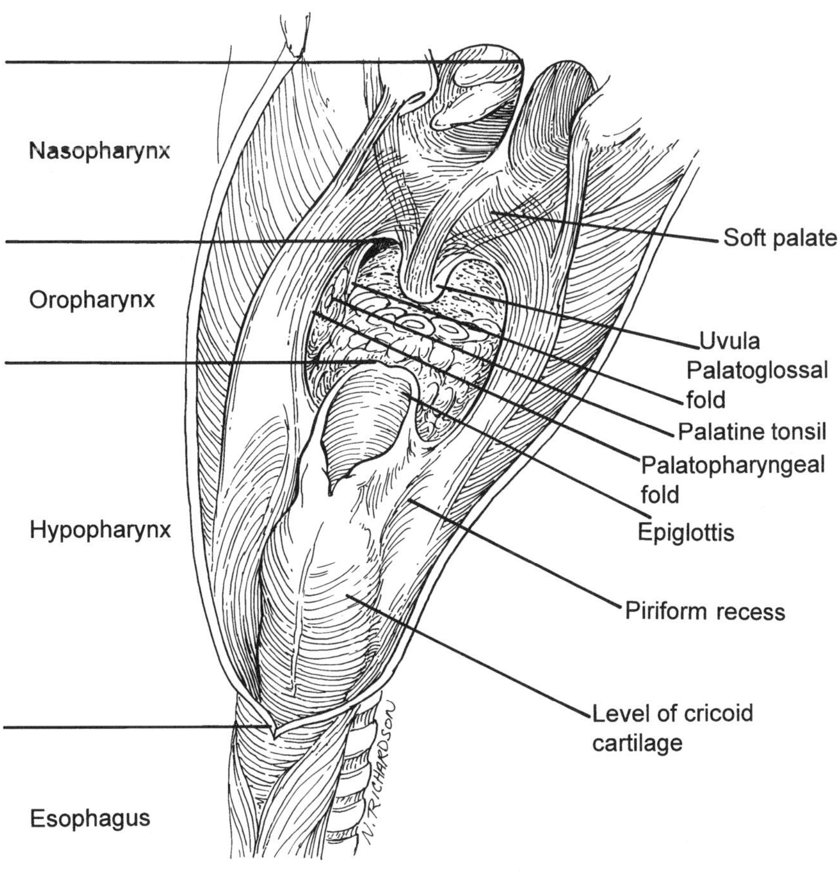

FIG. 9. Right posterior oblique view of the open pharynx depicting the relationship of the aryepiglottic folds, larynx, epiglottis, and piriform recesses.

Placement of a tracheal tube through the larynx interferes with these laryngeal functions. The intubated patient experiences loss of voice and possible aspiration of foreign material into the airway. In addition, the presence of the tube prevents the production of an adequate protective cough.

Laryngeal Skeleton

The laryngeal skeleton is formed predominantly by the thyroid and cricoid cartilages and the hyoid bone (Fig. 10A,B). These structures are readily palpated in the anterior midline of the neck. The thyroid cartilage is respon-

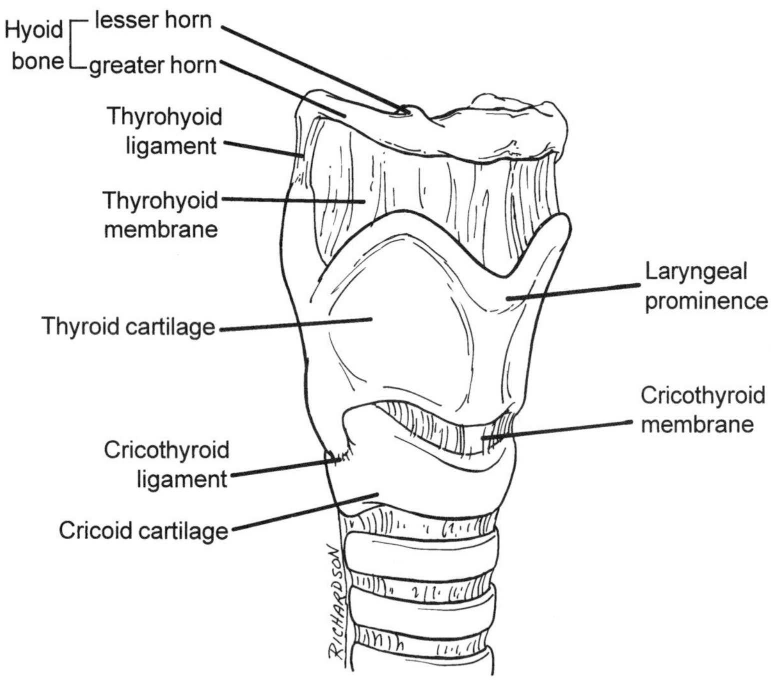

FIG. 10. A: Right anterolateral lateral view of the laryngeal skeleton.

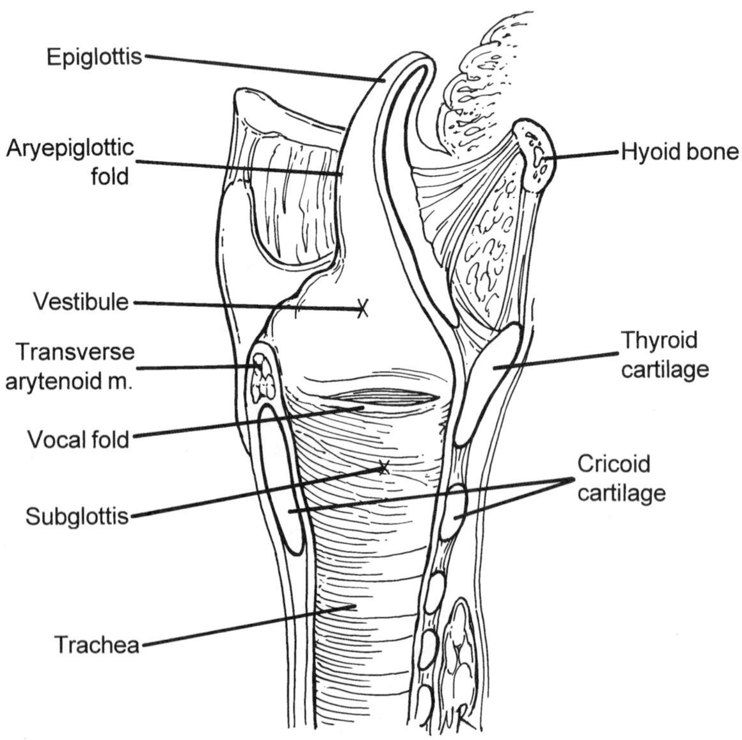

FIG. 10. B: Parasagittal view of the laryngeal skeleton showing the relationship of the epiglottis, thyroid and cricoid cartilages, and the glottis.

sible for the visible bulge (especially in male patients) known as the "Adam's apple."

The thyroid cartilage is composed of two superior horns, which aid in its suspension from the hyoid bone. The two horns join in the midline and remain open posteriorly. This forms an effective shield (Greek *thyrus*, "shield") for the opening of the airway and supports most of the soft tissue folds in the larynx. Two downward projections, inferior horns, articulate with the cricoid cartilage below.

Cricoid Cartilage

The cricoid cartilage (Greek *cricos*, "ring") is the only complete ring in the larynx and serves to support the posterior laryngeal structures. The anterior portion of the cricoid is short, measuring 5 to 7 mm in height, and the posterior portion of the cricoid is taller, measuring 2 to 3 cm in height. The posterior lamina is marked by a posterior ridge, which receives longitudinal fibers of the esophagus. The cricoid has two surfaces that articulate with the thyroid cartilage.

First Tracheal Ring

The first tracheal ring attaches to the cricoid cartilage by a dense cricotracheal ligament. The thyroid cartilage is attached above to the hyoid bone by the thyrohyoid membrane, and below to the cricoid cartilage by the cricothyroid membrane. Because of the relatively superficial location of the laryngotracheal complex, the cricothyroid membrane may be penetrated (cricothyroidotomy) to establish an airway in an emergency situation.

Epiglottis and Arytenoid Cartilages

Two additional cartilages contribute to the laryngeal skeleton. The epiglottic cartilage forms the anterior border of the laryngeal inlet and is attached to the hyoid bone and thyroid cartilage by several ligaments. The epiglottis is composed of cartilage and a covering mucous membrane. The bulk of the epiglottis projects posteriorly to the tongue and into the pharynx. The anterior surface of the epiglottis is concave; this feature, combined with laryngeal elevation, aids in airway protection during deglutition. The arytenoid cartilages are pyramidal in shape and articulate with the posterior parts of the cricoid cartilage. The intricate muscles of voice control are attached to the two arytenoid cartilages, and the vocal cords project anteriorly from the arytenoid cartilages to the thyroid cartilage. Movement of the cricoarytenoid joints from the action of the laryngeal muscles causes a change in size of the opening between the vocal cords.

Vocal Cords

The vocal cords are also called the "true vocal cords" or "vocal folds." They are composed of muscle, ligament, submucosal soft tissue, and mucous membrane covering. The vocal cords extend from the arytenoid cartilages posteriorly to the thyroid cartilage anteriorly. The laryngeal cavity begins at its entrance, the laryngeal aditus, and is bounded by the aryepiglottic folds. The laryngeal aditus leads into the vestibule, which in turn leads into the rima vestibuli. The rima vestibuli is bounded by two mucosal folds that are parallel and superior to the vocal folds; these are called the "ventricular folds," or "false vocal cords." The lateral spaces between the ventricular and vocal folds are called the "ventricles." The narrow space between the vocal folds is called the "rima glottidis," while the term "glottis" is used to refer to the rima glottidis and the adjacent true vocal cords. The space that leads from the rima glottidis to the trachea is the infraglottic cavity or subglottis.

Muscles of the Larynx

The intrinsic muscles of the larynx include the posterior cricoarytenoid (the only abductor of the vocal cords), lateral cricoarytenoid, transverse arytenoid, oblique arytenoid, thyroarytenoid, and the aryepiglottic muscles (Fig. 11). The intrinsic muscles and the solitary extrinsic muscle, the cricothyroid muscle, act synergistically and antagonistically to control the specialized functions of the larynx.

Nerve Supply of the Larynx

At the level of the hyoid bone, the vagus nerve gives off the superior laryngeal nerve, which immediately divides into internal and external laryngeal nerves. The larger, internal laryngeal nerve pierces the thyrohyoid membrane and supplies sensory fibers to the laryngeal mucosa down to the level of the vocal folds. The external laryngeal nerve courses on the lateral surface of the middle and inferior parts of the pharyngeal constrictor and finally reaches the level of the cricoid cartilage, where it supplies the cricothyroid muscle. The remainder of the intrinsic laryngeal muscles are supplied by the recurrent laryngeal nerve. On the right, the recurrent laryngeal nerve arises from the vagus nerve at the level of the right subclavian artery, and on the left the recurrent laryngeal nerve arises from the vagus nerve at the level of the aortic arch. A branch of the recurrent laryngeal nerve penetrates the cricothyroid membrane and supplies sensory fibers to the subglottic larynx up through the level of the vocal folds.

The false vocal cords, when viewed from above, overlap and parallel the course of the true vocal cords. These

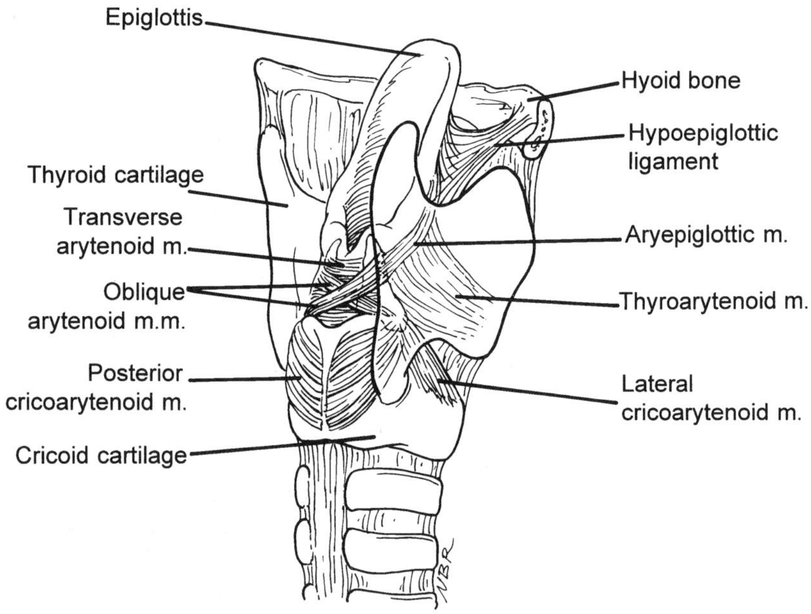

FIG. 11. Right posterior oblique view of the larynx showing the origin and insertion of the intrinsic and extrinsic laryngeal musculature.

cords are not as highly developed as the true vocal cords and do not approximate completely during phonation. They can close together, however, and act as a sphincter to protect the laryngeal inlet. When in spasmodic contraction, the false vocal folds obscure the view of the true vocal cords and glottis from above.

Pediatric Larynx

The infant larynx differs greatly from the adult larynx in appearance, location, and morphology. Several important differences should be noted.

Anatomy

The infant larynx is characterized by a funnel-shaped lumen whose point of greatest narrowing is about 1 cm below the cords. A tracheal tube that penetrates the glottis may be too large for the trachea. This funnel shape gradually disappears as the child grows and matures. The cartilaginous framework of the infant larynx is softer than its adult counterpart. In fact, the laryngeal cartilages undergo ossification throughout life, with resultant bony characteristics in adulthood. The pediatric epiglottis is proportionally narrower and longer, and in some infants the immature epiglottic cartilage may form an omega-shaped epiglottis. This configuration brings the aryepiglottic folds closer to the midline, narrows the laryngeal inlet, and increases the possibility of airway obstruction.

Position

The location of the larynx is higher in the neck of children than it is in adults. The tip of the epiglottis can frequently be seen through the open mouth of an infant. The epiglottis may be in contact with the soft palate, which contributes to the neonatal obligatory nasal respiration and assists the infant in swallowing.

Mucous Membranes

The laryngeal soft tissues and mucous membranes are loosely attached in the child. The loose attachment of the laryngeal soft tissues predisposes to swelling (edema), with resultant airway obstruction when the larynx is traumatized or infected. The insertion of an endotracheal tube or laryngeal manipulation with a laryngoscope may create edema that obstructs the upper airway. This obstruction is most marked in the subglottic region, where the narrow lumen and the restrictive cricoid ring can produce dangerous airway obstruction.

THE TRACHEOBRONCHIAL TREE

The trachea begins in the neck, where it is attached to the cricoid cartilage of the larynx. The trachea descends in the midline of the neck and thorax to the level of the fifth or sixth thoracic vertebra, where it bifurcates at the carina into the left and right main bronchi. The adult trachea is approximately 15 cm in length, and its lumen is supported by 16 to 20 C-shaped cartilaginous structures. The open ends of the tracheal cartilages face posteriorly. The posterior trachea is membranous and lies in contact with the anterior esophageal wall.

Right Main Bronchus

The right bronchus is shorter and straighter than the left bronchus. The right bronchus is a direct continuation

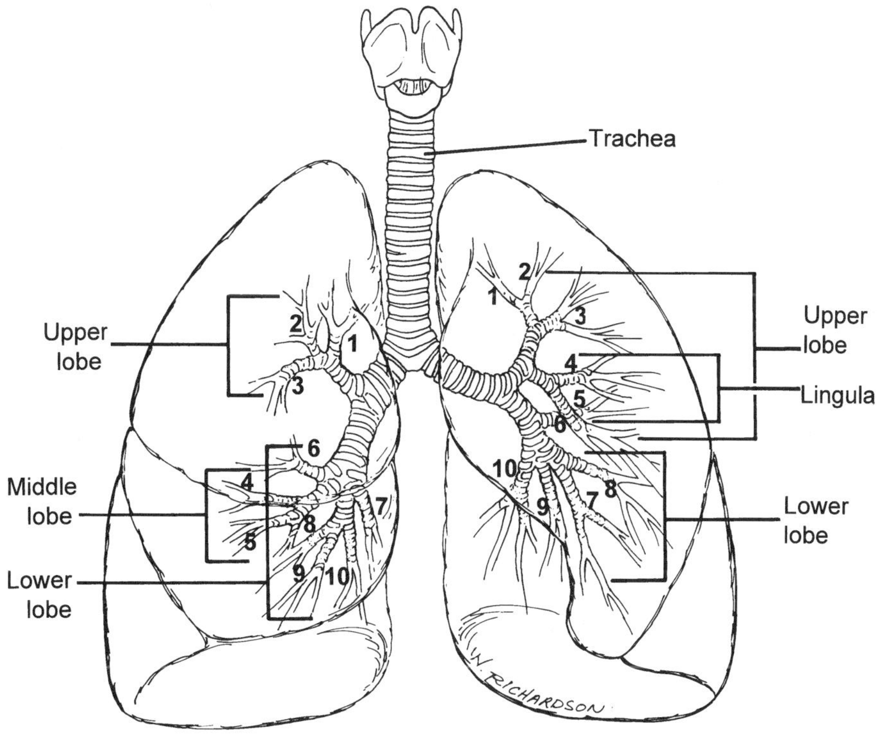

FIG. 12. Schematic diagram of the tracheobronchial tree showing the relationship of the trachea, main bronchi, and terminal bronchioles. In diagram of the right lung, note the segments of the right upper lobe **(1, 2, 3)**; right middle lobe **(4, 5)**; and the right lower lobe **(6, 7, 8, 9, 10)**. In the diagram of the left lung, note the segments of the upper division of the upper lobe bronchus **(1, 2, 3)**; the lingula **(4, 5)**; and the left lower lobe **(6, 7, 8, 9, 10)**.

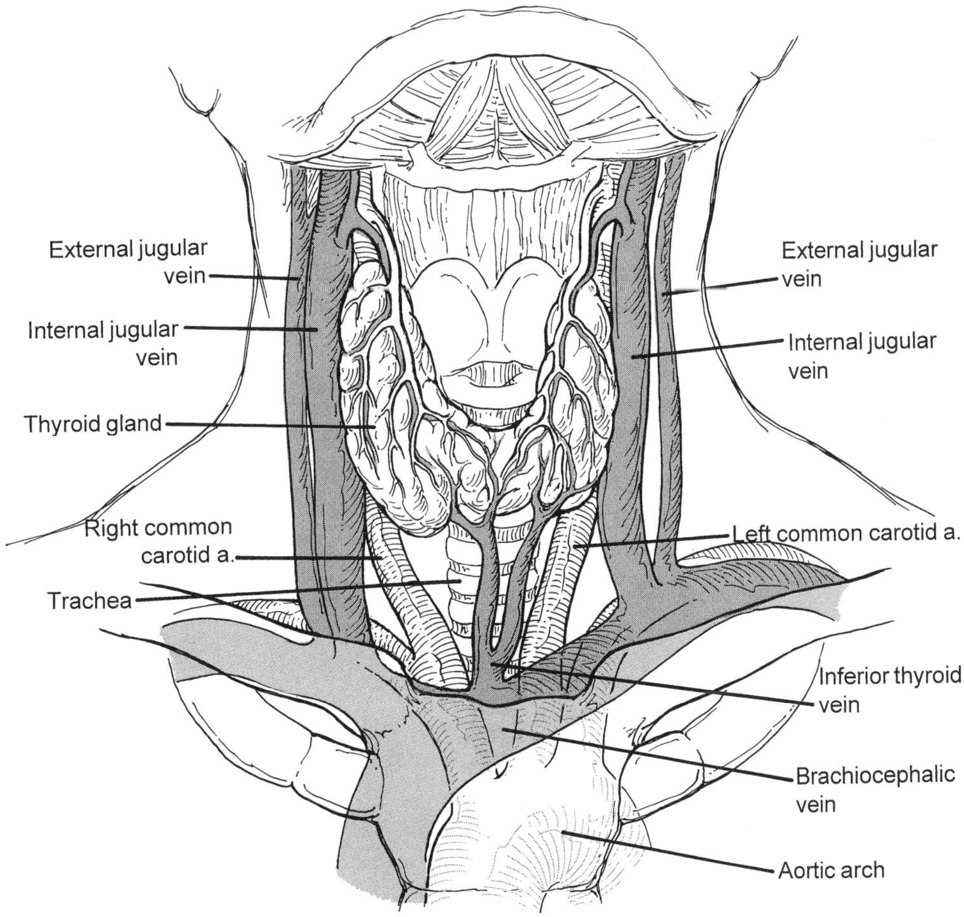

FIG. 13. Schematic diagram depicting the important vascular relationships of the anterior neck. Note the relationship of the primary vessels of the neck to the trachea and thyroid gland.

of the trachea (Fig. 12). Foreign body aspirates are more likely to become lodged in the right main bronchus. The right superior lobe bronchus arises above the pulmonary artery and supplies the right upper lobe of the lung. The right middle and inferior lobe bronchi continue and supply the middle and lower lobes of the lung, respectively.

Left Main Bronchus

The left bronchus is smaller in diameter but is longer than the right bronchus. The subcarinal angle between the two bronchi is approximately 60°, with the left bronchus diverging at approximately 35° angle and the right bronchus diverging at approximately 25° from the trachea. The left bronchus courses anteriorly to the esophagus and the thoracic aorta as it passes underneath the aortic arch. The left superior lobe bronchus supplies the left upper lobe and the lingula. The left inferior lobe bronchus disburses to the inferior lobe.

Distal Bronchi and Bronchioles

The distal bronchial tree has a complex course that becomes intimately associated with the lobular pulmonary vasculature. The C-shaped cartilages gradually become complete rings, encircling the bronchi fully in the peripheral portions. The terminal bronchioles do not contain cartilage in their walls, but they do contain a spiral muscle. The trachea and bronchi are lined by pseudostratified, ciliated respiratory mucosa, which gradually becomes a single cuboidal layer of epithelium in the terminal bronchioles.

Vascular Relations

There are several important vascular relationships to the trachea (Fig. 13). Superficially, the paired anterior jugular veins are located on the anterior tracheal surface and overlying strap muscles. These vessels frequently unite through a jugular venous arch in the low-midline. The inferior thyroid veins are located directly below the thyroid gland and communicate with the brachiocephalic veins. The brachiocephalic (innominate) artery crosses the trachea at the upper level of the sternum, although this artery may occasionally cross the trachea at a higher level. Lateral to the trachea are the internal jugular veins and the carotid arteries. Knowledge of these important vascular relations is mandatory for the performance of tracheotomy and for the management of posttracheotomy hemorrhage.

ACKNOWLEDGMENT

The authors wish to thank Nelva Richardson (medical illustrator) for her time, energy, and artistic creativity.

SUGGESTED READINGS

Hollinshead WH. Volume 1: The Head and Neck. In: *Anatomy for Surgeons*, 3rd ed. Philadelphia: JB Lippincott; 1982.

Tucker HM. *The Larynx*, 2nd ed. New York: Thieme Medical Publishers; 1993.

Woodburne RT. *Essentials of Human Anatomy*, 5th ed. New York: Oxford University Press; 1973.

Airway Management, edited by
L.H. Hanowell, M.D. and R.J. Waldron, M.D.,
Lippincott-Raven Publishers, Philadelphia © 1996.

CHAPTER 2

Monitoring Ventilation

Robert G. Loeb and William C. Santos

INTRODUCTION

The physician involved in airway management must assess the need for airway support, establish airway support if indicated, and confirm that the treatment is effective. Knowing how to monitor the ventilation system is essential to this process. The physician risks becoming a technician unless involved in the decision to establish airway support and in subsequent management.

Ventilation monitoring is discussed in this chapter. The first section presents methods to assess the adequacy of ventilation before and following airway support. In the second section, methods to confirm proper placement of an endotracheal tube are reviewed.

ASSESSING ADEQUACY OF VENTILATION

Clinical Signs

Physical examination of the respiratory system, which can be performed with little equipment, provides important information regarding the severity and cause of ventilation abnormalities. This section focuses on areas of examination that are pertinent before and after airway management. Clinical signs of increased respiratory work and decreased oxygenation are reviewed because airway management and ventilatory support are often needed to assist patients with these problems. The role of stethoscopy in diagnosing ventilation abnormalities is also discussed.

Indicators of Respiratory Work

Work of breathing is the amount of energy required over time to move gas into and out of the lungs (1). The respiratory muscles, consisting of the diaphragm, the intercostal muscles, and some of the muscles in the neck and abdomen, provide the force to move gas into the lungs during inspiration. In expanding the lungs, the muscles must overcome the elastic recoil of the chest (compliance) and shear forces as gas moves through the respiratory tract (resistance). Exhalation is usually passive, the force coming from the elastic recoil of the chest wall. However, active exhalation occurs during cough, exercise, and some disease states. The main impediment to exhalation comes from resistance, as gas moves through the airways.

Respiratory failure and hypoventilation ensue when the work of breathing exceeds the available force of the respiratory muscles. Respiratory work goes up with increases

R. G. Loeb: Department of Anesthesiology, University of California, Davis Medical Center, Sacramento, California 95817.
W. C. Santos: Department of Anesthesiology, University of California, Davis Medical Center, Sacramento, California 95817; and Central Anesthesia Service Exchange, Sacramento, California 95821.

in airway resistance, decreases in thoracic compliance, and increases in minute ventilation. Available respiratory muscle force diminishes when there is reduced central neural drive and respiratory muscle strength.

Tachypnea may be an indicator of increased work of breathing, especially when it is associated with dyspnea. Normal respiratory rate in a resting adult is 10 to 16 breaths per minute; in a newborn the rate is about 40 to 60, and the respiratory rate gradually decreases until it reaches adult levels during adolescence. Tachypnea is a nonspecific sign of increased work of breathing; other causes of tachypnea include fever, anxiety, pain, hypoxemia, and acidosis.

The breathing pattern can provide important clues in discerning the cause of respiratory distress. Rapid, shallow breathing is characteristic of patients with pulmonary restriction, such as those with pulmonary infiltrates, abdominal distention, pneumothorax, or weakness of the respiratory muscles. Prolongation of the inspiratory phase may indicate inspiratory obstruction, while prolongation of the expiratory flow phase is a sign of expiratory obstruction. Extrathoracic obstruction, such as in the upper airway, tends to result in inspiratory obstruction, while intrathoracic obstruction, such as in the trachea or bronchi, typically causes expiratory obstruction.

Inspection of the neck, chest, and abdomen can provide evidence of increased work of breathing. Tensing of the scalenus and sternocleidoid muscles during inspiration indicates that these accessory muscles are needed to overcome inspiratory work. Sternal and intercostal retractions may be observed with severe inspiratory obstruction. Complete respiratory obstruction causes a parodoxical motion of the chest and abdomen, in which the chest descends and the abdomen expands during inspiration.

Arterial blood pressure normally fluctuates by less than 10 mm Hg during the respiratory cycle. During inspiration, the decreased intrathoracic pressure causes expansion of the pulmonary vascular bed and diminished left atrial filling. *Pulsus paradoxus* is an abnormal finding in which the systolic blood pressure decreases by more than 10 mm Hg during the inspiratory period of a normal breath. Pulsus paradoxus may be a sign of increased work of breathing, as in asthma and upper airway obstruction, in which it occurs because of an abnormally low inspiratory intrathoracic pressure. However, pulsus paradoxus is a nonspecific sign that can also be caused by cardiac tamponade and pericardial effusion.

Indicators of Oxygenation

Although adequate oxygenation is a fundamental requirement for the survival of all tissues, there are few clinical signs of hypoxia. Nonspecific signs and symptoms of hypoxia occur when the oxygen supply to the more sensitive tissues, such as the brain and heart, falls below a critical level. Tachypnea and tachycardia are nonspecific signs of hypoxia. Both are caused by reflexes that serve to increase oxygen delivery to the tissues.

The hallmark sign of hypoxia is cyanosis, a blue color of the skin. With mild cyanosis, the skin looks slightly less pink, or dusky. In severe cyanosis, the skin may look almost purple. Generalized cyanosis is most readily observed in the lips, ears, mouth, and nail beds. Local cyanosis resulting from venous stasis does not indicate generalized hypoxemia. Desaturated hemoglobin in the skin causes cyanosis. For cyanosis to be visible, each 100 mL of blood must contain at least 5 g of reduced hemoglobin (2). For this reason, anemic patients may not appear cyanotic until desaturation is severe. The ability to detect cyanosis also depends on the patient's skin color and the room lighting. Pulse oximetry and blood gas analysis are much more sensitive measures of hypoxemia than is visible cyanosis.

Clubbing, a painless enlargement of the soft tissue of the terminal phalanges of the fingers or toes, may be a sign of chronic hypoxia. The diagnosis of clubbing is confirmed by 1) pressing on the skin over the base of the nail and demonstrating that the nail floats above the bone, or 2) finding that the angle between the bone and the nail bed is less than 20°. Clubbing may appear within 1 week of hypoxia and is a reversible finding that resolves with treatment of the underlying condition (3). It primarily occurs in patients with pulmonary or cardiovascular hypoxic disorders, but it can also be found in patients with cirrhosis and thyrotoxicosis.

Stethoscopy

Basics of Ausculation

Auscultation of the chest and neck yields important information about lung function and the adequacy of ventilation. Normal breath sounds vary in quality, depending on where the stethoscope is placed (Fig. 1). Breath sounds heard over the neck and upper sternum, called "tracheobronchial" sounds, come from the trachea and upper airway. They are loud and high-pitched because of the high velocity of gas through these air passages. A pause between inspiratory and expiratory sounds can normally be heard. Breath sounds heard over the lateral chest, termed "vesicular" sounds, come from the alveoli and distal bronchioles. They are quieter and of lower pitch. Here, no pause is normally heard between the inspiratory and expiratory phases, and only the initial third of the expiratory phase is audible. Normal breath sounds have yet a different quality over the lower sternum anteriorly and between the scapulae posteriorly. They have the same pitch as tracheobronchial sounds but are quieter as well as continuous from inspiration through expiration. Termed "bronchovesicular," they

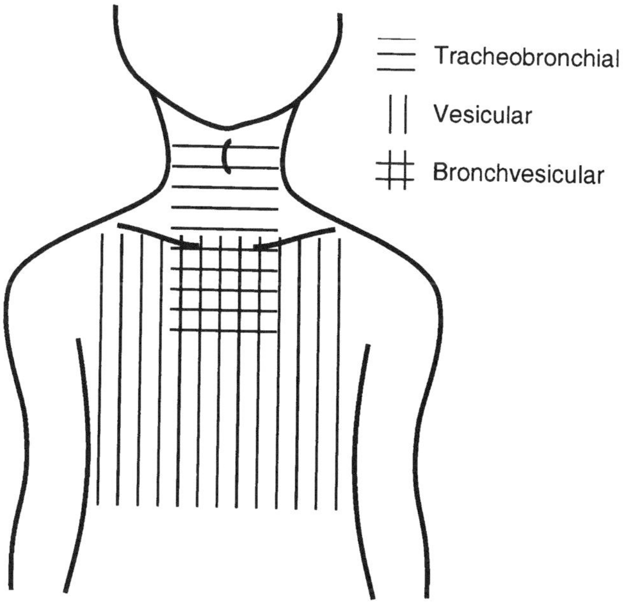

FIG. 1. Normal breath sounds, described as *tracheobronchial, bronchovesicular*, and *vesicular*, have distinct qualities over different areas of the body.

originate from gas flow through the main bronchi and central lung tissue.

Normal breath sounds, wherever they are heard, are smooth and even, similar to the sound of wind blowing through the trees. Abnormal breath sounds are characterized by an uneven or vibratory quality. There are a variety of abnormal sounds, including crackling, whistling, whining, gurgling, and bubbling. In the following sections, three major categories of abnormal sounds (Table 1) are discussed: wheezes, crackles, and stridor.

Wheezes and Rhonchi

Wheezes are vibratory sounds heard over the lung fields. In general, they indicate intrathoracic respiratory obstruction.

High-pitched wheezes have a whining or whistling quality. They are caused by air flow past secretions or areas of edema in the smaller airways. High-pitched wheezes are typically heard during expiration, when the airways are naturally smaller as they lose the tensile support of surrounding lung parenchyma. The characteristics of the wheezes may indicated the severity of the obstruction. Asymptomatic small-airway obstruction may cause wheezing only during forced exhalation. With mild small-airway obstruction, wheezes tend to be of medium pitch, quiet, and confined to end-expiration. More severe small-airway obstruction is associated with louder, higher-pitched wheezing that is heard throughout expiration and even during inspiration. Incongruously, wheezing may decrease with severe obstruction, as the patient tires and air flow decreases.

Low-pitched wheezes, also known as "rhonchi," have a bubbling or gurgling quality. They are caused by air flow past secretions in the larger airways. Rhonchi are often heard during inspiration and expiration and may decrease or resolve after vigorous cough. In the intubated patient, rhonchi may indicate a need for tracheal suctioning.

Crackles

Crackles, or inspiratory rales, are high-pitched popping sounds heard over the lung fields during inspiration. They are miniature explosions that occur when previously closed airways or collapsed alveoli suddenly open or expand. In older patients, crackles are normally heard at the lung bases on an initial deep inspiration. Notably, these "normal" crackles disappear on subsequent deep breaths or after a cough. Crackles that continue, or that are heard in less dependent areas of the lung, indicate abnormal collapse of alveoli or small airways. This occurs with pulmonary edema, pulmonary fibrosis, pneumonia, and chronic obstructive pulmonary disease (COPD). In general, crackles indicate abnormal lung compliance.

Stridor

Stridor is a vibratory sound heard over the neck but often transmitted to the lung fields. Typically heard during inspiration, stridor indicates extrathoracic airway obstruction. Stridor should not be confused with wheezing, which typically occurs during exhalation and is heard better over the lung fields than over the neck. Supraglottic obstruction, as in epiglottitis, is generally

TABLE 1. *Abnormal sounds of respiration*

Sound	Characteristic	Location	Timing	Causes
Wheezes	Musical, gurgling, vibratory	Lung fields	Typically exhalation	Asthma, bronchitis, anaphylaxis
Crackles	Fine popping or crackling	Lung bases	Typically inhalation	Pulmonary edema, fibrosis, pneumonia, COPD
Stridor	Harsh, vibratory	Neck	Typically inhalation	Epiglottitis, croup, tumor

COPD, chronic obstructive pulmonary disease.

sensitive to patient position. Glottic or subglottic obstruction, as in croup or vocal cord paralysis, generally is not affected by patient position. Stridor resolves with endotracheal intubation; however, the patient with stridor has a high risk for failed intubation and complete airway obstruction with sedation and anesthesia.

Arterial Blood Gas Analysis

Arterial blood gas analysis is a fundamental method for assessing ventilation. This is because the primary goals of the ventilation system are to provide adequate partial pressures of oxygen and carbon dioxide in the arterial blood. Arterial blood gas analysis indicates whether the ventilation system is meeting metabolic demand at a given point in time.

Methods for determining arterial pH and partial pressures of oxygen and carbon dioxide were developed from the 1900s through the 1950s (4). The pH electrode was the first ion-selective electrode; it was invented in the early 1900s. In the mid-1950s, Stow, and later Severinghaus, modified the pH electrode to measure partial pressure of carbon dioxide. The first practical polarographic oxygen electrode was developed by Heyrovski in 1925, and the modern oxygen electrode was invented by Clark in 1956. Clinical measurement of arterial blood gases became routine in the 1970s and has become progressively easier with the development of automated analyzers.

Measurement Principles

Laboratory blood gas analysis is performed by measuring pH, partial pressure of oxygen, and partial pressure of carbon dioxide at 37° C using electrochemical electrodes. Other commonly reported values, including bicarbonate concentration, base deficit, hemoglobin saturation, and blood gas concentrations at patient temperature, are calculated.

pH electrode

The pH electrode (Fig. 2) is also called the "glass-calomel" electrode. It measures the electric potential that is generated when solutions of different pH are separated by a special pH-sensitive glass membrane. The electrode consists of a sample cell and a reference cell. In the sample cell, a solution of known pH is placed on one side of the pH-sensitive glass membrane, and the blood sample, of unknown pH, is placed on the other side. In the reference cell, mercury and mercurous chloride sit in a solution of potassium chloride. The voltage across the two cells is proportional to the hydrogen ion concentration in the blood sample.

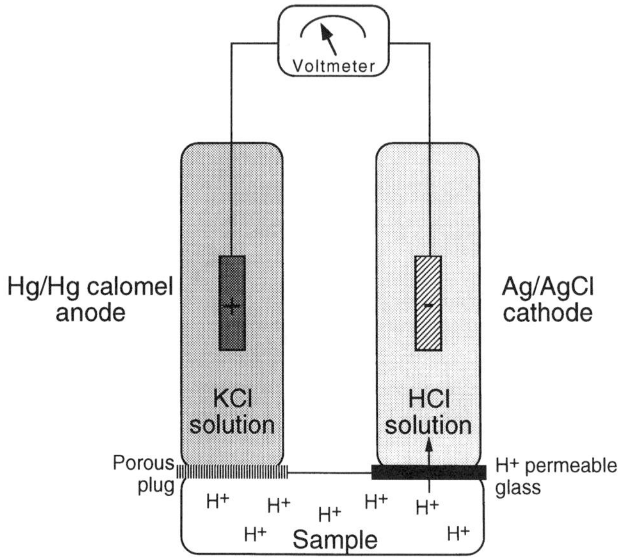

FIG. 2. Glass-calomel pH electrode.

Carbon Dioxide Electrode

Blood gas analyzers measure carbon dioxide partial pressure with a Severinghaus electrode (Fig. 3). This electrode is a modified pH electrode; a layer of bicarbonate buffer converts carbon dioxide concentration to hydrogen ion concentration. Carbon dioxide from the blood sample diffuses across a Teflon membrane into a bicarbonate buffer solution. The pH of the buffer solution drops as the carbon dioxide concentration increases. By measuring the pH of the buffer solution, the carbon dioxide concentration in the blood sample is determined. The

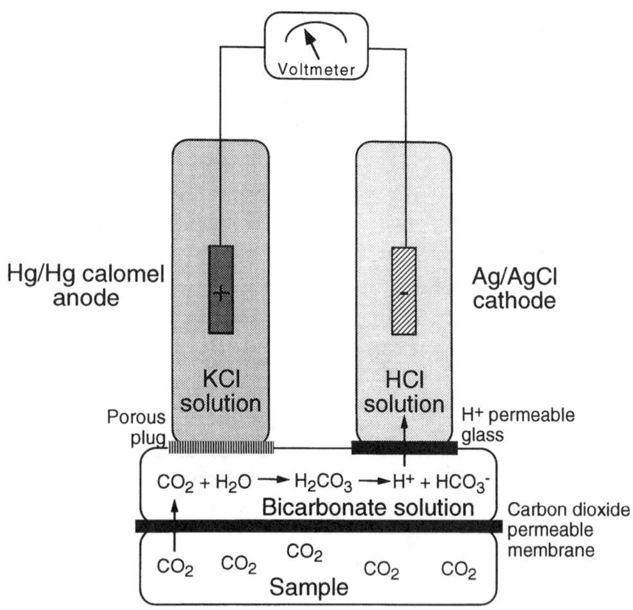

FIG. 3. Severinghaus carbon dioxide electrode.

Henderson-Hasselbalch equation relates the pH to the CO_2 concentration:

$$pH = pK_a - \log(PCO_2) + \log [(HCO_3)/S] \quad (1)$$

where S is the solubility of CO_2 and pK_a is the dissociation constant.

Oxygen Electrode

The oxygen electrode in a blood gas analyzer is a Clark electrode (Fig. 4). It is a polarographic sensor, similar in design to the polarographic oxygen analyzers found on anesthesia machines and ventilators. Oxygen diffuses from the blood sample into the electrode across an oxygen-permeable polypropylene membrane. The rate of diffusion, and thus the oxygen concentration within the electrolyte, is proportional to the oxygen partial pressure in the blood sample. Inside the electrode, oxygen undergoes a reaction with water that consumes electrons. This reaction accepts electrons from the platinum cathode. The current, which is proportional to oxygen concentration, is measured by a meter.

Bicarbonate and Base Excess

The bicarbonate concentration of the blood sample can be calculated from the measured pH and carbon dioxide concentration using the Henderson-Hasselbalch equation (in blood at 37° C, the pK_a is 6.1 and S is 0.03). The Siggaard-Andersen alignment nomogram (Fig. 5) is a graphic representation of the Henderson-Hasselbalch equation (5). The Siggaard-Andersen alignment nomogram additionally has a scale for determination of base excess. Base excess is an empirically derived value that represents the milliequivalents of base per liter of blood that would need to be subtracted to return the metabolic acid-base status to equilibrium. Therefore, a positive base excess suggests a metabolic alkalosis, while a negative base excess indicates metabolic acidosis.

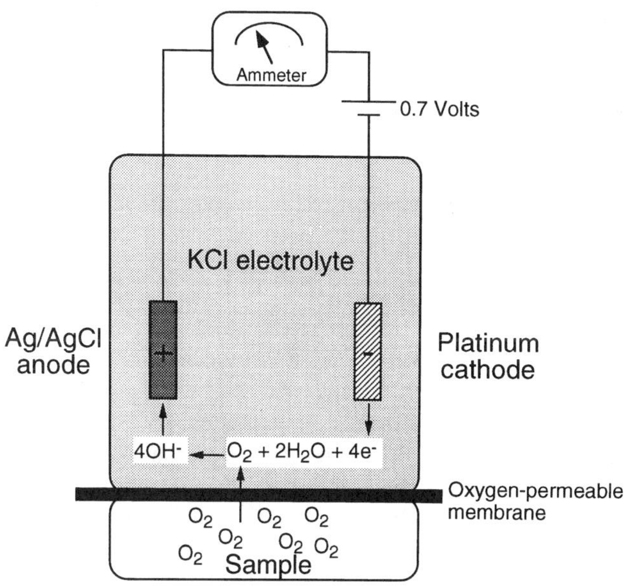

FIG. 4. Clark oxygen electrode.

Sample Collection

Blood gases are most commonly analyzed in arterial or mixed venous blood samples. Arterial blood is drawn from arteries, and mixed venous blood is drawn from the pulmonary arterial (PA) port of a Swan-Ganz catheter. Arterial blood gas analysis is most commonly used to investigate the functional status of the pulmonary system; the adequacy of tissue oxygen delivery is examined using mixed venous blood gas analysis. Both arterial and mixed venous blood gas values are necessary to calculate shunt.

A sample of heparinized whole blood is required for blood gas analysis. Minimal amounts of heparin should be used because heparin is acidic and an excessive amount lowers the pH of the blood sample. The sample should be collected anaerobically, and all the air should be expelled from the syringe after the sample is drawn. This prevents equilibration between the air bubbles in the syringe and the gases to be analyzed in the blood. If it is not analyzed immediately, the sample should be cooled on ice to decrease blood cell metabolic activity, which decreases oxygen partial pressure (PO_2) and increases carbon dioxide partial pressure (PCO_2) over time. Glass syringes are superior to plastic syringes in preserving samples with a high arterial oxygen partial pressure (PaO_2) (6). Management errors can occur if venous blood is mistaken for arterial blood. Unless arterial blood is withdrawn from an indwelling arterial cannula with an arterial waveform, a venous blood sample should be suspected when (what is presumed to be) the PaO_2 seems inappropriately low.

Interpretation

Arterial blood gases can be used to assess both oxygenation and ventilation quantitatively. PaO_2 is 100 mm Hg in a normal young person breathing room air. Normally, PaO_2 decreases with age. The normal PaO_2 of a subject breathing room air at sea level can be approximated with the following equation:

$$\text{Normal } PaO_2 \text{ (When } FIO_2 \text{ Is } 0.21) = 109 - (0.43 \times \text{age}) \pm 4 \quad (2)$$

Arterial carbon dioxide partial pressure ($PaCO_2$) is normally 40 mm Hg. This value does not change with age.

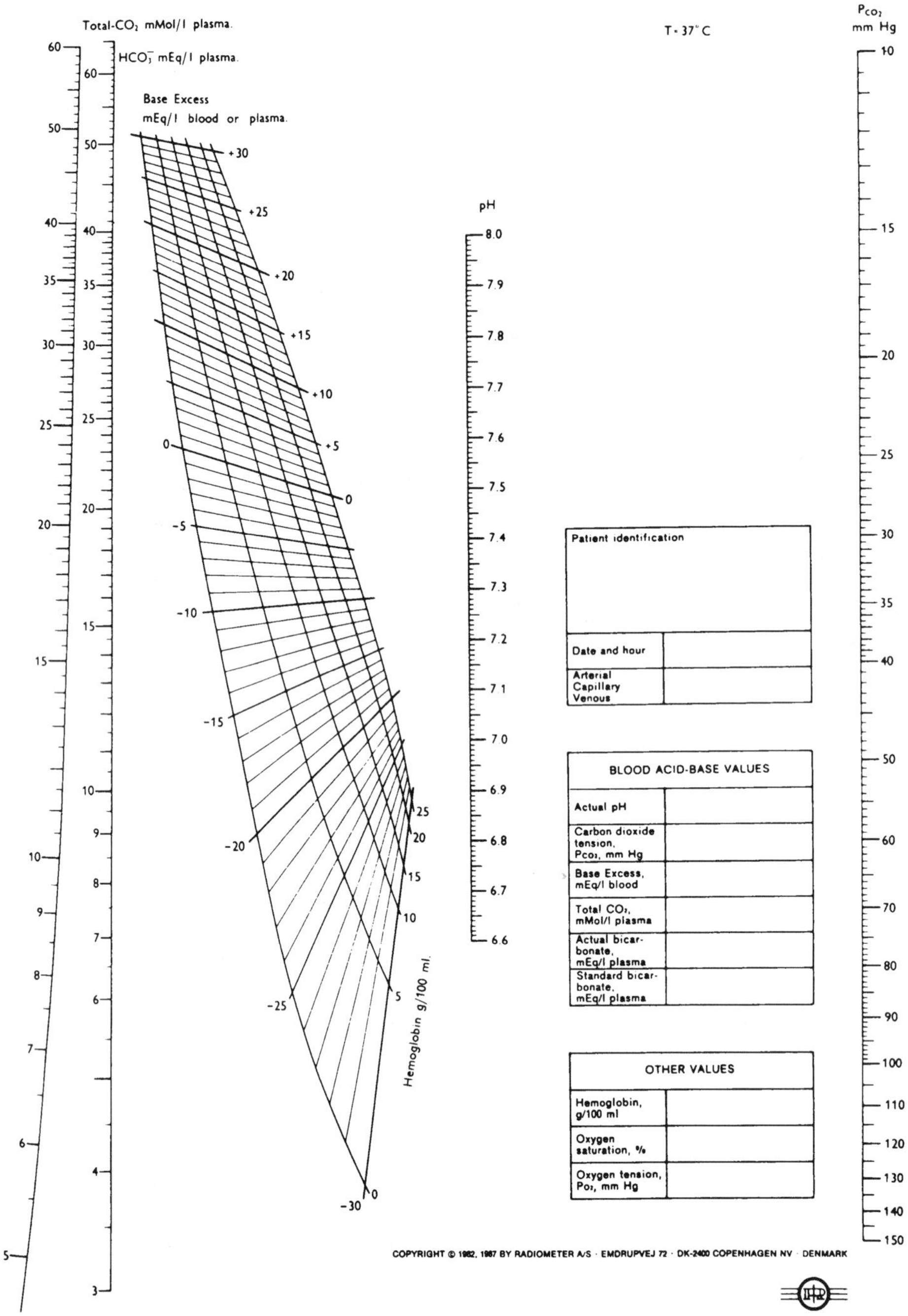

FIG. 5. Siggaard-Andersen alignment nomogram. (Reproduced with permission of Radiometer A/S, Copenhagen.)

Interpretation of Hypoxemia

A PaO_2 greater than 60 mm Hg is sufficient for adequate tissue oxygen delivery in most patients. Hypoxemia, defined as a PaO_2 of less than 60 mm Hg, may result from a number of conditions (Table 2). These conditions can be classified into five catagories: breathing hypoxic gas, hypoventilation, diffusion gradient, ventilation-perfusion mismatch, and shunt. Breathing hypoxic gas and hypoventilation cause hypoxemia by decreasing the oxygen concentration in the alveolar gas, whereas diffusion gradient, ventilation-perfusion mismatch, and shunt result in hypoxemia even when the partial pressure of alveolar oxygen is normal (or sometimes even elevated). Thus, knowing the alveolar concentration of oxygen is an important step in the differential diagnosis of hypoxemia. The alveolar gas equation is used to estimate the concentration of oxygen in the alveoli:

TABLE 2. *Causes of hypoxemia*

- Breathing hypoxic gas
  - Rebreathing (e.g., because of large apparatus dead space)
  - Breathing at high altitude
  - Respiratory support mishap (e.g., misfilled oxygen tank, gas crossover)
- Hypoventilation
  - Decrease or loss of ventilatory drive (e.g., drug overdose)
  - Decreased strength of respiratory muscles (e.g., myasthenia gravis)
  - Increased work of breathing (e.g., epiglottitis, asthma)
- Diffusion gradient
  - Alveolar thickening (e.g., pulmonary fibrosis)
  - Loss of total alveolar surface area (e.g, emphysema)
  - Extremely high cardiac output (e.g., exercise)
- Ventilation-perfusion mismatch
  - Partial bronchial obstruction (e.g., tumor, secretions, bronchospasm, COPD)
  - Low cardiac output
- Shunt
  - Cardiac right-to-left shunt (e.g., persistent fetal circulation, ventricular septal defect)
  - Nonalveolar pulmonary blood flow (e.g., bronchial, pleural, thebesian veins)
  - Alveolar shunt (e.g., main bronchial intubation, atelectasis, pneumonia, pulmonary edema)

$$P_AO_2 = [F_IO_2 \times (P_B - 47)] - [(P_aCO_2)/R] \quad (3)$$

where P_AO_2 is the partial pressure of alveolar oxygen, F_IO_2 is the fractional concentration of inspired oxygen, and P_B is the barometric pressure (760 mmHg at sea level). The vapor pressure of water, 47 mmHg, is subtracted from the barometric pressure. P_aCO_2 is the partial pressure of arterial carbon dioxide, and R is the respiratory quotient (normally 0.8). Thus, the P_AO_2 when breathing room air is approximately 100 mmHg ($[0.21 \times 713] - [40/0.8]$ from the above equation). Breathing a hypoxic gas causes hypoxemia by decreasing the F_IO_2; hypoventilation causes hypoxemia by increasing the P_aCO_2. Shunt causes hypoxemia by preventing the transfer of oxygen from the alveoli to the venous blood. Therefore, with shunt there is a discrepancy between the alveolar and arterial partial pressures of oxygen. This difference is referred to as the "A-a gradient." The A-a gradient is calculated using the following formula:

$$\text{A-a Gradient} = \text{Calculated } P_AO_2 - \text{Measured } PaO_2 \quad (4)$$

Normally, the A-a gradient increases with age and is approximately equal to age times 0.4. The A-a gradient increases at higher inspired concentrations of oxygen.

The a/A oxygen ratio is calculated below:

$$\text{a/A Ratio} = \text{Measured } PaO_2/\text{Calculated } P_AO_2 \quad (5)$$

This ratio is more constant with changes in inspired concentration. For this reason, the a/A oxygen ratio should be used at higher inspired oxygen concentrations to screen for oxygenation problems, and to predict a new PaO_2 when the inspired oxygen concentration is changed in a given patient (7). The normal a/A oxygen ratio decreases with age and can be estimated using the following equation:

$$\text{Normal a/A Ratio} = [110 - (0.43 \times \text{age})]/110 \quad (6)$$

Shunt must be calculated to track the severity of oxygenation problems accurately. Because arterial and mixed venous blood gas values are required to calculate shunt, the calculation is usually performed only in critically ill patients. The equation follows:

$$\text{Percent Shunt} = (CcO_2 - CaO_2)/(CcO_2 - C\bar{v}O_2) \quad (7)$$

where CcO_2 is the calculated oxygen content of alveolar capillary blood, CaO_2 is the calculated oxygen content of arterial blood, and $C\bar{v}O_2$ is the calculated oxygen content of mixed venous blood. Oxygen content is calculated using the following equation:

$$\text{Oxygen Content (mL/dL)} = (1.39 \times Hb \times SO_2) + (0.003 \times PO_2) \quad (8)$$

where SO_2 is the oxygen saturation and Hb is the hemoglobin concentration (g/dL).

Interpretation of Hypercapnia

Hypoventilation causes hypercapnia, defined as a $PaCO_2$ greater than 45 mm Hg. Hypercapnia can occur primarily, either acutely or chronically; however, it can also occur secondarily to compensate for a metabolic alkalosis (Table 3). Primary hypercapnia indicates a

TABLE 3. *Common causes of hypercapnia*

- Acute hypercapnia
  - Decrease or loss of ventilatory drive (e.g., drug overdose, head injury)
  - Decreased respiratory muscle strength (e.g., residual neuromuscular relaxation)
  - Increased work of breathing (e.g., acute asthma, upper airway obstruction)
  - Large dead space (e.g., apparatus dead space, pulmonary embolism, low cardiac output)
- Chronic hypercapnia
  - Decrease or loss of ventilatory drive (e.g., Pickwickian syndrome)
  - Decreased strength of respiratory muscles (e.g., myasthenia gravis)
  - Increased work of breathing (e.g., COPD)
  - Large dead space (e.g., emphysema)
- Metabolic alkalosis
  - Loss of hydrogen ion (e.g., nasogastric suction, vomiting, diuretics, steroids)
  - Exogenous bicarbonate

compromise of the ventilation system and is the focus of this discussion. Arterial blood gas analysis is a powerful tool for differentiating the mechanisms of hypercapnia.

The basis for differentiating the causes of hypercapnia lies in the underlying physiology of the acid-base system. The body tries to keep the extracellular fluid pH within the range of 7.35 to 7.45. It can manipulate two systems to achieve this goal: the lungs (or respiratory system) and the kidneys (or metabolic system). The lungs can cause *rapid* changes in extracellular pH by retaining or excreting carbon dioxide, which is an acid when dissolved in extracellular fluid. The kidneys can cause *slow* changes in extracellular pH by excreting or retaining dissolved acids and bases.

If the extracellular fluid has too low a level of dissolved acids or too high a level of dissolved bases, the pH will be greater than 7.45, indicating an alkalemia. The body compensates by retaining carbon dioxide, an acid, through hypoventilation. The body attempts to correct the alkalemia, but the level of hypercarbia it can achieve is limited; compensatory hypercapnia above 55 to 60 mm Hg is rare. Thus, a pH greater than 7.45 in the presence of hypercapnia indicates a primary metabolic alkalosis with compensatory hypercapnia and is not an indication of respiratory compromise. In this situation the base excess is abnormally high.

Primary hypercapnia results from acute or chronic respiratory insufficiency. Acute and chronic respiratory compromise can be differentiated by determining whether the kidneys have had time to respond to the altered pH. Acute hypercapnia causes, approximately, a decrease in pH of 0.05 for every increase of 10 mm Hg in $PaCO_2$. The dissolved carbon dioxide is buffered to yield bicarbonate; this leads to an increase of 1 mEq/L in HCO_3^- for every increase of 10 mm Hg in $PaCO_2$. During acute hypercapnia, the base excess is normal (Table 4).

The kidneys compensate for hypercapnia by retaining bicarbonate, a base. However, the response is slow, and maximal compensation may take more than 72 hours. In chronic respiratory acidosis, HCO_3^- increases by 0.4 mEq/L for every elevation of 1 mm Hg in $PaCO_2$. This retention of bicarbonate brings the pH toward normal levels, although total compensation is unusual. In chronic respiratory acidosis, the base excess is abnormally high (Table 4).

TABLE 4. *Expected arterial blood gas changes during hypercapnia*

Condition	$PaCO_2$	pH	HCO_3^-	Base excess
Acute hypercapnia[a]	↑10	↓0.05	↑1	0
Chronic hypercapnia	↑10	↓0.03	↑4.0	↑3
Metabolic alkalosis	↑ 6	↑0.07	↑10	↑9

[a] For instance, in acute hypercapnia, each increase in $PaCO_2$ of 10 mm Hg is associated with a decrease in pH of 0.05 and an increase in HCO_3^- of 1 mEq/dL.

Oximetry

Measurement Principles

Oximetry is absorption spectroscopy that quantifies the proportions of different types of hemoglobin in blood. It forms the basis of a number of clinical monitors, including the laboratory co-oximeter and the pulse oximeter. Laboratory co-oximeters, which have been used clinically since the 1960s, measure the concentrations of many hemoglobin moieties in a sample of hemolyzed blood. Pulse oximeters continuously measure the ratio of oxyhemoglobin to deoxyhemoglobin *in vivo*; they were introduced into clinical practice in the early 1980s and have rapidly become a monitoring standard.

Beer-Lambert Law and Oximetry

Absorption spectroscopy is the fundamental technique used in all oximeters. It is based on the Beer-Lambert law, which relates the amount of light that is absorbed in passing through a solution to the solute concentration, extinction coefficient of the solute, and distance through the solution:

$$\text{Absorbance} = \text{Concentration} \times \text{Extinction Coefficient} \times \text{Distance} \quad (9)$$

Only a single wavelength of light is needed to determine the solute concentration in a pure solution. A beam of monochromatic light is aimed through the solution and the percentage of transmitted light is measured. The solute concentration can be calculated if the distance through the solution and the extinction coefficient of the solute at the given wavelength are known.

To measure the concentrations of multiple solutes in a single solution, a number of monochromatic light sources are required—one wavelength for each solute. The extinction coefficient of each solute at each wavelength must be known to solve the multiple simultaneous equations. The absorption spectra of the four predominant hemoglobin species are shown in Figure 6. Multiple wavelength absorption spectroscopy is the basis of *in vitro* co-oximetry; modern co-oximeters analyze light transmission through a hemolyzed sample of whole blood to determine the concentrations of oxyhemoglobin (O_2Hb), deoxyhemoglobin (RHb), methemoglobin (MetHb), carboxyhemoglobin (COHb), and sulfhemoglobin (SHb). An assumption of absorption spectroscopy is that no unknown solutes are present. Since this may not be assumed in biologic samples, modern co-oximeters

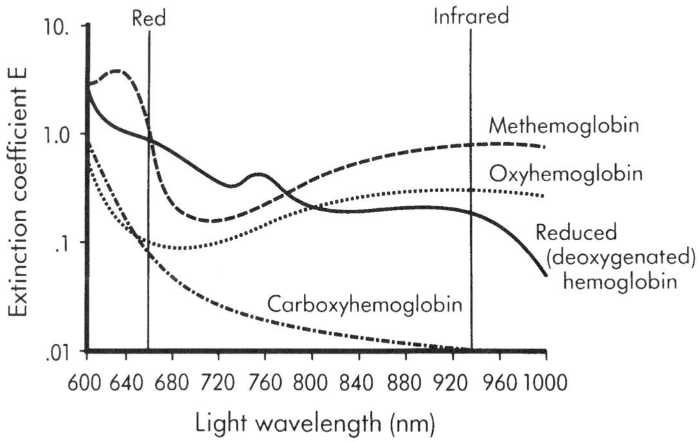

FIG. 6. Absorption spectra of the four predominant hemoglobin species. (From Barker SJ, Tremper KK. Pulse oximetry. In: Ehrenwerth J, Eisenkraft JB, eds. *Anesthesia Equipment.* St. Louis: Mosby-Year Book; 1993:249–263, with permission.)

use more than five wavelengths to correct for interference from bilirubin, turbidity, and dyes.

Pulsations and Pulse Oximetry

In vivo oximetry was first attempted in 1935. Two wavelengths of light were transmitted through tissue to measure the ratio of oxyhemoglobin to deoxyhemoglobin (with *in vivo* oximetry, solute *concentrations* cannot be determined because the distance through the solution is unknown). Although light absorption correlated with arterial hemoglobin saturation in this instrument, calibration was nearly impossible because of the presence of multiple unknown light absorbers in the tissue and venous blood. Two methods were eventually developed to correct for this interference: 1) oximeters were calibrated for background tissue absorption by taking measurements while compressing the tissue to remove the blood; and 2) the tissue was heated during measurements to "arterialize" the blood flow and reduce the effect of venous blood. Still, until the advent of pulse oximetry, oximeters were delicate, temperamental, and not used clinically except in pulmonary function laboratories.

The first pulse oximeter was developed in Japan in the 1970s (8). The inventor, Takuo Aoyagi, serendipitously discovered the technique while working on a method to measure tissue blood flow using dye-washout curves. By subtracting the baseline absorbance in a pulsating signal, he developed a method to isolate the light absorbance of arterial blood (Fig. 7).

Modern pulse oximeters measure light absorption at two wavelengths, red (660 nm) and infrared (940 nm). The light is generated by two light-emitting diodes (LEDs). The LEDs are switched on and off, in sequence, hundreds of times per second. In each cycle, the red LED is illuminated, then the infrared LED is illuminated, then both LEDs are extinguished. A broad-spectrum photodiode measures the transmitted light intensity under each condition, and a computer reconstructs the waveforms of red light, infrared light, and no light vs. time. The no-light waveform is subtracted from the red and infrared waveforms to correct for the presence of background light. Then, the resultant red-light-absorption and infrared-light-absorption waveforms are used to calculate the arterial hemoglobin saturation. Each waveform is first normalized by dividing the pulsatile component (AC) by the constant component (DC) (Fig. 7). Then the relative amplitudes of the normalized pulsatile components are compared with an empirically derived calibration curve to estimate the arterial oxygen saturation. The displayed saturation is a time-weighted average of the calculated

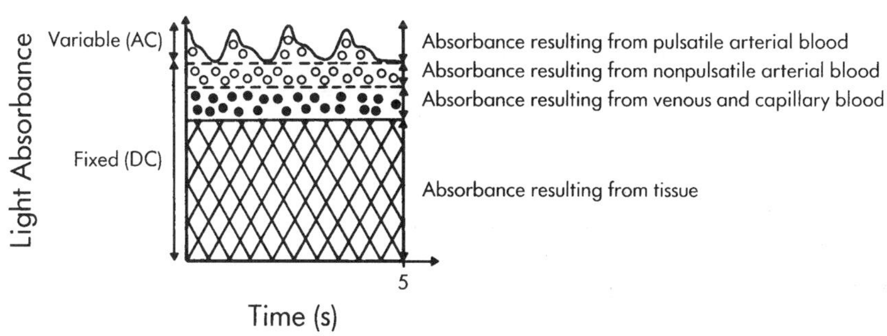

FIG. 7. The arterial component of the pulse oximeter's signal is pulsatile. (From Barker SJ, Tremper KK. Pulse oximetry. In: Ehrenwerth J, Eisenkraft JB, eds. *Anesthesia Equipment.* St. Louis: Mosby-Year Book; 1993:249–263, with permission.)

saturation. Differences in response time and accuracy between pulse oximeters of different manufacturers represent variations in calibration curves and calculation algorithms.

Interpretation of Oximetry

Two principles must be understood to interpret oximetry data correctly: the relationship between hemoglobin saturation and oxygen partial pressure, and the determinants of oxygen delivery.

Relationship Between Hemoglobin Saturation and Oxygen Partial Pressure

The correlation between hemoglobin saturation and oxygen partial pressure is well known as the oxygen-hemoglobin dissociation curve (Fig. 8). Hemoglobin is almost completely saturated ($SaO_2 = 100\%$) when the oxygen partial pressure is above 100 mmHg. Therefore, the oximeter cannot differentiate an arterial PO_2 of 100 mmHg from an arterial PO_2 of 500 mmHg. This limits its diagnostic usefulness, since a patient may have significant oxygenation abnormalities but still have a normal SaO_2 when breathing high oxygen concentrations. Hemoglobin oxygen saturation decreases slowly as oxygen partial pressure decreases from 100 to 60 mmHg; SO_2 is 90% at a PO_2 of 60 mmHg. Saturations in the range of 90% to 97% are not dangerous for most patients but are indicative of oxygenation problems. Hemoglobin oxygen saturation decreases rapidly below a PO_2 of 60 mmHg; small drops in oxygen partial pressure correspond to large drops in saturation. Arterial saturations below 85% are regarded as significant hypoxemia. The oxygen partial pressure of mixed venous blood is normally 40 mmHg, which corresponds to a saturation of 75%. Tissues cannot extract oxygen from blood below a saturation of 20%.

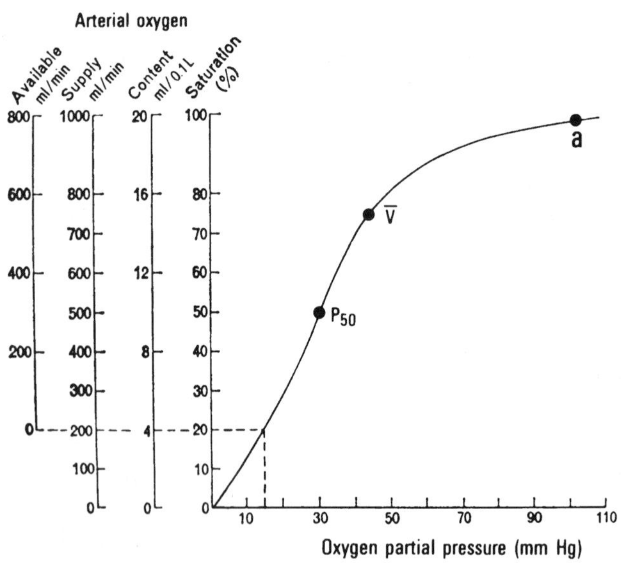

FIG. 8. The oxygen-hemoglobin dissociation curve depicts the relationship between partial pressure of oxygen and percentage saturation of hemoglobin. The additional y-axes in this figure, from *right* to *left*, extrapolate the relationships between oxygen partial pressure and oxygen content (assuming a normal hemoglobin concentration of 15 g/dL), oxygen supply (assuming a cardiac output of 5 L/min), and oxygen availability (assuming an inability of tissues to extract oxygen below a partial pressure of 20 mm Hg). a, normal arterial blood; v̄, normal mixed venous blood; P_{50}, blood with saturation of 50% and PO_2 of 27 mm Hg. (From Benumof JL. Respiratory physiology and respiratory function during anesthesia. In: Miller RD, ed. *Anesthesia*, 4th ed. New York: Churchill Livingstone; 1994:577–620, with permission.)

Determinants of Oxygen Delivery

Oxygen delivery is a function of oxygen content and blood flow. The oxygen content of blood depends on the the hemoglobin concentration, the hemoglobin saturation, and the partial pressure of oxygen:

$$\text{Oxygen Content (mL/dL)} = (1.39 \times \text{Hb} \times SO_2) + (0.003 \times PO_2) \quad (8)$$

Oxygen saturation is the only component of oxygen delivery that is measured by oximetry. The relationship between oxygen content and oxygen partial pressure at a normal hemoglobin concentration of 15 g/dL is demonstrated in Fig. 8 on the second rightmost y-axis. The amount of oxygen delivered is equal to the product of the oxygen content of blood and the blood flow (i.e., cardiac output). The relationship between oxygen delivery and oxygen partial pressure at a normal cardiac output of 5 L/min is demonstrated in Fig. 8 on the third rightmost y-axis.

Artifacts

One reason for the quick clinical acceptance of pulse oximetry is its ease of use. In most cases, accurate and continuous data are generated a few seconds after the sensor is applied to the patient. The most common pulse oximeter problem is a failure to display saturation, usually caused by an inadequate pulsatile signal. Inaccurate saturation values can usually be diagnosed because the pulse oximeter-derived pulse rate differs from the ECG-derived pulse rate. Inaccurate saturation values in the presence of an accurate pulse rate are rare. The reasons for pulse oximeter failure can be grouped into absorbance artifacts, pulsation artifacts, noise, and inaccurate calibration.

Absorbance Artifacts

The co-oximeter measures light transmission at multiple wavelengths and accurately measures the concentrations of oxyhemoglobin, deoxyhemoglobin, and a number of dyshemoglobins, even in the presence of interfering factors such as dyes, bilirubin, and turbidity. The pulse oximeter measures light transmission at only two wavelengths, and an assumption is made that all light that is not transmitted is absorbed by hemoglobin or deoxyhemoglobin. Absorption artifacts result when other factors interfere with the light transmission.

Dyshemoglobins. Oxyhemoglobin and deoxyhemoglobin are the normal hemoglobins. Oxyhemoglobin is reversibly bound to oxygen, and deoxyhemoglobin is capable of binding oxygen. Methemoglobin, carboxyhemoglobin, and sulfhemoglobin are the most common dyshemoglobins. Methemoglobin, hemoglobin oxidized to its ferric state, cannot bind oxygen; it may be inherited or induced by exposure to substances such as nitrates, nitrites, prilocaine, or benzocaine (a topical anesthetic commonly used in the airway). Carboxyhemoglobin is covalently bound to carbon monoxide and cannot carry oxygen; it is formed when carbon monoxide is inhaled, for instance, during exposure to smoke, automobile exhaust, or air pollution. Sulfhemoglobin is bound to sulfur and has a low affinity for oxygen. Each of these dyshemoglobins may be present in the normal population at concentrations up to 56%.

Dyshemoglobins interfere with the determination of hemoglobin saturation by pulse oximetry. This interference occurs at two levels: 1) Dyshemoglobins cause a discrepancy between fractional and functional saturation, and 2) dyshemoglobins result in erroneous readings, since they absorb light in the red and infrared spectra.

Hemoglobin saturation is the percentage of *all* hemoglobin that is oxyhemoglobin. This is referred to as "fractional saturation":

$$\text{Fractional Saturation} = [O_2Hb/Hb] \times 100 \qquad (10)$$

where Hb is the total hemoglobin concentration, including oxyhemoglobin, deoxyhemoglobin, carboxyhemoglobin, methemoglobin, and sulfhemoglobin. (Fetal hemoglobin and sickle hemoglobin are considered oxyhemoglobin and deoxyhemoglobin in their oxidized and reduced states, respectively). However, pulse oximeters measure only oxyhemoglobin and deoxyhemoglobin, yielding the functional saturation:

$$\text{Functional Saturation} = [O_2Hb/(O_2Hb + RHb)] \times 100 \qquad (11)$$

In the absence of dyshemoglobins, fractional and functional saturations are equivalent. However, when dyshemoglobins are present, functional saturation is high compared with fractional saturation.

Carboxyhemoglobin and methemoglobin cause pulse oximeters to determine functional saturation inaccurately because they absorb light in the red and infrared spectra (Fig. 6). Methemoglobin absorbs red and infrared light equally, and pulse oximeter-derived saturations decrease toward 85% as methemoglobin concentrations increase in the blood (9). Carboxyhemoglobin absorbs red light exclusively, and the pulse oximeter interprets it almost as oxyhemoglobin. Pulse oximeter-derived saturations decrease slowly, at approximately one-tenth the rate that carboxyhemoglobin concentrations rise (10). In the presence of either carboxyhemoglobin or methemoglobin, the pulse oximeter slightly underestimates functional saturation and greatly overestimates fractional saturation.

Dyes. Intravenous dyes may absorb light in the red or infrared spectra and cause inaccuracies in the pulse oximeter-derived saturation (11). Intravenous administration of methylene blue causes artifactual deep desaturation for 1 to 2 minutes; indigo carmine and indocyanine green cause smaller but noticeable effects.

Bilirubin. Bilirubinemia has no significant effects on pulse oximeter-derived or co-oximeter-derived saturation.

Nail Polish. Nail polish has variable effects on pulse oximeter-derived saturation. It usually causes no effect, but some colors, such as blue, green, brown, and black, can cause artificially low saturations. To avoid interference, nail polish should be removed or the probe should be positioned so that light is not transmitted across the polished nail.

Pulsation Artifacts

The pulse oximeter depends on a pulsatile signal to differentiate arterial blood from other tissues (Fig. 7). Pulsation artifacts result when pulsatile signals occur from factors other than the arterial plethysmogram.

Movement. Artifactual pulsation artifacts are most frequently caused by movement. This is rarely a problem during surgery or in the intensive care unit, but it can be a major difficulty in children, ambulatory patients, or patients who are shivering. The problem is usually easy to diagnose because the pulse oximeter will either fail to display a pulse rate and saturation or will display an inaccurate pulse rate (which can be confirmed in a number of ways). There are few options for the clinician in correcting this problem, aside from treating the agitation or shivering.

Venous Pulsations. Large venous pulsations have been reported to cause artifactual desaturation in a patient with severe tricuspid insufficiency. Venous pulsations are larger in the more dependent portions of the body and when the tissue is vasodilated (e.g., in hyperthermia). When venous pulsations are large compared with arterial pulsations, pulse oximeter-derived saturation decreases toward the hemoglobin saturation of the venous blood. Respiratory variations in the venous plethysmogram during positive-pressure ventilation may overwhelm the arterial pulsations in critically ill patients (12). In these cases, it may be necessary to interrupt ventilation intermittently to get a pulse oximetry reading.

Noise

With any monitor, artifacts occur when the noise-to-signal ratio becomes too large. The pulse oximeter is no exception. Artifacts of this type occur either because the pulsatile signal is too small or because the background noise is too great.

Low-Amplitude Pulsations. Low-amplitude pulsations are generally caused by vasoconstriction of the tissue at the measurement site. Pulse oximeters automatically attempt to maximize their signal by increasing either the LED brightness or the photodiode sensitivity. Because of this, pulse oximeters can determine saturations during low-perfusion states. For example, under experimental conditions, pulse oximeters continue to give readings at blood flows below 10% of baseline (13). Unfortunately, increasing LED brightness or photodiode gain tends to reduce the signal-to-noise ratio and degrade the saturation accuracy. The clinician can improve signal strength in a digit by performing a digital nerve block (14).

Anemia. Anemia decreases the amount of hemoglobin available to absorb the light of the pulse oximeter. As with low-amplitude pulsations, this decreases the pulsatile signal strength. There is a gradual increase in the loss-of-signal failure rate as the hematocrit decreases from 30% to 10%; below a hematocrit of 10%, the failure rate becomes very high. Pulse oximeter-derived saturations are accurate above a hematocrit of 15%, but at hematocrits below 10%, the calculated saturation becomes undependable and tends to underestimate the true saturation (15).

Penumbra Effect. The penumbra effect, also called "optical shunt," can cause pulse oximeter saturation errors via an improperly applied sensor. When the sensor is properly applied, all light from the LED passes through tissue before reaching the photodiode; when improperly applied, part of the light from the LED bypasses the tissue and travels directly to the photodiode. This situation can occur when an adhesive sensor is applied tangentially or when the sensor becomes partially dislodged during use. It is possible that the penumbra effect results from the shunted light drowning out the normal signal, depressing calculated saturation toward 85%. Artificially low saturations of 89% to 95% caused by this mechanism have been reported, and in each case the displayed heart rate was accurate (16). The effect is more pronounced when the tissue is vasodilated.

Light. Ambient light can interfere with a pulse oximeter, since the photodiode is a broad-spectrum detector. As discussed above (Pulsations and Pulse Oximetry), most pulse oximeters measure and correct for ambient light intensity. Still, bright or fluorescent lights can cause loss of signal or inaccurate saturations. Fluorescent lights are a particular problem because they flash. This can cause a false signal, caused by lack of synchronization between the flashing frequency of the light and the sampling frequency of the pulse oximeter (17). The clinician can resolve this problem by shielding the sensor from bright lights.

Electromagnetic Interference. Electromagnetic interference, either from an electrosurgery unit or a magnetic resonance imaging (MRI) scanner, can interfere with the pulse oximeter signal. MRI scanners also have the potential to cause patient burns at the sensor site, and only specially designed pulse oximeters should be used for that reason.

Inaccurate Calibration

Pulse oximeters do not require user calibration, but *two* factors may cause inaccurate readings through miscalibration. *First*, LEDs are manufactured with slight variations in the frequencies of light that they emit (average frequencies of 660 nm and 940 nm). Small changes in the transmitted frequency result in significant changes in calculated saturation, especially at low saturation values. Pulse oximeter manufacturers have largely overcome this problem by electronically coding the probes to indicate the emitted frequency and using a different calibration curve for each specific frequency. *Second*, pulse oximeter saturation is calculated from a calibration curve that is empirically, not theoretically, derived. Early curves were based on observed absorptions at high and moderately low saturations. A number of researchers found that the calibration curves were inaccurate at very low saturations, and many manufacturers have since updated their algorithms to improve accuracy at low saturations (18). Still, the proprietary algorithms result in discrepancies between instruments of different manufacturers, and accuracy is generally better at high saturations than at low ones.

Probe Location

Probe position is one of the few pulse oximeter factors that the clinician can control. Most commonly, probes are applied to a finger or toe, across the bridge of the nose, or across the pinna of an ear. Response times to sudden changes in saturation depend, in part, on the circulation time from the pulmonary veins to the probe site. The circulation time is variable between patients and is generally shorter at the ear and nose than at the finger or toe. However, venous pulsations tend to be more pronounced at the ear or nose than at the finger or toe. The probe must be positioned so that an adequate quantity of tissue is interposed between the LEDs and the photodiode; tangential application results in a penumbra effect. In small infants, the probe may be placed across the foot or hand. In the vasoconstricted patient, adequate pulsations are more commonly found in the more proximal locations, such as the ear or nose. Readings may be more readily obtained from the base of the finger than from the tip of the finger in these patients. A digital nerve block or application of topical nitroglycerin or local heat may improve the signal by decreasing vasoconstriction in a single digit.

Capnometry

Capnometry is the quantification of carbon dioxide in respiratory gases. It has been used clinically in operating rooms since the 1970s. In the early 1990s, the American Society of Anesthesiologists recommended capnometry as a standard intra-operative monitor to confirm endotracheal intubation and aid in the quantitative assessment of ventilation during general anesthesia (19).

A *capnometer* is a device that provides a quantitative display of carbon dioxide concentration, while a *capnograph* is a device that, additionally, provides a graphic display of carbon dioxide concentration over time. Stand-alone capnometers measure only carbon dioxide and are increasingly being used in intensive care units, emergency rooms, and other critical patient care areas. Respiratory gas analyzers, which measure other gases (oxygen, nitrogen, nitrous oxide, and the potent inhaled anesthetic agents) in addition to carbon dioxide, are more commonly used in the operating room.

Carbon dioxide concentration in respiratory gases is determined using either spectroscopy or colorimetry. The principles of spectroscopic monitoring and the interpretation of capnograms are discussed in this section. Colorimetric monitoring is discussed in a later section (Confirming Endotracheal Intubation).

Measurement Principles

Measurement Techniques

Clinical capnometers use one of three analytic methods: infrared spectroscopy, mass spectroscopy, or Raman spectroscopy. The method of analysis affects the cost of the instrument and the number of other gases that can be measured concurrently.

Infrared Spectroscopy. Infrared spectroscopy is by far the most common capnometric method and is the technique used in all stand-alone capnometers. Like pulse oximetry, its basis is the Beer-Lambert law of light absorption. In this case, carbon dioxide concentration is measured *in vitro* by quantifying the absorption of infrared light at a wavelength of 4.3 μm as it passes through a sample of gas. Only polar molecules absorb infrared light, and therefore infrared spectrometers cannot measure oxygen, nitrogen, or helium concentrations.

Nitrous oxide can interfere with some infrared capnometers (20). Capnometers that analyze at a broad spectral width may detect nitrous oxide, which absorbs infrared light at a wavelength of 4.5 μm, resulting in an artifactual increase. Nitrous oxide also reduces the optic density of carbon dioxide, an effect called "collision broadening"; this effect results in artificially low readings in capnometers that do not specifically correct for it. Some capnometers are not designed to be used in the presence of nitrous oxide, some require the user to indicate whether the gas contains more than 50% nitrous oxide, and others measure, and automatically correct for, nitrous oxide.

Mass Spectroscopy. Mass spectrometry can be used to quantify all respiratory gases. Mass spectrometers ionize a gas and measure the number of ions along the spectrum of mass-to-charge ratio. Laboratory instruments use a "sweeping detector" to analyze and quantify all the ions in a range of the spectrum, while clinical mass spectrometers quantify specific ions using multiple, fixed detectors.

Mass spectrometers are expensive, largely because of the high vacuum that must be maintained within the analyzer unit. As a result, clinical mass spectrometers are typically multiplexed to provide parallel monitoring of multiple patients within an intensive care unit or suite of operating rooms. Gas is continuously sampled from each patient and transmitted to a central analyzer. The central mass spectrometer sequentially samples a small amount of gas from each patient and transmits the results back to displays at each patient site.

A limitation of a multiplexed mass spectrometer is that continuous monitoring is not possible, because gas analysis is performed on each patient in sequence. Thus, there is an interval between analyses for a particular patient, the duration of which depends on the number of patients connected to the system and the duration of each patient's analysis (dwell time). In a worst-case scenario, two breaths may be analyzed every 3 minutes.

Raman Spectroscopy. One respiratory gas analyzer uses Raman spectroscopy to quantify carbon dioxide, nitrogen, oxygen, nitrous oxide, and the potent inhaled anesthetic agents (21). Raman spectroscopy measures the tiny fraction of light that is absorbed and re-emitted at a longer wavelength. Because of the small proportion of light that is scattered in this manner, the incident light is provided by an extremely bright laser. The high-power laser is relatively expensive.

Instrument Factors

Two instrument factors, the gas-sampling method and the response time, influence the clinical performance of all capnometers.

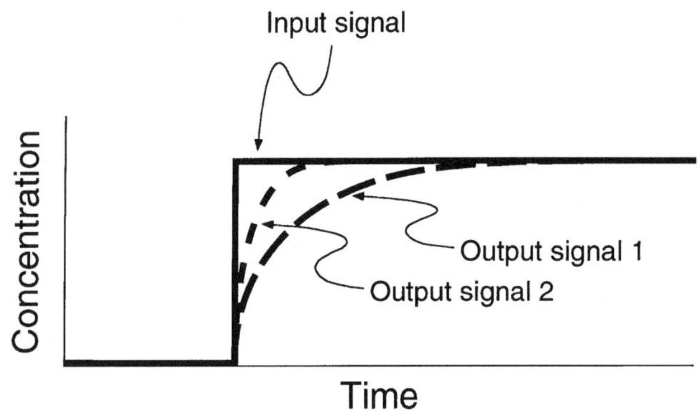

FIG. 9. Response time is a measure of how rapidly a monitor responds to a change in the input signal. *Output signal 1* is the output of a monitor with a long response time, whereas *output signal 2* is from a monitor with a relatively short response time.

Gas Sampling. A prerequisite for gas analysis is that the analyzer and respiratory gas be brought together. Mainstream capnometers bring the analyzer to the gas, whereas side-stream capnometers bring the gas to the analyzer.

Mainstream analyzers. In some infrared capnometers, the optics are located on a sensor that is connected to the endotracheal tube. An advantage of this approach is the absence of a delay between the breath and the analysis. A major limitation is that a heavy and bulky sensor must be attached to the endotracheal tube; also, essential components of the monitor are exposed to breakage. Mainstream capnometers tend to have fast response times (see below).

Side-stream analyzers. Most capnometers, and all multigas analyzers, continuously withdraw gas samples from the breathing circuit and analyze it within the monitor. An advantage of this technique is that gas can be sampled from an unintubated patient (e.g., by sampling at the nose). A limitation is that gas is continually lost from the breathing circuit. When anesthetic gases are being used, this sampled gas must either be returned to the breathing circuit or be disposed of in a scavenger system to avoid room pollution. Gas-sampling systems are also prone to problems, such as leaks and obstructions, that can cause failures or artifacts. Another disadvantage of side-stream capnometry is that the transit time of gas through the sampling system introduces a delay in analysis; also, mixing within the sample line tends to degrade the analyzer's response time (see below).

Response Time. Response time refers to the speed with which an analyzer responds to a change in the sensed parameter (Fig. 9). It is an important factor in a monitor that tracks an oscillating signal, such as a capnometer recording fluctuations in carbon dioxide concentration in the airway.

Capnometers have response times in the range of 0.05 to 0.9 second (50 to 900 milliseconds). The response time depends almost entirely on the design of the gas subsystems of the monitor, since the electric and optic components respond almost instantaneously.

The inherent response time of a capnometer is a function of the time required to wash gas out of the analyzer chamber and replace it with a fresh sample; this depends on the size of the analyzer chamber and the sampled gas flow rate (Fig. 10). Mass spectrometers and mainstream capnometers have fast inherent response times; side-stream infrared and Raman spectrometers are slower.

The gas-sampling system adds a delay and degrades the overall analyzer response time. The delay is the time it takes for a sample of gas to travel from the breathing circuit to the analyzer. The duration of the delay depends

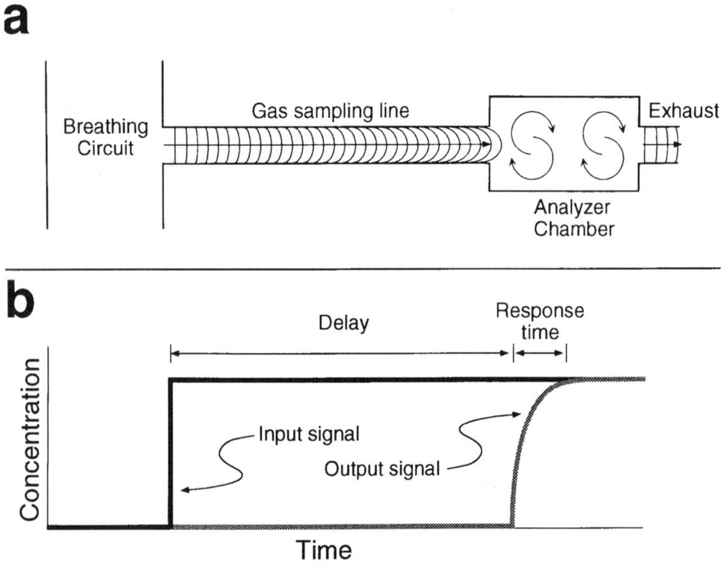

FIG. 10. A side-stream capnometer. **a:** The gas-sampling system; **b:** Graph of the input and output signals. The lag in output is divided into two components: transport delay and response time. The gas-sampling system influences both components. Transport delay is the time it takes for a sample of gas to travel from the breathing circuit to the analyzer. Response time is influenced by size of the analyzer chamber, sampled-gas flow rate, and amount of slurring that occurs in the gas-sampling line.

on the gas-sampling rate and on the caliber and length of the sample line. As gas travels through the sample line, flow patterns and diffusion cause gas mixing, which smears the boundaries and degrades response time.

A long response time impairs an analyzer's ability to track a rapidly changing signal (22). When the response time is too long, the end-tidal carbon dioxide concentration is underestimated. For a capnometer to determine the peak exhaled carbon dioxide concentration accurately, it must respond within the expiratory time. This may not occur when the response time is long or the respiratory frequency is high. To measure accurately the peak carbon dioxide concentration of a patient breathing 40 times per minute at an inspiratory-to-expiratory (I:E) ratio of 1:1 requires an analyzer with a response time under 250 milliseconds. Most dedicated capnometers have a response time shorter than this, but multiplexed mass spectrometers may not. However, even dedicated side-stream capnometers may not accurately track the capnogram of a neonate. Neonates have a high respiratory rate and small exhaled tidal volume. This decreases both the time and volume of gas available for the determination (23).

Interpretation of Capnometry

Capnometers display the peak (and sometimes the minimum) detected carbon dioxide concentration and usually the respiratory rate. Capnographs additionally display a graph of carbon dioxide concentration over time. Capnometers and capnographs are used to confirm endotracheal intubation, monitor respiratory rate, and noninvasively assess the arterial partial pressure of carbon dioxide. To interpret capnometry, the clinician must understand the relationships between arterial and exhaled carbon dioxide levels. By analyzing the shape of the capnogram, the clinician can gain additional information regarding the reliability of the sample and the state of the ventilation system.

Discrepancies Between End-tidal and Arterial Values

One must not incorrectly assume that the CO_2 concentration displayed on a capnometer is a reliable indicator of $PaCO_2$. The concentration displayed may not be reliable

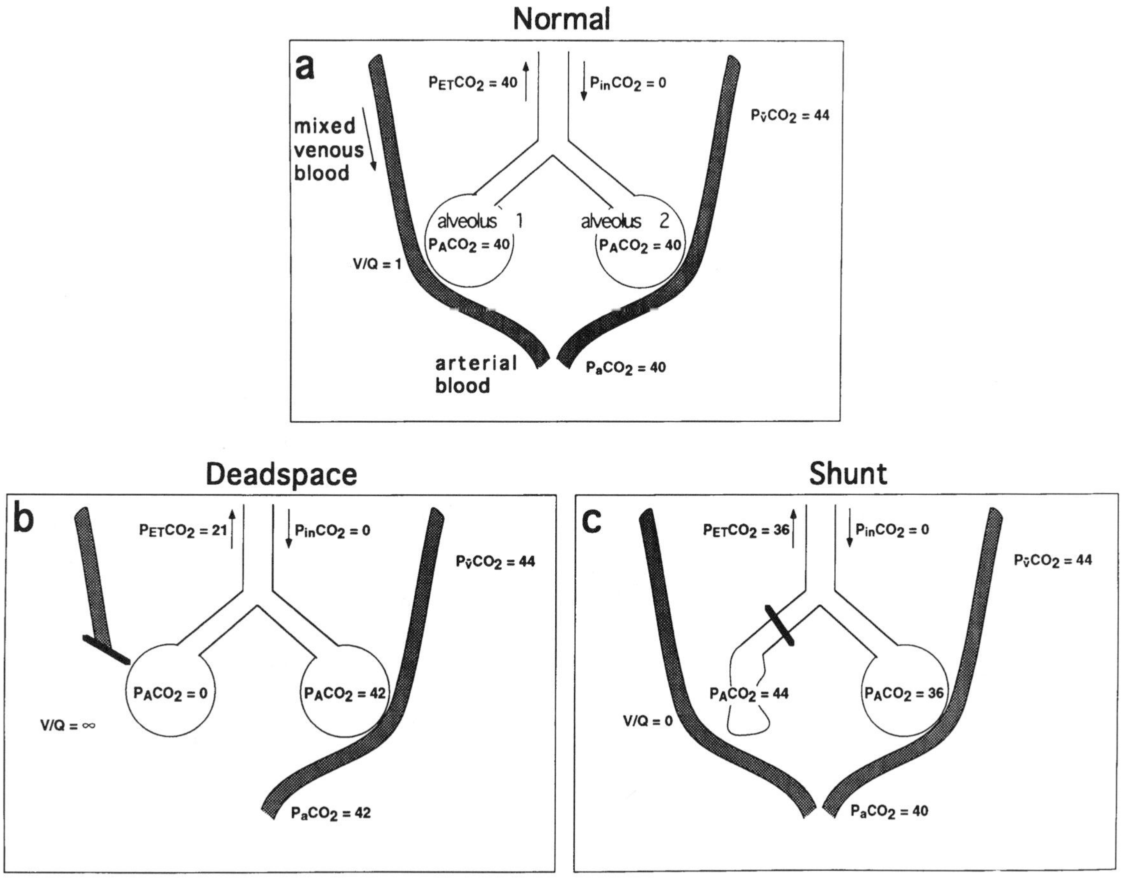

FIG. 11. A two-compartment lung model illustrates the effects of shunt and dead space abnormalities on exhaled CO_2. **a:** In the normal situation (V/Q = 1), end-tidal CO_2 approaches arterial CO_2. **b:** Alveolar dead space (V/Q = ∞) yields an end-tidal CO_2 that is much lower than arterial CO_2. **c:** Shunt (V/Q = 0) causes a small difference between end-tidal CO_2 and arterial CO_2. Note: all values given are in mmHg.

for two reasons: 1) Discrepancies may occur between the displayed CO_2 concentration and the end-tidal concentration, as discussed below (Artifacts), and 2) discrepancies may occur between end-tidal CO_2 and $PaCO_2$.

End-tidal gas is generally composed of mixed alveolar gas. By definition, alveolar CO_2 approaches arterial CO_2 when the ventilation-perfusion ratio (V/Q) is 1 (Fig. 11a). However, when V/Q is greater than 1, alveolar CO_2 is less than arterial CO_2; at the extremely high V/Q of infinity (dead space), alveolar CO_2 is 0 regardless of arterial CO_2 (Fig. 11b). Also, when V/Q is less than 1, alveolar CO_2 is slightly higher than arterial CO_2; at the extremely low V/Q of 0 (shunt), alveolar CO_2 is equal to mixed venous CO_2 (Fig. 11c). End-tidal CO_2 is the weighted average of the CO_2 concentration in each alveolus. The end-tidal CO_2 level is generally 1 to 3 mm Hg lower than arterial CO_2 in healthy patients, because more tidal volume usually goes to ventilate alveoli with a high V/Q than those with a low V/Q (24). The difference between end-tidal and arterial CO_2 is very high in patients with large areas of alveolar dead space (Fig. 11b), such as those with a pulmonary embolus (25). There is less discrepancy between end-tidal and arterial CO_2 in patients with large areas of shunt (Fig. 11c), such as those with an endobronchial intubation.

In rare instances, end-tidal CO_2 can be higher than arterial CO_2. This can occur when low V/Q alveoli empty more slowly than high V/Q alveoli, leading to a predominance of gas from the latter at the end of exhalation.

Interpretation of Waveforms

The capnogram has four phases: the inspiratory baseline (I), the expiratory upstroke (II), the expiratory plateau (III), and the inspiratory downstroke (IV) (Fig. 12). The inspiratory baseline is normally at 0, indicating that no carbon dioxide is being inhaled. The expiratory upstroke is normally steep, indicating that gas flow is swift as anatomic dead space gas, followed quickly by mixed alveolar gas, passes the sensor. The expiratory plateau is normally stable, indicating good mixing of gas from alveoli that empty evenly. The inspiratory downstroke is normally steep, indicating that fresh gas quickly replaces alveolar gas as it flows past the sensor.

Some patient and breathing circuit conditions have characteristic capnograms (Fig. 13). Elevation of the inspiratory baseline (Fig. 13a) indicates the presence of inspiratory CO_2, usually caused by rebreathing from a breathing circuit malfunction. An expiratory plateau that slopes upward (Fig. 13b) indicates uneven emptying of alveoli that have a wide V/Q range; this typically occurs during small-airway obstruction, as in asthma and COPD. Large-airway obstruction and endotracheal tube obstruction do not cause noticeable changes in the capnogram until the obstruction is almost complete, at which time decreases in the slopes of the expiratory upstroke and inspiratory downstroke may become apparent. Clefts in the expiratory plateau (Fig. 13c), sometimes called "curare clefts," are caused by small inspiratory tidal volumes superimposed on normal ventilation. This situation can be seen with hiccoughs, inadequate muscle relaxation (if the patient has a higher respiratory rate than the ventilator), and external forces applied to the patient (such as surgical manipulation of the abdomen to cause movement of the lungs). Oscillations in the expiratory plateau (Fig. 13d) are called "cardiac oscillations"; they are caused by small movements of gas in the breathing circuit caused by heartbeats during periods of low expiratory flow.

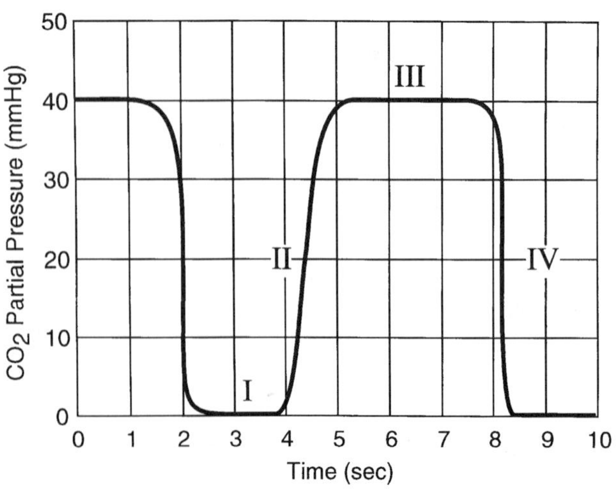

FIG. 12. The normal capnogram has four phases: *I*, inspiratory baseline; *II*, expiratory upstroke; *III*, expiratory plateau; *IV*, inspiratory downstroke.

Artifacts (Discordance Between Measured and True End-tidal Values)

The measured peak concentration of CO_2 is not always equal to the true end-tidal value. There are three common causes for a discrepancy: an inadequate end-tidal sample, a leak in the sampling system, and miscalibration of the monitor. An inadequate end-tidal sample should be suspected when the capnogram does not reach a plateau (Fig. 14a). This situation can occur during shallow ventilation, when tidal volumes are less than the anatomic dead space. However, as explained above (Response Time), it more commonly is caused by a respiratory rate that is too rapid for the response time of the capnometer. The measured end-tidal value is inaccurate when the capnogram does not reach a plateau; the true end-tidal value is higher by some unknown amount. With a leak in the sampling system, room air is entrained and the displayed values are artificially low. Leaks are difficult to detect, since the capnogram often looks normal during

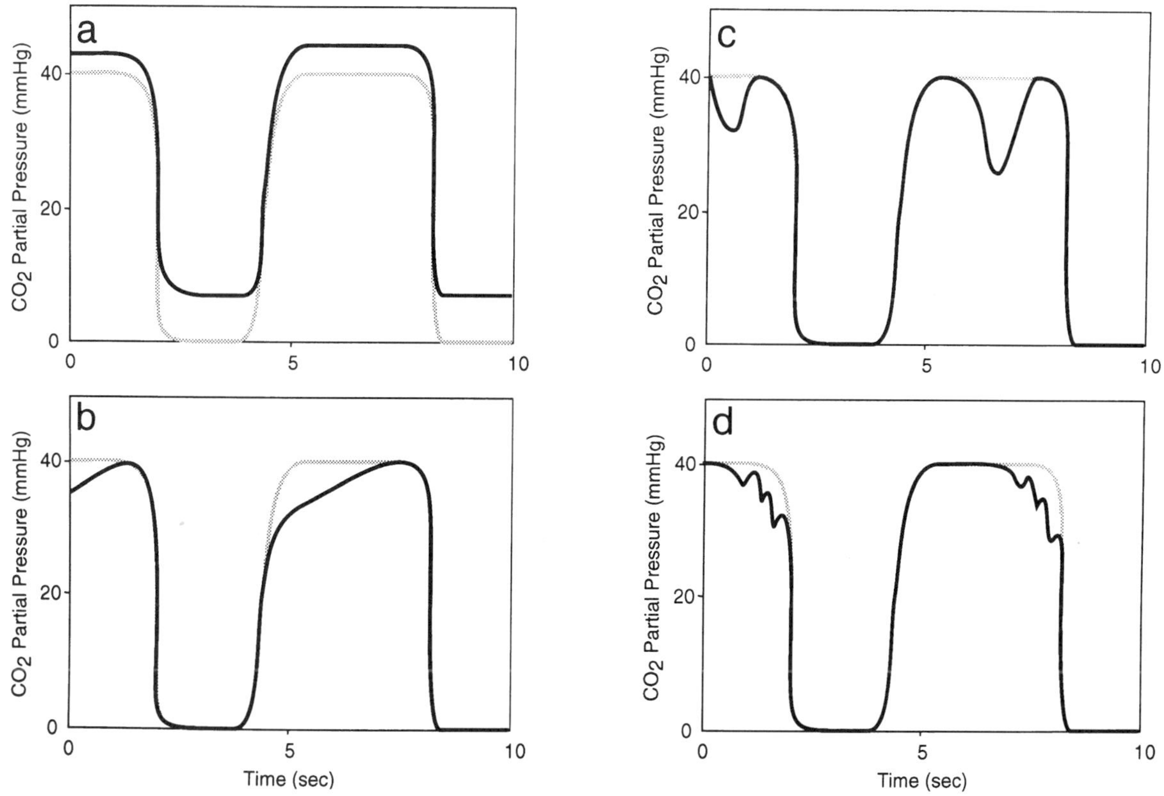

FIG. 13. Abnormal capnograms have characteristic shapes (normal capnogram shown in *gray* for comparison). **a:** The elevated baseline indicates the presence of inspired CO_2. This can be caused by exhaustion of soda lime or an incompetent exhalation valve in a circle breathing circuit. **b:** The sloping expiratory plateau indicates small-airway obstruction and is commonly seen in smokers and asthmatics. **c:** Curare clefts in the expiratory plateau can indicate superimposed spontaneous breaths during controlled ventilation. **d:** Cardiac oscillations are caused by heartbeats during periods of low expiratory flow.

spontaneous ventilation (Fig. 14b). However, during positive-pressure ventilation, a leak in the sampling line can cause a characteristic waveform (Fig. 14c). It is important that capnometers be properly calibrated. An uncalibrated monitor will display artificially low or high measured values. Most capnometers automatically calibrate to 0 during use; however, some require that the user initiate a 1-point calibration at another value.

Bedside Spirometry

A number of techniques are available to assess respiratory mechanics quantitatively at the bedside. These methods and their interpretation are discussed in this section.

Volume

Tidal volume is the volume of gas that is exchanged during a normal breath. To measure it, the patient breathes normally and a unidirectional valve directs the exhaled gas into a measuring device. For accuracy, a number of breaths are averaged to yield the tidal volume. Vital capacity is the largest volume of gas that can be voluntarily expelled from the lungs during a single breath. It represents the difference between the total lung capacity and the residual volume. To measure it, the patient forcefully exhales into a measuring device after inhaling maximally. Volume is measured either directly, by accumulating volume, or indirectly, by integrating flow.

The simplest device for measuring volume is the water seal respirometer, which has a vertical displacement that is proportional to the volume of gas that it contains. Water seal respirometers are reliable and accurate but are too awkward for bedside use; they have largely been replaced by more convenient methods. Rolling seal respirometers are an example of less bulky devices that are accurate at high and low rates of gas flow and are unaffected by gas composition. They measure gas volume directly with a system of revolving chambers that sequentially fill and empty in the gas stream.

Instantaneous gas flow can be integrated over time to calculate volume. Flowmeters used for this purpose must be highly accurate and have a rapid response to a chang-

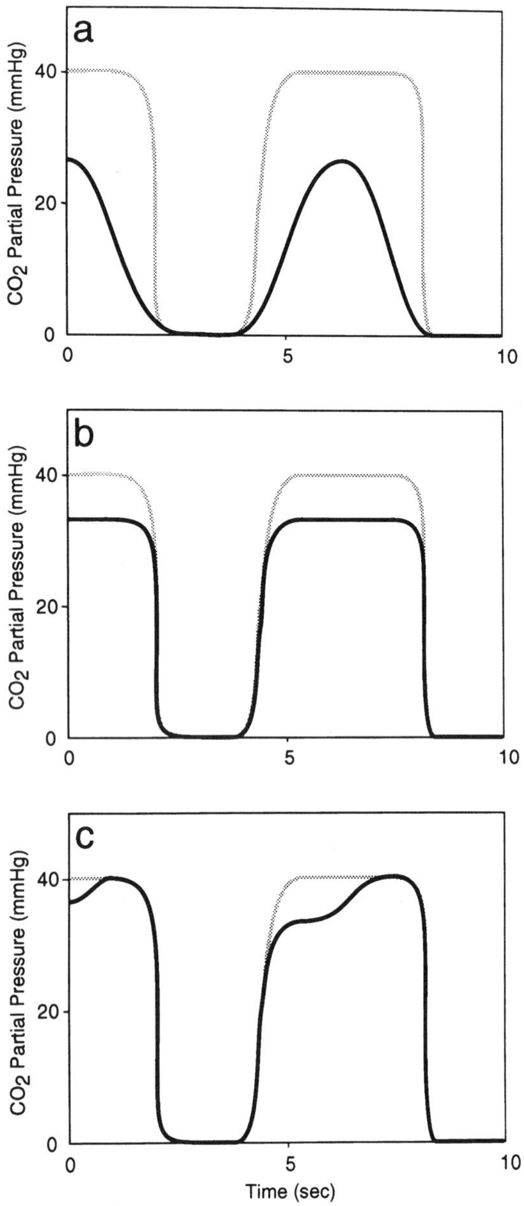

FIG. 14. Characteristic capnograms indicate the presence of an artifact (normal capnogram shown in *gray* for comparison). **a:** Measured end-tidal value is inaccurate when the capnogram does not reach a plateau. **b:** A leak in the sampling line during spontaneous ventilation is difficult to detect. **c:** A leak in the sampling line during positive-pressure ventilation causes a characteristic waveform.

ing flow rate, because small errors in instantaneous flow rate cause large errors when integrated to yield volume. A number of flowmeter technologies are commonly used; rotating-vane and pneumotachograph techniques are discussed here.

The Wright respirometer is an example of a device that uses rotating-vane technology; it counts the revolutions of a turbine vane that spins in the gas stream at a rate proportional to flow (26). Gas density as well as flow rate determines the force imparted to the vane, so the measurement is affected by gas temperature and composition. The rotating-vane technique is relatively inaccurate because of the inertia and friction of the mechanical vane; the vane does not move at low flow rates and is slow to respond to changing flow rates. However, rotating-vane spirometers are small, convenient, and often used for bedside measurements. The pneumotachograph is a more accurate method for measuring flow. It is commonly used in electronic spirometers. In this technique, differential pressure is measured across a flow resistor placed in the gas path. The flow resistor traditionally comprises a group of parallel tubes that have laminar flow within them; however, screens, variable-orifice resistors, or Pitot tubes, named after Henri Pitot (1695–1771), a French physicist who devised a method of flow-velocity measurement using a specially designed tube, may also be used. A sensitive pressure differential transducer measures the pressure signal, which is very small (under 1 cm H_20), since the resistance to flow must be kept low. Pneumotachographs respond rapidly to changing flow rates and can be very accurate. They are usually heated to prevent condensation of water, and gas composition and temperature must be compensated for, since gas viscosity significantly affects the relationship between the gas flow rate and the pressure signal (27).

The difference between tidal volume and vital capacity is an estimate of respiratory reserve; normally, the vital capacity is 10 times larger than the tidal volume. Normal vital capacity is strongly correlated with patient height. Vital capacity may be decreased by physical factors, such as muscle weakness or decreased respiratory system compliance, as well as by psychologic factors, such as pain and poor patient effort.

Peak Flow

Peak expiratory flow rate is a measure of the maximal flow rate that is generated during forced exhalation from total lung capacity. The first simple device to measure peak expiratory flow, the Wright peak flowmeter, was developed in 1959 (28). A number of simple, inexpensive, and often disposable peak flowmeters are now commercially available. Most measure either the peak pressure drop across a fixed resistance, or the minimal resistance with a fixed pressure drop. An independent test of eight different models of peak flowmeters found that they were generally accurate (29).

Peak flow is an indicator of the expiratory muscles' ability to overcome gas flow resistance during exhalation. Thus, it is affected by the strength of the respiratory muscles, the recoil of the respiratory system (lung and chest wall), and the airway resistance. Clinically, peak flow measurements are usually used to assess severity of bronchospasm.

Peak Pressure

Peak inspiratory and expiratory pressures indicate the maximal forces that can be applied for ventilation. They are important measures of respiratory muscle strength in patients with impaired neuromuscular function. Both are easily measured at the bedside with a simple aneroid gauge. Inspiratory pressure is an important factor in the ability to generate an adequate tidal volume, while expiratory pressure is an important factor in the ability to cough effectively. Peak inspiratory pressure is measured after forced exhalation because the inspiratory muscles generate maximal force at residual volume. Peak expiratory pressure is generated at vital capacity; therefore, it is measured after forced inhalation. Both measures depend on patient cooperation and may not be accurate in the sedated or disoriented patient.

Interpretation of Bedside Spirometry

Impaired respiratory mechanics stem from three potential causes: increased resistance, decreased compliance, or decreased muscle strength. Bedside spirometry differentiates among these and yields quantitative information that is useful for management decisions (Table 5). Increased resistance reduces peak flow rates, usually with preservation of normal peak expiratory pressure and vital capacity. Causes of increased airway resistance include breathing circuit or endotracheal tube obstruction, upper airway obstruction, tracheal obstruction, bronchospasm, airway secretions, and emphysema. Decreased compliance leads to decreased vital capacity, some decrease in peak inspiratory pressure, but preservation of normal peak expiratory flow rate. Causes of decreased compliance include abdominal distention (e.g., obesity, pregnancy, ascites, hepatomegaly, tumors), pleural or chest wall restriction (e.g., pleural effusion, pneumothorax, kyphoscoliosis), and decreased lung compliance (e.g., pulmonary edema, pneumonia, adult respiratory distress syndrome, pulmonary fibrosis). Decreased muscle strength decreases vital capacity, peak inspiratory and expiratory pressures, and peak expiratory flow rate. Causes of decreased muscle strength include neuromuscular relaxants, neuromuscular disease (e.g., Guillain-Barré syndrome, spinal injury, polio), pain, fatigue, and poor patient effort.

TABLE 5. *Differential diagnosis of hypoventilation using bedside spirometry*

Condition	Peak flow	Vital capacity	Peak expiratory pressure
Increased resistance	Low	Normal	Normal
Decreased compliance	Normal	Low	Normal or slightly low
Decreased muscle strength	Low	Low	Low

CONFIRMING ENDOTRACHEAL TUBE PLACEMENT

Perhaps the most critical step in the process of ventilating a patient is identifying correct placement of the endotracheal tube (ETT). Incorrect placement, though infrequent, can have disastrous consequences if undetected. Traditionally, methods for confirming placement include direct visualization of the airway (both during and following ETT placement), capnography, radiography, oximetry, and assessment of clinical signs. More recently, portable capnometry, the esophageal detection device, and computer algorithms have been described.

Clinical Signs

Perhaps the most frequently used method of determining proper ETT placement is the assessment of clinical signs. Indeed, the dictum "observe the patient" is nowhere more important than in confirming a patent airway. The observation of clinical signs should be one of the first steps a clinician performs after placing an ETT. Auscultation of breath sounds, followed by listening over the epigastrium for absence of sounds and gastric distention, is the commonly accepted procedure for initial confirmation of ETT placement. Other important clinical signs include chest expansion and the appearance of fog on the interior of the ETT. However, there have been reports of these methods failing to detect the esophageal placement of an ETT (30).

The anterior chest, although used frequently in practice, is not the best area for auscultation when determining ETT placement. Rather, listening for breath sounds at the right and left axillae while large tidal volumes are being delivered has been shown to be much more accurate (31). Although the so-called "educated hand" (the subjective "feel" of the reservoir bag during hand ventilation of a patient) has been described as a method of detection, it is very operator-dependent and has not been proved accurate, even among well-trained individuals.

The advantages of assessment of clinical signs for confirming ETT placement are availability and simplicity. A stethoscope can be carried easily to any location, requires no power, and can be used repeatedly. Stethoscopes are reliable, inexpensive, and readily available in most healthcare settings. However, because assessment of clinical signs is not entirely accurate, and because undetected ETT misplacement is a serious matter, one or more other methods should be used to confirm placement.

Capnometry

A very powerful and sensitive method for confirming endotracheal placement of ETTs became available with the advent of small, real-time detectors of end-tidal CO_2. The operation of these detectors is based on the fact that CO_2 gas is constantly excreted by the lungs, whereas only small amounts of the gas exist in the gastrointestinal tract.

The American Society of Anesthesiologists has recommended capnometry as a standard intra-operative monitor to confirm endotracheal intubation (19). Therefore, most operating rooms have capnography readily available for use by anesthesiologists and anesthetists. Many emergency departments and intensive care units also have capnometry available. In these locations, where intubating conditions may not be optimal, capnometry may be especially important.

Intubations in the prehospital setting are much more likely to be misplaced in the esophagus than those done in the hospital. Reasons for this include inexperience of healthcare providers, lack of muscle relaxation, trauma to the neck and/or airway, and poor intubating conditions in the field. Rapid and careful assessment of ETT placement by emergency department personnel is therefore crucial. If available, this should include clinical assessment, capnometry, and, if necessary, direct or fiberoptic laryngoscopy with the ETT in place.

Despite the widespread use of electronic capnometers, they are not available in some locations because of cost or logistics. A recently developed end-tidal CO_2 detector Easycap, (Nellcor Puritan Bennett, Pleasanton, Californa) is a useful tool for confirming endotracheal intubation in such locations (Fig. 15). The Easycap device was first marketed as the FEF device (Fenem, Inc., New York, New York). The Easycap device uses a colorimetric method to detect CO_2 tension continuously. A pH-sensitive colorimetric membrane within a clear plastic dome reversibly changes color in response to the CO_2 tension of the gas passing over it. The color of this membrane is then compared with a calibration color band located on the outside of the device. Dark purple to light purple indicates end-tidal CO_2 of less than 3.8 mm Hg; dark brown to light brown corresponds to end-tidal CO_2 tension in the range of 3.8 to 15 mm Hg; dark and light yellow represent an end-tidal CO_2 tension greater than 15 mm Hg. Since hemodynamically stable adults and children exhale CO_2 with a tension of 30 to 40 mm Hg, the yellow range is expected to confirm placement of an ETT in the trachea.

The Easycap device is lightweight (18.5 g), adds minimal dead space to the breathing circuit (38 mL), is disposable and inexpensive, and has a shelf life of approximately 15 months. Once activated, it functions for up to 5 hours; however, humidity in the circuit can decrease its life span to as little as 15 minutes. It is both sensitive (average minimum CO_2 detected is 4.1 mm Hg; CO_2 is detected in tidal

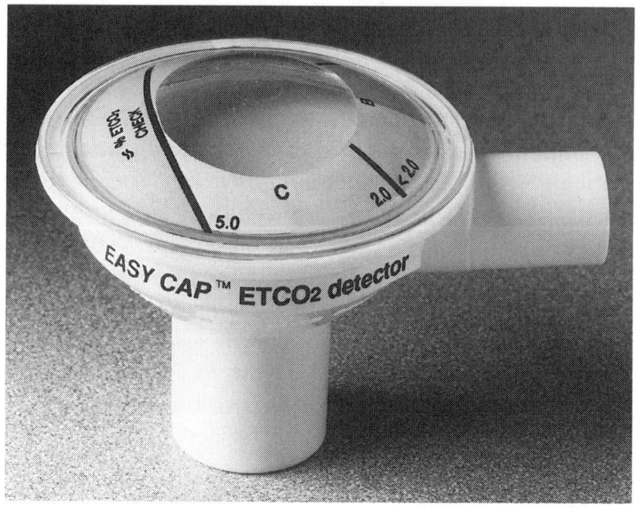

FIG. 15. The Easycap CO_2 detector device (reprinted with permission of Nellcor Puritan Bennett, Pleasanton, California).

volumes as low as 50 mL with end-tidal CO_2 greater than 15 mm Hg) and specific to CO_2. It provides rapid and accurate detection of end-tidal CO_2 both in hemodynamically stable adults (32) and children (33), whether they are breathing spontaneously or mechanically.

Another small CO_2 detection device, the MiniCAP III (MSA Catalyst Research, Owings Mills, Maryland), simply indicates the presence of CO_2 without any quantitative reading. It is a battery-operated capnometer that emits a flash and beep during each breath in which CO_2 is detected and an alarm signal in the absence of CO_2. The fact that it is small and reusable makes it unique. However, it does not give the additional semiquantitative information provided by the FEF CO_2 detector.

Regardless of the type of device, capnometry is an important tool for the detection of correct placement of ETTs. However, conditions that may lead to errors in interpretation warrant mentioning.

False-positives occur if CO_2 is detected when the ETT is not in the trachea. This occurs primarily during inadvertent esophageal intubation in a patient whose stomach contains CO_2. Normally the stomach contains little or no CO_2. However, the stomach may contain a significant amount of CO_2 after recent ingestion of a carbonated beverage; this is known as the "cola complication" (34). The cola complication causes a characteristic capnogram tracing, in which the end-tidal CO_2 decreases with each subsequent breath (35). There is concern that the cola complication may lead to inadequate detection of esophageal intubation when portable semiquantitative or qualitative devices, which do not display CO_2 waveforms, are used (36).

False-negatives occur when CO_2 is *not* detected, even though the ETT is properly placed in the trachea. In situations such as cardiac arrest and hypovolemic shock, cardiac output may not be adequate to produce normal end-tidal CO_2 levels. If profound enough, the low levels of CO_2 may be mistakenly interpreted as indicating an esophageal intubation. This is especially true if the capnogram is not displayed. The danger of a false-negative is that it exposes the patient to the risk of repeated direct laryngoscopy and intubation. Therefore, in patients with poor cardiac output, clinical signs and other adjunctive methods of detection should be used before deciding to reintubate.

Palpation of the Tracheal Balloon

Supplemental methods for determining placement of the endotracheal tube need not require special or expensive devices. One method requires nothing but the endotracheal tube and the clinician's hand. After placement of the ETT in the usual manner, and initial determination of placement by primary methods (see above), the ETT cuff is deflated and then reinflated briskly while the trachea is externally palpated above the sternum. In most patients, the inflation of the cuff is felt with the palpating hand. This maneuver confirms that the endotracheal tube is located at the proper depth within the trachea.

The usefulness of this technique is limited in obese patients and those with abnormalities of the neck or airway. As with any clinical exercise, it should be practiced in routine intubations, so that the clinician is comfortable with the positive and negative signs prior to its use in a difficult situation.

Visualization

Seeing is believing, and watching the ETT pass through the cords is considered one of the best indications of proper placement. Direct visualization is a reliable indicator for initial placement of an ETT. Repeated direct laryngoscopy, with the ETT in place, can be used to ascertain placement of a tube that may have been subsequently dislodged from its correct position.

The fiberoptic laryngoscope is also useful for confirming placement of the ETT. Here, positive confirmation is achieved by viewing the tracheal rings and carina below the level of the ETT. Knowledge of the segmental anatomy of the trachea and bronchi is helpful in detecting intended or inadvertent placement of the ETT in the right or left main bronchus.

It is worth mentioning that the anesthetist may be the first clinician to view a patient's airway, either by direct or fiberoptic laryngoscopy, and should therefore be attentive to any previously undiagnosed abnormalities of the airway. These may include tumors, trauma to the airway, fistulas, foreign bodies, abscesses, or abnormal tracheobronchial anatomy. Notation of these abnormalities in the medical record will serve to alert clinicians for future airway procedures. Consultation of appropriate medical and/or surgical specialists will insure proper treatment is received, if needed.

Esophageal Detector Device

A relatively new method for determination for ETT placement is aspiration of the ETT with the esophageal detector device (also known as the "syringe aspiration technique"). The technique is based on the fact that the esophagus is a collapsible structure, whereas the trachea is not. The esophageal detector device is simply a 50-mL Toomey syringe connected to a tracheal tube adapter via a 4-mm length of surgical tubing (Fig. 16). The device is connected to the ETT and the plunger of the syringe is withdrawn. If the ETT lies in the trachea, air is withdrawn easily. However, with the ETT in the esophagus, vacuum occurs and withdrawal of air with the syringe is not possible.

The esophageal detector device is more accurate than standard clinical methods of determining ETT placement. It is quicker than both determination of end-tidal CO_2 and clinical methods (37).

It is important to note that an air leak in the apparatus or an incompetent gastroesophageal junction may lead to false-positive results. Further, a foreign body in the airway, thick secretions, or a kinked or obstructed ETT may give false-negative results. Therefore, this device should not be the sole means of verifying correct ETT placement.

Oximetry

Oximetry is a direct measure of blood oxygenation, but it is often used clinically as an indirect indicator of proper ETT placement. This is appropriate, since hypoxia is the most life-threatening result of a misplaced ETT. However, there are two caveats when using pulse oximetry for this purpose. First, the value given by the pulse oximeter

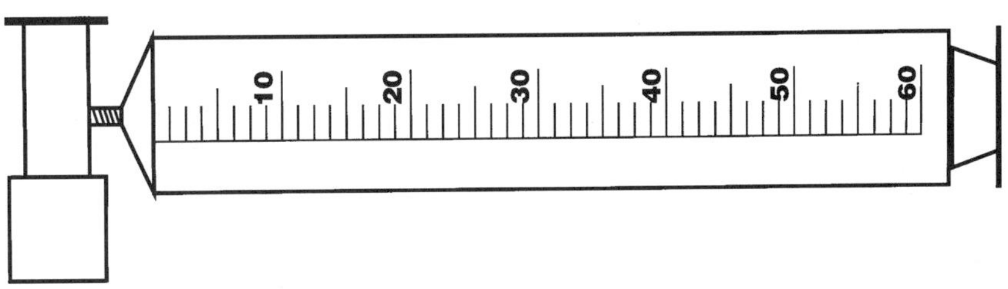

FIG. 16. The esophageal detector device.

is historical, in that the current pulse oximetry reading represents oxygenation at the lungs from some moments earlier. The delay, which can be as long as 30 seconds, is a function of the blood circulation time from the lungs to the measurement site. It is affected by probe site, cardiac output, and patient size. Because of this delay, the saturation may transiently decrease after a successful intubation. The second caveat is that pre-oxygenation limits the effectiveness of oximetry as a detector of failed intubation (38). If the patient has breathed 100% oxygen for an adequate time, it may take several minutes for oxygen stored in the functional residual capacity of the lungs to be depleted and for desaturation to occur.

Pulse oximetry is a sensitive monitor of bronchial intubation. The occurrence of main bronchial intubation should be considered whenever the maximum saturation is less than 97% while the patient is breathing oxygen-enriched gas.

Radiography

Although very useful in final confirmation of ETT placement, radiography has little use as an early technique for confirming ETT placement. The reason for this is purely logistic: Radiographs cannot be developed and delivered to the clinician quickly enough (an exception being fluoroscopy, which is bulky and expensive, requires specialized training, and is not usually available in most intubating locations). Further, radiographs are two-dimensional. Therefore, two views are necessary to determine proper ETT placement positively in the trachea. Radiography remains a standard method for detecting endobronchial intubation.

Artificial Intelligence

Artificial intelligence has been investigated as an aid in the detection of misplaced ETTs. One type of artificial intelligence device is called a "neural network." Neural networks can learn to recognize patterns in sets of data. A neural network that analyzes pressure-flow loops has been described. Once the neural network "learned" to recognize the characteristic pressure-flow signatures of tracheal and esophageal intubations, it was extremely accurate in identifying esophageal vs. tracheal placement of ETTs (39). In the future, neural networks may be integrated into ventilators and other airway monitors to aid in detection of esophageal intubation.

REFERENCES

1. Banner MJ, Jaeger MJ, Kirby RR. Components of the work of breathing and implications for monitoring ventilator-dependent patients. *Crit Care Med* 1994;22:515–523.
2. Lundsgaard C, Van Slyke DD. Cyanosis. *Medicine* 1923;2:1.
3. Sansores RH, Villalba-Caloca J, Ramirez-Venegas A, Salas J, Carrillo G, Chapela R, Selman M. Reversal of digital clubbing after lung transplantation. *Chest* 1995;107:283–285.
4. Severinghaus JW, Astrup PB. History of blood gas analysis. *Int Anesthesiol Clin* 1987;25:1–224.
5. Siggard-Andersen O. Blood acid-base alignment nomogram. *Scand J Clin Lab Invest* 1963;15:211–217.
6. Pretto JJ, Rochford PD. Effects of sample storage time, temperature and syringe type on blood gas tensions in samples with high oxygen partial pressures. *Thorax* 1994;49:610–612.
7. Peris LV, Boix JH, Salom JV, Valentin V, Garcia D, Arnau A. Clinical use of the arterial/alveolar oxygen tension ratio. *Crit Care Med* 1983;11:888–891.
8. Severinghaus JW, Astrup PB. History of blood gas analysis. VI. Oximetry. *J Clin Monit* 1986;2:270–288.
9. Barker SJ, Tremper KK, Hyatt J. Effects of methemoglobinemia on pulse oximetry and mixed venous oximetry. *Anesthesiology* 1989;70: 112–117.
10. Barker SJ, Tremper KK. The effect of carbon monoxide inhalation on pulse oximetry and transcutaneous PO_2. *Anesthesiology* 1987;66: 677–679.
11. Scheller MS, Unger RJ, Kelner MJ. Effects of intravenously administered dyes on pulse oximetry readings. *Anesthesiology* 1986;65: 550–552.
12. Scheller J, Loeb R. Respiratory artifact during pulse oximetry in critically ill patients. *Anesthesiology* 1988;69:165–166.
13. Lawson D, Norley I, Korbon G, Loeb R, Ellis J. Blood flow limits and pulse oximeter signal detection. *Anesthesiology* 1987;67:599–603.
14. Bourke DL, Grayson RF. Digital nerve blocks can restore pulse oximeter signal detection. *Anesth Analg* 1991;73:815–817.
15. Lee S, Tremper KK, Barker SJ. Effects of anemia on pulse oximetry and continuous mixed venous hemoglobin saturation monitoring in dogs. *Anesthesiology* 1991;75:118–122.
16. Kelleher JF, Ruff RH. The penumbra effect: vasomotion-dependent pulse oximeter artifact due to probe malposition. *Anesthesiology* 1989;71:787–791.
17. Hanowell L, Eisele JH Jr, Downs D. Ambient light affects pulse oximeters [Letter]. *Anesthesiology* 1987;67:864–865.
18. Severinghaus JW, Naifeh KH, Koh SO. Errors in 14 pulse oximeters during profound hypoxia. *J Clin Monit* 1989;5:72–81.
19. American Society of Anesthesiologists 1995 Directory of Members. *Standards for Basic Anesthetic Monitoring*, 60th ed. American Society of Anesthesiologists; 1995:384–385.
20. Kennell EM, Andrews RW, Wollman H. Correction factors for nitrous oxide in the infrared analysis of carbon dioxide. *Anesthesiology* 1973;39:441–443.
21. VanWagenen RA, Westenskow DR, Benner RE, Gregonis DE, Coleman DL. Dedicated monitoring of anesthetic and respiratory gases by Raman scattering. *J Clin Monit* 1986;2:215–222.
22. Brunner JX, Westenskow DR. How the rise time of carbon dioxide analysers influences the accuracy of carbon dioxide measurements. *Br J Anaesth* 1988;61:628–638.
23. Badgwell JM. Respiratory gas monitoring in the pediatric patient. *Int Anesthesiol Clin* 1992;30:131–146.
24. Whitesell R, Asiddao C, Gollman D, Jablonski J. Relationship between arterial and peak expired carbon dioxide pressure during anesthesia and factors influencing the difference. *Anesth Analg* 1981;60:508–512.
25. Drummond JC, Prutow RJ, Scheller MS. A comparison of the sensitivity of pulmonary artery pressure, end-tidal carbon dioxide, and end-tidal nitrogen in the detection of venous air embolism in the dog. *Anesth Analg* 1985;64:688–692.
26. Wright BM. A respiratory anemometer. *J Physiol (Lond)* 1955;127: 25P.
27. Yeh MP, Adams TD, Gardner RM, Yanowitz FG. Effect of O_2, N_2, and CO_2 composition on nonlinearity of Fleisch pneumotachograph characteristics. *J Appl Physiol* 1984;56:1423–1425.
28. Wright BM, McKerrow CB. Maximim forced expiratory flow rate as a measure of ventilating capacity. *Br Med J* 1959;2:1041–1047.
29. Gardner RM, Crapo RO, Jackson BR, Jensen RL. Evaluation of accuracy and reproducibility of peak flowmeters at 1,400 m. *Chest* 1992; 101:948–952.
30. Howells TH, Riethmuller RJ. Signs of endotracheal intubation. *Anaesthesia* 1980;35:984–986.
31. Andersen KH, Schultz-Lebahn I. Oesophageal intubation can be

undetected by auscultation of the chest. *Acta Anaesthesiol Scand* 1994;38:580–582.
32. Goldberg JS, Rawle PR, Zehnder JL, Sladen RN. Colorimetric end-tidal carbon dioxide monitoring for tracheal intubation. *Anesth Analg* 1990;70:191–194.
33. Kelly JS, Wilhoit RD, Brown RE, James R. Efficacy of the FEF end-tidal carbon dioxide detector in children. *Anesth Analg* 1992;75:45–50.
34. Zbinden S, Schüpfer G. Detection of oesophageal intubation: the cola complication. *Anaesthesia* 1989;44:81.
35. Good ML, Modell JH, Rush W. Differentiating esophageal from tracheal capnograms. *Anesthesiology* 1988;69:A266.
36. Petrioanu G, Widjaja B, Bergler WF. Detection of oesophageal intubation: can the "cola complication" be potentially lethal? *Anaesthesia* 1992;47:70–71.
37. Foutch RG, Maagelssen MD, MacMillan JG. The esophageal detector device: a rapid and accurate method for assessing tracheal versus esophageal intubation in a porcine model. *Ann Emerg Med* 1992;21:1073–1076.
38. McShane AJ, Martin JL. Preoxygenation and pulse oximetry may delay detection of esophageal intubation. *JAMA* 1987;79:987,991–992.
39. León MA, Räsänen J, Mangar D. Neural network-based detection of esophageal intubation. *Anesth Analg* 1994;78:548–553.

Airway Management, edited by
L.H. Hanowell, M.D. and R.J. Waldron, M.D.,
Lippincott-Raven Publishers, Philadelphia © 1996.

CHAPTER 3

Physiologic Aspects of Mechanical Ventilation

Russell T. Reid

INTRODUCTION

The 1980s witnessed a tremendous amount of interest in the subject of mechanical ventilation. Studies were performed that cast light upon many of the questions that had been of interest since the advent of mechanical ventilation in the early 1950s. These much-needed data, demonstrating relationships between important variables of interest, are the focus of this chapter, which summarizes current scientific knowledge regarding the physiologic effects of the application of mechanical ventilation.

The primary physiologic event that occurs, with respect to mechanical ventilation, is gas exchange or ventilation. The definition of ventilation—the exchange of fresh gas between the lungs and ambient air—identifies the primary purpose of the mechanical ventilator (1). The modern mechanical ventilator incorporates a full range of therapeutic modalities that contribute to optimal tissue oxygenation and ventilation. Accordingly, the information presented is categorized according to effect on ventilation and/or oxygenation.

In addition to the primary physiologic events of ventilation and oxygenation, the application of mechanical ventilation can alter a number of other physiologic variables. A partial listing of these physiologic variables includes hemodynamics, pulmonary mechanics, fluid balance, and pulmonary cellular integrity. This chapter also explores the effect of mechanical ventilation upon these physiologic variables and concludes with a discussion concerning the impact of mechanical ventilation upon lung injury.

R. T. Reid: Department of Respiratory Care, University of California, Davis Medical Center, Sacramento, California 95817.

VENTILATION AND CARBON DIOXIDE

Carbon Dioxide Production

Prior to examining mechanical ventilation and its physiologic effects, it may be beneficial to review the normal production, transport, and elimination of carbon dioxide (CO_2).

Carbon dioxide is produced as a by-product of glycolysis and the Krebs cycle (citric acid cycle) as illustrated in Fig. 1. The Krebs cycle breaks down pyruvic acid, produced during the initial steps of glycolysis, in order to produce energy for the cell. Each molecule of glucose that is glycolyzed results in the formation of two pyruvic acid molecules; in the presence of oxygen, these enter the Krebs cycle and are oxidized with the concomitant reduction of the coenzyme nicotinamide adenine dinucleotide (NAD) to $NADH^+$ and a hydrogen ion (H^+)(2,3).

During the oxidation of pyruvic acid, one of its three carbon molecules is lost as a molecule of CO_2. Keep in mind that there are two pyruvic acid molecules produced for every molecule of glucose that undergoes the process of glycolysis; therefore, two molecules of CO_2 have been produced thus far. The primary event in the Krebs cycle that is of importance, with respect to CO_2 production, is the entrance of acetylcoenzyme A.

Acetylcoenzyme A, which contains two molecules of carbon, combines with a four-carbon molecule of oxaloacetic acid to form citric acid (2,3). As citric acid progresses through the Krebs cycle and is further altered to isocitric acid, oxidation occurs, with the release of another molecule of CO_2 (2,3). The final molecule of CO_2 is produced when α-ketoglutaric acid, the product of the oxidation of isocitric acid, is itself oxidized to succinic acid (2,3). Thus, three molecules of CO_2 are produced as by-products for every molecule of pyruvic acid that enters the Krebs cycle. As two molecules of pyruvic acid are produced for every molecule of glucose that is glycolyzed, a total of six CO_2 molecules are produced.

Approximately 200 mL of CO_2 per minute is produced as a result of glucose metabolism and its subsequent entry into the Krebs cycle during aerobic metabolism (4). While total CO_2 production is usually of greater interest to the clinician, it is important to understand the metabolic pathways that result in the production of carbon dioxide, since the alteration of substrates used for metabolites or anaerobic metabolism alter CO_2 production.

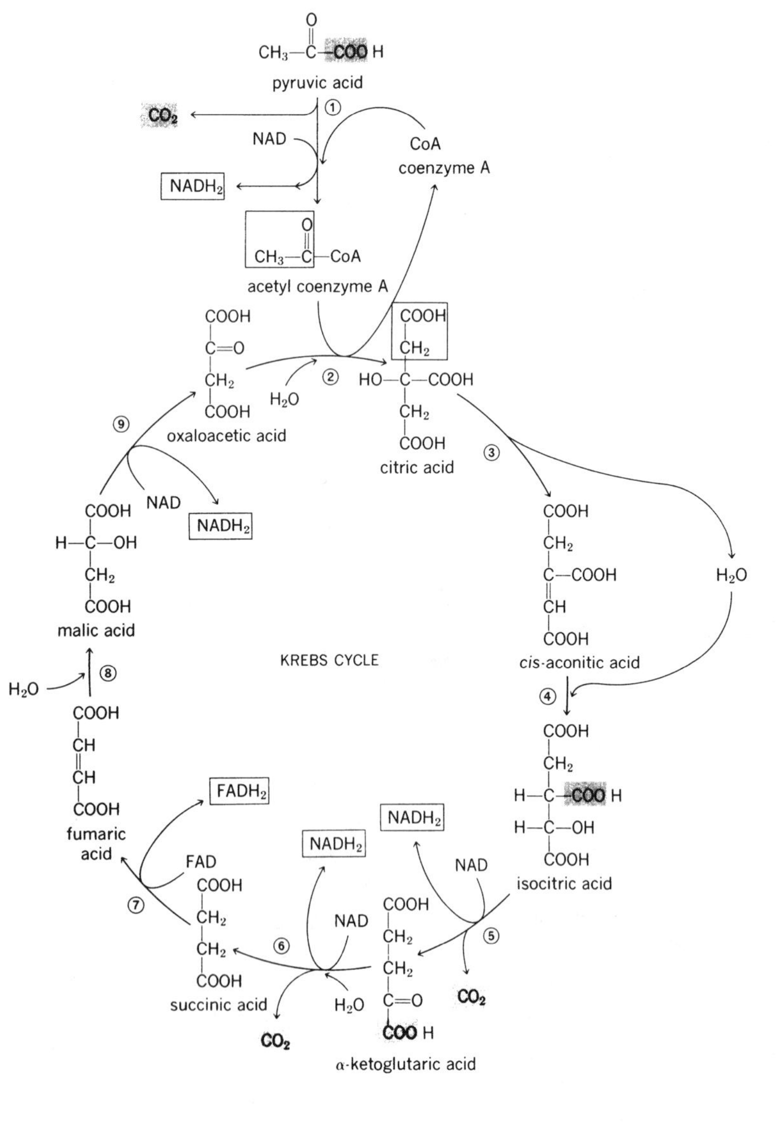

FIG. 1. The reactions of the Krebs cycle. (From Spence AP, Mason EB. Metabolism, nutrition, and temperature regulation. *Human Anatomy and Physiology.* Menlo Park: Benjamin Cummings; 1979:676. Reprinted with permission.)

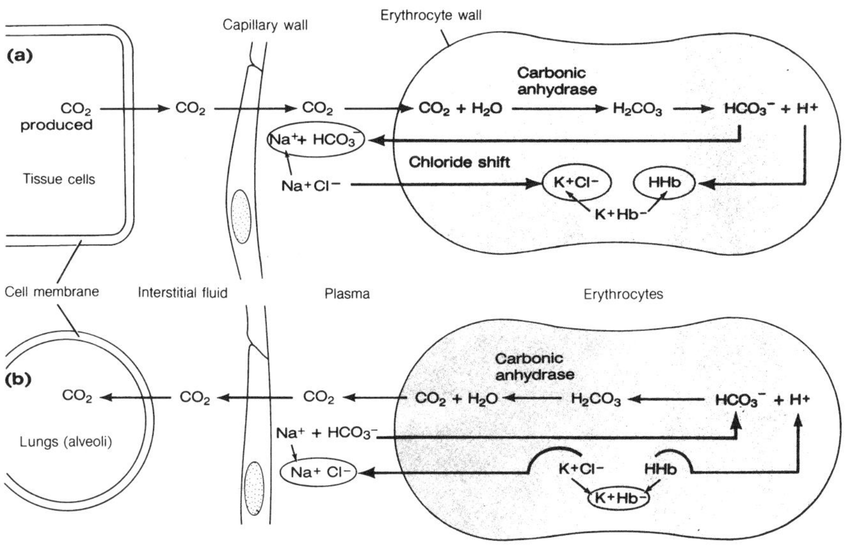

FIG. 2. Transport of carbon dioxide in the plasma as bicarbonate ions. **A:** Sequence of events that occurs in the tissues. **B:** Sequence of events that occurs in the lungs. *Hb*, hemoglobin. (From Spence AP, Mason EB. The respiratory system. *Human Anatomy and Physiology.* Menlo Park: Benjamin Cummings; 1979:603. Reprinted with permission.)

Carbon Dioxide Transport and Elimination

The transport of CO_2 in the blood, for subsequent elimination, occurs in a number of ways:

1. Small amounts, approximately 8%, are transported dissolved in the plasma.
2. Approximately 25% is carried in association with plasma proteins to form carbamino compounds, usually the globin moiety of hemoglobin.
3. More than 60% of CO_2 is carried as bicarbonate ions (HCO_3^-) after undergoing a reversible chemical reaction within the erythrocytes (5,6) (Fig. 2).

Carbon dioxide elimination occurs passively down its concentration gradient as it diffuses from the tissues (areas of high concentration) to the blood (areas of lower concentration). The circulation in turn carries blood that is high in CO_2 content through the pulmonary circulation via the pulmonary artery.

As oxygen molecules diffuse from the alveoli to the plasma and into the erythrocytes, there binding with hemoglobin, H^+ dissociates from globin. As illustrated in Fig. 2, chloride ions (Cl^-) leave the erythrocytes and HCO_3 re-enters and combines with H^+ to form carbonic acid ($H_2CO_3^-$); in turn, the enzyme carbonic anhydrase catalyzes the reaction whereby H_2CO_3 dissociates into CO_2 and H_2O. The CO_2 diffuses across the alveolar-capillary membrane and into the alveolus.

Minute Ventilation, Effective Alveolar Ventilation, and Dead Space Ventilation

Once CO_2 enters the alveolus, the rate of CO_2 elimination is normally proportional to the expired minute ventilation, as demonstrated in Fig. 3. Expired minute ventilation ($\dot{V}_E$) is calculated as the product of frequency and expired tidal volume as shown in equation 1:

$$\dot{V}_E = \text{Frequency (Breaths per Minute)} \times \text{Expired Tidal Volume } (V_{T_E}) \quad (1)$$

Tidal volume (the amount of gas inspired and expired during a normal breath) can be divided into the portion

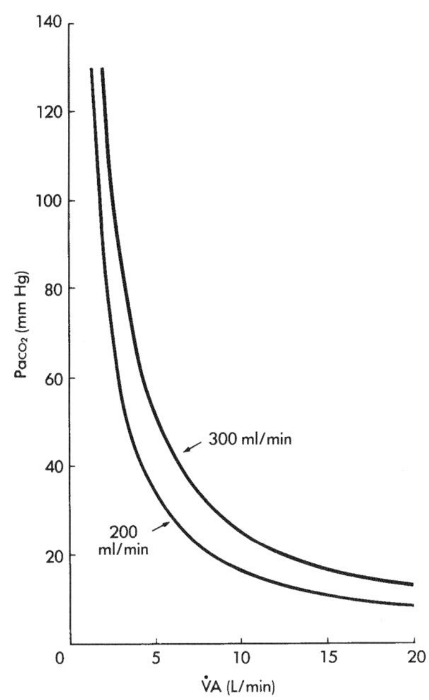

FIG. 3. $PaCO_2$ vs. alveolar ventilation ($\dot{V}A$). The relationship is shown for carbon dioxide production rates of 200 mL/min and 300 mL/min. A decrease in alveolar ventilation in the hypercapnic patient results in a greater rise in $PaCO_2$ than does the same change in alveolar ventilation when $PaCO_2$ is low or normal. Also, an increase in carbon dioxide production when alveolar ventilation is fixed results in an increase in $PaCO_2$. (From Martin L. PCO_2 and alveolar ventilation. *Pulmonary Physiology in Clinical Practice.* St. Louis: CV Mosby; 1987:83. Reprinted with permission.)

that participates in gas exchange (effective alveolar ventilation) and the portion that does not (dead space ventilation) (7). Dead space ventilation can be subdivided into anatomic and alveolar dead space, the sum of which represents physiologic dead space (8,9).

Anatomic dead space comprises the conducting airways (i.e., the trachea, main bronchi, and bronchioles), which are not perfused by the pulmonary capillaries; it is normally on the order of 2.2 mL/kg (1 mL/lb) and remains relatively constant (8). On the other hand, alveolar dead space, and thus physiologic dead space, can be markedly altered by such factors as disease states, including pulmonary emboli (10–12), modes of mechanical ventilation (13,14), and the application of positive end expiratory pressure (PEEP) (15), all of which affect the perfusion of alveoli.

The concepts of effective ventilation and dead space ventilation are typically described "per unit time," denoted by a dot over the $\dot{V}$ (16). Thus, effective alveolar ventilation is denoted as $\dot{V}_A$ and physiologic dead space is denoted as $\dot{V}_D$. The concept of dead space ventilation is described by equation 2:

$$\dot{V}_D = \left[V_{T_E} \times \frac{(PaCO_2 - P_ECO_2)}{PaCO_2}\right] \times \text{Frequency} \quad (2)$$

where P_ECO_2 is equal to the mixed expired pressure of CO_2.

The terms in equations 1 and 2 can be combined and rearranged to represent the concept of effective alveolar ventilation as shown in equation 3:

$$\dot{V}_A = (V_{T_E} - \dot{V}_D) \times \text{Frequency} \quad (3)$$

Figure 4 graphically illustrates the concept of effective alveolar ventilation and dead space ventilation. Even though total minute ventilation is unaltered, the percentage of each breath attributed to dead space increases as tidal volume decreases and respiratory rate increases.

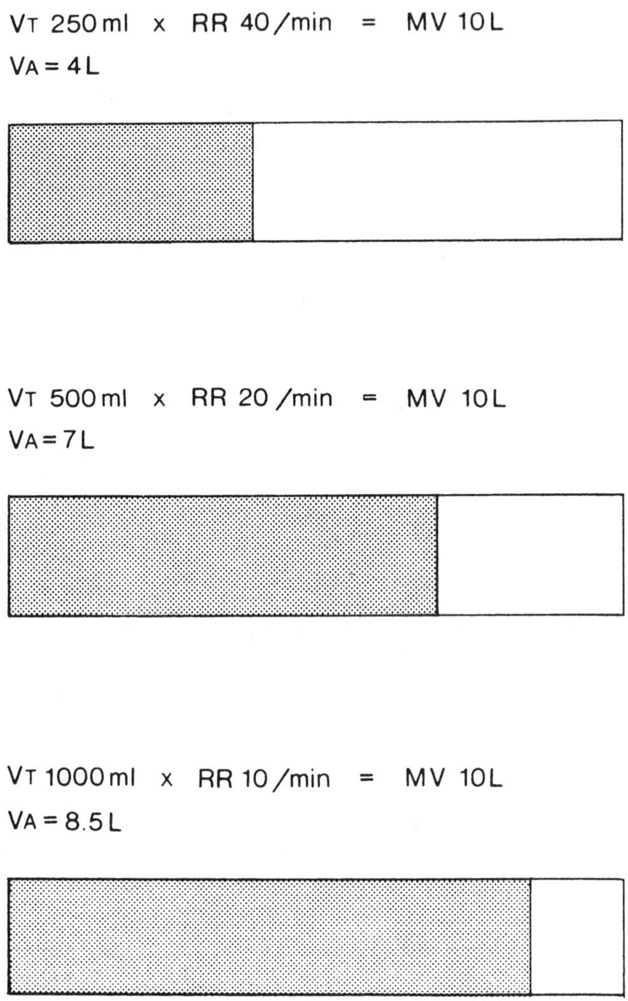

FIG. 4. The ventilatory pattern and alveolar ventilation. In all three examples, the minute ventilation is 10 L/min. Assuming an anatomic dead space of 150 mL, the alveolar ventilation (VA) varies markedly with changes in ventilatory pattern. Obviously, disease can add dead space other than the anatomic dead space and can cause even greater variances in alveolar ventilation. *VT*, tidal volume; *RR*, respiratory rate. (From Shapiro BA, Harrison RA, Walton JR. Arterial carbon dioxide tension. *Clinical Application of Blood Gases*, 5th ed. St. Louis: Mosby-Year Book; 1994; Fig. 3-3. Reprinted with permission.)

VENTILATION-PERFUSION ($\dot{V}_A/\dot{Q}c$) RELATIONSHIPS

The application of mechanical ventilation with or without PEEP, either applied or intrinsic, may increase alveolar dead space ventilation through either one of two mechanisms:

1. A situation is created whereby ventilation exceeds pulmonary perfusion; perfusion may remain unchanged while ventilation is redistributed.
2. Ventilation remains unchanged while pulmonary perfusion is decreased.

Shapiro (8) has coined the term "dead space effect" to describe these changes. The physiologic explanation for this phenomenon was elucidated by West and co-investigators in 1964 (17). Their work demonstrated that the lung can be conceptually divided into three regions or zones based upon relationships that exist between alveolar and pulmonary perfusion pressures.

The relationship existing among alveolar and pulmonary perfusion pressures within these three zones (in the normal, spontaneously breathing individual in the upright position) is illustrated in Fig. 5. Note the relationship of the three variables:

1. Alveolar pressure (P_A)
2. Pulmonary arterial pressure (Pa)
3. Pulmonary venous pressure (Pv)

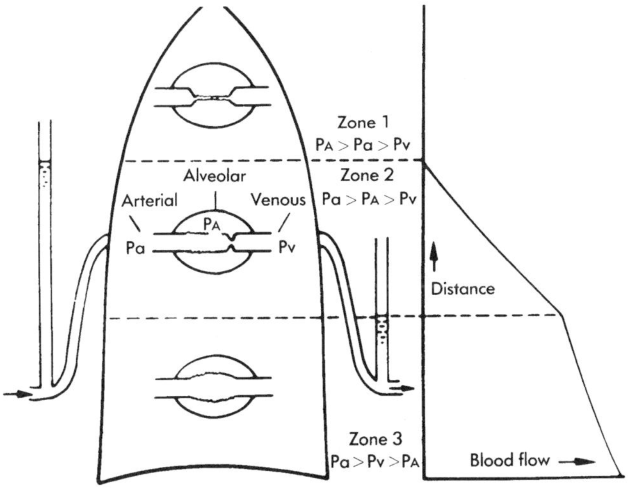

FIG. 5. Three zones of the lung in the upright position. (From West JB, Dollery CT, Naimark A. *J Appl Physiol* 1964;19: 713. Reprinted with permission.)

These pressure relationships are of great importance in establishing ventilation/perfusion ($\dot{V}_A/\dot{Q}_c$) relationships within the lung, ultimately culminating in gas exchange.

The theoretical relationship that exists in zone 1 ($P_A > Pa > Pv$), where blood flow past the alveolus is absent, is not present in the normal lung but may be created with the application of mechanical ventilation with or without PEEP. Zone 2 relationships ($Pa > P_A > Pv$) also serve to diminish or augment blood flow past alveoli located within these regions of the lung based upon alveolar-arterial pressure gradients. The greater the pressure gradient, the more diminished the blood flow past these areas; if alveolar pressure exceeds arterial pressure, then that area is converted to a high $\dot{V}_A/\dot{Q}_c$ area, resulting in increased alveolar dead space ventilation. The absolute extremes of $\dot{V}_A/\dot{Q}_c$ disturbances, either areas with ventilation and no perfusion (dead space ventilation) or areas with perfusion and no ventilation (shunt), would have ($\dot{V}_A/\dot{Q}_c$) ratios of infinity and zero, respectively (18).

Mechanical ventilation with either high peak airway pressures, high mean airway pressures, and/or the application of PEEP may convert areas of the lung that were previously zone 2 to zone 1. Additionally, zone 3 areas may be converted to zone 2 areas; the net effect of either conversion is an increase in alveolar dead space ventilation. This conversion may be cyclic, as during the inspiratory phase of the respiratory cycle with high peak airway pressures; alternatively, it may be continuous, as with relatively high mean airway pressures or with the application of PEEP. Figure 6 illustrates the concept of lung zone conversion in a supine patient being mechanically ventilated with 15 cm H_2O PEEP.

As previously mentioned, alveolar-arteriovenous pressure relationships may be further altered by mechanical ventilation via a redistribution of ventilation within the lung without an alteration in perfusion. In the spontaneously breathing individual in the upright position, intrapleural pressure is more positive near the lung bases primarily as a result of the hydrostatic pressures created by lung density (18,19). As shown in Fig. 7, the intrapleural pressure near the apex of the lung is more negative, resulting in a greater transpulmonary pressure; thus, the alveoli in the apices are more expanded in comparison to those in the bases.

When an individual inspires spontaneously, from functional residual capacity (FRC), the alveoli located within the apices of the lung quickly reach a point on the pressure-volume curve where further expansion is not possible because of the diminished transpulmonary pressure. Ventilation is now preferentially redirected to the lower lobes, which normally receive a greater proportion of

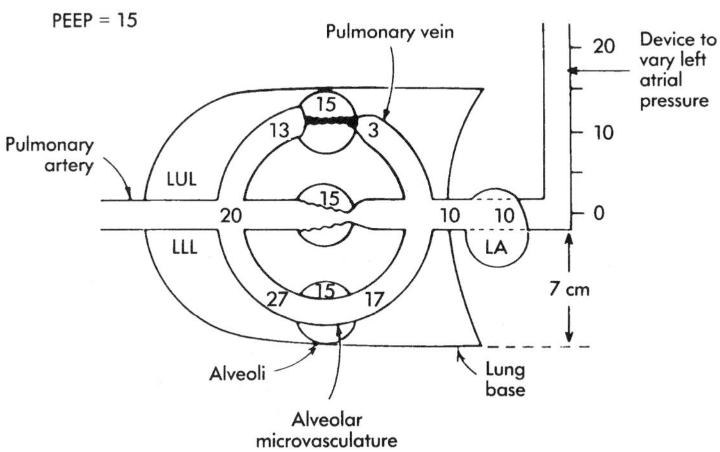

FIG. 6. Three zones of the lung in the supine position. This model assumes that a PEEP of 15 cm H_2O is transmitted to the alveoli and remains constant in all of the alveoli. Vascular pressures vary depending on the vertical height of the blood column (and are given in cm H_2O for comparison with alveolar pressures). Pulmonary artery pressure is 13 cm H_2O at the top of the lung, 20 cm H_2O in the middle of the lung, and 27 cm H_2O at the bottom of the lung. This difference in vascular pressure, in relation to the constant alveolar pressure, creates the three zones. At the top of the lung (zone 1), there is no blood flow since alveolar pressure (P_A) exceeds both pulmonary arterial pressure (Pa) and pulmonary venous pressure (Pv). A small zone 2 exists in the middle where Pa is greater than P_A, but where P_A is greater than, or close to, Pv. Finally, in zone 3, both Pa and Pv exceed P_A, and there is continuous blood flow. *LUL*, left upper lung; *LLL*, lower left lung; *LA*, left atrium. (From Tooker J, Butler J. *Am Rev Respir Dis* 1978;117:721–725. Reprinted with permission.)

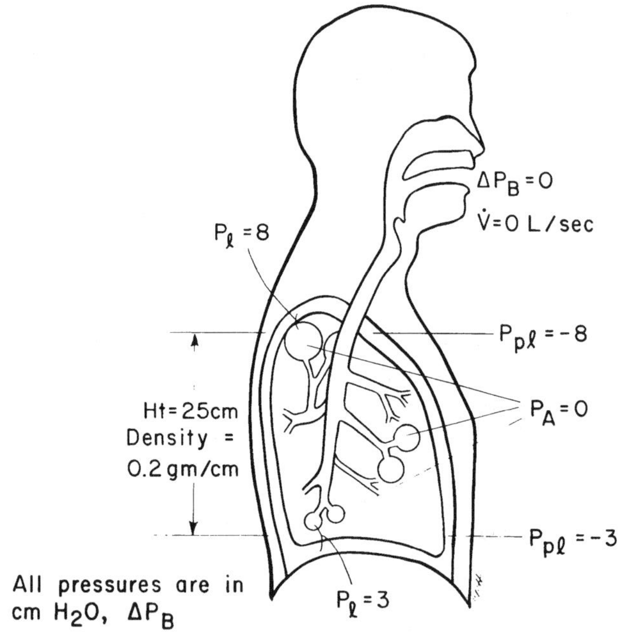

FIG. 7. The effect of hydrostatic pressure caused by lung density (0.2 gm cm vertical distance) on intrapleural pressure at different levels of lung height. Note that alveoli exposed to more "negative" pressure (toward the top) have greater transpulmonary pressure and are more expanded than those toward the bottom, where intrapleural pressure is less "negative." (From Slonim NB, Hamilton LH. Inspired air, pulmonary blood flow and ventilation-perfusion ratio. *Respiratory Physiology*, 5th ed. St. Louis: CV Mosby, 1987:124. Reprinted with permission.)

ventilation during normal spontaneous ventilation. Figure 8 demonstrates the relationship between transpulmonary pressure and lung volume. Additional factors that may contribute to the redistribution of ventilation within the lung, thereby increasing dead space ventilation, include underlying disease processes, patient position (20,21), anesthesia and muscle paralysis (30), and altered respiratory mechanics and modes of mechanical ventilation (13,14).

Valentine and co-workers (14) examined the $\dot{V}_A/\dot{Q}c$ relationship when patients who had cardiothoracic surgery were ventilated with one of three different modes of ventilation:

1. Synchronized intermittent mandatory ventilation (SIMV) (21,22)
2. Pressure support ventilation (PSV) (23)
3. Airway pressure release ventilation (APRV) (24)

This study utilized relatively sophisticated methodology in physiologic measurements, including (1) multiple inert gas elimination technique (MIGET), used for determination of $\dot{V}_A/\dot{Q}c$ ratios (25–28); (2) systemic arterial pressures; (3) catheterization of the right side of the heart with pressure data; (4) thermodilution cardiac outputs; and (5) arterial and mixed venous blood gas determinations.

Dead space to tidal volume ratio (V_D/V_T), which normally ranges from 28% to 33% in the nonintubated spontaneously breathing individual (16), was greatest in PSV (37.1 ± 2.7%) and SIMV (36.2 ± 1.5%); the lowest measurement was in APRV (30.1 ± 1.7%). Dead space measurements were positively correlated with peak airway pressures in this study; the greater the peak airway pressure, the greater the percentage dead space. These authors concluded that two probable mechanisms were responsible for the increase in dead space: (1) an increase in the volume of the conducting airways (increased anatomic dead space) and (2) decreasing perfusion to the alveoli in zone 1 (increased alveolar dead space). The explanation for the increase in anatomic dead space is that during ventilation with intermittent positive pressure, the conducting airways expand circumferentially and elongate, thus increasing their absolute volume.

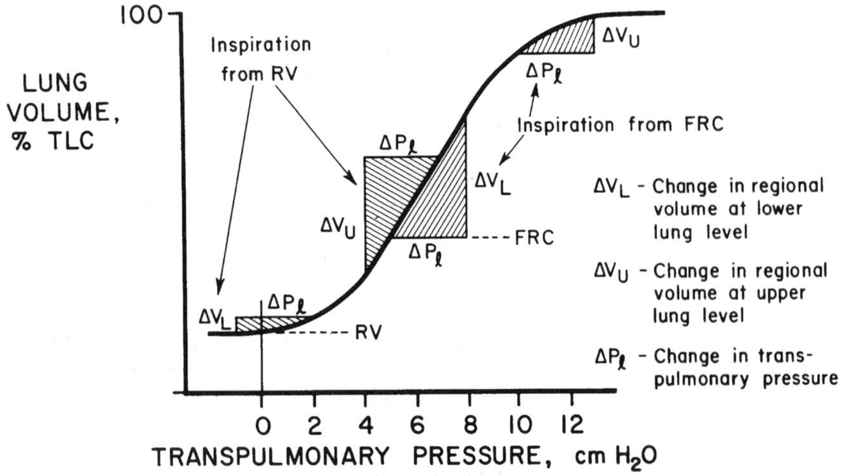

FIG. 8. Effect of the lung volume at the beginning of inspiration on the vertical distribution of inspired air and relationship of volume to regional lung compliance. (From Slonim NB, Hamilton LH. Inspired air, pulmonary blood flow and ventilation-perfusion ratio. *Respiratory Physiology*, 5th ed. St. Louis: CV Mosby, 1987:125. Reprinted with permission.)

Klingstedt and colleagues (20) demonstrated the effect of position changes on physiologic dead space using conventional ventilation with and without PEEP. Additionally, these investigators examined differential ventilation (DV) with 10 cm H_2O of PEEP. All studies were performed in surgical patients intubated with a double-lumen endobronchial tube in the left main bronchus (20). After induction of anesthesia, with patients in the supine position and using conventional ventilation without PEEP, gas exchange measurements and CT revealed atelectasis formation with no change in dead space ventilation.

Patients were then repositioned to the lateral position with conventional ventilation, without PEEP, as occurs during many surgical procedures. MIGET measurements indicated a subsequent redirection of ventilation towards areas with high $\dot{V}_A/\dot{Q}_c$; dead space to tidal volume ratio (V_D/V_T) increased from 43% (± 1%) to 50% (± 2%). Ventilation was redistributed to the nondependent portions of the lung, presumably because of airway closure and atelectasis in the dependent portions of the lung (29–32). No significant change in V_D/V_T occurred when 10 cm H_2O PEEP was applied.

The application of differential lung ventilation with 10 cm H_2O PEEP to the dependent lung, with the patient in the lateral position, demonstrated a further increase in V_D/V_T to 58% (± 2%). These investigators concluded that the selective increase in pressure caused by the application of PEEP in the dependent lung created a zone 1 situation (i.e., alveoli in the dependent lung compressing pulmonary capillaries and causing inadequate perfusion). This conclusion is supported by MIGET data indicating that when DV + 10 cm H_2O PEEP was used, there was a significant redistribution of ventilation to high $\dot{V}_A/\dot{Q}_c$ regions of the lung when compared with controlled ventilation both with and without PEEP.

Another recent clinical investigation examining V_D/V_T and the role of ventilator modes was conducted by Santak and co-workers (13). These investigators compared the influence of SIMV with pressure support (PS) vs. controlled mechanical ventilation (CMV) on $\dot{V}_A/\dot{Q}_c$ distributions during postoperative weaning. A significant increase in V_D/V_T from 37.2% (± 9.8) with CMV to 42.5% (± 8.5%) with SIMV-PS was observed. This was accompanied by an equally significant increase in patient minute ventilation requirements: 9.5 L/min (± 0.9) with CMV to 11.3 L/min (± 1.2) with SIMV-PS. Figure 9 illustrates a ventilation-perfusion ratio graph in a representative patient enrolled in this study. Note that the graph, generated by MIGET data, allows a quantitative analysis of $\dot{V}_A/\dot{Q}_c$ distribution and demonstrates a redistribution of ventilation toward lung regions of high $\dot{V}_A/\dot{Q}_c$, defined in this study as $10 < \dot{V}_A/\dot{Q}_c < 100$. There were no significant changes in measures of hemodynamics during this study.

Clinically, a significant increase in physiologic dead space may manifest itself as either (1) an increased $PaCO_2$ (14) or (2) an unchanging $PaCO_2$ with increased minute ventilation requirements (13). If the increase in $PaCO_2$ is significant, then the pH decreases correspondingly, leading to respiratory acidosis with its attendant problems.

Another potential problem associated with hypercapnia is a concomitant decrease in the partial pressure of alveo-

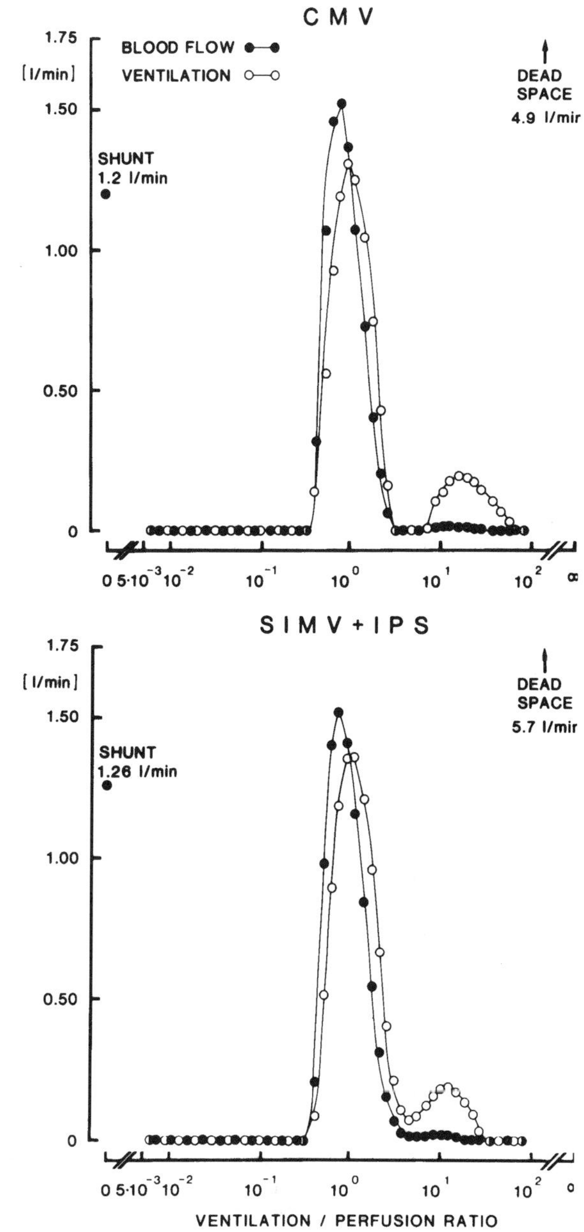

FIG. 9. Continuous ventilation-perfusion distributions of a representative patient during controlled mechanical ventilation (CMV) (*above*) and synchronized intermittent mandatory ventilation (SIMV) (*below*). The *open circles* represent alveolar ventilation, while the *closed circles* are pulmonary blood flow. Note that while inert gas dead space increased, the ventilation dispersion and the distribution of blood flow remained virtually unchanged. (From Santak B, Radermacher P, Sandmann W, Falke KJ. *Intensive Care Med* 1991; 17:138. Reprinted with permission.)

lar oxygen (P_AO_2), leading to a decrease in PaO_2. Dalton's law describes the mechanism for this phenomenon, stating in effect that in a mixture of gases at constant temperature and volume, the total pressure exerted is the sum of the partial pressures (33). As the P_ACO_2 increases, there is a simultaneous drop in P_AO_2, resulting in a drop in the PaO_2. Normally, increasing the F_IO_2 would lower the P_ACO_2 by raising the P_AO_2; this may be problematic when the patient is receiving an F_IO_2 approaching 100%.

Finally, if the patient has an increased minute ventilation requirement to maintain an acceptable $PaCO_2$, then there will be a corresponding increase in work. This is true in both assisted mechanical ventilation (AMV) (34, 35) and during "volume-controlled" SIMV breaths (35). The increased work results in an increase in oxygen consumption by the muscles of respiration that may be unsustainable in the critically ill patient, culminating in ventilatory failure.

DISTRIBUTION OF VENTILATION: PULMONARY MECHANICS AND MODES OF VENTILATION

The primary factors dictating distribution of gas within the lung of the mechanically ventilated patient are lung mechanics, inspiratory time, and the inspiratory flow waveform delivered by the mechanical ventilator. These factors may act in combination or singly to alter blood gas values in the critically ill patient significantly.

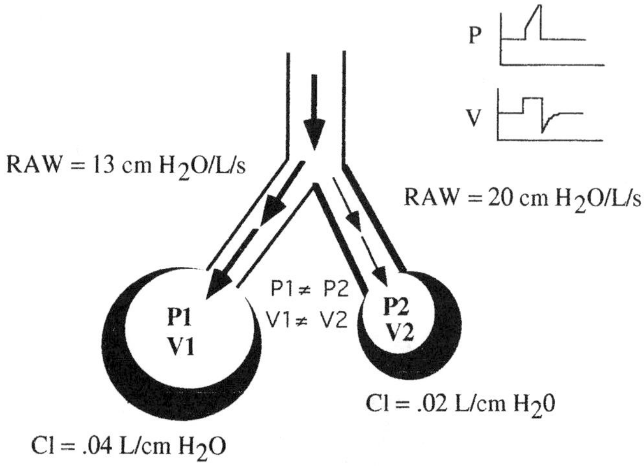

FIG. 10. A simple conceptual model of phasic gas distribution within the lungs of an ARDS patient. The lung unit *on the left* has a relatively low inspiratory airway resistance while the lung unit *on the right* has a greater resistance value. Also note that the lung unit *on the left* is twice as compliant as that *on the right*. This combination of mechanical abnormalities allows potential overdistention of the lung unit *on the left* while the lung unit *on the right* is hypoventilated. The final result is severe maldistribution of ventilation. The nonhomogenous nature of this disease process has been confirmed by Gattinoni and co-workers using CT (see text for further discussion). The dark alveolar areas represent end inspiratory volumes while the white alveolar areas represent end expiration. Note that neither the pressure nor volume equalizes during a typical breath, with a relatively short inspiratory time.

Airway Resistance, Compliance, and Time Constants

Airway Resistance

Two of the most frequently utilized measures of lung mechanics in the critically ill patient are airway resistance, which can be further partitioned into inspiratory (R_IAW) and expiratory airway resistance (R_EAW), and lung-chest wall compliance. Inspiratory airway resistance is the difference between mouth pressure and alveolar pressure (transairway pressure), divided by the flow rate of gas (V_I) entering the lung. In the mechanically ventilated patient, inspiratory airway resistance is the difference between peak inspiratory pressure and plateau pressure during a mechanical ventilator breath, divided by the flow rate of gas ($\dot{V}$) entering the lung. Inspiratory airway resistance is calculated as shown in formula 4:

$$R_IAW = [\text{Peak Inspiratory Pressure (PIP)} - \text{Plateau Pressure (Pl.Pressure)}]/\dot{V}_I \text{ (L/sec)} \quad (4)$$

Compliance

Static lung-chest wall compliance is a measure of the "stiffness" of the lung-chest wall described by the change in volume per unit change in pressure. To separate the components of airway resistance from lung-chest wall compliance, a "plateau maneuver" is performed in which gas flow is stopped and pressure is allowed to equilibrate across the endotracheal tube, between the patient's lung and ventilator circuit. Static compliance is calculated clinically as shown in formula 5:

$$C_{st} = \Delta\text{Volume}/(\text{Pl.Pressure} - \text{PEEP}) \quad (5)$$

Abnormal lung mechanics may affect the distribution of gas within the lung by (1) limiting the expansion of areas of the lung with relatively low compliance, thus potentially overdistending areas of the lung with relatively better compliance, and (2) redirecting gas flow away from areas of the lung with increased airway resistance to areas with relatively lower airway resistance, thus hypoventilating portions of the lung.

These factors may work in concert to magnify the maldistribution of ventilation and create the clinical picture of a patient with rapidly deteriorating gas exchange. Figure 10 illustrates the concept of abnormal lung mechanics and the effect on gas distribution in a disease process such as ARDS.

Respiratory Time Constants

The combination of the two previously discussed components of lung mechanics, airway resistance and static compliance, combine to form the basis for the concept of respiratory time constant, which is symbolized by the

Greek letter *tau* (τ). The respiratory time constant is useful since it allows the clinician to combine lung mechanics factors and conceptualize the effect on filling or emptying time created by abnormal lung mechanics.

The amount of time required for a 63% change in volume, pressure, and flow with a constant step change in pressure is 1τ. Multiplying τ by 2 is equivalent to an 86% change in volume, pressure, and flow with a constant step change in pressure, and multiplying τ by 3 is equivalent to a 95% change in volume, pressure, and flow with a constant step change in pressure (36). Clinically, the patient should be kept in the 95% range (3τ) to achieve adequate filling of the lung, unless hemodynamic complications warrant a reduction in inspiratory time. The formula used to calculate the respiratory time constant is described by equation 6:

$$\text{Respiratory Time Constant } (\tau) = C_{st}\,(\text{L/cm } H_2O) \times R_IAW\,(\text{cm } H_2O\text{/L/sec}) \quad (6)$$

After examining formula 6, it can be appreciated that changes in either compliance or airway resistances affect the filling and *emptying* of the lung. For example, a patient with a measured C_{st} of 0.040 L/cm H_2O and measured R_IAW of 20 cm H_2O/L/sec will have a respiratory time constant of 0.8 second. Achievement of a 95% equilibrium value would require that the time constant in this example (0.8 second) be multiplied by 3; the inspiratory time predicted for this set of lung mechanics would therefore be 2.4 seconds.

If this patient's R_IAW decreased to 5 cm H_2O/L/sec while C_{st} remained unchanged at 0.040 L/cm H_2O, then τ would change to 0.2 second. Again, to achieve a 95% equilibrium value in the lung would require that 0.2 second be multiplied by 3, indicating that the patient's predicted inspiratory time would be 0.6 second. This same concept can be applied to predict emptying of the lung for a given set of lung mechanics by substituting expiratory resistance (R_EAW) for R_IAW in equation 6.

When insufficient inspiratory time is given for a particular set of lung mechanics, maldistribution of ventilation results. Banner and co-workers (37), using a two-compartment lung model in which both C_{st} and R_IAW could be independently manipulated, demonstrated that CO_2 elimination was significantly altered when there was insufficient inspiratory time. When the time constant for their mechanical respiratory system was increased from 1τ to 3τ, the elimination of CO_2 was optimized and $PaCO_2$ was significantly reduced.

For example, a clinical illustration of this concept is the case in which a patient's airway resistance increases; if the patient is receiving a pressure-based mode of ventilation (i.e., pressure control), a drop in tidal volume occurs. If the length of the inspiratory time is increased, the tidal volume returns to near its original value. This is not true of changes in lung-chest wall compliance; regardless of the increase in inspiratory time, tidal volume does not return to its original value in pressure-controlled ventilation. Delivered tidal volume, in this case, is primarily dictated by lung-chest wall compliance. If lung-chest wall compliance decreases, then an increase in peak airway pressure (transairway pressure) is required to maintain the original tidal volume.

Inspiratory Flow Patterns

It is important to consider the mechanics of the underlying disease process in order to choose a rational venti-

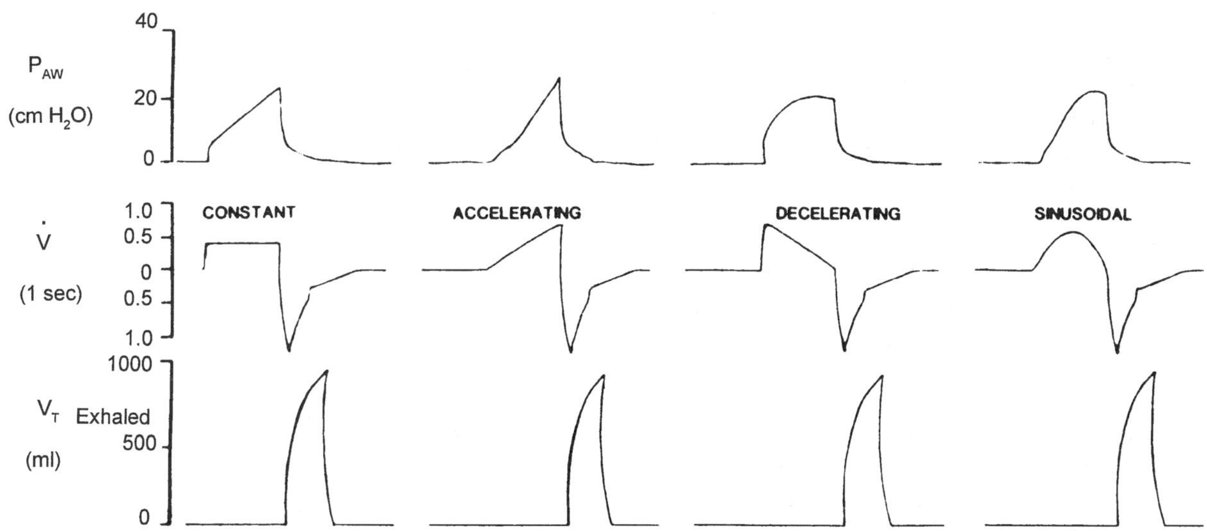

FIG. 11. Airway pressure (P_{AW}), flow rate ($\dot{V}$), and tidal volume (V_T) are shown for constant, accelerating, decelerating, and sinusoidal flow waveforms. Inspiratory time and V_T were held constant during the measurements. Peak inflation pressure was highest with the accelerating waveform and lowest with the decelerating waveform; however, mean airway pressure was highest with the latter waveform. (From Banner J, Lampotang S. Clinical use of inspiratory and expiratory waveforms. *Current Respiratory Care*. Philadelphia: BC Decker; 1988:138. Reprinted with permission.)

latory strategy. In disease processes such as chronic obstructive pulmonary disease (COPD), a primary concern is the emptying time of the lung. Connors and colleagues (38) studied the effects of increasing inspiratory flow rates on lung mechanics and gas exchange in two groups of patients, one with COPD and another group with other causes of respiratory failure.

These authors attributed significant improvements in lung mechanics and intrapulmonary gas distribution in the COPD group, 31.2% improvement in compliance of the respiratory system and a 23.7% decrease in V_D/V_T, to a redistribution of ventilation to low $\dot{V}_A/\dot{Q}_C$ areas. This occurred not as a result of the faster inspiratory flow rates but rather as a consequence of the increased time available for exhalation. The increased inspiratory flow rates allowed a greater proportion of the respiratory cycle to be used for exhalation; available expiratory time increased from 4.2 seconds to 6.1 seconds. This allowed time for hyperinflated areas of the lung to empty more completely. This is quite logical, in light of the fact that COPD patients have been shown to have increases in expiratory resistance of 10-fold above normal values (39).

The final major factor affecting gas distribution within the lung is the inspiratory waveform selected on the mechanical ventilator. Most modern microprocessor-controlled ventilators offer a variety of inspiratory flow waveforms. The four inspiratory flow waveforms typically available are as follows:

1. Square or constant flow waveform
2. Decelerating flow waveform
3. Accelerating flow waveform
4. Sine flow waveform.

Figure 11 illustrates the four types of waveforms and their associated pressure and volume waveforms. The peak airway pressures generated with these different waveforms can be appreciated.

As previously mentioned, Banner and co-workers (37) demonstrated that insufficient inspiratory time significantly altered CO_2 elimination. However, even when inspiratory time was sufficient, there were significant differences in CO_2 elimination between the different types of flow waveforms, as demonstrated in Fig. 12.

Numerous studies, using mechanical lung models (37, 40), computer and electric analog models (41,42), animal models (43,44), and human studies (45–47), have indicated that the decelerating inspiratory waveform provides improved distribution of ventilation. This inspiratory waveform additionally offers the advantages of improved respiratory system compliance (44,45,47,48), decreased peak inspiratory pressures (PIP) (41,42,44,47), decreased $PaCO_2$ (44,48), and decreased V_D/V_T (47,48).

The observations made using the decelerating waveform have predominantly been made using the pressure-controlled mode of ventilation. The decelerating waveform is also available as an option on many mechanical

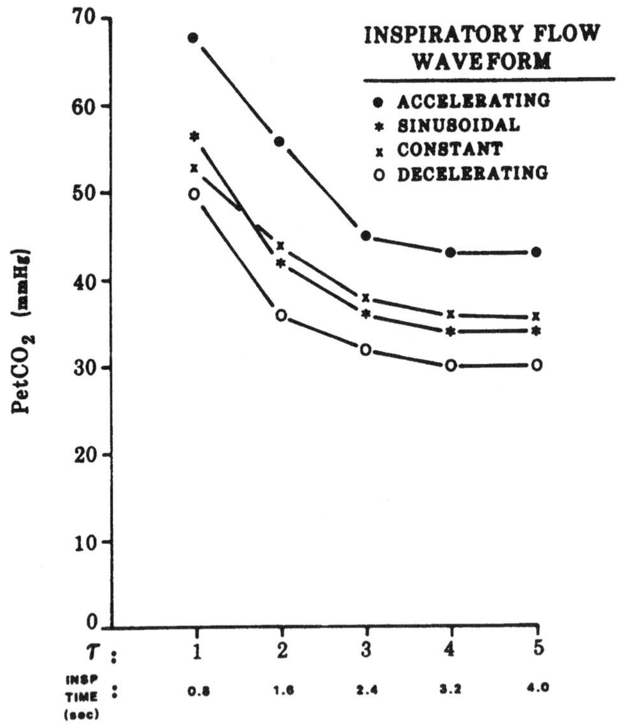

FIG. 12. Carbon dioxide elimination, as measured by partial pressure of end-tidal carbon dioxide ($P_{ET}CO_2$), with different inspiratory flow waveforms and times in a lung model with slow- and fast-filling compartments. The time constant (τ) of the lung model was 0.8 second (resistance = 16 cm H_2O per liter per second x compliance = 0.05 L/cm H_2O). When tidal volume and frequency were held constant, $P_{ET}CO_2$ decreased substantially when inspiratory time was increased; this effect was enhanced by a decelerating inspiratory flow waveform. At constant minute ventilation, $P_{ET}CO_2$ at inspiratory time 1τ reflects hypoventilation for all waveforms; at inspiratory time 3τ, ventilation is adequate with all waveforms except the accelerating type. Even at an inspiratory time of 5τ, $P_{ET}CO_2$ was abnormally high (reflecting hypoventilation) with an accelerating flow waveform. These data may be relevant in treating patients with chronic obstructive pulmonary disease. (All data are mean values.) (From Banner J, Lampotang S. Clinical use of inspiratory and expiratory waveforms. *Current Respiratory Care*. Philadelphia: BC Decker; 1988:139. Reprinted with permission.)

ventilators in the volume-controlled mode. The decelerating waveform coupled with a pressure-limited, time-cycled mode of ventilation appears to achieve clinical improvement through several mechanisms: (1) The rate of flow deceleration is an inverse function of both lung-chest wall compliance and airways resistance and is not controlled by the operator (49). Therefore, the flow waveform in effect attempts to optimize the deceleration profile to suit the patient's lung mechanics. (2) The decelerating flow waveform redistributes ventilation to previously underventilated areas of the lung with low $\dot{V}_A/\dot{Q}_C$, thereby decreasing V_D/V_T and serving to eliminate CO_2 more efficiently. (3) The use of a limited pressure (pressure control) prevents overdistention of relatively well-ventilated areas of the lung, thus serving to prevent the conversion of these areas to a zone 1 situation. A limited pressure additionally *may* reduce the incidence of "volutrauma," as is discussed in a subsequent section. (4) Lastly, the redistribution of ventilation also serves to improve compliance, thus allowing a reduction in peak airway pressures for a given tidal volume.

PEEP, Auto-PEEP, and Ventilation

While PEEP is normally employed as a therapeutic maneuver to increase oxygenation, it has been demonstrated that the application of PEEP, either intentionally (applied PEEP) or inadvertently (auto-PEEP) (50–52), may significantly influence ventilation through its effects on lung mechanics and hemodynamics. Auto-PEEP poses particular hazards because its presence may not be recognized.

The effects of applied PEEP have been well documented, one of the more significant complications being adverse hemodynamic effects. Several studies have demonstrated that mechanical ventilation with PEEP can result in reduced cardiac output (53,54). There have been a variety of mechanisms proposed to explain the observed reduction in cardiac output, including right ventricular dysfunction (55), an increase in pulmonary vascular resistance (55), a decreased left ventricular preload (56), and left ventricular dysfunction (56). The reduction in cardiac output can lead to a "dead space effect," as previously described, in addition to a reduction in oxygen delivery to the tissues. Applied PEEP may create or further aggravate perfusion problems when used in the hypovolemic patient (57) or the patient with elevated intracranial pressures (58).

Auto-PEEP is a phenomenon whereby a positive end expiratory pressure exists in the lung without the application of PEEP on the mechanical ventilator. Auto-PEEP may arise as a result of (1) expiratory muscle activity at end expiration *without* hyperinflation, (2) respiratory rates in excess of the respiratory system time constant, yielding insufficient expiratory time *with* hyperinflation, and (3) expiratory airflow limitation and collapse of conducting airways *with* hyperinflation.

Wright and Gong (52) studied 57 patients undergoing mechanical ventilation and discovered that 47% of them had auto-PEEP present that ranged from 1 to 6 cm H_2O. These patients comprised both medical and surgical patients. The authors concluded there was a significant increase in auto-PEEP when (1) V_E exceeded 18.4 L/min, (2) respiratory rate exceeded 27 breaths per minute, and (3) set PEEP exceeded 10 cm H_2O. Additionally, other factors that could logically be expected to contribute to the presence or worsening of auto-PEEP include (1) resistance of the mechanical ventilator expiratory valve, (2) patient I:E ratio, (3) changing lung mechanics (particularly expiratory resistance), and (4) endotracheal tube size.

The presence of undetected auto-PEEP may create a multitude of problems, which include increased V_D/V_T ratio and increased work of breathing (35). Auto-PEEP may also falsely elevate measures of hemodynamics, in particular central venous pressure and pulmonary capillary wedge pressure (59,60). Complications attributable to auto-PEEP may present a confusing clinical picture since the incidence of this phenomenon is greatly underappreciated.

An important component in the work of breathing is the sensitivity or "triggering" level required of the patient in order to initiate a breath from the mechanical ventilator (34). The sensitivity level is usually referenced to baseline airway pressure, although many newer ventilators also incorporate flow triggering. The patient must initiate a change in one of these parameters to receive a breath. Increased work of breathing results when the patient is hyperinflated and auto-PEEP is present. In these circumstances, the patient must not only drop airway pressure in excess of the sensitivity level but must additionally overcome the level of auto-PEEP that is present in the lung. Patients who are weak may be unable to trigger the ventilator because the respiratory muscles are unable to generate this level of work. Figure 13 illustrates this concept.

Recently, there has been increased interest regarding the application of PEEP in patients with COPD. Conventional wisdom held that the application of PEEP in these patients was contraindicated since hyperinflation, a hallmark of this disease, was already present and the appli-

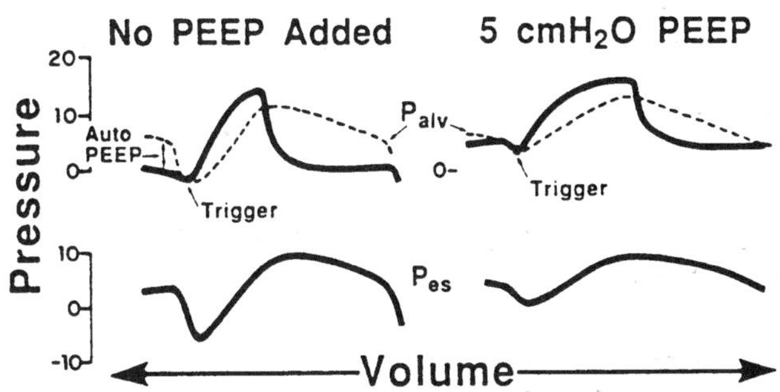

FIG. 13. Impact of auto-PEEP on trigger sensitivity and inspiratory effort. To trigger a machine cycle, alveolar pressure (P_A) must fall by the amount of auto-PEEP plus the set trigger sensitivity. The large dip in esophageal pressure (P_{ES}) reflects this effort. The addition of PEEP downstream from dynamically compressed airways reduces the P_A-P_{ES} gradient and attenuates the breathing workload without a significant increase in end inspiratory P_A. (From Marini JJ. Ventilatory management of COPD. In: Cherniak, ed. *Chronic Obstructive Pulmonary Disease*. Philadelphia: WB Saunders; 1990:495–507. Reprinted with permission.)

cation of PEEP would further increase FRC. It is now more widely appreciated that dynamic hyperinflation and auto-PEEP exist during tidal breathing in COPD as a direct result of expiratory flow limitation caused by critical closure of the airways (61,62).

Three recent clinical studies examined the issue of auto-PEEP and the effect of applied PEEP on lung mechanics in COPD (63–65). These studies confirmed that some level of auto-PEEP was present 100% of the time in their respective study populations. The mean auto-PEEP levels in mechanically ventilated patients in these three studies were 7.4 cm H_2O (63), 9.8 cm H_2O (64), and 9.6 cm H_2O (65).

As previously mentioned, the presence of auto-PEEP requires an increased workload to trigger the mechanical ventilator since the sensitivity threshold of the ventilator is uncompensated. For example, if the mean auto-PEEP in the lung was 9.6 cm H_2O and the pressure-sensitivity level of the mechanical ventilator was set at –2 cm H_2O, the patient would have to overcome both the auto-PEEP and the set pressure-sensitivity level. A negative pressure of 11.6 cm H_2O would have to be generated to initiate a breath from the ventilator under these circumstances.

It has been postulated that the addition of applied PEEP would in effect "unload" the respiratory muscles, thereby reducing the level of work required of these patients without increasing FRC; thus, hemodynamics and gas exchange should not suffer. Smith and Marini (66) demonstrated a reduced work of breathing in mechanically ventilated COPD patients with auto-PEEP when applied PEEP did not exceed auto-PEEP (66). Ranieri and colleagues (64) confirmed that judiciously applied PEEP, used in patients experiencing auto-PEEP and dynamic hyperinflation, caused no adverse effect on gas exchange and hemodynamics until applied PEEP exceeded 85% of the auto-PEEP. It would appear that in this particular study the critical pressure for airway closure was near 85% of auto-PEEP; further increases in applied PEEP resulted in increased FRC and worsening gas exchange and hemodynamics.

The Effect of Mechanical Ventilation on Cerebral Blood Flow

Cerebral blood flow (CBF) is very sensitive to changes in $PaCO_2$, which may be therapeutically manipulated to alter intracranial pressure (ICP). The relationship between CBF and $PaCO_2$ level is nearly linear within the $PaCO_2$ range of 20 to 60 mm Hg (67). Patients with closed head injuries are usually hyperventilated to a $PaCO_2$ level of 25 to 30 mm Hg to maintain an acceptable ICP (68). Arterial CO_2 manipulation by mechanical ventilation, with the goal of maintaining normal ICP (5 to 15 mm Hg) (69), has been used in many institutions.

However, caution should be exercised when manipulating $PaCO_2$ with mechanical ventilation. The use of high minute ventilation to lower $PaCO_2$, and subsequently ICP, to an acceptable level may raise mean airway pressure to the extent that ICP is actually increased via a reduction in venous return (impaired cerebral venous return). In this case, respiratory rate would be the *obvious* reason for the increase in mean airway pressure.

There may be another factor at work that also serves to increase mean airway pressure: auto-PEEP. As previously discussed, auto-PEEP may present a multitude of potential problems, the cause of which may not be readily apparent. The head-injured patient who is being hyperventilated should be monitored for the presence of auto-PEEP. This is especially true if the patient has a history of pre-existing obstructive lung disease.

Inadvertent hyperventilation may occur in a situation such as "autocycling" of the ventilator. This develops when the ventilator sensitivity mechanism is set at too great a sensitivity, or when a leak occurs within the ventilation system that causes the ventilator to cycle independently of any patient effort. Hyperventilation resulting in a $PaCO_2$ of less than 20 mm Hg causes maximal constriction of the cerebral vasculature and a precipitous reduction in CBF, with the possible consequence of hypoxic brain injury (70). It is imperative that care providers be vigilant in observing for "autocycling" of the mechanical ventilator.

OXYGENATION

Oxygenation is defined as "saturation with oxygen" (71). This is inadequate as a working clinical definition concerning the importance of adequate tissue oxygenation. Successful tissue oxygenation *does* depend upon saturating the arterial blood with oxygen. However, it is additionally dependent upon adequate cardiac output and utilization of oxygen by the tissues, factors which might be included in an expanded description termed "clinical oxygenation." The effect of mechanical ventilation upon clinical oxygenation will be discussed in this section.

Oxygen Content and Oxygen Delivery

Oxygen content, the sum of the oxygen dissolved in plasma and bound to hemoglobin, either in the venous or arterial blood, represents the total quantity of oxygen available to the tissues. Arterial oxygen content is calculated as shown in equation 7:

$$\text{Arterial } O_2 \text{ Content } (CaO_2) = (1.34 \text{ mL/g} \times \text{Hb g\%} \times SaO_2) + (PaO_2 \times 0.003) \quad (7)$$

where 1.34 is the maximum amount of oxygen in milliliters that 1 g of hemoglobin can carry when fully saturated and 0.003 is the solubility coefficient for oxygen in blood.

Normal oxygen content within the arterial blood is approximately 20.4 mL/100 mL blood (72). Calculation of O_2 content gives an appreciation for the small contribution of oxygen dissolved in plasma (PaO_2); this is normally less than 3% to 5% of the total quantity of oxygen available to tissues. The majority of oxygen available to the tissues is bound to hemoglobin. Therefore, abnormalities in hemoglobin level or abnormal hemoglobin species (i.e., methemoglobin) can have serious consequences with respect to optimal tissue oxygenation. The result of either inadequate oxygen supply to the tissues or inadequate utilization of oxygen by the tissues may be hypoxia with resultant cellular injury.

A normal oxyhemoglobin dissociation curve demonstrating the P_{50} (a measurement used to determine shifting of the oxyhemoglobin dissociation curve to either the right or the left), and $P\bar{v}_{O_2}$ is shown in Fig. 14. A number of factors cause the oxyhemoglobin dissociation curve to shift either left or right as shown in Table 1. If the oxyhemoglobin dissociation curve shifts to the left, hemoglobin has a greater affinity for oxygen; thus, abnormal release of oxygen to the tissues occurs. A rightward shift of the oxyhemoglobin dissociation curve results in a decreased affinity for oxygen, thereby releasing oxygen at the tissues more readily.

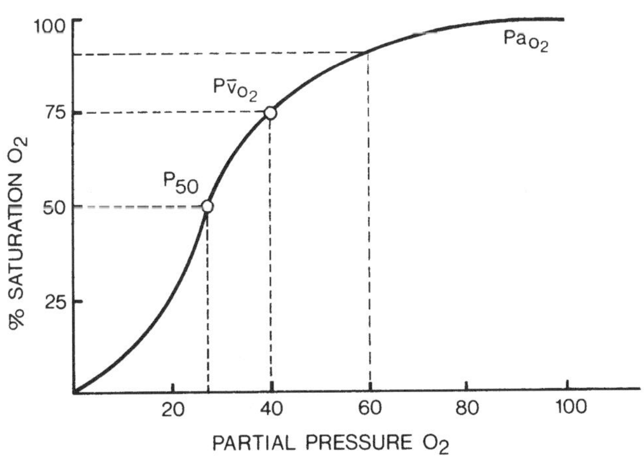

FIG. 14. The hemoglobin dissociation curve. This curve shows the relationship between plasma oxygen partial pressure and the degree to which potential oxygen-carrying hemoglobin sites have oxygen attached (oxygen saturation). This nonlinear relationship accounts for most of the oxygen reserves in the blood. Normally, hemoglobin is 50% saturated at a plasma PO_2 of approximately 27 mm Hg; this is designated P_{50}. Normal mixed venous blood has a partial pressure of oxygen (PO_2) of 40 mm Hg and an oxyhemoglobin saturation of 75%. A PO_2 of 60 mm Hg normally results in approximately 90% saturation. Normal arterial blood has a partial pressure of oxygen (PO_2) of 97 mm Hg and an oxyhemoglobin saturation of 97%. (From Shapiro BA, Harrison RA, Walton JR. Arterial oxygenation. *Clinical Application of Blood Gases*, 5th ed. St. Louis: Mosby-Year Book; 1994: Fig. 4-3. Reprinted with permission.)

TABLE 1. *Factors that shift the oxygen dissociation curve*

To the left	To the right
Alkalosis	Acidosis
Hypocapnia	Hypercapnia
Hypothermia	Fever
↓2,3-DPG	↑2,3-DPG
Hexokinase deficiency	Pyruvic kinase deficiency
Myxedema	Thyrotoxicosis
ACD-preserved bank blood	Hypoxia
	Anemia
Certain congenital hemoglobinopathies (e.g., hemoglobin Rainier)	Certain congenital hemoglobinopathies (e.g., hemoglobin Kansas)
Fetal hemoglobin	
Carboxyhemoglobin	

From Hodgkin JE. Measurements of oxygenation. In: Burton GG, Gee GN, Hodgkin JE, eds. *Respiratory Care: a Guide to Clinical Practice*, 1st ed. Philadelphia: JB Lippincott; 1977:238. Reprinted with permission.

Adequate oxygenation of the tissues not only depends upon adequate oxygen content but also upon adequate delivery of oxygen to the tissues. Oxygen delivery is the product of cardiac output and arterial oxygen content as shown in equation 8:

$$O_2 \text{ Delivery} = CaO_2 \times \text{Cardiac Output} \quad (8)$$

Normal oxygen delivery is approximately 1000 mL/min at rest, and 250 ml/min of the delivered oxygen is utilized by the tissues (73). Oxygen is extracted at different rates by the various tissues based upon the metabolic demand within those tissues. For example, the resting heart may extract up to 65% of the oxygen delivered, while the majority of tissues extract approximately 25% of the available oxygen (74).

Mismatching of Ventilation and Perfusion

As discussed previously, when uneven distribution of ventilation and/or perfusion ($\dot{V}A/\dot{Q}c$) results in alveolar ventilation in excess of pulmonary perfusion, there is an increase in alveolar dead space. When the opposite problem occurs (perfusion in excess of ventilation), the result is an area of low $\dot{V}A/\dot{Q}c$ which results in hypoxemia in the blood transiting such regions of the lung and ultimately venous admixture. Figure 15 depicts abnormalities of $\dot{V}A/\dot{Q}c$ using a computer model of the lung. In the most severe form, $\dot{V}A/\dot{Q}c$ abnormalities result in a shunt with a $\dot{V}A/\dot{Q}c$ of zero; there is essentially no ventilation, yet perfusion past this region continues.

Venous admixture can be separated according to three causes: (1) anatomic shunt, (2) physiologic shunt wherein no ventilation occurs but perfusion still persists, and (3) low ventilation-perfusion ratios (some ventilation with

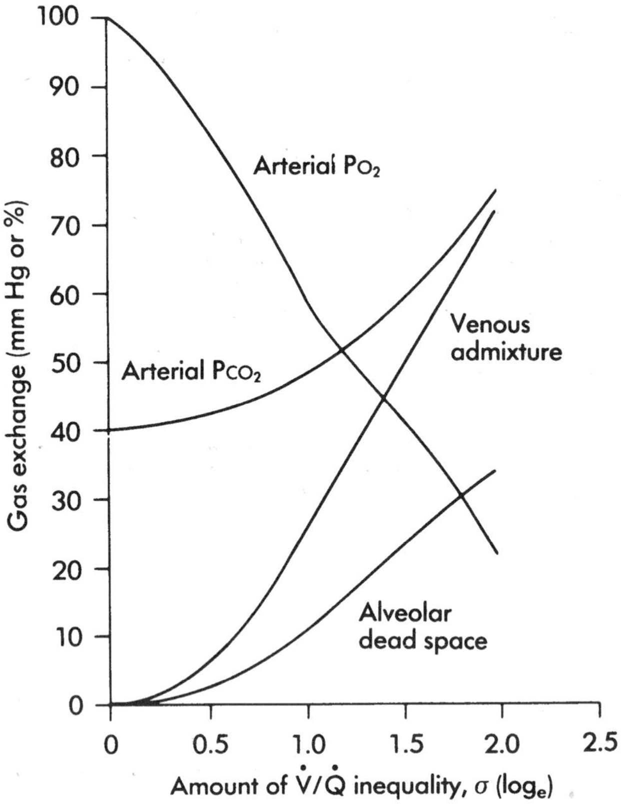

FIG. 15. Gas exchange effects from progressive $\dot{V}/\dot{Q}$ imbalance. Ventilation-perfusion inequality and overall gas exchange in computer model of the lung. For this model, oxygen uptake and carbon dioxide output were held constant. As the amount of $\dot{V}/\dot{Q}$ inequality increases (represented by a log scale on the abscissa), PaO_2 decreases and $PaCO_2$ increases; this change occurs because $\dot{V}/\dot{Q}$ inequality causes an increase in both venous admixture and alveolar dead space. (From Murray JF. *The Normal Lung*. Philadelphia: WB Saunders; 1976. Modified from West JB. *Respir Physiol* 1969;7:88–110. Reprinted with permission.)

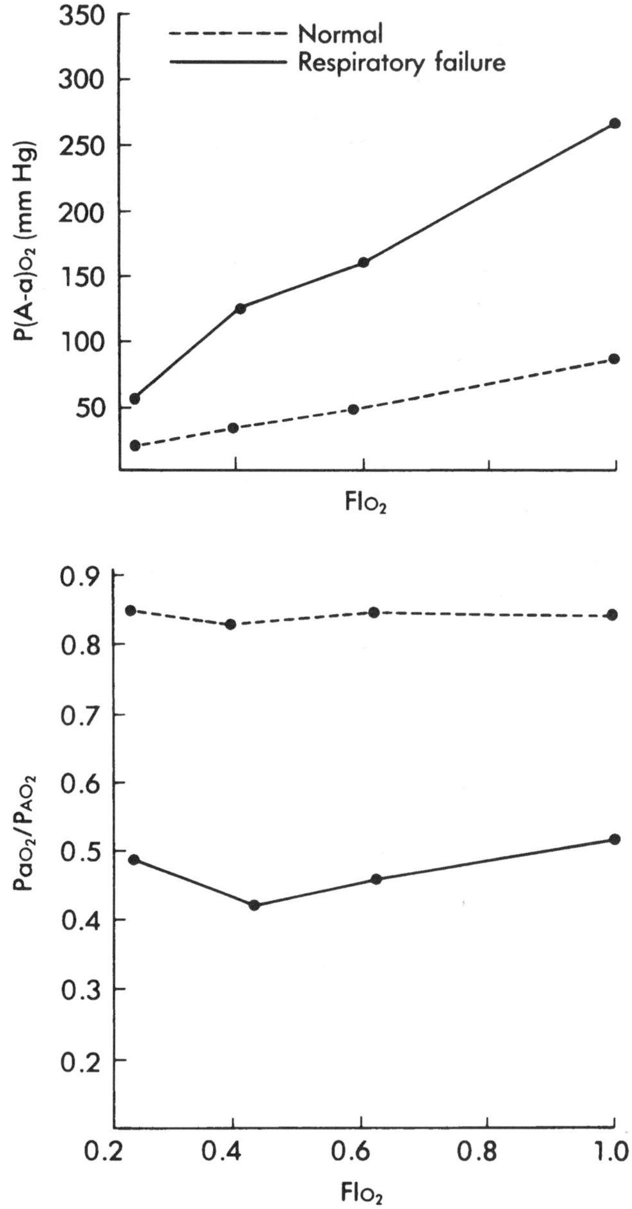

FIG. 16. Changes in $P(A\text{-}a)O_2$ and PaO_2/PAO_2 with increasing FIO_2, in a healthy subject and in a patient with respiratory failure. With increasing FIO_2, PaO_2/PAO_2 varies much less than $P(A\text{-}a)O_2$. (From Martin L. Oxygen transfer. *Pulmonary Physiology in Clinical Practice*. St. Louis: CV Mosby; 1987: 83. Reprinted with permission.)

adequate perfusion occurs in these units) (75). There is normally a 3% anatomic shunt present that occurs as a result of drainage of thebesian vessels and bronchial arteries, both carrying deoxygenated blood, into the left ventricle and left atrium, respectively. When hypoxemia occurs as a result of venous admixture, the resultant PaO_2 will be an average of all the oxygen *contents* that mix in the left side of the heart (75).

This concept is depicted in Fig. 15. If hypoxemia is a result of anatomic or physiologic shunt, then increasing the FIO_2 and supersaturating the plasma in the nonshunting areas will result in a PaO_2 much less then would be expected if the final PaO_2 were an average of all PaO_2s. Increasing the FIO_2 when hypoxemia results from low $\dot{V}A/\dot{Q}c$ results in significant improvements in PaO_2 and oxygen content since these units are still receiving ventilation. Shapiro and colleagues (72) have termed hypoxemia secondary to low $\dot{V}A/\dot{Q}c$ "shunt effect."

Another factor that can contribute to hypoxemia in the presence of shunting and/or low $\dot{V}A/\dot{Q}c$ is decreased mixed venous oxygen content ($C\bar{v}O_2$). Decreased $C\bar{v}O_2$ may result from reduced cardiac output, increased oxygen consumption, or decreased hemoglobin levels (72). As can be appreciated, the mechanisms associated with decreased $C\bar{v}O_2$ serve to limit the supply of oxygen to the tissues, or the tissues utilize a greater portion of the oxygen supplied. Either mechanism has the effect of worsening hypoxemia by contributing blood with a lower oxygen content to areas that are already abnormally exchanging gas.

Finally, an increase in the $PaCO_2$ can result in a decreased PaO_2 by raising P_ACO_2, thus decreasing the P_AO_2. Hypoventilation would also result in hypoxemia through the same mechanism as previously explained in the discussion concerning $\dot{V}_A/\dot{Q}c$ relationships, in accordance with Dalton's law (33).

Indices of Oxygenation

There have been several indices of oxygenation proposed to assess the degree of oxygenation deficit that may exist in the critically ill patient (76). The earliest index of oxygenation was the alveolar-arterial oxygen pressure difference $P(A\text{-}a)O_2$, or A-a gradient as it is sometimes labeled. To calculate this index, one first calculates the partial pressure of inspired oxygen (equation 9); using this value and information concerning $PaCO_2$, the alveolar air equation is calculated as shown in equation 10:

$$P_IO_2 = (P_B - 47) \times F_IO_2 \quad (9)$$

$$P_AO_2 = P_IO_2 - (PaCO_2 \times 1.25) \quad (10)$$

where P_B is barometric pressure, 47 mmHg is the partial pressure of water vapor present in the alveolus, and 1.25 is a constant representing the reduction in P_AO_2 owing to $PaCO_2$ partial pressure.

There are problems associated with the use of the $P(A\text{-}a)O_2$; it is age-dependent and has the shortcoming of changing when F_IO_2 is manipulated, without a corresponding worsening of the underlying pulmonary condition.

Another index of oxygenation that has been proposed for use is the PaO_2/F_IO_2 ratio. However, since neither of the components within this ratio considers the effect that a rising or falling P_ACO_2 has on PaO_2, this ratio changes when there is no actual change in the ability of the lung to diffuse oxygen.

Finally, the PaO_2/P_AO_2 ratio has been proposed as an index to assess oxygenation. This index has the relative advantages of being stable with changes in F_IO_2 unless there is a true change in underlying pulmonary condition, and the calculation of the P_AO_2 accounts for changes in P_ACO_2. Figure 16 compares the relative stability of the $P(A\text{-}a)O_2$ and PaO_2/P_AO_2 ratio in a normal patient and an acutely ill patient in respiratory failure. It would appear that the PaO_2/P_AO_2 ratio is the most advantageous when one is interested in changes in the underlying pulmonary condition with respect to oxygenation of the arterial blood.

Mechanical Ventilation and Oxygenation

Use of the modern mechanical ventilator to improve oxygenation is often one of the primary tasks of the clinician caring for the critically ill patient. The typical endpoints to be achieved with respect to oxygenation are (1) prevention of hypoxia, (2) reduction of hypoxemia and hypoxia, (3) reduction in cardiovascular work, and (4) reduction in the work of breathing. Foremost among these endpoints is prevention of hypoxia and associated cellular injury.

Modalities used to improve oxygenation include changes in the inspired concentration of oxygen and manipulation of various ventilatory parameters to increase mean airway pressure.

Oxygen Concentration

The fraction of inspired oxygen (F_IO_2) is typically one of the first variables manipulated in an effort to achieve acceptable oxygen saturation. The F_IO_2 concentration may be manipulated between 21% and 100% in an attempt to achieve the desired arterial oxygenation. It is widely recognized that high concentrations of oxygen are toxic and therefore every attempt to maintain acceptable oxygenation with minimal oxygen concentration is made. Oxygen toxicity is discussed in the section of this chapter addressing lung injury.

Mean Airway Pressure and Oxygenation

Mean airway pressure (P_{aw}) is a strong correlate of oxygenation. Mean airway pressure is defined as the area located beneath the pressure-time curve and reflects the average pressure exerted in the airway over time. Mean airway pressure can be calculated according to formula 11 when utilizing a square pressure waveform:

$$P_{aw} = \frac{[(f)(I.time)(PIP)] + [(PEEP)(60 - I.time)(f)]}{60} \quad (11)$$

where f is frequency, [(I.time)(PIP)] is the area under each positive pressure breath during inspiration, and [(PEEP)(60 – I.time)] is the area under the expiratory portion of the curve. A question certain to arise when one conceptualizes mean airway pressure is, "Is mean airway pressure the same as mean alveolar pressure?" This question is of importance since it is the influence of pressure, and the resulting pressure gradients, upon the gas-exchanging areas of the lung that dictate oxygenation. In addition, transmission of this pressure to structures such as the pleurae and pericardium influences hemodynamics, thus influencing oxygen delivery to the tissues.

The answer to this question was discussed at some length in a very thorough presentation by Marini and Ravenscraft (77,78). In essence, these authors concluded that mean airway pressure is equal to mean alveolar pressure when discrepancies between inspiratory and expiratory resistances are weighted by minute ventilation. This relationship can be described mathematically as shown in equation 12:

$$P_A = P_{aw} - (V_E/60) \times (R_E - R_I) \quad (12)$$

where P_A is mean alveolar pressure, P_{aw} is mean airway pressure, R_E is expiratory resistance, and R_I is inspiratory resistance. To illustrate the effect that differing inspiratory and expiratory resistances have upon this relationship, the above formula was used when estimating mean alveolar pressure with two different sets of inspiratory and expiratory resistance values.

The values for the various parameters incorporated in equation 12 follow in sets 1 and 2. Note that the only differences are the values for inspiratory and expiratory resistance:

Set 1: P_{aw}, 24 cm H_2O; V_E, 14 L/min;
R_E, 21 cm H_2O/L/sec; R_I, 18 cm H_2O/L/sec.
Set 2: P_{aw}, 24 cm H_2O; V_E, 14 L/min;
R_E, 26 cm H_2O/L/sec; R_I, 12 cm H_2O/L/sec.

When these values are used in formula 11, set 1 yields an estimated mean alveolar pressure of 24.7 cm H_2O while set 2 yields an estimated mean alveolar value of 27.2 cm H_2O. The effect that differences in inspiratory and expiratory resistance have upon estimated mean alveolar pressure, as other values are held constant, can be appreciated. In response to the question asked previously, it can now be answered, "The relationship between mean airway pressure and mean alveolar pressure primarily depends upon the difference between inspiratory and expiratory resistance weighted by minute ventilation."

Reynolds originally posited that mean airway pressure was a prime determinant of oxygenation (79–81). A number of studies have confirmed this theory and seem to indicate that the goal of increasing mean airway pressure is to recruit and stabilize alveoli, thereby keeping the lung open and optimizing oxygenation (82–87). Increases in mean airway pressure beyond the alveolar recruitment point demonstrate no further improvement in oxygenation and may result in adverse hemodynamic events (85,86).

Mean airway pressure may be altered by manipulation of any of the following five variables: (1) PEEP, (2) inspiratory time, (3) inspiratory flow waveform (thereby altering the pressure waveform), (4) respiratory rate, and (5) tidal volume. The question then becomes, "Is the manipulation of any one of these variables to achieve an increased mean airway pressure equivalent?"

COMPONENTS OF MEAN AIRWAY PRESSURE

PEEP

When PEEP is manipulated to achieve recruitment of alveoli, presumably by increasing functional residual capacity (FRC) (88,89), mean airway pressure is also increased. A variety of methodologies have been proposed to attain a level of PEEP that achieves the therapeutic goal of oxygenating the patient, while minimizing cardiovascular embarrassment. Included among these methodologies are end-tidal CO_2 gradient (90), supportive PEEP (91), optimum PEEP (92), pulmonary vascular resistance (PVR) index (93), and Pflex (85). Some of these methods use measures of pulmonary mechanics, such as the inflection point on a pressure-volume loop (85) or static compliance (92), while others use measures of physiologic variables (90,91,93). The best method remains debatable, with each method having proponents and detractors.

The creation of restrictive pulmonary disorders in animal models suggests there is a minimal level of PEEP necessary; below this level, suboptimal oxygenation occurs (85,90). The most probable explanation for this phenomenon is attainment of lung "closing volume," resulting in the collapse of terminal lung units during the expiratory phase of the respiratory cycle. The level of PEEP that maintains lung volume above closing volume appears to be the best choice for clinical application of PEEP. Once the optimal threshold for PEEP has been surpassed, the added PEEP has no further oxygenation benefit (85,90).

Existing evidence also indicates that high levels of PEEP applied in an attempt to maximize alveolar recruitment may have dire consequences. Carroll and co-investigators (91) conducted a randomized prospective clinical trial, involving 54 patients, to determine whether a difference existed between "supportive" or "recruitive" levels of PEEP. Either supportive PEEP or recruitive PEEP was applied in these study patients. Supportive PEEP was defined as the minimal PEEP required to maintain a PaO_2 greater than 60 mm Hg on 50% oxygen. Recruitive PEEP was defined as an increase in PaO_2 to more than 25 mm Hg from baseline or maintenance of a shunt fraction that was halved from the original value and maintained between 10% and 25%. Twenty-two of the patients received recruitive PEEP, with the distribution of complications representing hypotension (55%), pneumothorax (20%), and death during treatment (27%). This compared with no incidents of hypotension in the supportive PEEP group, and only one death during treatment (4%).

As discussed in a previous section (PEEP, Auto-PEEP, and Ventilation), the application of PEEP may reduce oxygen delivery to the tissues by reducing cardiac output (53–56). This adverse effect of PEEP relates to the fluid status of the patient, the compliance of the lung, and the absolute level of PEEP that is applied. Studies indicate that in the normal lung approximately half of the pressure from applied PEEP levels greater than 15 cm H_2O is transmitted to the pericardium; however, the proportion of pressure transmitted to the pericardium is markedly diminished when lung compliance is reduced (94).

Since the degree of pressure transmission to structures within the thorax is related to compliance of the lung, there are times when therapeutic interventions designed to improve oxygenation and lung mechanics may have the opposite effect. For example, consider the case in which a patient suffers a decrease in lung compliance secondary to pulmonary edema, resulting in an increased work of breathing and decreased oxygenation. The application of PEEP may be a therapeutic maneuver the clinician employs to improve oxygenation and decrease the work of breathing. As the underlying cause for the pulmonary edema becomes clear (for example, congestive heart failure), the patient receives diuretic therapy. As the patient undergoes diuresis, there is a significant improvement in lung compliance; however, the applied PEEP has remained unchanged, resulting in a greater proportion of pressure being transmitted to the pericardium. The patient may now present with a reduced cardiac output and actual worsening of oxygen delivery and oxygenation. If cardiac output is not being followed, the clinician may be tempted either to increase FIO_2 or PEEP to improve oxygenation. In fact, what is needed is a reduction in the PEEP level.

It is generally recognized that applied PEEP elevates several measures of hemodynamics, including pulmonary arterial pressure, right atrial pressure, pulmonary vascular resistance, and pulmonary capillary wedge pressure. These values should be interpreted in light of the effects of applied PEEP on measures of hemodynamics. Significant consequences regarding the fluid management of the patient are at stake. Auto-PEEP is particularly worrisome if it goes undetected since many of the measures of hemodynamics will be skewed upwards, indicating that the patient should receive a minimal amount of fluid when in fact the patient may be hypovolemic. Routine measurement of auto-PEEP in patients that are at clinical risk for development of this phenomenon is highly recommended.

There appears to be some confusion, with good reason, regarding the effect of PEEP with respect to fluid filtration rate (FFR) and development of pulmonary edema. A number of studies have indicated that the application of PEEP increases the measured lung water within isolated lung preparations (95–97), while other studies have indicated that the application of PEEP decreases measured lung water (98–100).

These conflicting data are most probably the product of variables that differed between these studies. For example, some of these studies applied PEEP at different times: (1) prior to the development of edema, (2) during development of edema, or (3) after development of edema. Blomqvist and colleagues (101) demonstrated that the application of PEEP after edema development actually slowed the resolution of pulmonary edema. Studies additionally varied in the models used (normal lungs vs. oleic acid-induced injury vs. hydrostatic pulmonary edema), the PEEP levels, the range of tidal volumes during mechanical ventilation, and the length of time mechanical ventilation with PEEP was employed. Therefore, direct comparison of these studies becomes quite difficult.

A recent study by Zabner and colleagues (101a) may shed light on the effect that mechanism of injury has upon the relationship of PEEP and pulmonary edema. This study is worthy of mention since it compares three different lung conditions with all other variables held constant. These investigators used isolated rabbit lungs that were either normal, had hydrostatically induced edema, or had oleic acid-induced edema. There was significant positive correlation ($r = +0.94$) between PEEP and FFR in normal lungs, indicating that the application of PEEP in normal lungs may create pulmonary edema. The application of PEEP, when hydrostatic pulmonary edema was created, led to a significant negative correlation ($r = -0.94$), demonstrating a reduction in FFR and subsequent pulmonary edema. There was no correlation present between PEEP and FFR when injury was caused by oleic acid.

The authors' explanation for the increase in pulmonary edema with the application of PEEP in the normal lung relies on the following three factors: (1) The vessels within the intra-alveolar walls are compressed, leading to an increase in hydrostatic pressure, pulmonary vascular resistance, and mean pulmonary arterial pressure. (2) The increase in alveolar pressure leads to an increase in the extra-alveolar vessel surface area (93,102) and increases blood volume within the lung. (3) Lastly, since the increase in PEEP increases intravascular hydrostatic pressure, there is a relative decrease in interstitial pressure favoring fluid flux into the interstitium and the alveolus.

The authors' explanation for the observation that PEEP reduced edema development when injury was caused by hydrostatic pulmonary edema depended primarily on two mechanisms. The first mechanism is the transmission of alveolar pressure, increased by the application of PEEP, to the interstitium. The transmission of alveolar pressure occurs more readily because interstitial pressure is already increased. It rises once interstitial water content exceeds 25% to 50% (103,104); compressing the fluid within the interstitium serves to elevate the interstitial pressure. The increased interstitial pressure serves to oppose the FFR, thereby serving to reduce pulmonary edema. The second mechanism involves a loss of effective vascular surface within zone 3 regions, caused by increasing transpulmonary pressure. Increasing transpulmonary pressure has previously been demonstrated to reduce edema development (98).

Lastly, there is evidence that mechanical ventilation with PEEP exerts an influence on neurohormonal systems, including the sympathetic nervous system (105, 106), renin-angiotensin-aldosterone system, atrial natriuretic factor (ANF) system (107,108), and brain natriuretic factor (BNF) (109). The primary response of these differing systems to mechanical ventilation with PEEP is fluid retention, although the mechanisms through which this occurs are markedly different.

Andrivet and co-investigators (110) examined the role of mechanical ventilation with PEEP and the effect of infused synthetic ANF in eight patients. The application of mechanical ventilation with PEEP induced a decreased plasma ANF level in four of the patients, while the remaining four patients had no reduction in plasma ANF levels. However, all patients experienced a reduction in renal excretory function, an increase in plasma renin activity, and only minor changes in renal hemodynamics. ANF infusion normalized renal function without altering renal hemodynamics. It was noted to increase diuresis and natriuresis to a lesser degree than in the control group, which received no PEEP. The authors concluded that this may demonstrate that water retention occurs independently of reductions in ANF.

Inspiratory Time

Inspiratory time is a variable that can be manipulated to either increase or decrease mean airway pressure. As inspiratory time is increased, mean airway pressure is also increased. Inverse ratio ventilation makes use of increased inspiratory time as a mainstay of this ventilatory strategy (111–113). The inspiratory time is increased in an attempt to recruit alveolar units and allow for optimal gas distribution within the lung. There is evidence that increasing the inspiratory time may improve collateral ventilation (114).

It is difficult to predict the optimal inspiratory time for a given set of lung mechanics. The concept of respiratory time constant was discussed earlier in this chapter and should not be confused with optimal inspiratory time. Respiratory time constant addresses the predicted *filling* time of the lung for a constant step change in pressure; however, this does not always equate with an optimal inspiratory time. The diseased lung may have great interregional variances in respiratory time constants; the number that is predicted from mechanics measurements provides an average value for these interregional variances of the lung. Therefore, the optimal inspiratory time is clinically determined by adjustments that optimize oxygen delivery to the tissues.

The choice of lengthening inspiratory time vs. raising applied PEEP has implications for particular modes of ventilation. For example pressure-controlled ventilation (PCV), sometimes referred to as pressure-preset ventilation (PPV), behaves differently if PEEP is increased vs. increased inspiratory time for a given mean airway pressure. If PEEP is increased, the driving pressure or ΔP (difference between end expiratory pressure and peak airway pressure) of the system is reduced, resulting in a reduction in expired tidal volume. This may necessitate an increase in peak airway pressure to maintain the same tidal volume. However, the increase in PEEP and set inspiratory pressure may result in a greater mean airway pressure than would be realized if inspiratory time alone were increased.

Caution must be exercised when increasing mean airway pressure through the reversal of I:E ratios for three primary reasons: (1) Excessive increases in inspiratory time resulting in high mean airway pressures, like increases in PEEP, may have adverse consequences on hemodynamics (115). (2) Long inspiratory times reduce the time available for exhalation. This may lead to significant auto-PEEP, which will not be reflected in the mean airway pressure displayed by the mechanical ventilator. Thus, the true mean airway pressure will be underestimated in this situation. (3) The reduction in driving pressures caused by auto-PEEP, in modes such as pressure control, may lead to decreasing tidal volumes and require higher peak airway pressures.

Inspiratory Waveforms

Differing inspiratory flow waveforms have a corresponding set of inspiratory pressure waveforms, as shown in Fig. 11. These differing inspiratory pressure waveforms are an important factor affecting mean airway pressure. The associated pressure waveforms differ both in the peak airway pressures achieved and their integral area. In general, the greatest mean airway pressure results from use of the decelerating flow waveform followed by accelerating, sine, and square flow waveforms.

Several prospective randomized studies, usually with small numbers of patients, have been performed comparing different modes of mechanical ventilation and their respective effects upon peak airway pressure, mean airway pressure, ventilation, and oxygenation and oxygen delivery. The majority of these studies have compared the decelerating flow waveform of pressure-controlled ventilation with the constant flow waveform of volume-controlled ventilation.

Studies comparing decelerating vs. square inspiratory flow waveform using conventional I:E ratios, in patients with acute respiratory failure or undergoing anesthesia, demonstrated significant improvements with the decelerating waveform. These included improvements in oxygenation (i.e., oxygen delivery) and tissue oxygen consumption, reductions in peak airway pressure (93,116, 117), improvements in lung-chest wall compliance (116, 117), and fewer days of mechanical ventilation (117).

Although the complete explanation for the observations in these studies may not yet be fully appreciated, reasonable hypotheses based upon existing evidence have been proposed. The key elements that explain the observed improvements with the use of a decelerating flow pattern appear to be as follows: (1) a change within the lung to redistribute gas to areas that were previously hypoventilated (in effect recruiting alveolar units and improving compliance); (2) high initial flow rates, which allow gas to fill areas of the lung with the lowest resistances rapidly followed by deceleration to promote even gas distribution still further; (3) limited expansion of the areas of the lung with the best mechanical properties by utilizing a pressure limit (thereby avoiding further tissue injury); (4) reduction in peak airway pressure, which occurs as a result of the improved lung-chest wall compliance; and (5) increased mean airway pressure.

Respiratory Rate

An increase in respiratory rate, with other factors held constant, results in an increased mean airway pressure. The increase in mean airway pressure may occur through two mechanisms as follows:

1. A reduction in the total respiratory cycle time, by an increase in respiratory rate, increases the area under the collective inspiratory pressure-time curves while simultaneously decreasing the corresponding area under the expiratory curves. This is illustrated by equation 11:

$$P_{aw} = \frac{[(f)(I.time)(PIP)] + [(PEEP)(60 - I.time)(f)]}{60} \quad (11)$$

2. As the absolute time for exhalation is diminished, there may be an increase in or creation of auto-PEEP.

The manipulation of respiratory rate to obtain the desired mean airway pressure or reduce potential complications entails a wide spectrum of techniques. At one end of the spectrum, there are those that advocate the use of extracorporeal carbon dioxide removal with low-frequency positive-pressure ventilation ($ECCO_2R$-LFPPV) (118–120) and permissive hypercapnia utilizing low-frequency ventilation (121,122). These strategies are primarily directed at minimizing lung injury, which is discussed in the final portion of this chapter. At the opposite end of the spectrum are those who advocate the use of high respiratory rates with relatively low tidal volumes, using what is known as high-frequency positive-pressure ventilation (HFPPV) (123–127) and the use of ultrahigh-frequency ventilation (UHFV) (128).

Extracorporeal carbon dioxide removal with low-frequency positive-pressure ventilation ($ECCO_2R$-LFPPV) has been employed as a strategy to provide adequate physiologic support of oxygenation and ventilation while attempting to reduce further lung injury induced by the mechanical ventilator. This strategy uses a veno-venous bypass to remove blood high in CO_2 and low in O_2. The blood is passed through a diffusing membrane to return blood high in O_2 and low in CO_2 to the venous system.

Oxygenation can be further enhanced by a catheter placed just above the carina, through the endotracheal tube, flowing 100% oxygen at a rate equal to oxygen consumption (118). Small tidal volumes (approximately 300 mL) and low frequencies (4 cycles per minute) are used to inflate the lungs. The most recent study using this technique, reported by Brunet et al. (118), demonstrated a 50% survival rate in 23 ARDS patients. Hemorrhage was a serious complication of this technique, resulting in 4 deaths (17%). Mean airway pressure was maintained using PEEP.

Permissive hypercapnia can be achieved through either the use of low tidal volumes or low respiratory rates. Darioli and Perrett (121) studied 26 asthmatics who required mechanical ventilation. These investigators chose to employ low respiratory frequencies (6 to 10 cycles per minute) with relatively normal tidal volumes (8 to 12 mL/kg). Carbon dioxide levels were allowed to climb in these patients as long as they remained below a level of 90 mm Hg. There were no deaths or pneumothoraces in this study. This was remarkable considering the fact that the reported mortality for status asthmaticus ranges from a low of 9.5% (129) to a high of 38% (130) upon the initiation of mechanical ventilation. This strategy seems particularly logical during severe acute airway obstruction since it serves to limit dynamic hyperinflation with its attendant risk of "volutrauma" and worsening $\dot{V}A/\dot{Q}c$ relationships.

The opposite end of the spectrum comprises both HFPPV and UHFV. Both of these strategies make use of respiratory rate to manipulate mean airway pressure and prevent the lung from reaching closing volume, attempting to improve oxygenation by preventing alveolar collapse. High-frequency positive-pressure ventilation is a ventilatory strategy that makes use of high respiratory rates (60 to 100 cycles per minute) and small tidal volumes (approximating anatomic dead space) to maintain ventilation and oxygenation.

A recent study conducted by Lichtwarck-Aschoff and colleagues (86), using a porcine model of respiratory distress, compared pressure-controlled high-frequency positive-pressure ventilation (PC-HFPPV) with four other modes of ventilation. These modes included volume-controlled ventilation (VCV) with 8 or 15 cm H_2O PEEP, pressure-controlled inverse-ratio ventilation (PC-IRV), and high-frequency ventilation with inspiratory pulses superimposed, identified as combined high-frequency ventilation (CHFV).

These investigators observed that peak airway pressure was significantly lower in the PC-HFPPV and the CHFV modes of ventilation. A greater minute ventilation was required in the PC-HFPPV mode to maintain an acceptable $PaCO_2$, and PaO_2 did not differ between the modes as long as a sufficient level of PEEP, defined as 15 cm H_2O in this study, was maintained to "keep the lung open." Oxygen delivery was greatest in the PC-HFPPV mode and least in the PC-IRV mode.

Finally, ultrahigh-frequency ventilation (UHFV) is a relatively new development, introduced in 1987 for use in ARDS. It utilizes small volumes of gas pulsed at *ultra*-high frequencies. These frequencies approach the natural resonant frequency of the adult lung, approximately 5 Hz or 300 breaths per minute. This is the frequency at which the impedance of the lung is overcome, resulting in a consistent pressure in the peripheral airways (131). Carlon and colleagues (132) conducted the largest prospective, randomized clinical study to date examining the role of high-frequency jet ventilation (HFJV) in ARDS. These investigators concluded that HFJV did not offer improved efficacy in the treatment of ARDS compared with conventional ventilation. However, it must be noted that the ventilation frequency employed in their trial was 100 breaths per minute. This rate is far below the frequency approaching the predicted resonant frequency of the lung, at which it has been speculated optimal gas exchange would occur (133).

Gluck and associates (128) conducted a prospective nonrandomized multicenter trial examining the use of UHFV in ARDS. This trial involved 111 patients with confirmed ARDS who were placed on UHFV when they were failing conventional ventilation. These investigators demonstrated that over a 24-hour period there were significant improvements in required mean $F_{I}O_2$ (85% to 61%) and $PaO_2/P_{A}O_2$ ratio (.14 to .25). PEEP was decreased by 5 cm H_2O and mean airway pressure was decreased by 4 cm H_2O. Complications reported in this study included pneumothorax after placement on UHFV (15%), mucus desiccation (15%), and tracheitis (n = 1), probably resulting from inadequate gas humidification or mucosal ischemia.

Overall survival in this study was 54%. Keep in mind that these patients were placed upon UHFV *after* they were deemed to be failing conventional ventilation. Further stratification of the data revealed that 28 patients were placed on UHFV after less than 48 hours on conventional ventilation; the survival rate for this group was 79%. This has led to speculation that early placement of the ARDS patient on UHFV may lead to a decreased mortality rate. Further study is required to determine if early intervention does change mortality.

Tidal Volume

The final component of mean airway pressure is tidal volume, which may be manipulated to achieve desired mean airway pressure. Mean airway pressure increases when tidal volume is increased as a result of increased peak airway pressure.

Using CT, Gattinoni et al. (134) demonstrated that ARDS is a nonhomogenous disease process. Accordingly, there are areas of the lung that have much more favorable mechanical characteristics; conceptually, some investigators have viewed the ventilation of the patient with ARDS as the ventilation of a "small lung" rather than a lung that is entirely abnormal. This has led to the investigation of the use of small tidal volumes in an attempt to ventilate areas of the lung effectively participating in gas exchange without overdistending these areas to create further parenchymal damage.

Hickling and co-investigators (135) have used this strategy to ventilate ARDS patients since 1984 in an attempt to minimize peak airway pressures. A retrospective analysis of 50 patients admitted to the ICU with lung injury scores greater than 2.5 demonstrated a significantly lower mortality (16%) than would be predicted by APACHE II (39%; $p < 0.001$) (136). The tidal volumes employed in this study were as low as 5 mL/kg, with the tidal volumes being manipulated in an attempt to keep peak pressures less than 30 cm H_2O and always less than 40 cm H_2O. The mean maximum PCO_2 in these patients was 65 mm Hg, with the maximum PCO_2 being 129 mm Hg. The mean pH was 7.23 (range, 7.02 to 7.38). These data are quite intriguing. Unfortunately, no control group existed, and a number of potential pitfalls are associated with retrospective analysis. However, the underlying rationale for this ventilatory strategy, reduction of iatrogenic lung injury, certainly has a sound foundation.

In a randomized, prospective clinical trial examining the effect of differing tidal volumes, Lee and co-investigators (137) randomized 113 surgical patients to be ventilated with either 12 mL/kg (n = 56) or 6 mL/kg (n = 47). There were no significant differences in APACHE II scores between the two groups. Findings included a significantly lower mean airway pressure and lower $PaO_2/F_{I}O_2$ in the 6 mL/kg group. These investigators concluded that differences in oxygenation between the two groups were not clinically significant. More interestingly, there was a trend towards a lower incidence of pulmonary infection, duration of intubation, and duration of surgical ICU stay in the low-volume group. Again, these data need to be confirmed through larger multicenter trials or meta-analysis of multiple trials.

MECHANICAL VENTILATION AND LUNG INJURY

Lung injury has been an area of continued controversy in relation to mechanical ventilation. The earliest studies performed to elucidate the cause of extrapulmonary air were performed in 1944, prior to the advent of mechanical ventilation (138). It is now known that the occurrence of barotrauma correlates with overall mortality in the ICU (139). During the mid-1980s considerable debate existed concerning the role of pressure as it related to lung injury. Some investigators believed that high mean airway pressures were responsible for lung injury associated with mechanical ventilation, while others believed it was high peak inspiratory pressures that were the decisive factor. Even the description traditionally used for lung injury, barotrauma defined as injury caused by pressure, left little doubt that some form of pressure was responsible for ventilator-induced lung injury (140). It now is clear that this premise was only partially correct.

An important study performed by Dreyfuss and colleagues (141) in 1988 provided considerable insight into the mechanisms of injury related to mechanical ventilation. These investigators demonstrated that severe lung injury occurred in animals with previously normal lungs when alveolar overdistention was present. Animals ventilated with high positive pressure and large tidal volumes, as well as animals ventilated with *negative* pressure and large tidal volumes, exhibited diffuse pulmonary edema and parenchymal injury. Conversely, animals that were ventilated with high peak airway pressure and low tidal volumes, obtained by restricting chest wall movement, had little pulmonary edema or parenchymal injury.

Pressure undoubtedly plays a role in lung injury since pressure cannot be divorced from volume changes in the lung; there is no volume change in the lung when a transpulmonary pressure gradient (alveolar-pleural pressure) does not exist. Transpulmonary pressure, a major determinant of alveolar expansion, appears to be the pressure of greatest importance. The relationship of transpulmonary pressure to lung expansion in ARDS patients (the single largest group at risk for barotrauma) is further complicated by the fact that this disease process has been demonstrated to be nonhomogenous (134). Therefore, areas of the lung exist that have relatively normal lung compliance curves, while other areas exist where the compliance curve has been shifted to the right (i.e., a greater transpulmonary pressure is required to achieve the same degree of alveolar expansion). The primary determinants of lung compliance in the collapsed alveolus are surface tension and diameter of the alveolar duct. Elasticity becomes the primary factor once the collapsed alveolus has reached critical opening pressure (142).

The importance of transpulmonary pressure is also supported in a more recent study by Dreyfuss and colleagues (143). These investigators studied the effects of tidal volume, FRC, and PEEP in the development of pulmonary edema. Ventilation of animals with large tidal volumes (39 mL/kg) and zero end expiratory pressure (ZEEP) resulted in profuse permeability pulmonary edema. A second group of animals ventilated with increased FRC (PEEP of 10 cm H_2O) and moderate tidal volumes (12 mL/kg) experienced increases in pulmonary edema but, unlike the group ventilated at high volumes, demonstrated no alveolar flooding. Two other groups of animals were ventilated with ZEEP and tidal volumes of 12 mL/kg or PEEP of 10 cm H_2O and low tidal volumes of 7 mL/kg; neither group experienced pulmonary edema. The final two groups of animals were ventilated with negative pressure, generating large tidal volumes and returning to atmospheric pressure during end expiration (i.e., no increase in FRC) or low tidal volumes and continuous negative pressure (increased FRC). These two groups of animals demonstrated marked pulmonary edema with alveolar flooding and less marked pulmonary edema, respectively.

Prima facie evidence supplied by both of Dreyfuss' investigations (141,143) support the theory that transpulmonary pressure, a determinant of alveolar expansion, is a primary factor in mediating ventilator-induced lung injury. As transpulmonary pressure increases, alveolar distention also increases when compliance is held constant. Figure 7 illustrates transpulmonary pressure for spontaneous breaths in the normal lung. When alveolar pressure is equal to proximal airway pressure, then gas flow stops and a given transpulmonary pressure relationship exists. Equilibrium exists during positive-pressure breaths when forces opposing alveolar expansion (elastic recoil and increasing pleural pressure) equal the forces favoring alveolar expansion (positive pressure and chest wall expansion). This relationship exists until approximately 70% of total lung capacity (TLC) has been reached.

When large transpulmonary pressure gradients, which may be created by high mean alveolar pressures, exist, the result may be overdistention of alveolar units with subsequent endothelial and epithelial disruption. When chest wall motion is restricted, even though peak airway pressures are high, transpulmonary pressures are lower, resulting in less alveolar distention and lower tidal volumes (i.e., the forces opposing alveolar expansion reach equilibrium at a lower point on the pressure-volume curve).

Dreyfuss and colleagues (142) also demonstrated that the lung volume from which ventilation begins, FRC, is an important factor associated with lung injury. The application of PEEP, with subsequent increase in FRC, increases the transpulmonary pressure, thus favoring expansion of alveoli to a new equilibrium FRC. Supraphysiologic tidal volumes (i.e., volumes greater than 5 to 6 mL/kg) delivered on top of an elevated FRC, further increasing transpulmonary pressure and alveolar distention, resulted in pulmonary edema in the study animals. In light of these findings, the word "volutrauma" has emerged and would appear to be a more accurate description of the mechanisms involved in lung injury secondary to mechanical ventilation.

Data with similar results have also been reported in other animal studies (143–147). Based upon animal data, The American College of Chest Physicians consensus conference recommended that plateau pressure (i.e., alveolar pressure) be kept at less than 35 cm H_2O. When a value greater than 35 cm H_2O occurs, then the tidal volume should be decreased to as low as 5 mL/kg (68). Peak pressure is not a true reflection of alveolar pressure when airway resistance values are elevated, as previously discussed in this chapter. The lung damage created by alveolar overdistention also appears to be a threshold phenomenon, although the exact value at which damage occurs is unknown at the present time.

Gammon and co-investigators (139) conducted a retrospective study of risk factors for the development of barotrauma. A total of 139 intubated patients were screened, with barotrauma diagnosed in 34 patients. The initial manifestation of barotrauma was mediastinal emphysema in 24 patients. A total of 10 patients went on to develop pneumothorax, yielding a positive predictive value of 42%. In this study, increased levels of PEEP and peak inspiratory pressure (PIP) were associated with the development of barotrauma, with only one case of pneumothorax occurring at a PIP less than 40 cm H_2O. Respiratory rate and minute ventilation were also correlated with barotrauma.

These authors concluded that since respiratory rate and minute ventilation correlated with barotrauma and tidal volume did not, there must be other factors associated with barotrauma. It may be quite true that other factors predispose to barotrauma; however, the correlation of respiratory rate and minute ventilation with barotrauma may be explained by another factor—auto-PEEP. The presence of auto-PEEP was not measured in this study. Yet, based upon the work of Wright and Gong (52), one would conclude that the probability of auto-PEEP was very high. Wright found a significant increase in auto-PEEP when (1) V_E exceeded 18.4 L/min, (2) respiratory rate was more than 27 breaths per minute, and (3) set PEEP was greater than 10 cm H_2O. The ARDS patients in Gammon's study had a mean applied PEEP of 10.3, mean V_E of 22.5 L/min, and mean respiratory rate of 27 breaths per minute. The presence of auto-PEEP could have led to alveolar overdistention and ultimately "volutrauma." Both respiratory rate and minute ventilation have been found to correlate with auto-PEEP. It therefore would not be surprising for correlation between respiratory rate, minute ventilation, and barotrauma to exist.

The toxic potential of high concentrations of oxygen is widely recognized. Oxygen toxicity appears to be a result of the partial pressure of oxygen, concentration of oxygen, duration of exposure, and host tolerance (148). The calculation of the partial pressure of inspired oxygen is shown in equation 9 and may be used as an index to oxygen toxicity:

$$P_{IO_2} = (P_B - 47) \times F_{IO_2} \qquad (9)$$

It would appear that oxygen concentrations of 50% or less are relatively safe for moderate duration of exposure. This would equate to a P_{IO_2} of 356 mm Hg at 1 atmosphere (atm). It has been demonstrated that symptoms of oxygen toxicity occur rapidly when subjects are exposed to greater pressure (P_{IO_2} of 1,473 mm Hg or 2 atm) for shorter duration (12 hours) (149). Additionally, animals exposed to high levels of oxygen demonstrate a significant decline in mortality when exposure is interrupted for a few minutes several times a day (150).

Oxygen toxicity can be divided into early and late phases, with distinct symptomology representing each component. During the early phase, a mild irritation of the trachea occurs, which then spreads to the bronchi. This is followed by severe cough, pain on inspiration, and finally severe shortness of breath. It has also been demonstrated that a significant reduction in vital capacity occurs after exposure to 100% oxygen, or P_{IO_2} of 713 mm Hg at sea level, for 24 hours (151).

The late phase of oxygen toxicity is characterized by involvement of the pulmonary capillary membrane with noncardiogenic pulmonary edema, diffuse patchy infiltrates on chest x-ray, possible alveolar atelectasis with copious secretions, and finally complete consolidation and pulmonary fibrosis (148).

The use of high oxygen concentrations may also result in absorption atelectasis (152). This occurs as a result of nitrogen being washed out of alveolar areas with low $\dot{V}_A/\dot{Q}_c$ through collateral channels. As nitrogen is washed and replaced by oxygen within these poorly ventilated areas, the oxygen is absorbed into the pulmonary capillaries with subsequent alveolar collapse, thereby converting areas of low $\dot{V}_A/\dot{Q}_c$ to 0 $\dot{V}_A/\dot{Q}_c$. This serves to worsen the venous admixture, with the end result being a worsening of patient oxygenation.

Adequate humidification of the airways during mechanical ventilation is very important, although it is often an underappreciated factor. Inadequate humidification of the airways can lead to significant airway damage. Chalon et al. (153) developed a cellular scoring system and using tracheobronchial washings assessed changes that occurred in the airway of 202 patients under three humidification conditions: group 1, dry anesthetic gas; group 2, 60% relative humidity (RH) at room temperature (20° to 23° C); and group 3, 100% RH at 32° C (154). Anesthesia and mechanical ventilation lasted approximately 4 hours. There were cellular changes and significant differences in mean cellular scores ($p < 0.0005$) in both the dry gas and 60% RH groups. No changes were demonstrated in the 100% RH group. Additionally, it was found that there were significant changes in the mean body temperature of these three groups. Mean body temperature fell in group 1 by 3.31° C (± 1.7) and in group 2 by 1.8° C (± 0.5), while in group 3 it fell only 0.3° C (± 0.5). This resulted in no postanesthetic shivering in group 3 patients. Based upon these data as well as the data of others (154,155), standards developed by the American National Standards Institute (ANSI) currently recommend that humidification of inspired gases deliver a minimum of 30 mg H_2O/L at 30° C (156).

Lastly, mechanical ventilation has been associated with an incidence of pneumonia ranging from 9% to 21%, with resultant mortality of 55% to 71% (157,158). The clinical diagnosis of pneumonia has proved difficult because of concurrent pathophysiologic processes occurring in many patients undergoing mechanical ventilation (159,160). These concurrent pathophysiologic processes include atelectasis, congestive heart failure, and fluid overload (161,162). Criteria that have been proposed for the confirmation of pneumonia in patients undergoing mechanical ventilation include (1) appearance of new or progressive pulmonary infiltrates on chest x-ray, (2) fever, (3) leukocytosis, (4) purulent tracheobronchial secretions, and (5) Gram stain with more than 25 leukocytes and fewer than 10 squamous cells per low-power field and confirmation of a pathogen by stain or culture (157,158).

These proposed criteria were tested in a prospective study of 147 patients (163). The results demonstrated that 93% of the patients met three of the first four proposed criteria and 51% of the patients met all of the first four criteria. However, pneumonia was documented in only 52 cases. Additionally, these authors analyzed 15 clinical variables without successfully identifying any combination of variables that could effectively identify pneumonia. Identification and treatment of pneumonia may be particularly important in the treatment of ARDS. The mortality rate in ARDS with multiple organ failure in one clinical study was 67%, while the death rate in the same population of patients without pneumonia was 7% (164). There has been speculation that the pneumonia may even lead to multiple organ failure and sepsis. Meduri (164a) has concluded that perhaps the most reliable method of diagnosing pneumonia in the mechanically ventilated patient is to obtain specimens from the lower respiratory tract by either protected spectrum brushing (160,165–167) or bronchoalveolar lavage (168,169). The available data would seem to support this contention.

CONCLUSION

An attempt has been made to present a summary of the scientific information regarding the physiologic effects of mechanical ventilation. Information is of value only if used to improve a measurable outcome for the patient. The value of the information presented can be judged only by the reader. Many of the ideas presented may suggest a change in the current management of mechanically ventilated patients within the reader's institution. As can be appreciated by all, change is at best difficult. However, change has always been a cornerstone of medicine and will continue as long as progress occurs.

REFERENCES

1. Ventilation. *Dorland's Illustrated Medical Dictionary*, 25th ed. Philadelphia: WB Saunders; 1974:1706.
2. Spence AP, Mason EB. Metabolism, nutrition, and temperature regulation. *Human Anatomy and Physiology*. Menlo Park: Benjamin Cummings; 1979:673–699.
3. Vander AJ, Sherman JH, Luciano DS. Energy and cellular metabolism. *Human Physiology*, 2nd ed. New York: McGraw-Hill; 1975: 61–90.
4. Slonim NB, Hamilton LH. Respiration and metabolism. *Respiratory Physiology*, 4th ed. St. Louis: CV Mosby; 1981:11–19.
5. Spence AP, Mason EB. The respiratory system. *Human Anatomy and Physiology*. Menlo Park: Benjamin Cummings; 1979:583–617.
6. Slonim NB, Hamilton LH. Blood gas transport. *Respiratory Physiology*, 4th ed. St. Louis: CV Mosby; 1981:121–138.
7. Tidal volume. *Dorland's Illustrated Medical Dictionary*, 25th ed. Philadelphia: WB Saunders; 1974:1724.
8. Shapiro BA, Harrison RA, Walton JR. Arterial carbon dioxide tension. *Clinical Application of Blood Gases*, 3rd ed. Chicago: Year Book; 1982:67–75.
9. Hodgkin JE. Specialized pulmonary function tests. In: Burton GG, Gee GN, and Hodgkin JE, eds. *Respiratory Care: a Guide to Clinical Practice*, 1st ed. Philadelphia: JB Lippincott; 1977:215–233.
10. Hodgkin JE. Pulmonary embolism and infarction. In: Burton GG, Gee GN, and Hodgkin JE, eds. *Respiratory Care: a Guide to Clinical Practice*, 1st ed. Philadelphia: JB Lippincott; 1977:732–747.
11. Fischer SR. Comparative changes in ventilatory deadspace following micro and massive pulmonary emboli. *J Surg Res* 1976;29:195.
12. Duranceau A. Ventilatory deadspace in diagnosis of acute pulmonary embolism. *Surg Forum* 1974;25:229.
13. Santak B, Radermacher P, Sandmann W, et al. Influence of SIMV plus inspiratory pressure support on VA/Q distributions during post-operative weaning. *Intensive Care Med* 1991;17:136–140.
14. Valentine DD, Hammond MD, Downs JB, et al. Distribution of ventilation and perfusion with different modes of mechanical ventilation. *Am Rev Resp Dis* 1991;143:1262–1266.
15. Hammon JW, Wolfe WG, Moran JF, et al. The effect of positive end expiratory pressure on regulated ventilation and perfusion in the normal and injured primate lung. *J Thorac Cardiovasc Surg* 1976;72: 683–689.
16. Martin L. PCO_2 and alveolar ventilation. *Pulmonary Physiology in Clinical Practice*. St. Louis: CV Mosby; 1987:74–87.
17. West JB, Dollery CT, Naimark A. Distribution of blood flow in isolated lung: relation to vascular and alveolar pressures. *J Appl Physiol* 1964;19:713.
18. Slonim NB, Hamilton LH. Inspired air, pulmonary blood flow and ventilation-perfusion ratio. *Respiratory Physiology*, 4th ed. St. Louis: CV Mosby; 1981:121–138.
19. Burton G. Respiratory gas exchange mechanisms. In: Burton GG, Gee GN, and Hodgkin JE, eds. *Respiratory Care: a Guide to Clinical Practice*, 1st ed. Philadelphia: JB Lippincott; 1977:185–204.
20. Klingstedt G, Hedenstierna G, Baehrendtz S, et al. Ventilation-perfusion relationships and atelectasis formation in the supine and lateral positions during conventional mechanical and differential ventilation. *Acta Anaesthesiol Scand* 1990;34:412–429.
21. Coonan TJ, Hope CE. Cardio-respiratory effects of change of body position. *Can Anaesth Soc* 1983;30:424–437.
22. Downs JB, Klein EF Jr, Desautels D, et al. Intermittent mandatory ventilation: a new approach to weaning patients from mechanical ventilators. *Chest* 1973;64:331–335.
23. Downs JB, Perkins HM Jr, Modell JH. Intermittent mandatory ventilation: an evaluation. *Arch Surg* 1974;109:519–523.
24. McIntyre NR. Respiratory function during pressure support ventilation. *Chest* 1986;89:677–683.
25. Stock MC, Downs JB, Frolicher DA. Airway pressure release ventilation. *Crit Care Med* 1987;15:462–466.
26. Wagner PD, Nauman PF, Laravuso RB. Simultaneous measurement of eight foreign gases in blood chromatography. *J Appl Physiol* 1974; 36:600–608.
27. Wagner PD, Saltzman HA, West JB. Measurement of continuous distributions of ventilation-perfusion ratio: theory. *J Appl Physiol* 1974; 36:588–599.
28. Wagner PD, Laravuso RB, Uhl RR, et al. Continuous distributions of ventilation-perfusion ratios in normal subjects breathing air and 100% O_2. *J Clin Invest* 1974;54:54–68.
29. Evan JW, Wagner PD. Limits on VA/Q distribution from analysis of experimental inert gas elimination. *J Appl Physiol* 1977;42:889–898.
30. Rehder K, Hatch DJ, Sessler AD, et al. The function of each lung of anesthetized and paralyzed man during mechanical ventilation. *Anesthesiology* 1972;37:16–26.
31. Rehder K, Sessler AD, Rodarte JR. Regional intrapulmonary gas distribution in awake and anesthetized-paralyzed man. *J Appl Physiol* 1977;42:391–402.
32. Klingstedt C, Baehrendtz S, Bindsley L, et al. Lung and chest wall

mechanics during differential ventilation with selective PEEP. *Acta Anaesthesiol Scand* 1985;34:716–721.
33. Newell SB. Gases. *Chemistry: an Introduction*. Boston: Little, Brown; 1977:231–258.
34. Marini JJ, Capps JS, Culver BH. The inspiratory work of breathing during assisted mechanical ventilation. *Chest* 1985;87:612–618.
35. Marini JJ. Strategies to minimize breathing effort during mechanical ventilation. *Crit Care Clin* 1990;6:635–661.
36. Otis A, McKerrow C, Bartlett R, et al. Mechanical factors in distribution of pulmonary ventilation. *J Appl Physiol* 1956;8:427–432.
37. Banner MJ, Boysen PG, Lampotang S, et al. End tidal CO_2 affected by inspiratory time and flow waveform—time for a change. *Crit Care Med* 1986;14:374.
38. Connors AF Jr, McCaffree R, Gray BA. Effect of inspiratory flow rate on gas exchange during mechanical ventilation. *Am Rev Respir Dis* 1981;124:537–543.
39. Mead J, Lindgren I, Gaebsler EA. The mechanical properties of the lungs in emphysema. *J Clin Invest*;34:1005–1016.
40. Hedenstierna G, Johansson H. Different flow patterns and their effect on gas distribution in a lung model study. *Acta Anaesthesiol Scand* 1973;17:190–196.
41. Jannson L, Jonson B. A theoretical study on flow patterns of ventilators. *Scand J Respir Dis* 1972;53:237–246.
42. Bergman NA. Fourier analysis of effects of varying pressure waveforms in electrical lung analogs. *Acta Anaesthesiol Scand* 1984;28: 174–181.
43. Modell HI, Cheney FW. Effects of inspiratory flow pattern on gas exchange in normal and abnormal lungs. *J Appl Physiol* 1979;46: 1103–1107.
44. Lachman B, Jonson B, Lindroth M, et al. Modes of artificial ventilation in severe respiratory distress syndrome: lung function and morphology in rabbits after wash out of alveolar surfactant. *Crit Care Med* 1982;10:724–732.
45. Johansson H. Effects of different inspiratory flow patterns and their effect on thoracic compliance during respiratory treatment. *Acta Anaesthesiol Scand* 1975;19:190–196.
46. Johansson H. Effects on breathing mechanics and gas exchange of different inspiratory gas flow patterns in patients undergoing respirator treatment. *Acta Anaesthesiol Scand* 1975;19:19–26.
47. Al-Saady N, Bennett ED. Decelerating inspiratory flow wave form improved lung mechanics and gas exchange in patients on intermittent positive pressure ventilation. *Intensive Care Med* 1985;11:68–75.
48. Baker AB, Collins JE, Cowie RW. Effects of varying inspiratory flow wave form and time in intermittent positive pressure ventilation: II. Various physiological variables. *Br J Anaesth* 1977;49:1221–1233.
49. Blanch PB, Jones M, Layon AJ, et al. Pressure-preset ventilation—part 1: physiologic and mechanical considerations. *Chest* 1993;104: 590–599.
50. Rossi A, Gottfried SB, Zocchi L, et al. Measurement of static compliance of the total respiratory system in patients with acute respiratory failure during mechanical ventilation: the effect of intrinsic positive end expiratory pressure. *Am Rev Respir Dis* 1985;131:672–677.
51. Scott LR, Benson MS, Pierson DJ. Effect of inspiratory flow rate and circuit compressible volume on auto-PEEP during mechanical ventilation. *Respir Care* 1986;31:1075–1079.
52. Wright J, Gong H. "Auto-PEEP": incidence, magnitude and contributing factors. *Heart Lung* 1990;19:352–357.
53. Hemmer WL, Suter PM. Treatment of cardiac and renal effects of PEEP with dopamine in patients with acute respiratory failure. *Anesthesiology* 1979;50:399–403.
54. Kumar A, Falke KJ, Geffin B, et al. Continuous positive pressure ventilation in acute respiratory failure. Effects on hemodynamics and lung function. *N Engl J Med* 1970; 283:1430–1436.
55. Cassidy SS, Eschenbacher WL, Robertson CH, et al. Cardiovascular effects of positive-pressure ventilation in normal subjects. *J Appl Physiol* 1979;47:453–461.
56. Calvin JE, Driedger AA, Sibbald WJ. Positive end expiratory pressure (PEEP) does not depress left ventricular function in patients with pulmonary edema. *Am Rev Respir Dis* 1981;124:121–128.
57. Harken AH, Brennan MF, Smith B, et al. The hemodynamics response to positive end expiratory ventilation in hypovolemic patients. *Surgery* 1974;76:786–793.
58. Luce JM, Huseby JS, Kirk W. Mechanisms by which positive end expiratory pressure increases cerebrospinal fluid pressure in dogs. *J Appl Physiol* 1982;52:231–235.
59. Chapin JC, Dawn JB, Douglas ME, et al. Lung expansion, airway pressure transmission, and positive end expiratory pressure. *Arch Surg* 1979;114:1193–1197.
60. Pepe PE, Marini JJ. Occult positive end-expiratory pressure in mechanically ventilated patients with airflow obstruction: the auto-PEEP effect. *Am Rev Respir Dis* 1982;126:166–170.
61. Hyatt RE. The interrelationship of pressure, flow and volume during respiratory maneuvers in normal and emphysematous subject. *Am Rev Respir Dis* 1961;83:676–683.
62. Haluszka J, Chartrand DA, Grassino AE, et al. Intrinsic PEEP and arterial CO_2 in stable patients with chronic obstructive pulmonary disease. *Am Rev Respir Dis* 1990;141:1194–1197.
63. van den Berg B, Stam H, Bogaard JM. Effects of PEEP on respiratory mechanics in patients with COPD on mechanical ventilation. *Eur Respir J* 1991;4:561–567.
64. Ranieri VM, Giuliani R, Cinnella G, et al. Physiologic effects of positive end expiratory pressure in patients with chronic obstructive pulmonary disease during acute ventilatory failure and controlled mechanical ventilation. *Am Rev Respir Dis* 1993;147:5–13.
65. Tan IKS, Bhatt SB, Tam YH, et al. Effects of PEEP on dynamic hyperinflation in patients with airflow limitation. *Br J Anaesth* 1993; 70:267–272.
66. Smith TC, Marini JJ. Impact of PEEP on lung mechanics and work of breathing in severe airflow obstruction. *J Appl Physiol* 1988;65: 1488–1499.
67. Hewlett RI. Respiratory care of the neurological/neurosurgical patient. In: Burton GG, Gee GN, and Hodgkin JE, eds. *Respiratory Care: a Guide to Clinical Practice*, 1st ed. Philadelphia: JB Lippincott; 1977:748–763.
68. Slutsky AS. ACCP consensus conference: mechanical ventilation. *Respir Care* 1993;38:1389–1417.
69. Frost EAM. Preoperative management of central nervous system trauma. In: Stene JK, Grande CM, eds. *Trauma Anesthesia*, 1st ed. Baltimore: Williams & Wilkins; 1991:250–265.
70. Slonim NB, Hamilton LH. Chemical regulation of pulmonary ventilation. *Respiratory Physiology*, 4th ed. St. Louis: CV Mosby; 1981: 168–178.
71. Oxygenation. *Dorland's Illustrated Medical Dictionary*, 25th ed. Philadelphia: WB Saunders; 1974:1115.
72. Shapiro BA, Harrison RA, Walton JR. Arterial oxygenation. *Clinical Application of Blood Gases*, 3rd ed. Chicago: Year Book; 1982: 77–92.
73. Martin L. Is the patient adequately oxygenated? *Pulmonary Physiology in Clinical Practice*. St. Louis: CV Mosby; 1987:88–111.
74. Spence AP, Mason EB. Special circulatory pathways. *Human Anatomy and Physiology*. Menlo Park: Benjamin Cummings; 1979:567–579.
75. Martin L. Oxygen transfer. *Pulmonary Physiology in Clinical Practice*. St. Louis: CV Mosby; 1987:112–128.
76. Hess D, Maxwell C. Which is the best index of oxygenation—$P(A\text{-}a)O_2$, PaO_2/PAO_2, or PaO_2/FIO_2? *Respir Care* 1985;30:961.
77. Marini JJ, Ravenscraft SA. Mean airway pressure: physiologic determinants and clinical importance—part 1: physiologic determinants and measurements. *Crit Care Med* 1992;20:1461–1472.
78. Marini JJ, Ravenscraft SA. Mean airway pressure: physiologic determinants and clinical importance—part 2: clinical implications. *Crit Care Med* 1992;20:1604–1616.
79. Reynolds EOR. Management of hyaline membrane disease. *Br Med Bull* 1975;31:18.
80. Reynolds EOR. Effect of alterations in mechanical ventilator settings on pulmonary gas exchange in hyaline membrane disease. *Arch Dis Child* 1971;46:152.
81. Reynolds EOR, Herman S. Methods for improving oxygenation in infants mechanically ventilated for severe hyaline membrane disease. *Arch Dis Child* 1973;48:612.
82. Ratner I, Hernandez J, Accurso F. Low peak inspiratory pressures for ventilation with hyaline membrane disease. *J Pediatr* 1982;100:802–804.
83. Boros SJ. Variations in inspiratory:expiratory ratio and airway pressure wave form during mechanical ventilation: the significance of mean airway pressure. *J Pediatr* 1979;94:114–117.
84. Ciszek TA, Modanlou HD, Owings D, et al. Mean airway pressure—significance during mechanical ventilation in neonates. *J Pediatr* 1981;99:121–126.
85. Presenti A, Marcolin R, Prato P, et al. Mean airway pressure vs. pos-

itive end expiratory pressure during mechanical ventilation. *Crit Care Med* 1985;13:34–37.
86. Lichtwarck-Aschoff M, Nielsen JB, Sjostrand UH, Edgren EL. An experimental randomized study of five different ventilatory modes in a piglet model of severe respiratory distress. *Intensive Care Med* 1992;18:339–347.
87. Gallagher TJ, Banner MJ. Mean airway pressure as a determinant of oxygenation. *Crit Care Med* 1980;8:244 (abst).
88. Katz JA, Ozanne AM, Zinn JE, et al. Time course and mechanisms of lung volume increase with PEEP in acute pulmonary failure. *Anesthesiology* 1981;54:9.
89. Falke KJ, Pontoppidan H, Kumar A, et al. Ventilation with end expiratory pressure in acute lung disease. *J Clin Invest* 1972;51:2315.
90. Murray IP, Modell JH, Gallager TJ, et al. Titration of PEEP by the arterial end-tidal carbon dioxide gradient. *Chest* 1984;85:100–104.
91. Carroll GC, Tuman KJ, Braversman B, et al. Minimal positive end-expiratory pressure (PEEP) may be "BEST PEEP." *Chest* 1988;93: 1020–1025.
92. Suter PM, Fairley HB, Isenberg MD. Optimum end-expiratory pressure airway pressure in patients with acute pulmonary failure. *N Engl J Med* 1975;292:284–289.
93. Canada E, Benumof JL, Tousdale FR. Pulmonary vascular resistance correlates in intact normal and abnormal canine lungs. *Crit Care Med* 1982;10:719.
94. Prewitt RM, Wood LDH. Effects of positive end expiratory pressure on ventricular function in dogs. *J Appl Physiol* 1980;48:670.
95. Toung TJ, Saharia P, Mitzner WA. The beneficial and harmful effects of positive end expiratory pressure. *Surg Gynecol Obstet* 1978;147: 518–522.
96. Demling RH, Staub NC, Edmonds LH. Effect of end expiratory airway pressure on accumulation of extravascular lung water. *J Appl Physiol* 1975;38:907–911.
97. Miller WC, Rice DL, Linger KM. Effect of PEEP on lung water content in experimental noncardiogenic pulmonary edema. *Crit Care Med* 1981;9:7–17.
98. Golberg HS, Mitzner W, Batra G. Effect of transpulmonary and vascular pressures on rate of pulmonary edema formation. *J Appl Physiol* 1977;431:14–26.
99. Blomqvist H, Frostell C, Pieper R, et al. Measurement of dynamic lung fluid balance in the mechanically ventilated dog: theory and results. *Acta Anaesthesiol Scand* 1990;34:370–376.
100. Frostell C, Blomqvist H, Wickerts CJ. Effects of PEEP on extravascular lung water and central blood volume in the dog. *Acta Anaesthesiol Scand* 1987;31:711–716.
101. Blomqvist H, Wickerts CJ, Berg B, et al. Does PEEP facilitate the resolution of extravascular lung water after experimental hydrostatic pulmonary edema. *Eur Respir J* 1991;4:1053–1059.
101a. Zabner J, Angeli LS, Martinez RR, et al. The effects of graded administration of positive end expiratory pressure on the fluid filtration rate in isolated rabbit lungs, using normal lungs, hydrostatic oedema lungs and oleic acid induced oedema. *Intensive Care Med* 1990;16:89–94.
102. Hauge A, Nicholaysen G. Studies on transvascular fluid balance and capillary permeability in isolated lung. *Bull Physiopathol Respir* 1971;7:1197–1203.
103. Lai-Fook SJ. Perivascular interstitial fluid pressure measured by micropipettes in isolated dog lungs. *J Appl Physiol* 1982;521:9–15.
104. Staub NC. Pulmonary edema. *Physiol Rev* 1974;54:678–758.
105. Morita H, Vatner SF. Effects of volume expansion on renal nerve activity, renal blood flow and sodium and water excretion in conscious dogs. *Am J Physiol* 1985;249:F680–687.
106. DiBona GF. Update on renal neurology: role of the renal nerves in formation of edema. *Mayo Clin Proc* 1989;64:469–472.
107. Leithner C, Frass M, Pacher R. Mechanical ventilation with positive end expiratory pressure decreases release of alpha-atrial natriuretic peptide. *Crit Care Med* 1987;15:484–488.
108. Frass M, Watshinger B, Triaindi O. Atrial natriuretic peptide release in response to different positive end expiratory pressure levels. *Crit Care Med* 1993;21:343:47.
109. Shirkami G, Magaribichi T, Shingu K. Positive end expiratory pressure ventilation decreases plasma atrial and brain natriuretic peptide levels in humans. *Crit Care Trauma* 1993;77:1116–1121.
110. Andrivet P, Adnot S, Sanker S. Hormonal interactions and renal function during mechanical ventilation and ANF infusion in humans. *J Appl Physiol* 1991;70:287–292.
111. Abraham E, Yoshihara G. Cardiorespiratory effects of pressure controlled inverse ratio ventilation in severe respiratory failure. *Chest* 1989;96:1356–1359.
112. Tharratt RS, Allen RP, Albertson TE. Pressure controlled inverse ratio ventilation in severe adult respiratory failure. *Chest* 1988;94:755–762.
113. Gurevitch MJ, Van Dyke J, Young ES, et al. Improved oxygenation and lower peak airway pressure in severe adult respiratory distress syndrome. *Chest* 1986;89:211–213.
114. Terry PB, Traystman RJ, Neball HH, et al. Collateral ventilation in man. *New Engl J Med* 1978;298:10–15.
115. Mercat A, Graini L, Tieboul JL, et al. Cardiorespiratory effects of pressure controlled ventilation with and without inverse ratio in adult respiratory distress syndrome. *Chest* 1993;104:871–875.
116. Johansson H, Lofstrom JB. Effects on breathing mechanics and gas exchange of different inspiratory gas flow patterns during anesthesia. *Acta Anaesthiol Scand* 1975;19:8–18.
117. Rappaport SH, Shipner R, Yoshihara G. Randomized, prospective trial of pressure limited versus volume-controlled ventilation in severe respiratory failure. *Crit Care Med* 1994;22:22–32.
118. Brunet F, Belghith M, Mira JP, et al. Extracorporeal carbon dioxide removal and low frequency positive-pressure ventilation. *Chest* 1993; 104:889–898.
119. Kolobow T, Gatinoni L, Tomilson T, et al. An alternative to breathing. *J Thorac Cardiovasc Surg* 1978;75:261–266.
120. Gatinoni L, Presenti A, Mascheroni D, et al. Low frequency positive-pressure ventilation with extracorporeal CO_2 removal in severe acute respiratory failure. *JAMA* 1986;256:881–886.
121. Darioli R, Perret C. Mechanical controlled hypoventilation in status asthmaticus. *Am Rev Respir Dis* 1984;129:385–387.
122. Menitove SM, Godring RA. Combined ventilator and bicarbonate strategy in the management of status asthmaticus. *Am J Med* 1983;74: 898:901.
123. Oberg PA, Sjostrand U. Studies in blood pressure regulation I: common carotid artery clamping in studies of the carotid-sinus baroreceptor control of the systemic blood pressure. *Acta Anaesthesiol Scand* 1969;75:276.
124. Sjostrand U. Review of the physiological rationale for the development of high frequency positive pressure ventilation: HFPPV. *Acta Anaesthesiol Scand* 1977;64(Suppl):7.
125. Sjostrand U, Erikson I. High rates and low tidal volumes in mechanical ventilation—not just a matter of ventilatory frequency. *Anesth Analg* 1980;59:567.
126. Bjerager K, Sjostrand U, Wattwil M. Long term treatment of two patients with respiratory insufficiency with IPPV/PEEP and HFPPV/ PEEP. *Acta Anaesthesiol Scand* 1977;64(Suppl):55.
127. Villar J, Winston B, Slutsky AS. Non-conventional techniques of ventilatory support. *Crit Care Clin* 1990;6:579–603.
128. Gluck E, Heard S, Patel C, et al. Use of ultrahigh frequency ventilation in patients with ARDS. *Chest* 1993;103:1413–1420.
129. Westerman DE, Benatar SR, Potgieter PD, et al. Identification of the high risk asthmatic patient: experience with 39 patients undergoing ventilation for status asthmaticus. *Am J Med* 1979;66:565–572.
130. Scoggin CH, Sahn SA, Petty TL. Status asthmaticus: a nine year experience. *JAMA* 1977;238:1158–1162.
131. Gluck E, Frey T, Ostram M. Airway pressure measurements in pigs during UHFV. *Chest* 1987;VOL(Suppl):92;1075.
132. Carlon CC, Howland WS, Ray C, et al. High frequency jet ventilation. *Chest* 1983;84:551–558.
133. Fredberg JJ. Augmented diffusion in the airways can support pulmonary gas exchange. *J Appl Physiol* 1980;49:232–238.
134. Gattinoni L, Presenti A, Avalli L, et al. Pressure-volume curves of total respiratory system in acute respiratory failure: computed tomographic study. *Am Rev Respir Dis* 1987;136:730–736.
135. Hickling KG, Henderson SJ, Jackson R. Low mortality associated with low volume pressure limited ventilation with permissive hypercapnia in severe adult respiratory distress syndrome. *Intensive Care Med* 1990;16:372–377.
136. Murray JF, Mathay MA, Luce JM, et al. An expanded definition of the adult respiratory distress syndrome. *Am Rev Respir Dis* 1988;138: 720–723.
137. Lee PC, Helsmoortel CM, Cohn SM, et al. Are low tidal volumes safe? *Chest* 1990;97:430–434.
138. Macklin MT, Macklin CC. Malignant interstitial emphysema of the lungs and mediastinum as an important occult complication in many respiratory diseases and other conditions: an interpretation of the

clinical literature in light of laboratory experiment. *Medicine* 1944; 23:281–358.
139. Gammon RB, Shin MS, Buchalter SE. Pulmonary barotrauma in mechanical ventilation: patterns and risk factors. *Chest* 1992;102: 568–572.
140. Barotrauma. *Dorland's Illustrated Medical Dictionary*, 25th ed. Philadelphia: WB Saunders; 1974:186.
141. Dreyfuss D, Soler P, Basset G, et al. High inflation pressure pulmonary edema: respective effects of high airway pressure, high tidal volume, and positive end-expiratory pressure. *Am Rev Respir Dis* 1988; 137:1159–1164.
142. Slonim NB, Hamilton LH. Mechanics of breathing. *Respiratory Physiology*, 4th ed. St. Louis: CV Mosby; 1981:66–86.
143. Dreyfuss D, Saumon G. Role of tidal volume, FRC, and end-inspiratory volume on the development of pulmonary edema following mechanical ventilation. *Am Rev Respir Dis* 1993;148:1194–1203.
144. Kolobow T, Moretti MP, Fumagalli R, et al. Severe impairment in lung function induced by high peak airway pressure during mechanical ventilation. *Am Rev Respir Dis* 1987;135:312–315.
145. Thornton D, Ponhold H, Butler J, et al. Effects of pattern of ventilation on pulmonary metabolism and mechanics. *Anesthesiology* 1975; 42:4–10.
146. Tsuno K, Miura K, Takeya M, et al. Histopathologic pulmonary changes from mechanical ventilation at high peak airway pressures. *Am Rev Respir Dis* 1991;143:1115–1120.
147. Carlton DP, Cummings JJ, Scheerer RG, et al. Lung overexpansion increases pulmonary microvascular protein permeability in young lambs. *J Appl Physiol* 1990;69:577–583.
148. Menn SJ, Tisi GM. Oxygen as a drug: chemical properties, benefits, and hazards of administration. In: Burton GG, Gee GN, and Hodgkin JE, eds. *Respiratory Care: a Guide to Clinical Practice*, 1st ed. Philadelphia: JB Lippincott; 1977:386–399.
149. Clark JM, Lambersten CJ. Development of pulmonary O_2 toxicity in man during O_2 breathing at 2.0 atm. *J Appl Physiol* 1971;30:739.
150. Wright RA. Risk of mortality in interrupted exposure to 100% O_2: role of air vs. lowered PO_2. *Am J Physiol* 1966;210:1015.
151. Fischer AB. Effect of oxygen at 2 atmospheres on pulmonary mechanics of normal man. *J Appl Physiol* 1968;24:529.
152. Martin L. Oxygen therapy. *Pulmonary Physiology in Clinical Practice*. St. Louis: CV Mosby; 1987:175–196.
153. Chalon J, Patekl C, Ali M, et al. Humidity and the anesthetized patient. *Anesthesiology* 1979;50:195.
154. Mercke U. The influence of varying air humidity on mucociliary activity. *Acta Otolaryngol* 1975;79:133–139.
155. Dahlby RW, Hogg JC. Effect of breathing dry air on structure and function of airways. *J Appl Physiol* 1980;6:312–317.
156. American National Standards Institute. Standard for humidifiers and nebulizers for medical use. *ANSI* 1979;Z79;9.
157. Johanson WG Jr, Pierce AK, Sanford JP, et al. Nosocomial respiratory infections with gram-negative bacilli: the significance of colonization of the respiratory tract. *Ann Intern Med* 1972;77:701–706.
158. Craven DE, Kunches LM, Kilinsky V, et al. Risk factors for pneumonia and fatality in patients receiving continuous mechanical ventilation. *Am Rev Respir Dis* 1986;133:792–796.
159. Andrews CP, Coalson JJ, Smith JD, et al. Diagnosis of nosocomial bacterial pneumonia in acute, diffuse lung injury. *Chest* 1981;80:254–258.
160. Chastre J, Viau F, Brun P, et al. Prospective evaluation of the protected specimen brush for the diagnosis of pulmonary infections in ventilated patents. *Am Rev Respir Dis* 1984;130:924–929.
161. Bryant LR, Mobin-Uddin K, Dillon ML, et al. Misdiagnosis of pneumonia in patients needing mechanical respiration. *Arch Surg* 1973; 106:286–288.
162. Joshi M, Ciesla N, Caplan E. Diagnosis of pneumonia in critically ill patients. *Chest* 1988;94:4S.
163. Fagon JY, Chastre J, Hance AJ. Detection of nosocomial lung infection in ventilated patients: use of a protected specimen brush and quantitative culture techniques in 147 patients. *Am Rev Respir Dis* 1988;138:110–116.
164. Bell RC, Coalson JJ, Smith JD, et al. Multiple organ failure, system failure and infection in adult respiratory distress syndrome. *Ann Intern Med* 1983;99:293–298.
164a. Meduri GU, Chastre J. The standardization of bronchoscopic techniques for ventilator-associated pneumonia. *Chest* 1992;102:557–564s.
165. Fagon JY, Chaster J, Domart Y, et al. Nosocomial pneumonia in patients receiving continuous mechanical ventilation: prospective analysis of 52 episodes with use of a protected specimen brush and quantitative culture techniques. *Am Rev Respir Dis* 1989;139:877–884.
166. Wimberly N, Faling LJ, Bartlett JG. A fiberoptic bronchoscopy technique to obtain uncontaminated lower airway secretions for bacterial culture. *Am Rev Respir Dis* 1979;119:299–303.
167. Johanson WG Jr, Seidenfield JJ, Gomez P, et al. Bacteriologic diagnosis of nosocomial pneumonia following prolonged mechanical ventilation. *Am Rev Respir Dis* 1988;137:259–264.
168. Chastre J, Fagon JY, Soler P. Quantification of BAL cells containing intracellular bacteria rapidly identifies ventilated patients with nosocomial pneumonia. *Chest* 1989;95:190S–92S.
169. Chastre J, Fagon JY, Soler P. Diagnosis of nosocomial bacterial pneumonia in intubated patients undergoing ventilation: comparison of the usefulness of bronchoalveolar lavage and the protected specimen brush. *Am J Med* 1988;85:499–506.

Airway Management, edited by
L.H. Hanowell, M.D. and R.J. Waldron, M.D.,
Lippincott-Raven Publishers, Philadelphia © 1996.

CHAPTER 4

Assessment of the Airway

Jan M. Davies and Christopher J. Eagle

INTRODUCTION

Why Is Airway Assessment So Important?

Early techniques of inhaled anesthesia required the patient to breathe spontaneously to maintain oxygenation while breathing room air. Additionally, the alveolar concentration of the anesthetic agent (and the depth of anesthesia) was determined by the patient's minute ventilation. In turn, this ability to breathe depended on central nervous system drive, peripheral neuromuscular power, and an unobstructed airway. In regard to airway management, the early practitioners of anesthesia recognized the importance of a clear airway. In 1881, Lyman (1) recounted an apparent death from chloroform. He noted that the patient was restored by drawing forward the tongue. The patient's pulse was noted to stop suddenly, as did her breathing. The "surgeon then passed his finger into the pharynx, raised the epiglottis, and drew forward the tongue. This excited an inspiration. As soon as the tongue was released, it fell back, and respiration stopped again. The same traction was now repeated, and the tongue was held out of the mouth; respiration began again, and the patient quickly recovered."

Also in that era, "pulmonary insufflation" was recommended in the treatment of apnea during anesthesia. Mouth-to-mouth ventilation was described in the late 19th century as "a vulgar method"; however, it was noted to be efficacious for resuscitation of infants. Mouth-to-mouth ventilation was criticized because of the risk of abdominal distention and paradoxical respirations. Insufflated air could pass from the pharynx, through the esophagus, and into the stomach. Another technique, analogous to modern-day airway intubation, consisted of passing a "flexible tube, like a gum catheter of large size," through the larynx into the trachea.

Lyman (1) noted that in this way the lungs could be easily inflated. He also described difficulties with intubation and recommended artificial respiration and tracheotomy if intubation was delayed.

Many other authors have commented on the contribution of the airway to the process and outcome of anesthesia. Although John Snow's evaluation in 1850 of two deaths recognized the "want of sufficient air to the lungs" (2), the importance of the airway in anesthetic mortality was not appreciated for some years. In 1881, Lyman (1) detailed the number of fatal cases resulting from surgical anesthesia performed during the period from 1846 to

J.M. Davies and C.J. Eagle: Department of Anaesthesia, Foothills Hospital and University of Calgary, Calgary, Alberta, Canada T2N 2T9.

1881. The rate of death ranged from 1 in 300 to 1 in 36,500 to 0 (with great variation in the period of study and the agent used). Lyman analyzed outcome and found 1 in 16,542 deaths associated with ether anesthesia and 1 in 5,860 deaths related to chloroform anesthesia. He also added that "when the patient ceases to breathe during the administration of anesthetics—other complicating or possible causes of death being excluded—it is easy to assign the cause of the unfortunate result" (1).

One way to analyze airway management problems is to consider the role they play in the course of delivering a general anesthetic. The performance of the anesthesiologist is never perfect; we are all subject to human error. During anesthesia care, many errors of both omission and commission are made. Consider the patient with a *difficult airway*. If, for example, the anesthesiologist has completed a preoperative evaluation of the patient but has not mastered airway assessment, he or she may omit several steps in evaluation. One may, therefore, make an *error* in judgment. Consider the instance in which, after induction of general anesthesia, the anesthesiologist performs laryngoscopy but is unable to view the vocal cords. This unplanned but common event is an *incident*. The anesthesiologist might then reposition the patient's head, repeat laryngoscopy, and insert the endotracheal tube inadvertently into the esophagus. The presence of the tube in the esophagus is not inherently harmful, but has the potential for harm, thus making this scenario a *critical incident*. If the anesthesiologist immediately recognizes the esophageal intubation, removes the tube, and then successfully oxygenates and ventilates the patient, then no harm will have occurred. (A similar situation exists if the anesthesiologist fails to intubate the patient's trachea but provides bag-and-mask oxygenation/ventilation, or if the patient resumes spontaneous ventilation.) However, if the anesthesiologist does not recognize esophageal intubation, or makes repeated attempts at tracheal intubation without adequate oxygenation and ventilation, then the patient will suffer hypoxic brain damage, a *complication* (3).

With these definitions in mind, let us consider those reports in which difficulty with the airway was an important factor.

Incidents

The actual incidence of difficulties with management of the airway is not known. However, useful results have come from large epidemiologic studies, such as that by Rose and Cohen (4). They assessed methods, risk factors, and outcomes of airway management in all patients (excluding obstetric patients) managed by anesthetists at a busy teaching hospital over 27 months. Tracheal intubation was attempted in 18,558 of 29,145 patients. Intubation was graded as easy, awkward (requiring two or fewer attempts at laryngoscopy), or difficult (requiring more than two attempts at laryngoscopy); the use of any alternative approach was documented. Almost 95% of laryngoscopies were graded as easy and 2.5% were considered awkward.

However, any study must necessarily examine not only the patients but also the anesthesiologists and their expertise. Obviously, trainees experience more problems than staff anesthesiologists. For example, Rocke and colleagues (5) reported their prospective analysis of factors associated with difficult intubation in 1,500 obstetric patients. If two anesthesiologists were managing a case, assessment was performed by the senior clinician, and management of the airway was performed by the junior member of the team. No other description of the degree of expertise was given. Intubations were graded as easy, somewhat difficult, very difficult, and failed. In this study, 89.9% of patients were judged to be easy to intubate and 7.9% of patients were judged to pose some difficulty during intubation attempts (5).

Critical Incidents

Also in the report by Rocke et al. (5), 2.0 % of intubations required "removal of the laryngoscope, further oxygenation by mask ventilation and subsequent intubation with or without the use of an introducing stylet, an alternative laryngoscope blade or intubation by a senior colleague." In a further 0.1% of patients, failed intubation occurred. A slightly greater incidence of failed intubation was noted in a study from a teaching hospital maternity unit in Yorkshire (6). Between 1978 and 1983 in that unit, 2,331 general anesthetics were given. Eight cases of failed intubation were reported, for an incidence of 1 in 291 or 0.34%. A similar percentage (0.3%) was found in the study by Rose and Cohen (4). In 1983, 4,260 general anesthetics were given for obstetric cases in the Yorkshire region. Two cases of failed intubation were reported, for an incidence of 1 in 2,130 or 0.05 % (7). In a retrospective study of failed intubation cases between 1982 and 1985, Samsoon and Young (8) found 7 of 1,980 obstetric patients and 6 of 13,380 surgical patients who could not be intubated. This represented an incidence of 1 in 280 (0.36%) for obstetric patients, in contrast to 1 in 2,230 (0.04%) for surgical patients (8).

Complications: Fatal vs. Nonfatal

Fatal

Data about fatalities related to difficult intubation are available from a long-term study of maternal mortality in the United Kingdom. Maternal deaths are detailed in the Reports on Confidential Inquiries into Maternal Deaths in the United Kingdom. These reports review each death associated with pregnancy and childbirth. The number of maternal deaths is then related to the number of mothers delivered (rather than to the number of births). For the triennium 1982 through 1984, 243 women died either during pregnancy or the 42 days postpartum, out of a total 1,883,753 parturients delivered. Of these 243 deaths, 18 were related to anesthetic problems. Ten women died because of difficulty with tracheal intubation, and five others as a result of pulmonary aspiration of gastric contents. These deaths represented 79% of anesthetic-related deaths (9), an increase from 55% in the previous report (10). Fortunately, the most recent report (11) shows an improvement, with 238 deaths occurring in 2,360,309 women who delivered. Only five deaths were directly related to anesthesia; one women died of hypoxia consequent to difficulty with airway intubation, and the others succumbed to aspiration of gastric contents (11).

In the United States, similar national obstetric data are not available. One report, from Michigan in 1988, described "failure to secure a patent airway" as the "predominant cause of anesthesia-related maternal death" since 1980 (12). However, national data relating to closed claims analysis do provide useful information. In 1991, Cheney and colleagues (13) reviewed 762 cases in which adverse respiratory events led to a malpractice suit. The "overall incidence of severe injury (permanent brain damage or death)" in five major categories of problems was 47%. The authors emphasized the critical nature of airway management in providing patient safety during anesthesia.

Nonfatal

Nonfatal complications can be divided into those associated with difficult tracheal intubation and those directly related to a traumatic intubation. The former include myocardial and cerebral damage from hypoxia and hypertension, and respiratory difficulties from aspiration of gastric contents. The latter include trauma to the lips, temporomandibular joints, teeth, swelling of the uvula (14), and perforation of the esophagus (15).

How does this litany of complications relate to assessment of the airway? After all, are difficulties with the airway not simply part of the normal process of anesthesia? Although it is impossible to cite an exact incidence, many problems can be avoided by better preoperative evaluation and preparation. Endler et al. (12) asserted that complications caused by difficult or failed intubation, "many including death, could be avoided by careful and unhurried evaluation of all patients." This chapter details the methods of airway assessment that are essential to preparedness and optimal airway management.

ASSESSMENT TECHNIQUES

As described above, estimation of ease of intubation is critical to safe anesthetic care. To this end, the patient's history, physical examination, and laboratory investigations may all provide relevant information. Although it is necessary to concentrate on the airway, practitioners should remember that the airway does not exist in isolation from the rest of the body. Together, the history and focused physical examination may provide clues about a number of congenital, developmental, and acquired conditions that are associated with difficult intubation (Table 1). Some of these conditions may pose straightforward anatomic difficulties for the anesthesiologist. Other conditions, such as congenital or chronic instability of the cervical spine, may become manifest as a result of intubation; positioning of the neck for or during laryngoscopy in certain patients may result in fracture or subluxation of the cervical spine, with resultant cord compression and injury (16).

History

A comprehensive history is the basis of all good medical care. The general health may provide important clues. For example, the patient with rheumatoid arthritis who has been forced to discontinue anti-inflammatory drugs because of gastric or renal side effects may have increased symptoms attributable to neck movement. Important points to be noted in the past history include previous awake intubation, cancellation of surgery following induction of anesthesia, prolonged sore throat in the postoperative period (i.e., longer than 48 hours), dental damage (particularly to the apical surfaces of the front

TABLE 1. *Examples of Conditions associated with difficult intubation*[a]

Congenital
Pierre Robin syndrome
Fetal alcohol syndrome
Acquired
Degenerative: osteoarthritis
Infectious: submandibular or retropharyngeal abscesses
Endocrine: acromegaly; Cushing's syndrome
Inflammatory: rheumatoid arthritis; ankylosing spondylitis
Traumatic: facial trauma/fracture

[a]The reader is directed to the following references for more details regarding conditions associated with a difficult airway:

1. Steward D. *Manual of Pediatric Anesthesia*, 2nd ed. New York: Churchill Livingstone, 1985.
2. McIntyre JWR. The difficult tracheal intubation. *Can J Anaesth* 1987;34:204.
3. Crosby ET, Lui A. The adult cervical spine: implications for airway management. *Can J Anaesth* 1990;37:77.

maxillary teeth), postoperative discussions with the anesthesiologist, or advice to wear a Medic Alert bracelet or pendant (17). Following a difficult intubation, some anesthesiologists provide the patient with a letter describing the nature of the problem.

An anesthetic history may also be obtained from the hospital chart, as well as from the patient. In many cases, review of previous anesthetic records can confirm or refute the possibility of airway difficulty. If no previous difficulty can be identified, the patient should be questioned about changes that might have occurred since the last anesthetic. In particular, major dental work, facial trauma, temporomandibular joint or cervical spine disease, pregnancy, and excessive weight gain may adversely affect ease of intubation.

In addition, documentation of a patient's history is important. For example, a report from the Harvard Risk Management Foundation reported that 29% of anesthetic claims were for dental damage and that tracheal intubation was the principal factor in producing such damage (18). In contrast, a review of closed claims in the state of Washington revealed that 19% were for dental damage. Solazzi and Ward (19) found that dental damage was as commonly caused by patients biting down on oral airways in the postoperative period as by traumatic tracheal intubation. Similarly, patients' reports of unspecified difficulties ("Something happened but I can't remember.") should be further defined if possible (patient chart transmission by fax and discussion with previous care providers).

Physical Examination

The physical examination may also provide clues about ease of intubation. General inspection should not be forgotten. For example, the middle-aged man who rotates his body to turn his head and the young woman who stands 5 feet tall and weighs 400 pounds may each present unique difficulties with airway management. Also, the anesthesiologist must not only look but listen. The patient with dyspnea, hoarseness, or stridor may have significant *upper airway* disease.

Bedside Assessment Techniques

A variety of bedside assessment techniques, based on physical examination findings, have been used to evaluate the airway. As indicated below, many of these tests, while easy to perform, have been plagued by failure to predict the difficult airway consistently. Research continues to be done to make these tests more reliable and has taken two approaches (20). The first is identification of the underlying abnormalities associated with difficult intubation (21), and the second is development of simple bedside tests (22,23).

TABLE 2. *Four-point grading systems of laryngoscopy*

Grade	Cormack & Lehane (25)	Samsoon & Young (8)
I	Most of the glottis	Full view of the glottis
II	Only the posterior extremity of the glottis	Only the posterior commissure
III	No part of the glottis but only the epiglottis	Only tip of epiglottis
IV	Not even the epiglottis	No glottis structure

The underlying objective of all of these tests is to aid the anesthesiologist in predicting difficulty of intubation. However, in studies of the utility of these tests, difficulty of laryngoscopy rather than of intubation has generally been measured. The reason for this is that difficult intubation is not easy to define and occurs infrequently (20). Even difficult laryngoscopy is not well defined. For example, in 1988 Wilson and colleagues defined difficult laryngoscopy as "failure to see even the arytenoids" (24). In 1993, Wilson noted that most researchers had defined "difficult laryngoscopy" as failure to see beyond the epiglottis (20). However, he added that the widespread use of the gum elastic bougie had "quietly but radically altered anesthetic practice," with the consequence that "difficult laryngoscopy" implied "failure to see the epiglottis." The first widely used, standard grading system for laryngoscopy was that of Cormack and Lehane (25). This four-point grading system was based on the visibility of laryngeal structures at laryngoscopy. The views ranged from a full view of the laryngeal aperture (grade I), to a partial view (grade II), to only the epiglottis (grade III), to only the base of the tongue (grade IV) (Table 2.)

The original method of airway evaluation is that of Mallampati (22). In this system, visibility of the faucial pillars and uvula is assessed when the patient is seated and has the tongue fully protruded with the mouth opened widely (Fig. 1A,B). Mallampati noted that the finding of concealment of the faucial pillars and uvula was helpful in predicting the difficulty of intubation. In patients in whom the faucial pillars and uvula were readily seen, exposure of the glottis by direct laryngoscopy was easily accomplished.

Mallampati and co-authors then conducted a prospective study of the *clinical sign* of concealment of the faucial pillars and uvula by the tongue (23). Based on this observa-

TABLE 3. *Classification of visibility of pharyngeal structures (23)*

Class 1	Faucial pillars, soft palate, and uvula could be visualized.
Class 2	Faucial pillars and soft palate could be visualized, but uvula was masked by the base of the tongue.
Class 3	Only soft palate could be visualized.

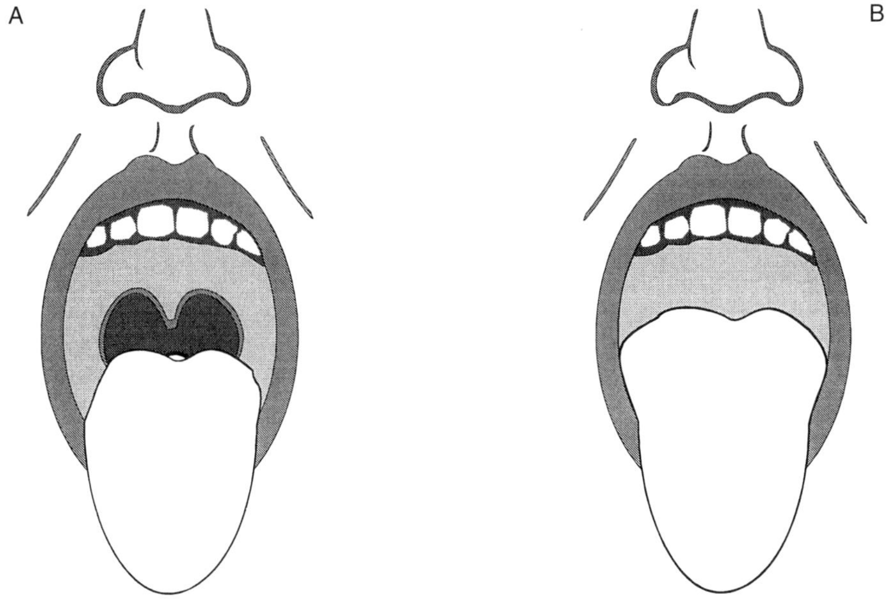

FIG. 1. A: Normal visibility of faucial pillars and uvula. **B:** Concealment of faucial pillars and uvula by base of tongue. (From Mallampati SR. Clinical sign to predict difficult tracheal intubation [hypothesis]. *Can Anaesth* Soc J 1983;30: 316.)

tion, patients could be divided into three classes (Table 3). In addition to a preinduction classification, the authors reported degree of difficulty with four grades of laryngoscopy. Good correlation was noted between the classification of pharyngeal structures and difficulty in visualization of the larynx. Roughly three-quarters of patients classified as class I had a grade I or II laryngoscopy.

Samsoon and Young (8) subsequently modified Mallampati's three-level classification system into a four-level classification. Their modification was based on a retrospective study of patients who were impossible to intubate tracheally on a previous occasion. The authors re-examined 7 of 1,980 obstetric patients and 6 of 13,380 surgical patients. Of the 7 obstetric patients, 6 had class IV airways. The one exception was assessed as class II, but that patient had tracheal stenosis. All of the surgical patients were class IV. The authors also included a grading of laryngoscopy. The descriptions were essentially the same as those of Cormack and Lehane, as shown in Table 2. However, what Samsoon and Young added was a useful pictorial classification of pharyngeal structures aligned with the (presumed) correlating pictorial grading of laryngoscopy (Fig. 2A,B). The classification and grading systems of Samson and Young are now commonly used by many anesthesiologists, although the term "Mallampati classification" is frequently used.

Despite the common use of this classification, many problems have been found with observer variability, fail-

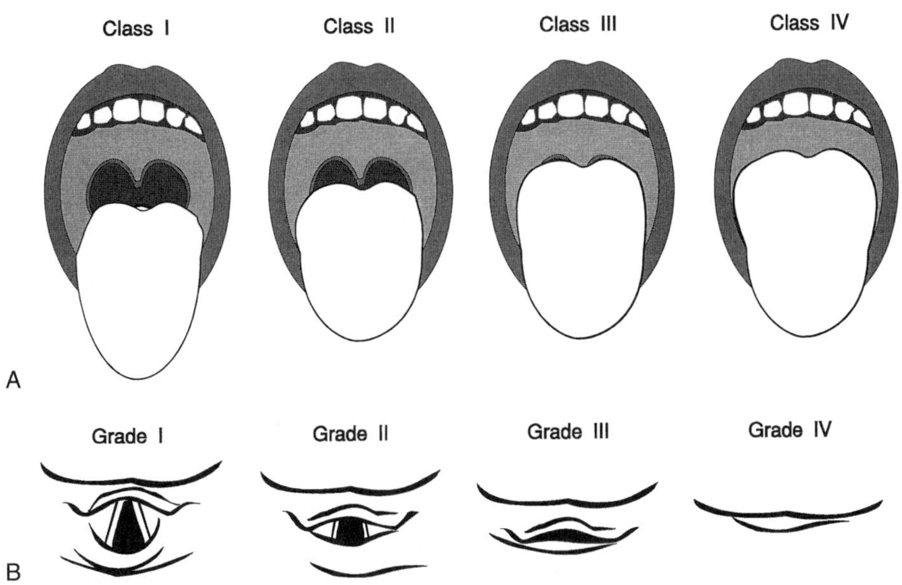

FIG. 2. A: Pictorial classification of the pharyngeal structures. **B:** Pictorial classification of the laryngoscopic views. (From Samsoon GLT, Young JRB. Difficult tracheal intubation: a retrospective study. *Anaesthesia* 1987:42:487.)

ure to consider factors such as head or cervical spine mobility, and false-positive and false-negative test results. (A false-positive result implies that the test predicts intubation difficulty when there is none. A false-negative test implies that there is no difficulty when, indeed, there is.) In addition, the test has not been uniformly applied. In 1983, Mallampati's original description of the method of assessment involved "directing the seated patient to open the mouth widely and to fully protrude the tongue" (22). In their 1985 prospective study, Mallampati and colleagues (23) instructed each patient to open the mouth and protrude the tongue maximally while in the sitting position. They directed each patient to perform the maneuver at least twice to reduce the likelihood of erroneous observation. Samsoon and Young, in their 1987 retrospective study, had the patients sit upright with a neutral head position. They asked patients to open their mouth as widely as possible and protrude the tongue maximally. They recommended that the observer sit opposite the patient at eye level and inspect the pharyngeal structures with the aid of a pen-light (8).

Another, albeit unusual, problem with the Mallampati score is a reported change in classification during labor. Farcon et al. (26) described a healthy primiparous patient who was assessed as class I–II in early labor. At 5-cm cervical dilation, she "began to bear down strenuously with every contraction. Advised that early pushing was hazardous, she alternated screaming with continued bearing down." At 8-cm cervical dilation, preparation was made for a possible cesarean section. Reassessment of the airway by the same observer "revealed marked oedema of the lower pharynx giving rise to a Mallampati score of III–IV, a finding which was confirmed by the attending anesthetist." Immediately postpartum the classification was still III–IV, but 12 hours later it had reverted to class I–II.

A more complex assessment was carried out by Wilson and colleagues (24). In a study of 633 adult patients, they attempted to determine a *simple rule* to predict difficulty of intubation. An additional 38 patients who had been previously difficult to intubate were also assessed. The authors prospectively assessed 14 different measurements of the airway, as well as patient height and weight, and combined these to give 20 different factors (e.g., weight/neck length). They then correlated these factors with difficulty of laryngoscopy, based on the laryngeal view obtained. Five grades of difficulty were used: grade 1, almost all of cords; 2, only half of cords; 3, only arytenoids; 4, only epiglottis; and 5, not even epiglottis (24). Two groups of patients were found: "normal" and "difficult." From the features that might predict difficulty with intubation, only *five useful risk factors* were identified. A very simple scoring system, based on the five factors at three levels of severity, was developed (Table 4) and tested prospectively on 778 consecutive patients. Laryngoscopy was difficult in 1.5%. Use of this risk-sum scoring system revealed difficulties with false-positive predictions. For example, if the system was adapted to identify 75% of difficult patients prospectively (total score ≥2), then there would be a false-positive rate of 12.1%. However, the authors concluded that because the incidence of difficult laryngoscopy was so low, a test would need to be so predictive as to be *clearly unattainable*.

TABLE 4. *Risk-sum scoring system for five risk factors (24)*

Risk factor	Score
Weight (kg)	
< 90	0
90–110	1
> 110	2
Head and neck movement	
Above 90°	0
About 90° (±10°)	1
Below 90°	2
Jaw movement	
IG ≥ 5 cm or SLux ≥ 0	0
IG < 5 cm and SLux = 0	1
IG > 5 cm and SLux ≤ 0	2
Receding mandible	
Normal	0
Moderate	1
Severe	2
Buck teeth	
Normal	0
Moderate	1
Severe	2

IG, interincisor gap; SLux, maximal forward protrusion of the lower incisors beyond the upper incisors.

Three studies have subsequently evaluated these earlier works. Oates and colleagues (27) prospectively compared the classification of Mallampati and the risk-sum scoring system of Wilson. The difficulty of laryngoscopy was assessed using Wilson's method of grading the laryngoscopic view. A total of 751 patients were studied, with complete data available for 675 patients (27). The incidence of difficult laryngoscopy was 1.8%. Both tests identified only 5 of 12 difficult laryngoscopies (more than 50% of difficult laryngoscopies were not predicted using either system). Using the risk-sum scoring system, the positive predictive value was only 8.9%. (The positive predictive value is the proportion of patients with positive bedside test results who actually have the problem.) In other words, only 8.9% of patients predicted to be difficult to intubate actually proved to be difficult. Use of the Mallampati classification achieved a positive predictive value of only 4.4%. Both tests achieved high negative predictive value (a high proportion of patients with negative bedside tests had easy laryngoscopy). Another way of summarizing these results is to say that the tests had high specificity (the tests were good when the disorder was absent), but low sensitivity (the tests were poor when the disorder was present). The authors concluded by expressing a preference for the risk-sum scoring system because of lower interobserver variability.

The next evaluation was a prospective study of 244 patients comparing a modified Mallampati test with a measurement of thyromental distance (28). In this study by Frerk, the thyromental distance was defined as the distance between the "prominence of the thyroid cartilage and the bony point of the chin" with the head fully extended (28). Patients in whom the posterior pharyngeal wall could not be seen below the soft palate (Mallampati grade 3) and who had a thyromental distance of less than 7 cm were significantly more likely to present difficulty with intubation. This combination of tests is easy to perform at the bedside, but the result has not been independently verified.

Another study was that by Savva (29), who prospectively examined the value of five simple tests to predict difficulty of intubation in 350 consecutive patients. The five tests were (1) the Samsoon and Young modification of the Mallampati test (with four classes); (2) the thyromental distance, measured with the head fully extended and the mouth closed; (3) the sternomental distance, measured with the head fully extended and the mouth closed; (4) the interincisor gap, measured with the mouth opened as far as possible; and (5) the ability to protrude the mandible, such that the lower incisors were anterior to the upper incisors. Laryngoscopy was scored using the four-grade system of Cormack and Lehane (25). The incidence of difficulty at tracheal intubation was 4.9%. The results showed that the modified Mallampati test and thyromental distance lacked the sensitivity and specificity needed for routine use. Measurement of sternomental distance was more sensitive and specific than these two tests. However, the author noted that a larger sample size would be required to minimize statistical error. Forward protrusion of the mandible lacked sensitivity, and there was no correlation between interincisor gap and laryngoscopic view.

As indicated above, there has been little consistency from one study to the next. Inconsistencies include positioning of body, head, and tongue, use of phonation (saying "ahh"), and other details of assessment (hyoid vs. thyroid cartilage, and inside vs. outside of the mentum). To overcome some of these problems, Lewis and colleagues (30) assessed 213 adults for 24 different method combinations, based on (1) visibility of oropharyngeal structures and (2) length of the mandibular space. These investigators found that oropharyngeal structures were best assessed with the "patient sitting, head in extension, tongue out, with or without phonation." The length of the mandibular space was best measured from the inside of the mentum to the thyroid cartilage when the patient was sitting with the head in extension (30). Consistent with previous studies, this evaluation showed that these two tests, used alone or in combination, would fail to predict a *few difficult laryngoscopies*. In addition, these tests would predict difficult laryngoscopy in a "significant number of patients" who presented no difficulty (30).

What is therefore required is a bedside test of high sensitivity and high positive predictive value. Unfortunately, no such bedside test has been designed to date. In their absence, experts have suggested use of multiple tests to assess the airway. Benumof (31) suggested that patients should be examined for ability to open the mouth widely, structures visible on mouth opening, size of the mandibular space, and ability to assume the sniffing position. We would also add the ability to subluxate the mandible, as this maneuver (i.e., jaw thrust) is also essential in maintenance of the airway. While all this appears logical, further evaluation is necessary to prove whether the approach is optimal. As commented by Wilson, "The clearest and simplest version is: If you cannot see any of the posterior pharyngeal wall, predict 'difficult' "(20).

Laboratory Investigations

Laboratory investigations are most frequently used to assess patients with known airway disease. In patients with upper airway abnormalities, especially malignancies, pulmonary function tests and radiographic investigation may be performed. Other tests are under review.

Pulmonary Function Tests

Of the currently available pulmonary function tests, flow-volume loops provide a graphic representation of gas flow rates and volumes, allowing the easiest recognition of airway obstruction. As shown in Fig. 3, the shape of the loop may be helpful in identifying the site and

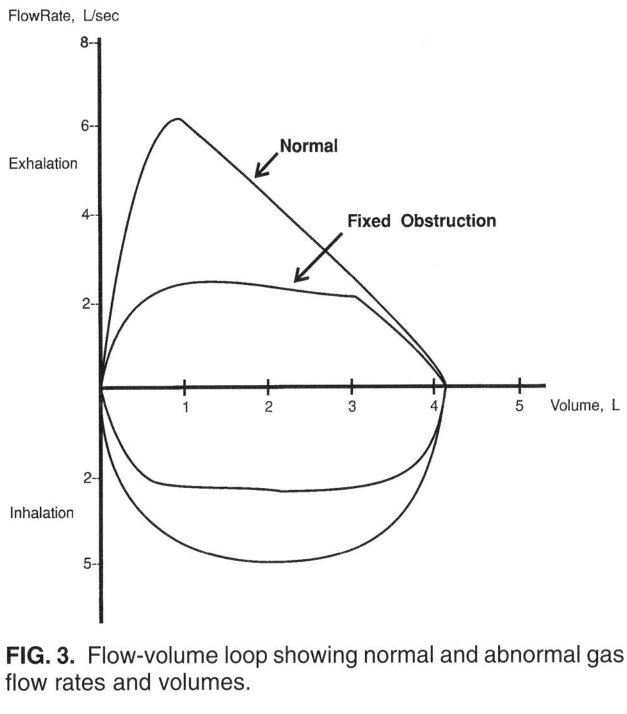

FIG. 3. Flow-volume loop showing normal and abnormal gas flow rates and volumes.

nature of the obstruction. Obstructions can be identified as intrathoracic or extrathoracic, and then as either fixed or variable. In addition, obstructive defects of pulmonary mechanics can be distinguished from restrictive ones. Nevertheless, there are limitations in the generation and interpretation of flow-volume loops. One important factor is that patient cooperation is required to produce an accurate tracing. Also, when upper airway obstruction co-exists with disease of the lower airways, such as chronic bronchitis or emphysema, the characteristic shape of the flow-volume loop may be obscured.

Radiologic Examinations

Patients with malignancies of the upper airway frequently undergo CT or MRI as part of their preoperative work-up. Both CT and MRI scans can give excellent axial views of laryngeal and subglottic tumors. MRI additionally provides sagittal and coronal views, which are potentially of greater value to the anesthesiologist. Recently developed computer imaging techniques allow information derived from CT or MRI of the airway to be processed into three-dimensional representations. Such imaging may allow difficult airway problems to be assessed in detail before intubation. Unfortunately, such techniques are not yet routinely clinically available.

More traditional investigations, such as lateral-view roentgenograms of the soft tissues of the neck, cervical spine films, and routine chest roentgenograms, can also provide useful information about the upper airway and surrounding structures. C-arm fluoroscopy has also been used to evaluate cervical spine mobility and temporomandibular joint motion directly.

White and Kander (21), at a hospital specializing in ear, nose, and throat procedures, carried out radiologic examination of 13 patients in whom direct laryngoscopy had proved difficult. Thirteen control patients were also examined (edentulous patients were excluded). Radiographs of the lateral, posteroanterior, and submental vertical views were obtained. Airway measurements were made after pharmacologic neuromuscular relaxation. The most important factor determining ease of laryngoscopy was the posterior depth of the mandible, determined by measuring the distance from the alveolus immediately behind the third molar tooth to the lower border of the mandible. The authors concluded that an increase in this measurement would "hinder displacement of the soft tissues by the laryngoscope blade"(21). Three other measurements that would adversely affect laryngoscopy were (1) increased anterior depth of the mandible, (2) reduced distance between the occiput and the C1 spinous process, and (3) a reduced C1-2 interspinous gap. The presence of protruding upper teeth was irrelevant. One factor of importance was reduced mandibular range of motion associated with temporomandibular joint arthritis or trismus. Readers should note that the investigators studied adults in a hospital where the incidence of difficult laryngoscopy was 1 in every 65 anesthetics (21).

Bellhouse and Dore (32) studied lateral radiographs of the head and neck of 19 patients in whom tracheal intubation proved difficult and compared them with films of 14 patients in whom intubation was relatively easy. Patients were selected from the anesthetic practice of one of the authors (Bellhouse), in which the incidence of difficult intubation was 0.5%. All patients were awake and ambulatory when studied. Views were taken both with head erect and mouth closed and with the head fully extended and mouth fully open. Stepwise discriminant analysis was performed on 22 measurements and 5 ratios. Three variables were found to be most reliable in predicting difficulty: reduced atlanto-occipital extension, increased anteroposterior thickness of the tongue, and reduced mandibular space. Atlanto-occipital extension, normally 35°, was graded on the extent of limitation. Grade 1 has normal movement; grade 2, a one-third reduction; grade 3, a two-thirds reduction; and grade 4, no movement. Good extension of this joint allows the axes of the mouth and trachea to be brought to close approximation. Increased thickness of the tongue was assessed according to the description of Samsoon and Young (8). Mandibular space was estimated by observing the lateral profile of the head and neck and attempting to construct a "line of vision" (Fig. 4). A retrognathic jaw is clearly associated with a decreased mandibular space. A system of prediction, based on an 18-month clinical experience, was developed

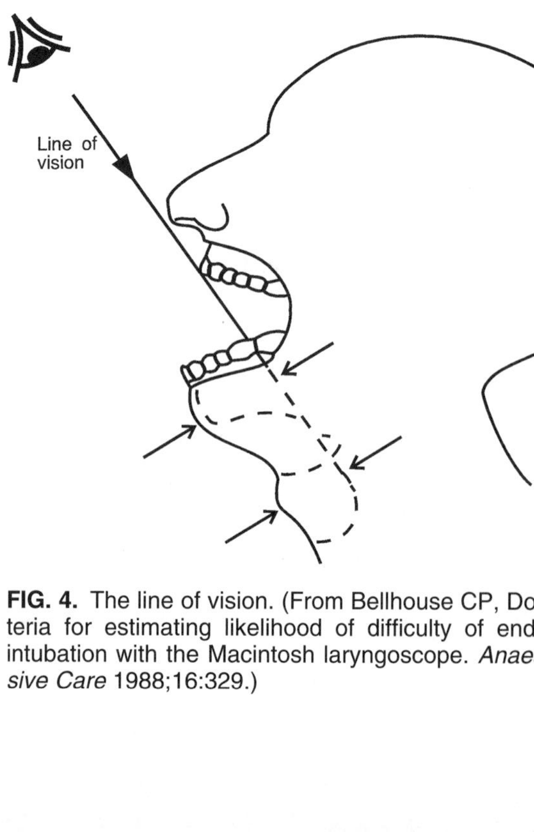

FIG. 4. The line of vision. (From Bellhouse CP, Dore C. Criteria for estimating likelihood of difficulty of endotracheal intubation with the Macintosh laryngoscope. *Anaesth Intensive Care* 1988;16:329.)

by Bellhouse and Dore (32). While easy to employ, the system has not been subjected to formal evaluation nor compared with other methods.

A similar study by Chou and Wu (33) compared the radiographic findings in 11 patients in whom direct laryngoscopy had been difficult. The films were compared with those of 100 control (general population) subjects. These authors determined that patients in whom tracheal intubation was difficult had an increase in the mandibulohyoid distance. They suggested that a short mandibular ramus or a relatively caudal larynx could be significant and unfavorable factors in laryngoscopy. Again, no independent prospective assessment of these recommendations has been performed.

Other Tests

Reissel and colleagues (34) assessed laryngoscopic conditions of 62 Type I diabetics (mean duration of diabetes, 24 years) who underwent renal transplantation or vitrectomy. Laryngoscopy was graded on a three-point scale. Postoperatively, palm prints were obtained by painting the dominant hand with black paint and then applying the hand, with fingers spread, on white paper. Palm prints were scored by an individual unaware of the laryngoscopic grading. Analysis focused on the extent to which the metacarpophalangeal and proximal interphalangeal joints of the fifth and fourth fingers were visible in the palm print. A score of 0 was assigned when all phalangeal areas were visible, 1 when areas were only partly visible, 2 if areas were barely visible, and 3 when only fingertips were printed. The incidence of difficult laryngoscopy in this highly selected population was 31%, and higher scores correlated with more difficult laryngoscopy (correlation coefficient, 0.60; $p < 0.001$). The investigators postulated that tissue glycosylation leading to joint rigidity could also involve the laryngeal and cervical regions, resulting in a difficult laryngoscopy.

TABLE 5. *Requirements for standardization of studies of laryngoscopy (44)*

Requirement	Comment
Standardized intubating condition	Positioning should be monitored during laryngoscopy as it may change.
Controlled mouth opening	Mouth should be closed around blade.
Choice and technique of blade	Blade determines mouth closure position.
Controlled position of larynx	Avoid pulling or tilting larynx forward.
Allowance of very long epiglottis	Position blade tip below epiglottis for consistency.
Accurate record of view	Use photographic techniques.

Recently, Charters (35) has suggested that any future studies should be standardized to allow logical and meaningful comparisons to be made. Six requirements (with comments) for such standardization are shown in Table 5.

Comprehensive Evaluation

Assessment of a patient presenting for surgery with a known *difficult* airway can be a time-consuming process. Tasks to be completed include routine preanesthetic workup and acquisition of old charts, but may also include indirect or fiberoptic evaluation of the larynx and radiologic investigation. A comprehensive approach to these issues may be advantageous. These activities can be integrated into a special clinic, such as the one described at the University of Michigan (36).

COMMUNICATION OF FINDINGS

Communication of details of airway assessment should be made to two individuals: the anesthetic practitioner who will provide care in the future and the patient.

Communication to the Practitioner

The Anesthetic Chart: MOUTHS

Many anesthetic records have a section devoted to preoperative assessment, and some allow details of the

TABLE 6. *An acronym for airway assessment (37)*

Components		Descriptors	Assessment activities
M	Mandible	Length and subluxation	Measure mental-hyoid distance and anterior displacement of mandible.
O	Opening	Ease, symmetry, and range	Assess and measure mouth opening in centimeters.
U	Uvula	Visibility	Assess pharyngeal structures and classify.
T	Teeth	Dentition	Assess for presence of loose teeth and dental appliances.
H	Head	Flexion, extension, rotation of head and cervical spine	Assess all ranges of movement.
S	Silhouette	Upper body abnormalities, both anterior and posterior	Identify potential impact on control of airway of large breasts, buffalo hump, and kyphosis, etc.

airway assessment to be recorded. However, having a space on the record may not be enough to prompt a complete notation. A systematic method for description of the airway is required. Davies and Eagle (37) recommended the use of the acronym "MOUTHS," which is discussed below (Table 6).

Mandible

With the patient standing or sitting upright, observe the patient head on and in profile. Assess the length of the mandible. Note the receding mandible with poorly defined mandibular angles. Assess the ability of the patient to subluxate the mandible. The mandible should move forward at least 5 mm, such that the apical surfaces of the mandibular teeth rest anterior to the apical surfaces of the maxillary teeth. If the patient is not able to comprehend the instruction to slide the lower jaw forward, then a demonstration (by the anesthesiologist) may be helpful. Alternatively, asking the patient to bite the upper lip may demonstrate adequate movement of the mandible. If the patient is edentulous, then palpation of the mandibular angles as the jaw is protruded may indicate good mobility.

Opening

Anything less than a distance of 27 mm between the apical surfaces of the teeth (in adult patients) suggests a problem. Assess also any disease/dysfunction of the temporomandibular joints. Although a patient may, when requested, be able to open the mouth widely preoperatively, problems may occur after muscle relaxation. In some patients it may be necessary to unlock or manually protract the mandible to achieve maximal opening (38). In addition, the architecture of the palate (Romanesque vs. Gothic) should be noted. A "Gothic" palate is usually associated with a narrow mouth and overlapping maxillary incisors.

Uvula

Ideally, the entire uvula should be visible when the patient opens the mouth and protrudes the tongue. Allowing the patient to extend the head may improve visibility.

Teeth

Note all teeth, including their position, alignment, and condition. Draw a picture and indicate any preoperative problems (Fig. 5). Note specifically the condition of the anterior maxillary and mandibular teeth, especially if protruding, inward-pointing, loose, severely decayed, damaged, or absent.

Head

Observe the degree of mobility of the patient's head. Before examining the patient, ask about symptoms of neurovascular compromise associated with neck movement. Ask patients to move only within their normal range of motion, and to report any abnormal sensations. Have the patient flex (with mouth closed), extend (with teeth locked closed), and laterally rotate (without tilting) the neck. These movements can be described in degrees from the starting position. Observe also the presence or absence of scars over the thyroid and trachea, which may suggest previous surgery with resultant deviation of underlying structures, including tracheal stenosis.

Silhouette

Observe the patient in profile, noting the general shape. Note specifically obesity, head position, kyphosis, large breasts, and thyroid goiter.

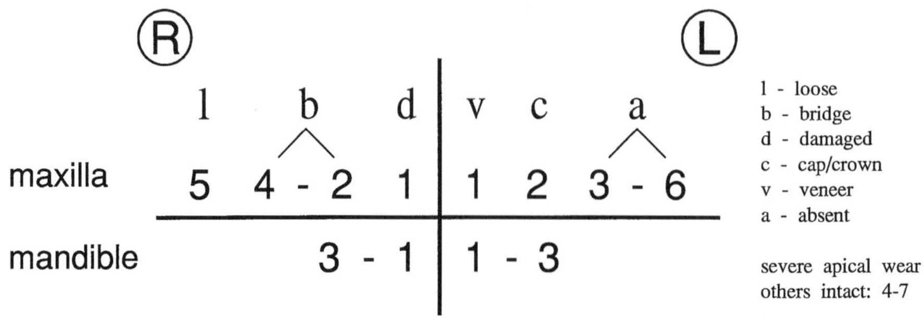

FIG. 5. Schematic representation of dentition, with teeth numbered sequentially from midline. Abnormalities are indicated by abbreviations shown. (From Davies JM, Eagle CJ. M.O.U.T.H.S. *Can J Anaesth* 1991:38;687.)

Medic Alert

In addition, the practitioner may recommend to the patient that a Medic Alert notification be obtained (17). This is particularly important if the patient plans to travel or engages in hazardous activities, e.g., rodeo bull riding. Registration forms for Medic Alert may be obtained at most pharmacies. In addition, the Medic Alert Foundation has created The National Registry for Difficult Airway/Intubation. The objective of this registry is "to develop mechanisms for uniform documentation of critical information and to maximally protect patients identified through the Medic Alert emergency response system, in the event that the patient re-enters the health care system" (17).

Communication to the Patient

Letter of Explanation

Another consideration is communicating information to the patient. This should be done if difficulties are encountered with actual management of the airway, particularly if no difficulties were anticipated preoperatively. As described above, providing a letter for the patient may be invaluable, especially if old anesthetic records are not available. The information should be detailed in language that the patient can understand.

Copies of the letter should be given to the patient or the patient's guardian, with instructions to carry one in the wallet or purse as well as in the glove compartment of the car, if appropriate (as suggested for patients with a genetic predisposition to malignant hyperthermia). Additional copies may be sent to the patient's family practitioner and surgeon.

Medic Alert

Although Medic Alert notification is described above as a form of communication to the practitioner, we include mention of it here as a form of communication to the patient. (Even just a decade ago, patients espoused the attitude towards doctors that could be summed up by the phrase, "Whatever you say, doc." Today, patients are more informed. Indeed, some patients with chronic illnesses, such as renal failure or rheumatoid arthritis, can recount the results of laboratory tests and current and future therapies. Thus, the patient with the compromised airway in many cases may be capable of describing the problem and even the possible management. For example, the patient who requires hand surgery, and who knows that the last fiberoptic-assisted tracheal intubation took 90 minutes to achieve, may rightly say, "I wish the procedure to be done under block."

Medic Alert notification provides general reassurance to a group of patients who have had significant adverse outcomes, such as tracheostomy. The Registry for Difficult Airway/Intubation described above surveyed the first 120 patients enrolled. All "identified an overall sense of comfort that future health care providers would understand the significance of their difficult airway and the concept of the Medic Alert emergency response system" (17).

THE REAL WORLD

Preparedness

The first step in the prevention of problems with the airway is acceptance that there may be a problem. Bellhouse (39) recommended that anesthesiologists be guided in their practice by the results of any tests that indicate that a patient's trachea could be difficult to intubate. He further recommended that the "very first attempt at laryngoscopy should always be the best that one can make it." In addition, the anesthesiologist should recognize that the view at laryngoscopy does not always correlate with difficulty of tracheal intubation. Benumof (40) noted that pathologic conditions (laryngeal web, laryngeal tumors, tracheal stenosis, other conditions) may dissociate ease of laryngoscopy from difficulty of tracheal intubation. Being prepared, which includes having a plan (41), is the basis by which all anesthesiologists, no matter what their level of training, should practice. This leads to the next stage, which is expertise.

Expertise

The preoperative assessment form states "possible difficult intubation," yet the anesthetic proceeds without difficulty. Is there an explanation for this discrepancy between prediction and actual outcome? One answer is that the methods of prediction, as described above, are imperfect. However, another answer is that anticipation of problems subtly alters the behavior of the anesthesiologist such that no difficulties are encountered. Take the case of a patient who has been described as having a grade III–IV Mallampati airway and who requires a general anesthetic. From the moment the patient arrives in the operating room, the behavior and activity of the anesthesiologist will be directed to minimizing difficulties. The patient will be positioned carefully with the head in the correct degree of flexion/extension, the "sniffing" position described by Magill in 1930 (42). This requires that the head "should be the same in the recumbent as in the erect position; this may involve the insertion of a pillow below the occiput. When the position on the table is correct, the cervical vertebrae are in normal relation to the dorsal vertebrae and are not extended. . . . These, in fact, are the relative positions of the air passages instinc-

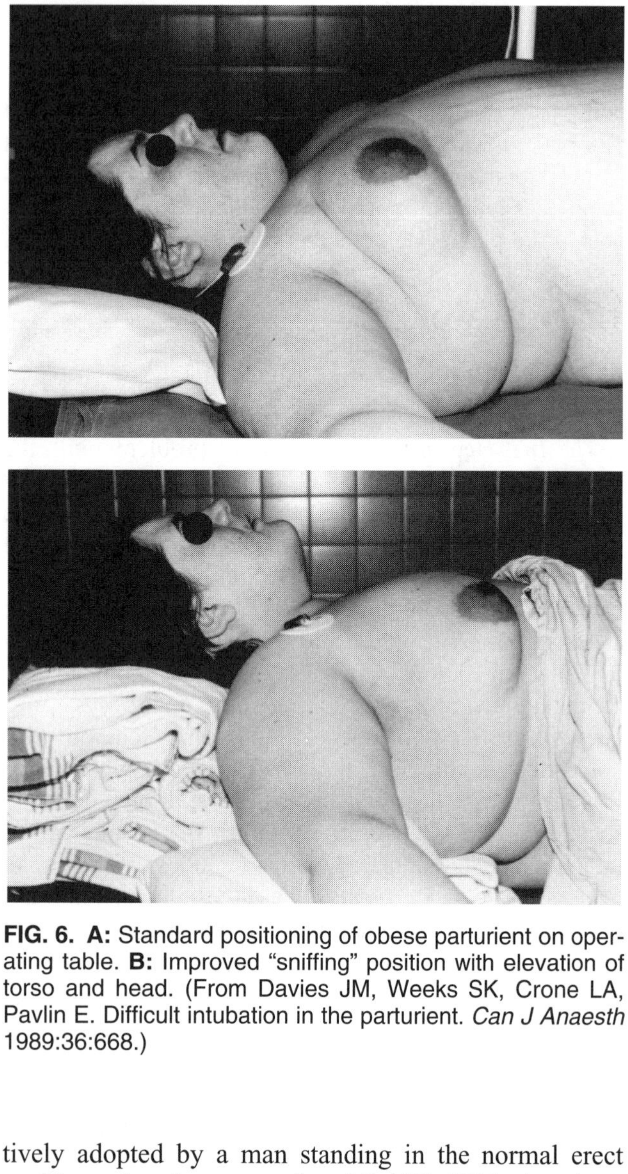

A

B

FIG. 6. A: Standard positioning of obese parturient on operating table. **B:** Improved "sniffing" position with elevation of torso and head. (From Davies JM, Weeks SK, Crone LA, Pavlin E. Difficult intubation in the parturient. *Can J Anaesth* 1989:36:668.)

tively adopted by a man standing in the normal erect position when he scents the air" (42). With the obese patient, achieving this position may require that the neck, shoulders, and upper body, as well as the head, be supported by a ramp of blankets and pillows (Fig. 6).

An assistant to the anesthesiologist will be directed to stand to the right of the patient, with no other tasks or duties except to help the anesthesiologist. Monitors will be attached, checked, and the values from them charted on the anesthetic record. The anesthesiologist, having made an assessment of ability to maintain the airway by face mask, chooses to proceed with induction and paralysis. Preoxygenation will proceed, for not just three breaths but three minutes, to allow denitrogenation of the lungs. An intravenous dose of an anesthetic induction agent will be sufficient to ensure rapid and deep loss of consciousness. A dose of succinylcholine will provide complete neuromuscular blockade. No attempts at laryngoscopy will be made until complete blockade is achieved. Having chosen the appropriate shape and size of blade, the anesthesiologist will insert the laryngoscope and will exert maximum force to protrude the mandible. The well-trained assistant will be ready to provide external pressure on the larynx, as demonstrated by the anesthesiologist's right hand. The tube will have been prepared and a lubricated stylet inserted through it. Tracheal intubation will be accomplished on the first attempt. The anesthesiologist will put aside the laryngoscope and note "easy intubation—first attempt" on the anesthetic record. The anesthesiologist may even think "What problem?" However, each of these activities was probably carried out without active conscious thought. This is the nature of "expertise."

The above scenario assumes that with expertise the anesthesiologist is certain the airway can be intubated as described above. Overconfidence and inadequate expertise are a potentially lethal combination during airway management.

CONCLUSION

Failure to assess the airway properly may lead an anesthesiologist to remove from a patient the ability to breathe "God's good air." If tracheal intubation is attempted, repeated attempts to secure the airway "increase the incidence of hypoxia, gastric acid aspiration and trauma" (43). Failed tracheal intubation does not lead to hypoxia and death, but unrecognized intubation of the esophagus and failure to oxygenate and ventilate do. Assessment of the airway must be considered the cornerstone of every anesthetic. Subsequent chapters will address further strategies and techniques in managing the difficult airway.

REFERENCES

1. Lyman HM. *Artificial Anaesthesia and Anaesthetics.* New York: William Wood & Company; 1881.
2. Snow J. *On Chloroform and Other Anaesthetics.* London: Churchill; 1858:74.
3. Davies JM. Critical incidents during anesthesia. In: Healy TEJ, Cohen PJ, eds. *Churchill-Davidson's a Practice of Anesthesia.* Boston: Edward Arnold; 1995:924–937.
4. Rose DK, Cohen MM. The airway: problems and predictions in 18,500 patients. *Can J Anaesth* 1994;41:372.
5. Rocke DA, Murray WB, Rout CC, Gouws E. Relative risk analysis of factors associated with difficult intubation in obstetric anesthesia. *Anesthesiology* 1992;77:67.
6. Lyons G. Failed intubation. Six years' experience in a teaching maternity unit. *Anaesthesia* 1985;40:759.
7. Lyons G, Macdonald R. Difficult intubation in obstetrics. *Anaesthesia* 1985;40:1016.
8. Samsoon GLT, Young JRB. Difficult tracheal intubation: a retrospective study. *Anaesthesia* 1987:42:487.
9. *Report on Confidential Enquiries into Maternal Deaths in England and Wales 1982–1984.* London: Her Majesty's Stationery Office; May 1989.
10. *Report on Confidential Enquiries into Maternal Deaths in England and Wales 1979–1981.* London: Her Majesty's Stationery Office; May 1986.
11. *Report on Confidential Enquiries into Maternal Deaths in the United*

Kingdom 1988–1990. London: Her Majesty's Stationery Office; May 1994.
12. Endler GC, Mariona FG, Sokol RJ, Stevenson LB. Anesthesia-related maternal mortality in Michigan, 1972 to 1984. *Am J Obstet* Gynecol 1988;159:187.
13. Cheney FW, Posner KL, Caplan RA. Adverse respiratory events infrequently leading to malpractice suits. *Anesthesiology* 1991;75:932.
14. Davies JM. Complications of general anesthesia. In: Nimmo W, Rowbotham DJ, Smith G, eds. *Anaesthesia*. Oxford: Blackwell Scientific Publishers; 1994.
15. Norman EA, Sosis M. Iatrogenic perforation due to tracheal or nasogastric intubation. *Can Anaesth* Soc J 1986;33:222.
16. Crosby ET, Lui A. The adult cervical spine: implications for airway management. *Can J Anaesth* 1990;37:77.
17. Cheriat M, Mark L, Schauble J, et al. The National Medic Alert Difficult Airway/Intubation Registry: patient safety and patient satisfaction. *Anesthesiology* 1994;81:A1232.
18. Holzer JF. Current concepts in risk management. *Int Anesthesiol Clin* 1984;22:91.
19. Solazzi RW, Ward RJ. The spectrum of medical liability cases. *Int Anesthesiol Clin* 1984;22:43.
20. Wilson ME. Predicting difficult intubation. *Br J Anaesth* 1993;71:333.
21. White A, Kander PL. Anatomical factors in difficult direct laryngoscopy. *Br J Anaesth* 1975;47:468.
22. Mallampati SR. Clinical sign to predict difficult tracheal intubation (hypothesis). *Can Anaesth Soc J* 1983;30:316.
23. Mallampati SR, Gatt SP, Gugino LD, et al. A clinical sign to predict difficult tracheal intubation: a prospective study. *Can Anaesth Soc J* 1985;32:429.
24. Wilson ME, Spiegelhalter D, Robertson JA, Lesser P. Predicting difficult intubation. *Br J Anaesth* 1988;61:211.
25. Cormack RS, Lehane J. Difficult tracheal intubation in obstetrics. *Anaesthesia* 1984;39:1105.
26. Farcon EL, Kim MH, Marx GF. Changing Mallampati score during labour. *Can J Anaesth* 1994;41:50.
27. Oates JDL, Macleod AD, Oates PD, Pearsall FJ, Howie JC, Murray GD. Comparison of two methods for predicting difficult intubation. *Br J Anaesth* 1991;66:305.
28. Frerk CM. Predicting difficult intubation. *Anaesthesia* 1991;46:1005.
29. Savva D. Prediction of difficult tracheal intubation. *Br J Anaesth* 1994;73:149.
30. Lewis M, Keramati S, Benumof JL, Berry CC. What is the best way to determine oropharyngeal classification and mandibular space length to predict difficult laryngoscopy? *Anesthesiology* 1994;81:69.
31. Benumof JL. Management of the difficult adult airway: with special emphasis on awake tracheal intubation. *Anesthesiology* 1991;75:1087.
32. Bellhouse CP, Dore C. Criteria for estimating likelihood of difficulty of endotracheal intubation with the Macintosh laryngoscope. *Anaesth Intensive Care* 1988;16:329.
33. Chou HC, Wu TL. Mandibulohyoid distance in difficult laryngoscopy. *Br J Anaesth* 1993;71:335.
34. Reissel E, Orko R, Maunuksela EL, Lindgren L. Predictability of difficult laryngoscopy in patients with long-term diabetes mellitus. *Anaesthesia* 1990;45:1024-27.
35. Charters P, Marks RRD, Hill S, Hancock R. Accurate record of view at laryngoscopy. *Br J Anaesth* 1993;71:758P.
36. Norton ML, Brown ACD. Difficult airway clinic. In: Norton ML, Brown ACD, eds. *Atlas of the Difficult Airway*. St. Louis: Mosby-Year Book; 1991:33.
37. Davies JM, Eagle CJ. M.O.U.T.H.S. *Can J Anaesth* 1991;38:687.
38. Tey HK. Difficult tracheal intubation as a result of unsuspected abnormality of the temporomandibular joint. *Anaesthesia* 1986;41:436.
39. Bellhouse CB. Predicting difficult intubation. *Br J Anaesth* 1994;72:494.
40. Benumof JL. Difficult laryngoscopy: obtaining the best view. *Can J Anaesth* 1994;41:361.
41. Eagle CJ. The compromised airway: recognition and management. *Can J Anaesth* 1992;39:R40.
42. Magill IW. Technique in endotracheal anesthesia. *Br Med J* 1930:2:817.
43. Davies JM, Weeks S, Crone LA, Pavlin E. Difficult intubation in the parturient. *Can J Anaesth* 1989;36:668.
44. Charters P. Analysis of mathematical model for osseous factors in difficult intubation. *Can J Anaesth* 1994;41:594.

PART II

Basic Airway Techniques

Airway Management, edited by
L.H. Hanowell, M.D. and R.J. Waldron, M.D.,
Lippincott-Raven Publishers, Philadelphia © 1996.

CHAPTER 5

Normal Laryngoscopy and Intubation

Marcus W. Skinner, Richard J. Waldron, and Malcolm B. Anderson

HISTORY

Instrumentation of the upper airway and trachea has a long history. The following is a brief summary of some of the more important events:

1555 Tracheal insufflation in animals is described by Andreas Vesalius of Padua.

1667 Robert Hooke, in his publication "Philosophical Transactions with an Account of an Experiment Made by Hooke," describes a dog being kept alive for over an hour by the use of "reciprocal blowing up of his lungs with bellows."

1754 Benjamin Pugh describes the use of an "air pipe" in resuscitation of the newborn. It was 10 inches long and was inserted by finger into the larynx.

1788 Charles Kite, in his essay "On the Recovery of the Apparently Dead," used a tube that passed beyond the glottis via oral and nasal routes.

1806 The French obstetrician Chaussieur used rounded tubes for intubation of the larynx in a case of asphyxia neonatorum. In the same year Bozzini developed the endoscope.

1871 To facilitate operations in the mouth and pharynx, Friedrich Trendelenburg passed three-cornered vulcanite tubes into the human trachea, occluding the trachea by an inflatable cuff.

1878 William MacEwen of Glasgow reported in the British Medical Journal clinical observations on introducing tracheal tubes by mouth instead of performing tracheostomy or laryngotomy. The tube was passed from the mouth into the trachea using fingers as a guide in the conscious patient. Advantages included administration of chloroform and air during surgery, relief of upper airway obstruction, protection of the airway from

M. W. Skinner: Department of Anaesthetic Services, Fremantle Hospital, Perth, Western Australia 6160.
R. J. Waldron: Department of Anaesthetic Services, Royal Hobart Hospital; and University of Tasmania, Hobart, Tasmania, Australia 7001.
M. B. Anderson: Department of Anaesthetic Services, Royal Hobart Hospital; and University of Tasmania, Hobart, Tasmania, Australia 7001.

contamination, and providing a monitor of patient respiration.

1892 Eisenmenger used a hard rubber tube with an inflatable cuff and pilot balloon (to indicate the cuff was inflated).

1889 Annandale used a gum elastic tube for tracheal insertion.

1895 Alfred Kirstein designed the "autoscope" for examining the larynx and trachea.

1907 Chevalier Jackson of Philadelphia published a book on the subject of intubation.

1928 Magill published his results of blind nasal intubation with a single wide-bore tube. The first blind nasal intubation was performed by Stanley Rowbotham. Both of them had gained significant clinical experience during World War I and later at the Queen's Hospital for Facial and Jaw Injuries at Sidcup.

1941 Macintosh described his laryngoscope.

PHYSIOLOGIC EFFECTS OF DIRECT LARYNGOSCOPY AND INTUBATION

The larynx is richly innervated by parasympathetic (via the vagus and glossopharyngeal nerves) and sympathetic nerve fibers. Direct laryngoscopy and endotracheal intubation are noxious stimuli that produce marked physiologic responses. Irritation and injury to these areas trigger a combination of autonomic reflexes and brain stem activation. These responses have important ramifications for the medically or surgically compromised patient, and an understanding of the normal physiologic responses allows one to anticipate and attenuate any problems that may occur in patients with certain pre-existing conditions.

Cardiovascular Responses

The principal effects of direct laryngoscopy and intubation are a marked sympathoadrenal response, which produces an increase in heart rate, systemic vascular resistance, arterial and ventricular filling pressures, and plasma catecholamine levels (1). Depending on the individual patient, this may cause an increase in cardiac output or impair left ventricular function (2). The exact neurohumoral mechanisms by which these changes occur have not been fully elucidated, but they clearly involve cardiac and sympathetic adrenal and stress hormone release. Sensory impulses from the root of the tongue, epiglottis, and trachea are carried to the brain stem to stimulate the vasomotor and cardioaccelerator system to produce a hyperdynamic circulation.

Reflex vasoconstriction occurs within a few seconds, followed by sinus tachycardia, which reaches a peak in 2 minutes and lasts about 5 minutes. Transient hypertension and tachycardia are probably well tolerated in the healthy patient, but hypertensive patients often show an exaggerated response. Unfortunately, the increase in cardiac output, oxygen consumption, filling pressures, and ventricular afterload may cause myocardial ischemia, arrhythmias, and impaired left ventricular function in susceptible patients. Because these effects are relatively transient, they may be missed if one is not monitoring invasive pressures, cardiac rhythm, or ST segment changes until after successful intubation. By contrast, parasympathetic/vagal reflexes seem to be more pronounced in children, and even spraying the larynx may precipitate bradycardia. This may occur as a baroreflex to the increase in systemic vascular resistance or be part of a nonspecific autonomic reflex to stimulation, especially as the parasympathetic nervous system is relatively more developed in this age group.

Attenuation of Cardiovascular Effects

The aim of attenuating the cardiovascular changes is to avoid the following:

1. Excessive swings in blood pressure, which may stress certain important circulations (myocardial and cerebral)
2. Worsening of any pre-existing increased intracranial pressure
3. Anesthetic-induced myocardial ischemia (3)

Known or suspected ischemic heart disease is by far the most common condition necessitating modification of the hemodynamic response to intubation (4,5). Although the brain is obtunded by general anesthetic agents, the level of anesthesia required for intubation is often greater than that required for surgery. The ideal technique should be short-acting (for the duration of laryngoscopy and intubation) with optimum cardiovascular stability, i.e., allowing normal pressures and heart rates to be maintained as far as possible. Some suggested techniques include the following:

1. Ensuring level of anesthesia is adequate or deep, either with inhalational agents or by giving a small intravenous bolus of an induction agent or opiate (6) 30 to 60 seconds prior to laryngoscopy and intubation.

2. Using high-dose opioids for induction (e.g., fentanyl 5 to 10 μg/kg up to 50 to 100 μg, depending on the procedure and other patient factors). Because this technique requires high doses of opiates, it is often impractical in short surgical procedures.

3. Applying topical anesthesia to the larynx and trachea with nebulized lidocaine, gargle or spray. Remember that using direct laryngoscopy to facilitate the application of topical lidocaine (4% or 10%) often precipitates the physiologic responses one is trying to avoid.

4. Administering an intravenous bolus of lidocaine (1 to 2 mg/kg) about 30 to 60 seconds prior to laryngoscopy.

5. Using short-acting cardiac agents such as glyceryl trinitrate, alpha blockers, or beta blockers. If esmolol (100 to 200 mg) is used, it should be combined with another agent, e.g., fentanyl (7,8).

6. Avoiding stimulation with the laryngoscope by using fiberoptic or blind nasal intubation.

Respiratory Responses

The stimulation of laryngoscopy produces an increase in ventilatory drive (i.e., increased respiratory rate and tidal volume) in the spontaneously ventilating patient. Laryngospasm may occur if the patient is not paralyzed and too "light," and bronchospasm may occur once instrumentation of the trachea has been performed. Bronchospasm is common in patients in whom the airway is already irritable or reactive (e.g., individuals with asthma, chronic bronchitis, or cystic fibrosis).

In addition, in some patients in whom laryngoscopy is difficult and prolonged, there may be a significant time between intravenous induction and successful intubation. Inadequate ventilation during this time may lead to hypoxemia and hypercapnia (9). Hypoxemia occurs more rapidly in obese, pediatric, and obstetric patients, in whom oxygen consumption is high and lung reserves are low (10). Pre-oxygenation (or denitrogenation) with 100% oxygen 1 to 3 minutes prior to induction should be carried out whenever a difficult intubation is anticipated. We would recommend pre-oxygenation for *any* patient requiring intubation or control of the airway. In certain situations (e.g., emergency cesarean sections), it may not be practicable to spend time pre-oxygenating the patient; in these situations, three maximal inspiratory breaths of 100% oxygen will suffice (9,11).

Central Nervous System Responses

The most significant changes that occur are increased intracranial pressure (ICP) and intraocular pressure (IOP). The mechanism of raised ICP is primarily increased systemic arterial and venous filling pressure, but hypoxia and hypercapnia amplify this problem. Raised ICP is detrimental to patients with either pre-existing raised ICP (e.g., subjects with head injuries, cerebral tumors) or cerebral aneurysms; transient hypertension during intubation may either worsen ICP or cause the aneurysm to rupture. Attenuation of this response is imperative in such patients (see Attenuation of Cardiovascular Effects). The same principles apply for patients with either pre-existing raised IOP or penetrating eye injuries, which create the risk of extrusion of the eye contents.

INDICATIONS FOR AND COMPLICATIONS OF DIRECT LARYNGOSCOPY AND INTUBATION

Like any medical procedure, laryngoscopy and intubation are associated with certain risks of morbidity or mortality. Clinicians contemplating intubation should therefore be familiar with both the indications and complications (Tables 1 and 2).

Cardiorespiratory arrest is perhaps one of the most common emergency indications for intubation. Respiratory arrest/failure leading to complete cardiorespiratory arrest is common in children, whereas the opposite is true in adults (i.e., cardiac arrest precedes respiratory arrest). Certain drugs (lidocaine, atropine, epinephrine, isoprenaline, naloxone) may be given in these situations via an endotracheal tube when intravenous access has not been achieved. Note that the absorption of these drugs is erratic and requires twice the recommended intravenous dose and a larger volume (as there is such a large surface area).

There are many procedures in which the clinician may have remote access to or share the airway (faciomaxillary, neurosurgical, and dental procedures). Intubations in such circumstances allows a secure, definitive airway where there is an otherwise constant threat to ventilation. Other individuals who may require intubation include pediatric patients requiring MRI under general anesthesia and patients requiring surgery in the prone position or undergoing prolonged procedures (more than 2 hours) under general anesthesia.

Most of the complications occur during or immediately after laryngoscopy, and fortunately the more serious ones

TABLE 1. *Common indications for intubation*

Resuscitation
Cardiac or respiratory failure/arrest
e.g., cardiac arrest, chest trauma, flail chest, pneumothorax, pulmonary embolus, obstructed airway (epiglottitis, croup, bilateral recurrent laryngeal nerve palsy)
Control of carbon dioxide
e.g., head injuries, raised intracranial pressure
Protection of the airway
Unconscious patient
e.g., stroke, drug overdose, diabetic coma, other causes of coma
Full stomach, bleeding in the airway
e.g., general anesthesia for cesarean section, inadequate fasting, faciomaxillary trauma, epistaxis
Paralysis (chemical or traumatic)
Surgical access to site of operation
Faciomaxillary surgery/remote diagnostic procedures
e.g., MRI, CT
Shared airway procedures
e.g., microlaryngoscopy, rigid esophagoscopy, tonsillectomy
Patient positioning (prone, lateral)
Prolonged surgery

TABLE 2. *Complications of intubation*

Problems with insertion
Inability to intubate
Esophageal/endobronchial intubation
Trauma to the teeth, mouth, pharynx, nerves, eyes
Autonomic response to intubation, e.g., hypertension, tachycardia, raised intracranial pressure
Vomiting/regurgitation, aspiration, laryngospasm, laryngobronchospasm
Laryngeal trauma, pneumothorax, pneumomediastinum, dislocated arytenoids
Manipulation of the cervical spine
Problems with short-term use (after insertion)
Unrecognized esophageal intubation
Endotracheal tube movement or blockage, distention of cuff causing tracheal tear/rupture
Circuit disconnection, accidental extubation
Problems with prolonged intubation
Trauma to the vocal cords
Laryngeal edema, laryngomalacia, tracheal ulceration
Distention of cuff
Lack of humidification
Atelectasis
Problems at extubation
Autonomic responses
Straining/coughing (Valsalva effects, e.g., decreased venous return, decreased cardiac output, elevated intracranial pressure, hypoxemia)
Trauma from failure to deflate cuff
Laryngospasm
Aspiration
Dental trauma
Dysphonia

are rare events (Table 2). Proper vigilance and monitoring for correct placement and functioning of the endotracheal tube during its use can prevent many immediate serious problems.

PREPARATION FOR DIRECT LARYNGOSCOPY AND INTUBATION

Some patients of apparently normal appearance may present great difficulties at intubation. As a result, there are several methods that attempt to identify patients who will be difficult or impossible to intubate with the usual techniques. The techniques of assessment are described in more detail in Chapter 4 (Assessment of the Airway). However, none of these methods identifies *all* patients who will be difficult/unsuccessful intubations.

Intubations in 1% of normal anesthetic practice are either difficult or unsuccessful. Certain patient populations have a higher incidence than this. For example, Samsoon and Young (12) reported an incidence of 1 in 280 in obstetric patients, as compared with 1 in 2,230 in the general surgical population. In the emergency room, most intubations are difficult because of urgency, lack of patient history and examination, and the nature of the injuries. In intensive care units, critically ill patients may require urgent intubation because of impending cardiorespiratory arrest. Appendix A gives a list of some of the conditions that should alert the clinician to a potentially difficult intubation. If such circumstances present, the supervising clinician must be familiar with failed intubation drills and ensure the availability of adequate facilities to perform these (see later in this chapter).

Clinicians who are learning the techniques of direct laryngoscopy and intubation should practice in a controlled environment (e.g., perform simulated intubations on mannequins or in the operating room), in which intubation is normally a relatively uncomplicated procedure, prior to working under emergency conditions. Any clinician who attempts direct laryngoscopy and intubation must be aware of and prepared for the difficult airway. The best way to prepare for this contingency is to perform as many intubations as possible with skilled supervision available.

This section outlines the preparation for normal laryngoscopy and intubation.

Pre-anesthetic Airway Assessment

Whenever possible, an ample history should be obtained. Particular points to elicit are previous problems

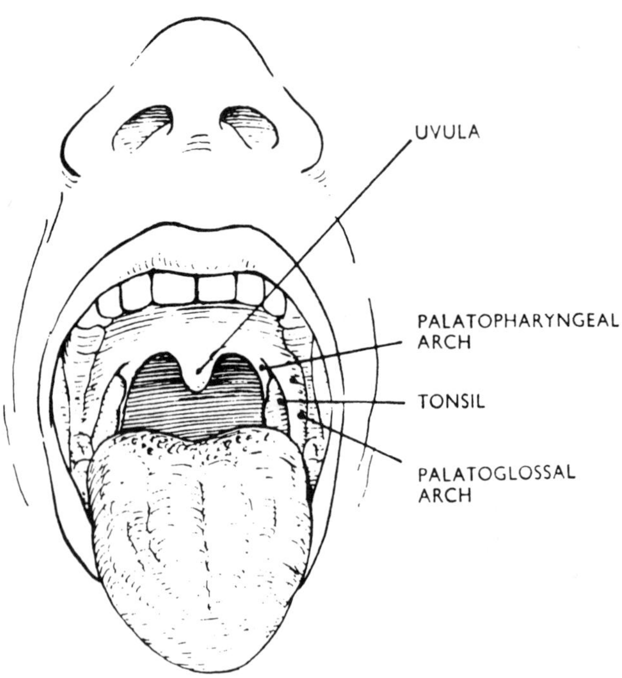

FIG. 1. Anatomic features relevant to the Mallampati assessment of the airway. Labelled anatomic features are important for this clinical assessment technique (see text for details) (From Ellis H and Feldman S. *Anatomy for Anaesthetists, 5th Edition.* London: Blackwell Scientific Publications Pty. Ltd.; 1988, with permission).

with anesthesia (there may have been previous difficulty with the patient's airway), any arthritis that may limit neck movement or mouth opening, or congenital syndromes (e.g., Pierre Robin). The reason for operation (e.g., fractured mandible, drainage of tonsillar abscess) should always be elicited. Fasting status and the likelihood of vomiting and/or regurgitation should also be assessed (see Chapters 4 and 7).

Pre-assessment and Laryngoscopic Grades

Figures 1 and 2 depict the anatomy of the upper airway. Figure 1 is particularly relevant when using the Mallampati (13,14) assessment technique. This open-mouth view is obtained simply by asking patients to open their mouth and poke their tongue out maximally (*don't* ask them to say "ahh"). The various classes are shown in Table 3, along with description of the structures seen.

It is essential for anyone performing direct laryngoscopy and intubation to be familiar with the anatomy of the upper airway (Figs. 3 and 4). No single anatomic factor determines the ease of laryngoscopy. One must be able to insert a laryngoscope into the mouth and subsequently obtain a clear view of the vocal cords. The mobility of all soft tissues and bony structures involved in the process of opening the mouth and extending the neck therefore needs to be examined. The effect of soft tissues in a difficult intubation has generally been underestimated, especially regarding the mobility of the base of the tongue.

TABLE 3. *Classifications of Mallampati and of Cormack and Lehane*

Oral assessment (Mallampati)	Description
Class 1	Faucial pillars, soft palate, and uvula seen
Class 2	Faucial pillars and soft palate seen, but uvula masked by base of tongue
Class 3	Only soft palate seen
Laryngoscopic grade (Cormack and Lehane)	**Description**
Grade 1	Glottis (including anterior and posterior commissures) can be fully exposed
Grade 2	Glottis can be partly exposed (anterior commissure not visualized)
Grade 3	Glottis cannot be seen (only corniculate cartilages visualized)
Grade 4	Glottis including corniculate cartilages cannot be exposed

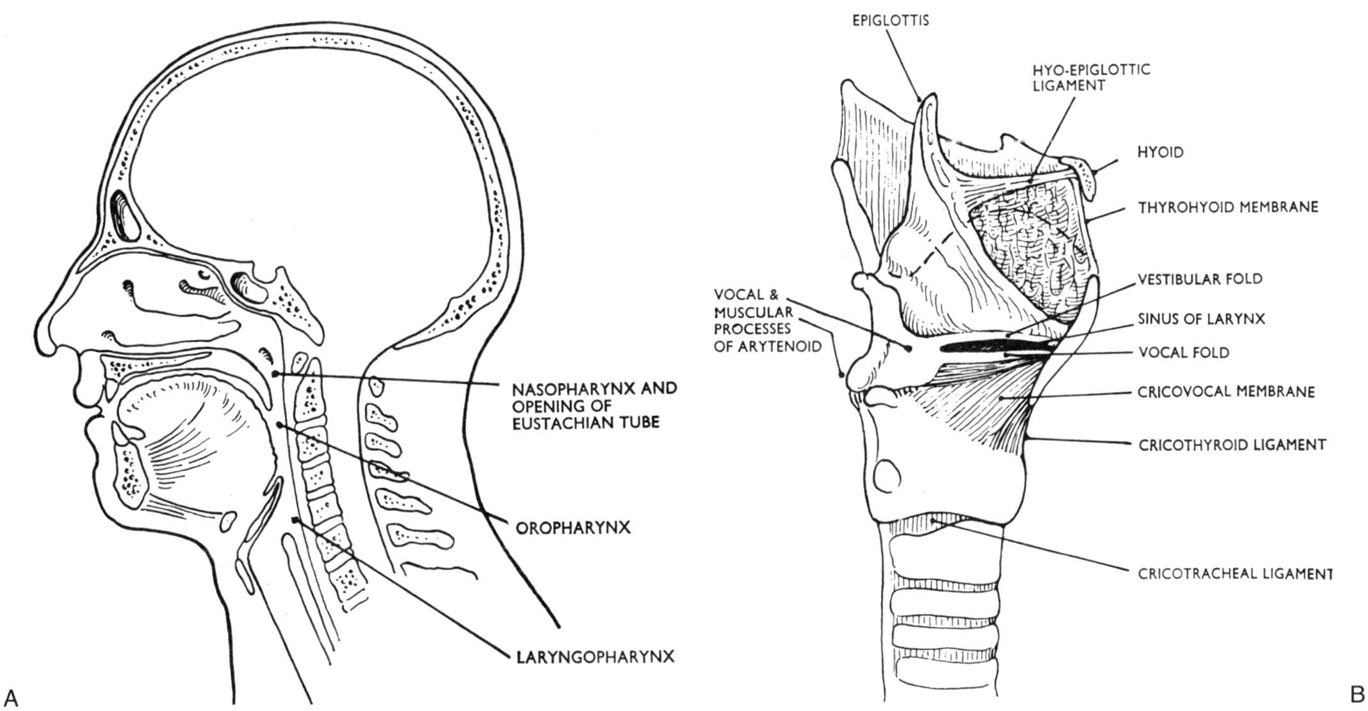

FIG. 2. Lateral view of the upper airway. **A:** Distinction between nasopharynx, oropharynx, and laryngopharynx. **B:** Detailed diagram of the larynx and related structures (From Ellis H and Feldman S. *Anatomy for Anaesthetists, 5th Edition.* London: Blackwell Scientific Publications Pty. Ltd.; 1988, with permission).

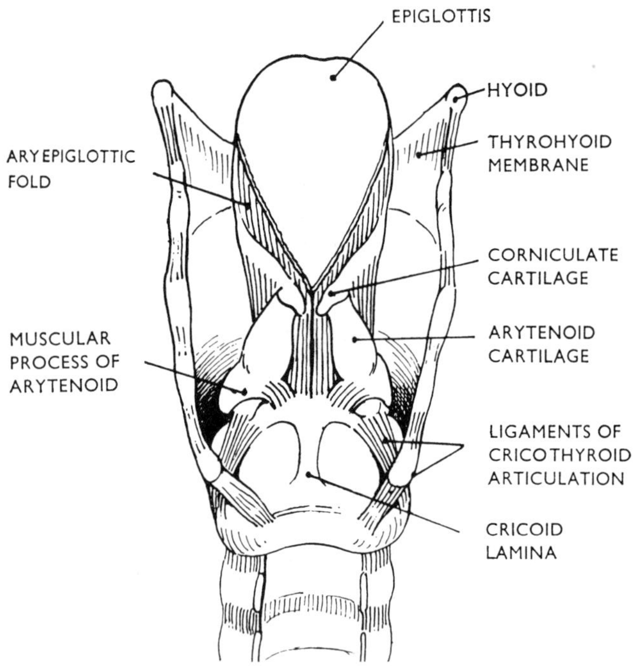

FIG. 3. Posterior view of the epiglottis, larynx, and upper trachea, detailing cartilaginous structures and muscles (From Ellis H and Feldman S. *Anatomy for Anaesthetists, 5th Edition.* London: Blackwell Scientific Publications Pty. Ltd.; 1988, with permission).

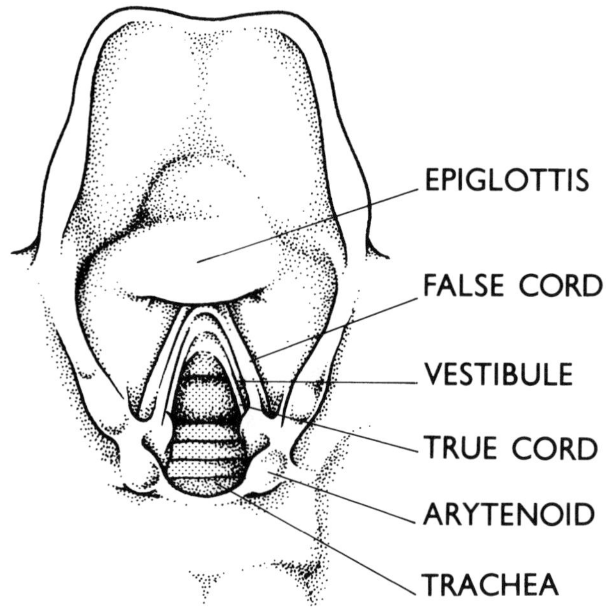

FIG. 4. Laryngoscopic view of the larynx and vocal cords (From Ellis H and Feldman S. *Anatomy for Anaesthetists, 5th Edition.* London: Blackwell Scientific Publications Pty. Ltd.; 1988, with permission).

The importance of the pre-anesthetic assessment of the patient is shown in Table 4 and Fig. 5. In Table 4 and Fig. 5, the Mallampati classification is correlated to the laryngoscopic view. According to the table, the more difficult laryngoscopic views (which increase the difficulty of intubation) occur only with the higher Mallampati classes.

Classic signs at the pre-anesthetic examination suggestive of difficult intubation include the following:

1. Small mouth or poor mobility of the mandible (trismus, or arthritis at the temporomandibular joint)
2. Short muscular neck with a full set of teeth
3. Receding mandible with obtuse mandibular angles (especially note patients with beards)
4. Protruding maxillary incisors with relative maxillary overhang
5. Long, arched palate associated with a long, narrow mouth
6. Thyromental distance of less than 6 cm (the measured distance between the lower border of the chin and the thyroid notch with the neck fully extended)

Anesthetic Equipment Check

Patient morbidity and critical incidents can be reduced by being adequately prepared for all eventualities. Once the patient is asleep and apneic, the problem is not whether intubation can be performed but whether adequate ventilation is possible; for this reason, if there is any doubt about maintaining the airway, anesthesia should not be induced and the airway should be secured by some other means (see Chapter 8).

The preoperative history and examination usually identify patients whose airways are potentially difficult to maintain or intubate, but it is the unexpectedly difficult airway that causes most concern. It is a good philosophy *always* to be prepared for a difficult intubation and have the minimum of necessary equipment available to be able

TABLE 4. *Correlation between Mallampati classification and laryngoscopic grades*

Class	Visibility of pharyngeal structures, No. (%)	Laryngoscopy grade, No. (%)			
		1	2	3	4
1	155 (73.8)	125 (59.5)	30 (14.3)	—	—
2	40 (19)	12 (5.7)	14 (16.7)	10 (4.7)	4 (1.9)
3	15 (7.4)	—	1 (0.5)	9 (4.3)	5 (2.4)

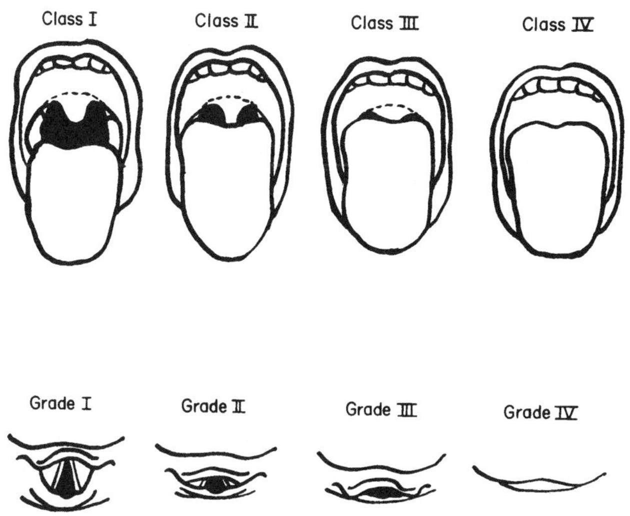

FIG. 5. Correlation between Mallampati pre-assessment and laryngoscopic views (From ref. 12).

to ventilate and oxygenate the patient. There is nothing worse than having a malfunctioning laryngoscope or requiring a bougie that has not been replaced at a critical moment; one cannot overemphasize the importance of thoroughly checking the anesthetic "cockpit" before every procedure. This is particularly relevant in busy operating rooms, where circuits, suckers, and laryngoscopic blades are constantly being replaced between cases.

Before *every* procedure, ensure that you are in an area with ready access to the following:

- A checked and fully functioning anesthetic machine or breathing circuit with the ability to provide adequate oxygen and positive-pressure ventilation (e.g., Ambu or Laerdel bags, a ventilator)
- A range of face masks, endotracheal tubes, oropharyngeal and nasopharyngeal airways
- Two functioning laryngoscopes with appropriate blades
- Intubating stylets and bougies
- Suction (preferably from the wall), with Yankaeur and tracheal suction catheters
- A stethoscope, tape, and scissors
- Emergency airway devices in case of failed intubation/ventilation (e.g., laryngeal masks, Combitubes, transtracheal jet ventilation)
- Anesthetic drugs drawn and clearly labeled
- Routine patient monitors (oxygen saturation, blood pressure, electrocardiogram, end-tidal carbon dioxide)
- A tilting trolley or operating table
- An anesthetic assistant (another doctor, nurse) who is familiar with your requirements

Positioning the Patient

Correct positioning of the patient is vital in order to obtain the best view of the cords. The aim is to bring the oral, pharyngeal, and tracheal axes into alignment with the laryngoscope blade, sweeping the tongue to the left of the mouth and elevating the epiglottis.

Pregnant women with large breasts or morbidly obese patients often produce difficulties when laid flat, either because the chest interferes with the handle of the laryngoscope or because mouth opening and neck extension are limited by compression of the shoulders, chest, and neck structures. Elevating the upper body by placing a wedge of sheets under the back of such patients generally improves the angles and line of vision.

Macintosh (15) originally described the position of the head as being similar to that when sniffing the morning breeze, i.e., with the neck flexed on a pillow and extended at the atlanto-occipital joint. Subsequent work has defined a standard intubating position for research and intubating purposes as 35° of lower neck flexion and 15° of extension of the facial plane.

Inability to extend the head is an important cause of difficult intubations, with the amount of extension limited by the abutment of the occiput against the posterior tubercle of the atlas. It is important that the correct position be adopted before the patient is anesthetized, particularly with rapid-sequence inductions, as this avoids time wasted in trying to reposition the patient if the first attempt at intubation proves difficult.

Types and Choice of Laryngoscopic Blades

The laryngoscope is simply a device used to expose and visualize the larynx and surrounding structures, with the principal purpose of inserting a tube into the trachea. It is a left-handed instrument and consists of a handle containing batteries for the light source connected to a blade, which may be fixed or detachable. If a globe device is used, ensure that the bulb is firmly attached for electrical contact and to prevent the globe from suddenly falling into the pharynx at the crucial moment! Most modern laryngoscopic blades now use fiberoptic technology.

The blade is inserted into the mouth with the tip either directly or indirectly raising the epiglottis. Anatomic variation or disease can produce marked differences in the human airway that can make laryngoscopy difficult, and it is not surprising that more than 50 different designs have evolved over the years to make intubation simpler, each with its own claimed advantage (see Chapter 15). The most significant and beneficial development in recent times has been the refinement and widespread use of the flexible fiberoptic laryngobronchoscope (see Chapter 16).

Despite the large number of blades available, there are three basic types of blades (Fig. 6), namely:

1. Curved (e.g., Macintosh, Polio angled)
2. Straight (e.g., Jackson-Wisconsin, Flagg, Guedel)
3. Straight with curved tip (e.g., Miller)

There is no one blade that suits every situation, and often the choice of blade is an individual preference based on personal experience. In general, straight blades often have the advantage of providing greater exposure of the glottic opening, allowing better visualization of the tube being passed through the cords. Straight blades are generally preferred in neonatal and pediatric intubations, mainly because of an infant's relatively long and floppy epiglottis. In these situations, the blade is passed beyond the epiglottis and larynx into the upper esophagus and then slowly withdrawn, aiming to catch and elevate the epiglottis directly.

The curved blades are said to provide less view, and for this reason a stylet-loaded tube is preferred prior to induction. They range in size from 1 to 4, with a size 3 being used for most adults. The curved blades are generally thought to promote less epiglottitis, soft tissue, and dental trauma and allow more room for the endotracheal tube. Both produce a marked cardiosympathetic response, with severity depending on the relative difficulty of intubation, and thus the duration and pressure required to visualize the cords.

Endotracheal Tubes

Types

There are many types of endotracheal tube (ETT) available, some of which are shown in Figs. 7 and 8. Smooth polyvinyl chloride (PVC) ETTs are now standard and have replaced rubber tubes because of cost and the need for a sterile, disposable, single-use device. Although most ETTs have a curve to assist introduction, anatomically shaped tubes (S-shaped) have been developed that show some promise in reducing the incidence of pressure-related tracheal trauma (16).

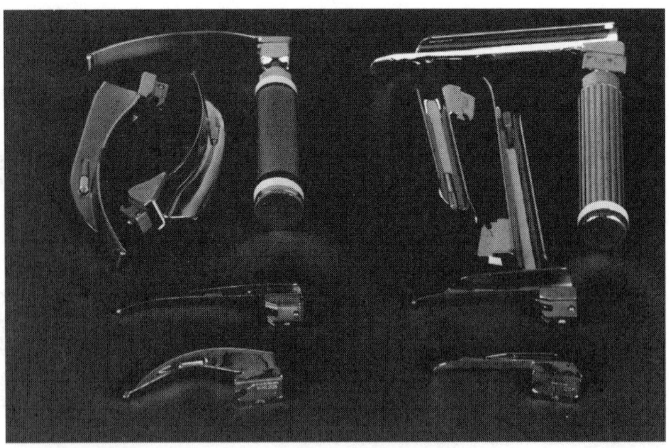

FIG. 6. Different laryngoscopic blades. **Left:** Various curved blades, including Macintosh blades (*top*), which come in several sizes. **Right:** An assortment of straight blades, including Miller blades (*top*).

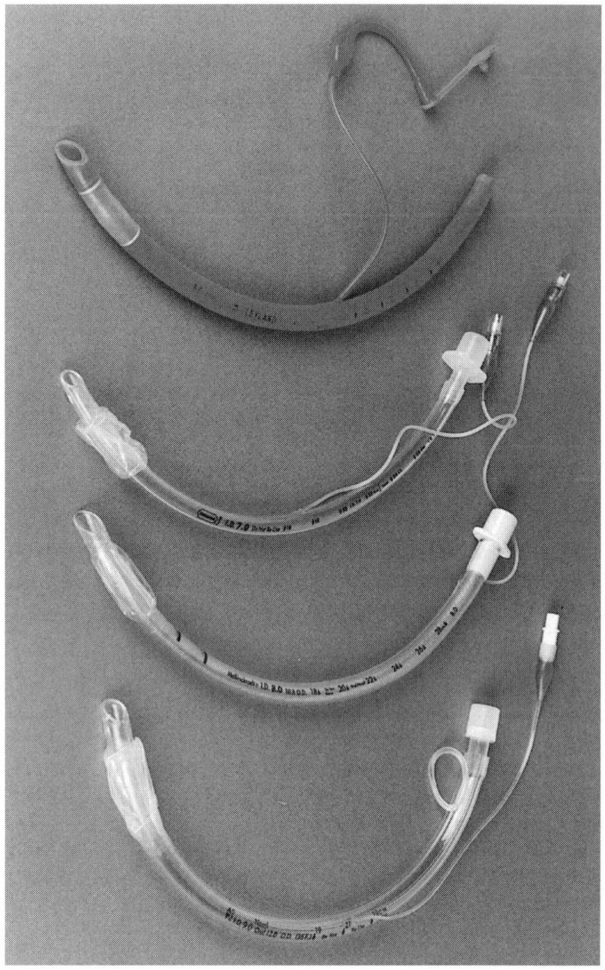

FIG. 7. Endotracheal tubes. **Top to bottom:** Red rubber (Magill), ordinary PVC tube, and reinforced (armored) and Endotrol endotracheal tubes.

The complete range of ETTs is discussed in Chapter 6, but in general tubes can be classified as cuffed or uncuffed and can be used for both oral and nasal intubations. The standard (Magill) ETT (Fig. 9) has a rounded tip, a left-facing bevel when the tube is viewed from the concave surface, and usually a hole opposite the bevel, known as the "Murphy eye" and first described by F.J. Murphy in 1941 (17). The purpose of this hole is to allow gas to flow freely should the bevel become occluded or abut against the tracheal mucosa.

A few other ETTs have particular characteristics that are worthy of mention. The armored (reinforced, compression-resistant) ETTs have a spiral cable (metal wire or fiber filament) incorporated into their wall so that they cannot be compressed or kinked; they are often used in patients who are prone or in whom head movement may cause distortion of the tube (Fig. 7)

The RAE endotracheal tubes (designed by Ring, Adair, and Elwyn) are preformed for either oral or nasal intubations. The oral RAE is used primarily for head, eye, and ear-nose-throat (e.g., tonsillectomy) surgery; the nasal

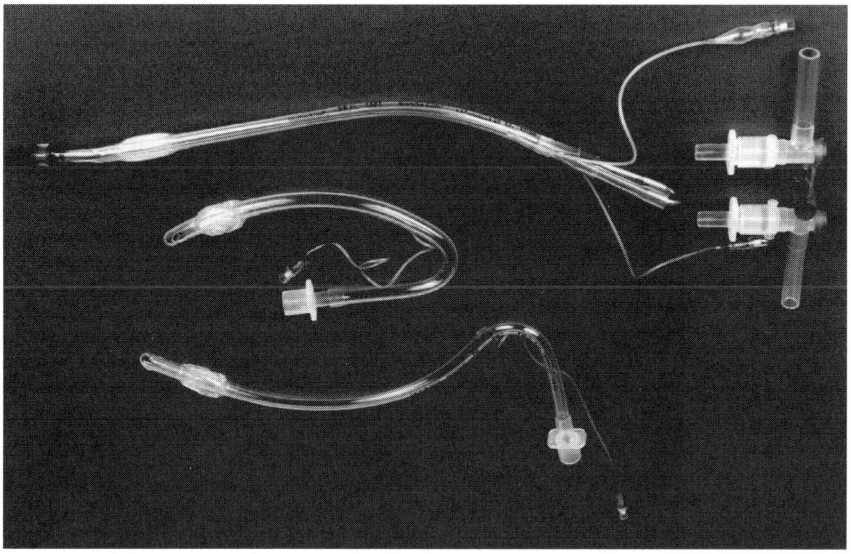

FIG. 8. Endotracheal tubes. **Top to bottom:** Double-lumen, oral RAE (Ring, Adair, and Elwyn), and nasal RAE endotracheal tubes.

RAE (with its curve directed back over the forehead) is used primarily for oral/faciomaxillary surgery (Fig. 8). This ETT was originally designed for pediatric intubations, but it is now also used in adults. Care should be taken to select a correctly sized tube in children (often half a size less than anticipated) in order to avoid endobronchial intubation.

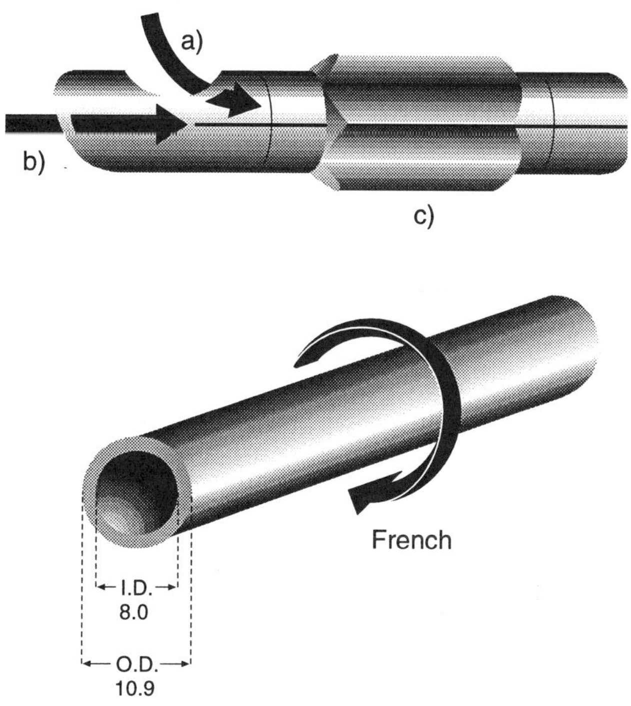

FIG. 9. Diagram of a typical endotracheal tube. Features highlighted include Murphy eye (**a**), left-facing bevel (**b**), and cuff (**c**), which is inflated via a pilot balloon (not shown). The lower diagram indicates the various measurements. *ID*, inner diameter; *OD*, outer diameter; *French*, $\pi \times$ OD).

With the use of lasers in surgery, plastic tubes are unsuitable, as they are incapable of withstanding intense focal heat without igniting. The alternatives are flexible metal tubes (which have a relatively higher incidence of trauma to the airway) or silicon tubes impregnated with metal particles. The cuffs (some have double cuffs) should be filled with sterile saline solution rather than air.

Tube Size and Depth of Insertion

Clinical Significance

Gas flow, resistance, and the work of breathing are primarily dependent on the internal diameter of the ETT. These factors are important in pediatric patients, spontaneously breathing (via ETT) patients, and critically ill patients. Additionally, the length of the ETT and its internal diameter in critically ill patients requiring long-term ventilation impact on dead space and ease of pulmonary toilet. For these reasons, tracheostomies are usually performed on such patients (Chapters 18 and 26).

In general, the critical flow (generally described in liters per minute of fresh gas flow) at which laminar flow becomes turbulent through the ETT has approximately the same numeric value as the internal diameter of the airway (in millimeters). For example, the flow in a size 9.0 ETT becomes turbulent when the flow exceeds 9 L/min (18). The internal diameter can be reduced by external compression or kinking of the tube, or the build-up of secretions within the lumen. Similarly, right-angled connectors, humidifiers, and filters can significantly increase resistance and alter flow characteristics. In spontaneously breathing and pediatric patients, this may prevent adequate ventilation.

In normal anesthetic practice, the length of the ETT in adults has little clinical influence on airway resistance or

TABLE 5. *Average dimensions and insertion distance of endotracheal tubes*

Age	Internal diameter, mm	External diameter, mm	Insertion distance at teeth (at nose), cm
Adult (14 y)	8.0–9.0	10.8–12.1	20–21 (24–25)
10 y	6.5	8.9	17 (21)
6 y	5.5	7.5	15 (19)
4 y	5.0	6.9	14 (17)
1 y	4.0	5.6	11 (14)
3 mo	3.5	4.9	10 (12)
Newborn (3 kg)	3.0	4.9	6 (7.5)

dead space volume. The length of the tube has been made far in excess of the average tracheal length according to age. If the ETT is fully inserted, it will usually pass into the right main bronchus, as this is the larger and straighter of the two bronchi. Subsequent endobronchial intubation is associated with the problems of desaturation, pneumothorax, and left-lobar collapse. Whenever an ETT is inserted, correct depth of insertion must be confirmed.

Calculation of Tube Size and Depth of Insertion

The size of ETTs is classified by their internal diameter and produced in specific lengths according to patient age and size. ETT size is designated as internal tube diameter in millimeters; manufacturers produce ETTs varying usually by increments of 0.5 mm, the most common sizes being between 2.5 and 9.0 mm. "French size" refers to the external circumference in millimeters. This type of sizing is commonly used for double-lumen ETTs. For example, the size of an ETT with an internal diameter of 8.0 mm is roughly 32F. The ETT contains a radio-opaque strip along the side to allow depth and position determination after chest radiograph. The average dimensions and insertion distance are shown in Table 5. There is controversy regarding the use of uncuffed ETTs in children. Some authors advocate uncuffed ETTs in children up to 5 to 6 years and others up to 11, while there are those who use uncuffed ETTs in children up to puberty. Chapter 19 examines these issues more closely.

Most adult women accept a 7.5- to 8.0-mm ETT, and an 8.5-to 9.0-mm ETT is acceptable for adult men. The selection of tube size and depth of insertion are clearly very important for pediatric patients. The following formulas may be applied in children older than 1 year (see also Table 5):

$$\text{ETT Size (internal diameter in mm)} = 4 + \text{age (y)}/4$$

$$\text{ETT Insertion Distance at Lip (cm)} = 12 + \text{age}/2$$

$$\text{ETT Insertion Distance at Nose (cm)} = 15 + \text{age}/2$$

Endotracheal Tube Cuffs

The earliest use of cuffed tubes (Fig. 9) was in 1871 by Trendelenburg. They allow positive-pressure ventilation and positive end expiratory pressure at lower corresponding pressures and flow rates, as well as the prevention of pulmonary contamination from the stomach or upper airway. Cuffs on ETTs also have secondary uses. They help to center the ETT in the trachea so that the tip does not cause trauma to the mucosa. In the study by Van Elstraete et al. (19), the authors demonstrated that an inflated ETT in the oropharynx increases the success rate of blind nasal intubations.

Modern ETT cuffs are generally classified as high-pressure (low-volume) or high-volume (low-pressure). Even though the incidence of sore throat is lower with high-pressure (low-volume) cuffs because of their small area of contact, they are considered dangerous because they require a high internal pressure to obtain a satisfactory seal. Some of this pressure is transmitted to the surrounding mucosa, and even with short exposure it may cause mucosal ischemia and damage, leading to hoarseness or tracheal stenosis (20).

The low-pressure (high-volume) cuffs generally require intraluminal pressures of 15 to 30 mm Hg; these decrease, but do not remove, the incidence of tracheal injury (21). In clinical practice, for intubations of short duration, cuff pressures can be estimated from the feel of the pilot balloon. It should be remembered that with nitrous oxide use and rising temperature, there is gas expansion and increased cuff volume. A similar problem develops in the cuffs of patients who are to undergo aeromedical transfer in craft not pressurized to sea level (e.g., helicopters). These, and patients requiring longer-term intubations, should have their cuff pressures measured accurately and regularly (22). In situations in which the cuff volume is likely to change (e.g., changing ambient pressure, prolonged use of nitrous oxide), it may be useful to inflate the cuff with saline solution rather than air.

Pilot Balloons

The purpose of the pilot balloon is to provide an indication of the state of inflation of the cuff. Its free end is fitted with a self-sealing, inflating valve, and with introduction of air both the cuff and the pilot balloon expand. Ideally, the pressure should be adjusted to approximately 20 to 30 mm Hg to prevent aspiration and still maintain mucosal perfusion. With the use of the McGinnis balloon system (23), end expiratory cuff pressure remains relatively constant at 20 to 25 mm Hg and adjusts automatically for changes in cuff volume and pressure caused by heat and nitrous oxide.

Ancillary Equipment

Stylets and Forceps

A stylet is a semirigid guiding catheter that fits inside the ETT to allow the tube to be bent and held in a desired shape to facilitate insertion. It should always be available when intubations are performed. Because airway trauma may occur with the use of stylets, the tip should never protrude beyond the end of the ETT. Lighted stylets are also available and have met with mixed success.

Of more benefit in difficult situations is the use of a blunt, flexible gum elastic bougie, which can be passed behind the epiglottis into the trachea; the ETT is subsequently "railroaded" into position in a manner similar to the Seldinger technique for venous access.

The Magill forceps is useful for guiding the tip of the ETT between the cords during nasotracheal intubation, as well as for inserting nasogastric tubes and throat packs.

Oropharyngeal/Nasopharyngeal Airways

The oropharyngeal or Guedel airways are useful devices for maintaining a patent airway during hand/mask ventilation, especially in patients without teeth. They are hard plastic devices, and although they prevent the patient from biting and compressing the endotracheal tube or laryngeal mask, they are a major cause of dental trauma.

A nasopharyngeal airway is an alternative that is much softer and better tolerated in the lightly sedated patient but may cause epistaxis. It is important to remember that both devices can elicit laryngeal spasm or a gag reflex if inserted too early in a lightly anesthetized patient.

TECHNIQUE OF INTUBATION

Normal Orotracheal Intubation

The oral route is the easiest, fastest, and most common approach for tracheal intubation. It is the preferred route for emergency intubations in resuscitation and other short-term procedures requiring rapid control and protection of the airway.

Once the patient is correctly positioned with a pillow under the head (Figs. 10A and 11) and routine monitoring applied, the patient is anesthetized after a short period of pre-oxygenation designed to avoid hypoxemia at induction. Once anesthesia has been induced by an intravenous or gas technique, it is recommended that ventilation be assessed with bag and mask before the muscle relaxant is administered.

Sufficient time should pass to enable full effect of the muscle relaxant before laryngoscopy is attempted in order to avoid coughing or laryngospasm. Gentle hand/mask ventilation during this stage maintains adequate oxygenation and anesthesia and prevents hypercapnia ($PaCO_2$ rises approximately 3 mm Hg/min with apnea). Intubation can be achieved without muscle paralysis, but a deeper level of anesthesia is required to obtund the airway reflexes and avoid laryngospasm and coughing. A topical local anesthetic or induction with propofol and alfentanil can be used for this purpose, but these methods may not be completely reliable (24,25).

The head is then extended at the atlanto-occipital joint in the classic sniffing position (Fig. 11), thereby increasing the flexion of the lower cervical spine and aligning the oral, pharyngeal, and tracheal axes. The head is held in this position with the right hand on the vertex of the skull or with the right index finger under the hard palate. The laryngoscope is held in the left hand close to the blade, with the palm helping to protect the lips and reduce leverage on the teeth. The lips are then separated with the fingers and thumb of the right hand and the blade is gently introduced into the right corner of the mouth (Fig. 10B). By sliding the blade over the back and base of the tongue, aiming to the right of the midline, the soft palate, uvula, and tonsillar bed are brought into view (Fig. 10C).

The natural curve of the Macintosh blade sweeps the tongue to the left and out of the way. After reaching the back of the tongue, gently lift the left forearm up and forward keeping the wrist straight (along the axis of the laryngoscope handle). This maneuver pushes the tongue anteriorly into the submandibular space and allows vision of the posterior pharynx and the tip of the epiglottis (a leaflike structure). The key of the technique is to identify the epiglottis (Fig. 10D), not the larynx and vocal cords. (The epiglottis is the signpost of the upper airway, directing you to the larynx.) Once the epiglottis has been identified, continue to slide the blade into the pharynx so that it rests in the vallecula, anteriorly and superiorly to the epiglottis. Repeat the thrust of the left forearm, thus moving the epiglottis upwards and anteriorly; the glottic inlet, pyriform fossae, and cords should come into view (Fig. 10D).

It is extremely important to minimize rotation or leverage motion that may damage the teeth and upper airway. Having identified the vocal cords, insert the ETT under direct vision with your right hand. An assistant may be useful at this stage to stabilize the head and to pull on the corner of the patient's mouth in order to improve the view (Fig. 10E). Pass the ETT into the trachea about 3 to 4 cm so that the cuff just disappears beneath the cords, and note its position adjacent to the upper teeth (or upper alveolar margin), e.g., 22 cm. Hold the ETT steady and gently remove the laryngoscope.

By ventilating the lungs and slowly inflating the pilot tube until the gas leak around the endotracheal tube disappears, overinflation of the cuff is avoided. Secure the endotracheal tube using cotton ribbon ties or tape applied to the maxilla (not the mandible as it is mobile), ensuring that the tube does not move in or out from the desired position recorded at the upper alveolar margin. Finally, ensure bilateral lung inflation by auscultation and confirm correct position of the ETT. The trachea is only 15 cm long in adults, and endobronchial insertion is avoided by placing the tube cuff only 1 to 2 cm beyond the vocal cords. In patients older than 1 year the following formula can be used:

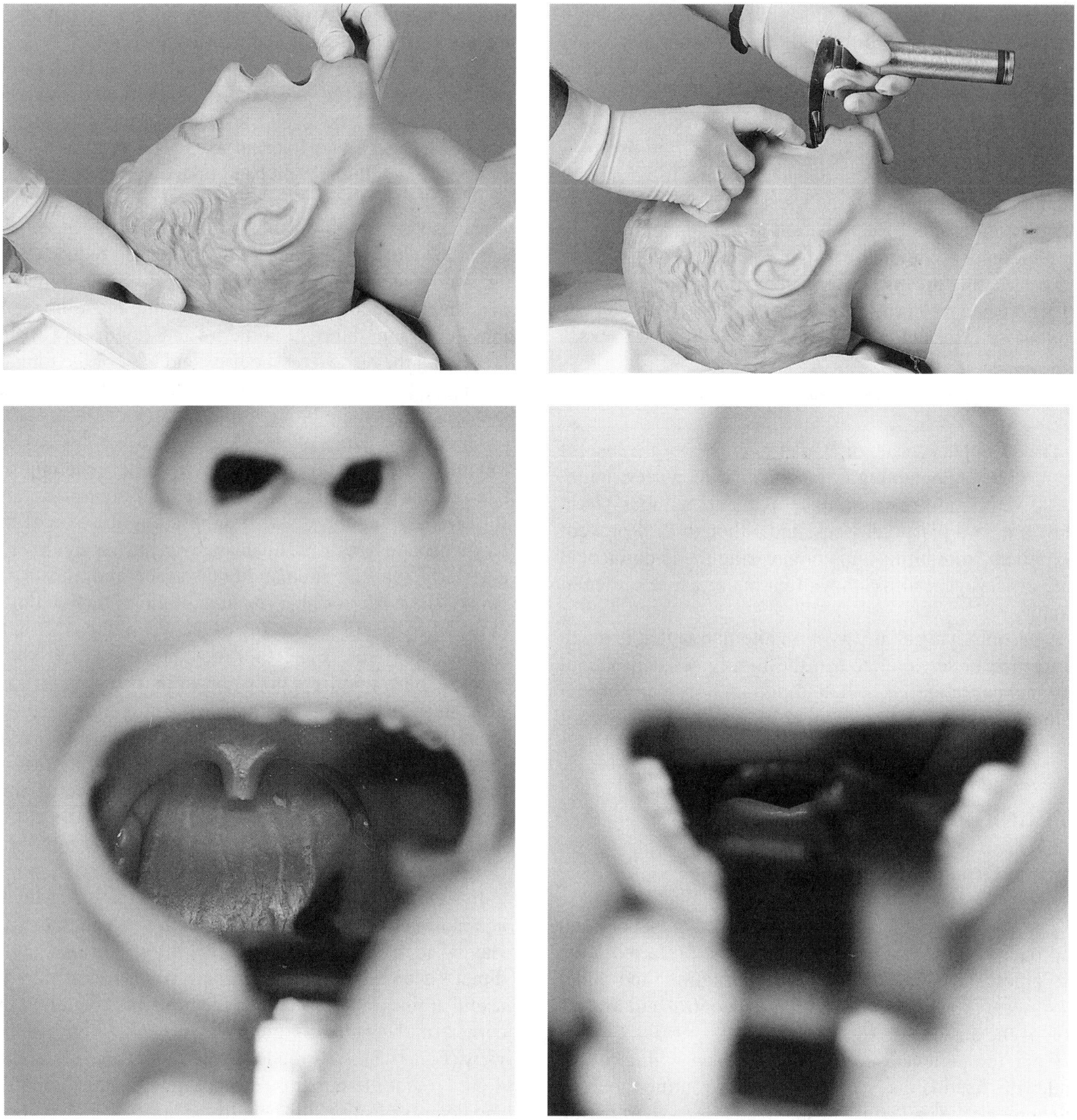

A B C D

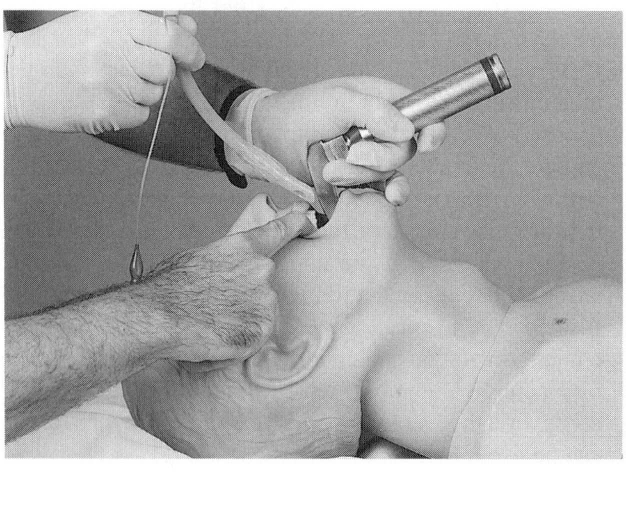

E

FIG. 10. Oral intubation. **A:** The patient's head is positioned on a small pillow with the head extended. **B:** The laryngoscope is introduced into the mouth while the patient's position is maintained. **C:** The laryngoscope is introduced, allowing identification of oral structures (soft palate, uvula, posterior paryngeal wall). **D:** The laryngoscope is advanced until the epiglottis is identified. The laryngoscope is then lifted forward (do not rotate backwards) along the axis of its handle to improve the view. **E:** Cricoid pressure or retraction of the corner of the mouth by an assistant improves the view to allow intubation.

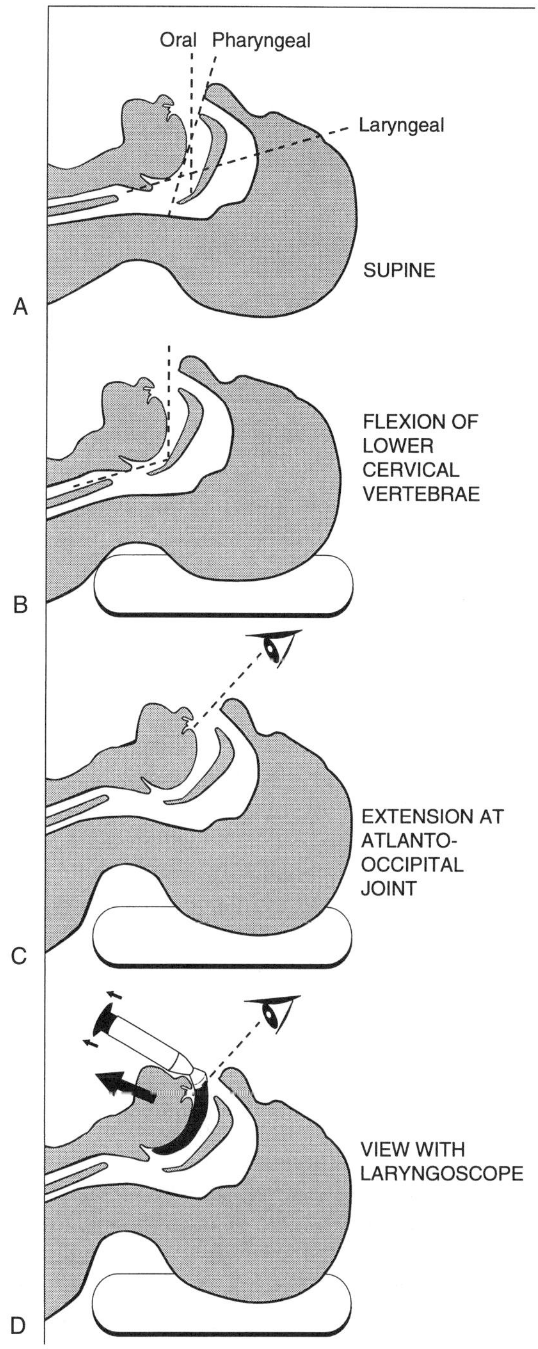

FIG. 11. Correct positioning of the patient is important in optimizing the laryngoscopic view. **A:** Illustration of the various planes. **B:** Simple flexion of the lower cervical spine. **C:** Extension of the head at the atlanto-occipital joint. **D:** Use of the laryngoscope.

Length at the Lips (cm) = 12 + Age (y)/2

Normal Nasotracheal Intubation

This route is less common, more difficult, produces a greater degree of bacteremia, and is associated with a high incidence of epistaxis. It can be performed with the patient awake using topical anesthesia, with the patient under general anesthesia using direct laryngoscopy, or as a blind technique. Table 6 lists the indications for nasotracheal intubations and Table 7 the contraindications.

TABLE 6. *Indications for nasotracheal intubation*

- Certain intra-oral and plastic operations on the head
- Repair of fractured mandible
- Ankylosis of the temporomandibular joint
- Conditions that make laryngoscopy and oral intubations difficult
- Some intubations in the intensive care setting

After assessing which is the largest and most patent nostril (ask the patient if there is any difficulty breathing through one nostril and use the other), the nose should be pretreated with a vasoconstricting agent and well lubricated (e.g., 0.5% phenylephrine, 4% cocaine, 4% lidocaine with phenylephrine). Select an ETT 1 to 1.5 sizes smaller than would be recommended for oral intubation and soften it with sterile hot water. This makes the ETT more flexible and causes less trauma to the nasopharynx.

Once the patient is anesthetized and paralyzed, insert the ETT directly posterior and parallel to the floor of the nose (the hard palate), and gently slide the ETT around the nasopharyngeal bend (Fig. 12A). Under direct laryngoscopic vision, the tube is then passed through the cords by flexing the neck, using cricoid pressure, or using the Magill forceps (Fig. 12B). The ETT should be suctioned before ventilation is performed in order to avoid any blood, tissue, or lubricant being blown into the lungs. As the procedure takes longer to perform than the oral method, it is prudent to administer 100% oxygen first and hyperventilate the patient in order to avoid hypoxemia and hypercapnia.

During the blind nasal technique, the patient remains spontaneously breathing; once the ETT is positioned in the oropharynx, the operator listens over the proximal end while it is steadily advanced towards the glottis or connects an end-tidal carbon dioxide monitor and watches the capnograph. When the breath sounds appear loudest, the tube is quickly advanced during inspiration, with the purpose of sliding it between the cords when they are fully abducted. Flexing the neck helps improve

TABLE 7. *Contraindications for nasotracheal intubation*

- Choanal atresia
- Coagulopathy
- Fractured base of skull (otorrhea, bleeding from ear after trauma)
- Presence of cerebrospinal fluid, rhinorrhea (anterior cranial fossa fracture)
- Severe intranasal disease
- Fractured middle third of face (Le Forte)

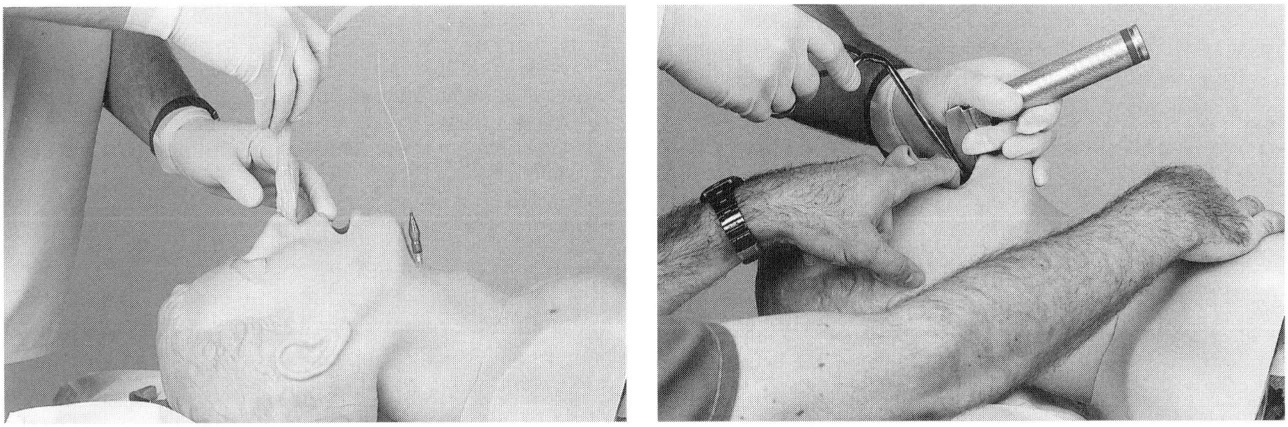

A B

FIG. 12. A: Positioning at the start of a nasotracheal intubation is the same as for orotracheal intubation. Remember that the hard palate (floor of the anterior nasal cavity) goes straight back. **B:** Insertion of the nasal tube through the vocal cords may be assisted by either cricoid pressure, flexion of the head and neck, or by the use of Magill forceps.

the plane of insertion, but often the epiglottis causes persistent obstruction to insertion. An absence of breath sounds indicates either laryngospasm or esophageal intubation. Inflating the cuff of the ETT once it is in the oropharynx increases the success rate of entering the glottic aperture, but remember to deflate the cuff to advance the ETT into the trachea (19).

Once the tube is secured with tape or ribbon ties, the nasotracheal route is more stable and better tolerated than the oral route for longer-term intubations. Nasal secretions are a problem with prolonged intubations when tape is used, as the adhesive properties are quickly removed and the patient is at risk for accidental extubation.

Nasotracheal tubes used in children should be approximately 3 cm longer than the length provided by the formula for orotracheal tube length.

Length at the Nose (cm) = 15 + age (y)/2

Cricoid Pressure

Often the larynx lies anterior to the plane of sight despite good head and neck position; this is most obvious in people with long necks and prominent incisors. Backward pressure on the cricoid and thyroid cartilage during laryngoscopy can often move the posterior commissure into position and turn a grade 4 view into a grade 2 view and enable successful intubation.

Backward pressure on the cricoid cartilage also compresses the esophagus against the sixth cervical vertebra and thus prevents gastroesophageal reflux. This maneuver was originally described by Sellick in 1961 (26), and it is now universally used to assist in preventing regurgitation of stomach contents into the trachea. Having identified the thyroid cartilage and cricothyroid membrane, the thumb and index finger are placed over the cricoid cartilage and directed posteriorly. Studies by Howells et al. (27) showed that a pressure of up to 64 newtons (N) (mean tested was 46.4 N) was required to occlude the esophagus but that in practice there was an unacceptably wide variation in operator performance. In this study, 47% of subjects failed to achieve the value of 44 N.

Cricoid pressure prevents reflux even with high gastric pressures of 94 cm H_2O (17 kPa), and hence it should be sufficient to overcome the 40 to 60 cm-H_2O (7.2 to 10.9 kPa) pressures in pregnant women in the lithotomy position. When correctly used, cricoid pressure should prevent aspiration of gastric contents in most cases or at least reduce reflux.

The timing of application of cricoid pressure is debatable. Correct technique is an uncomfortable experience for the patient, and although some authors advocate application before induction, we believe cricoid pressure should be applied the moment consciousness is lost.

Incorrect application of cricoid pressure can make intubation difficult by moving the larynx laterally, and the need for skilled assistants to provide cricoid pressure is imperative. Excessive pressure over the larynx may also damage the thyroid cartilage and cause airway trauma, and even with correctly applied cricoid pressure, fatal aspiration has been reported (28).

Rapid-Sequence Induction and Intubation

The rapid-sequence induction (inappropriately named "crash induction") is used to secure endotracheal intubation in the shortest possible time in order to reduce the risk of tracheal soiling from either gastrointestinal reflux or from the oropharynx once the protective airway reflexes are lost. Indications would include patients who have not fasted, have full stomachs or symptomatic esophageal reflux, or in whom the risk of reflux is high, such as pregnant women, the morbidly obese, or those with bowel obstruction. Similarly, it can be used in patients with bleeding tonsils or facial trauma to avoid aspiration of blood. Any patient (particularly a child) who has sustained trauma shortly after eating and requires narcotic analgesia should be considered nonfasted even after 24 hours.

As before, after having checked that the anesthetic machine and suction and ancillary equipment are working correctly, the routine monitors are applied and the patient is correctly positioned. An assistant experienced in applying cricoid pressure identifies the anatomic landmarks and applies gentle pressure over the cricoid cartilage (Figs. 10 and 12).

The patient is then pre-oxygenated with 100% oxygen for 3 minutes to optimize PaO_2 and to ensure that a small oxygen reservoir (functional residual capacity) is present in the lungs once apnea has occurred. An intravenous induction agent is administered, and with loss of consciousness cricoid pressure is immediately applied and paralysis produced with 1 to 1.5 mg succinylcholine. The trachea is intubated after fasciculations end and relaxation has occurred, usually after about 40 to 60 seconds. The cuff is inflated and **cricoid pressure maintained until endotracheal intubation has been confirmed**, particularly by observing a normal capnographic waveform. No attempt should be made to ventilate the patient until the trachea has been secured in case the stomach is unintentionally inflated. Because of its speed of action, succinylcholine remains the muscle relaxant of choice for this procedure, despite its side effects, until the latest competitive drug becomes available for general use.

In patients in whom succinylcholine is contraindicated, an alternative is to use a priming dose followed 2 minutes later by 1.5 times the usual intubating dose of a short-acting agent. (e.g., vecuronium 0.01 mg/kg, then 0.15 mg/kg). Unfortunately, some patients may experience muscle weakness with the priming dose and risk loss of airway protection before they are induced and cricoid pressure applied. Rocuronium (0.9–1.2 mg/kg) may also be used.

In the event of a failed intubation, cricoid pressure should be maintained and the failed intubation/ventilation drill performed (see below).

Confirmation of Successful Endotracheal Intubation

Failure to accomplish tracheal intubation is not a disaster, but failure to ventilate or to recognize unintentional esophageal intubation can be fatal. Signs indicating that successful intubation has been accomplished include observing a combination of the following:

- The tube passing through the cords
- A normal capnographic waveform
- The chest expanding and falling with ventilation
- Moist gas escaping from the tube during expiration
- Breath sounds heard when auscultating both lung fields in the midaxillary line/no breath sounds over epigastrium
- Movement of the reservoir bag when the patient inspires
- Identification of tracheal rings with a flexible fiberoptic scope
- Maintenance of blood saturation
- Radiographic evidence

Securing the Endotracheal Tube

Securing the ETT to the patient's face or mouth is one of the most important requirements following intubation. The ideal technique prevents accidental extubation and facial or mouth trauma, and allows the tube to be adjusted or removed easily (29). Most commonly, the tube is fastened by tape that encircles the tube and is then secured to the skin. It is preferable to run the tape over the skin of bony areas, such as the maxilla and the mandible, in order to limit tube movement. Securing the tube in patients with beards or oily, exfoliated, or traumatized skin is particularly difficult. Cotton ribbon ties are preferred in this situation, with a double throw or round turn, which are used to prevent the tube from sliding under the knot. Metal tube holders and small wire frames taped to the forehead are used in some pediatric units, but the ideal technique varies with each case.

FAILED INTUBATION/VENTILATION DRILL

Ideally, the can't intubate/can't ventilate situation should not arise. Whenever possible, patients with known difficult airways who require surgical procedures should have them performed under local or regional anesthesia. When intubation is required, a variety of techniques and other devices (see relevant chapters in Advanced Airway Techniques) may be appropriate. If one is unable to intubate a patient, first ensure that the patient can be easily ventilated by hand before attempting further maneuvers to secure the airway. If ventilation is possible and the surgical procedure is not life-saving, hand ventilate and allow the patient to wake up and demonstrate adequate return of neuromuscular function. If the situation is life-threatening, attempts are made to maintain the airway by any technique possible until the condition has stabilized or been overcome. It is in this last scenario that a failed intubation drill should be initiated. A suggested failed intubation drill is as follows:

1. **Maintain cricoid pressure** if there is a risk of aspiration, e.g., emergency surgery, cesarian section.
2. **Get help.**
3. **Ventilate with 100% oxygen.** Use jaw thrust or Guedel airway to ventilate, or have an assistant ventilate

while you maintain the airway with two hands. Suction the oropharynx as required. If ventilation is successful and intubation is not required, allow the patient to regain spontaneous ventilation. If unable to ventilate or if intubation is required, then proceed to point 4 or 5.

4. **Make two attempts using a bougie (gum elastic, flexible) or intubation stylet.** This should be attempted only if a view of the epiglottis has been obtained and the patient is still oxygenated. Ensure correct head position before attempting further direct laryngoscopy and adjustment of cricoid pressure, as each attempt may cause trauma. If this technique is unsuccessful, proceed to either point 5, 6, or 7.

5. **Insert laryngeal mask or Combitube.** This should be attempted only if the operator is familiar with the use of these devices. Remember that these devices currently do not guarantee protection of the airway, but they do allow ventilation.

6. **Perform percutaneous needle cricothyroidotomy and lung insufflation.** This technique is discussed in Chapter 17. This technique allows oxygenation but not necessarily optimal ventilation. Definitive airway control is still required.

7. **Perform cricothyroidotomy or tracheostomy.** This can be achieved either surgically or by the use of emergency devices designed for such situations. The operator again should be familiar with these devices before using them for urgent airway access.

Different institutions have variations of this basic drill. Remember that the primary goal is to achieve oxygenation of the patient, followed by restoration of gaseous exchange. It is important to become familiar with and practice the various techniques involved in optimizing the airway. Obviously, the worst time to learn about a failed intubation drill is when a failed intubation occurs.

SUMMARY

This chapter has presented an overview of the factors involved with laryngoscopy and normal intubation. Even though the procedure normally requires less than 3 to 4 minutes, the manner in which it is carried out has profound implications for the patient's overall well-being. It is important to become familiar with the equipment and the technique in a controlled environment before attempting it under emergency conditions.

REFERENCES

1. Brossy MJ, James MF, Janicki PK. Haemodynamic and catecholamine changes after induction of anesthesia with either thiopentone or propofol with suxamethonium. *Br J Anaesth* 1994;72:596–598.
2. Millard Forbes A, Dally FG. Acute hypertension during induction of anesthesia and endotracheal intubation in normotensive man. *Br J Anaesth* 1970;42:618–624.
3. Stoelting RK. Endotracheal intubation. In: Miller RD, ed. *Anesthesia*, 2nd ed. New York: Churchill Livingstone; 1986:523–552.
4. Thomson IR. The haemodynamic response to intubation: a perspective [editorial]. *Can J Anaesth* 1989;36:367–369.
5. Fusciardi J, Godet G, Bernard JM, et al. Roles of fentanyl and nitroglycerine in the prevention of myocardial ischaemia associated with laryngoscopy and tracheal intubation in patients undergoing operations of short duration. *Anesth Analg* 1986;65:617–624.
6. Cork RC, Weiss JL, Hameroff SR, Bentley J. Fentanyl preloading for rapid-sequence induction of anesthesia. *Anesth Analg* 1984;63:60–64.
7. Chung KS, Sinatra RS, Halevy JD, Paige D, Silverman DG. A comparison of fentanyl, esmolol, and their combination for blunting the haemodynamic responses during rapid-sequence induction [see comments]. *Can J Anaesth* 1992;39:774–779.
8. Miller DR, Martineau RJ, Wynands JE, Hill J. Bolus administration of esmolol for controlling the haemodynamic response to tracheal intubation: the Canadian multicentre trial. *Can J Anaesth* 1991;38: 849–858.
9. Kung MC, Hung CT, Ng KP, Au TK, Lo R, Lam A. Arterial desaturation during induction in healthy aduts: should pre-oxygenation be a routine? *Anaesth Intensive Care* 1991;19:192–196.
10. Norris MC, Dewan DM. Preoxygenation for caesarian section: a comparison of two techniques. *Anesthesiology* 1985;62:827–829.
11. Thorpe CM, Gauntlett IS. Arterial oxygen saturation during induction of anesthesia. *Anesthesia* 1990;45:1012–1015.
12. Samsoon GLT, Young JRB. Difficult tracheal intubation: a retrospective study. *Anesthesia* 1987:42;487–490.
13. Mallampati SR. Clinical sign to predict difficult tracheal intubation (hypthosis). *Can Anaesth Soc J* 1983;30:316.
14. Mallampati SR, Gatt SP, Gugino LD, et al. A clinical sign to predict difficult tracheal intubation: a prospective study. *Can Anaesth Soc J* 1985;32:429.
15. Macintosh RR. A new laryngoscope. *Lancet* 1943:1:205.
16. Alexopoulous C, Larsson SG, Lindholm CE. The conformity of an anatomically shaped endotracheal tube to the shape of the airway. *Acta Anaesthesiol Scand* 1983;27:235.
17. Murphy FJ. Two improved intratracheal catheters. *Anesth Analg* 20: 102–104 1941.
18. Parbrook GD, Davis PD, Parbrook EO. Fluid flow. *Basic Physics and Measurement*, 3rd ed. Oxford: Butterworth-Heinemann; 1990:14–28.
19. Van Elstraete AC, Pennant JH, Gajraj NM, Victory RA. Tracheal tube cuff inflation as an aid to blind nasotracheal intubation. *Br J Anaesth* 1993;70:691–693.
20. Loeser EA, Hodges M, Gliedman J, Stanley TH, Johansen RK, Yonetani D. Tracheal pathology following short-term intubation with low- and high-pressure endotracheal tube cuffs. *Anesth Analg* 1978;57: 577–579.
21. Cooper JD, Grillo HC. Analysis of problems related to cuffs on endotracheal tubes. *Chest* 1972;62:21–27.
22. Lewis FR, Schlobohm RM, Thomas AN. Prevention of complications from prolonged tracheal intubation. *Am J Surg* 1979;135:452–457.
23. McGinnis GE, Shively JG, Patterson RL, Magovern GJ. An engineering analysis of of intratracheal tube cuffs. *Anesth Analg* 1971;50: 557–564.
24. Beck GN, Masterson GR, Richards J, Bunting P. Comparison of intubation following propofol and alfentanil with intubation following thiopentone and suxamethonium. *Anaesthesia* 1993;48:876–880.
25. Scheller MS, Zornow, MH, Saidman LJ. Tracheal intubation without the use of muscle relaxants: a technique using propofol and varying doses of alfentanil. *Anesth Analg* 1992;75:788–793.
26. Sellick RA, Cricoid pressure to control regurgitation of stomach contents during induction of anesthesia: preliminary communication. *Lancet* 1961;2:404–406.
27. Howells TH, Chamney AR, Wraight WJ, Simons RS. The application of cricoid pressure: an assessment and a survey of its practice. *Anaesthesia* 1983;38:457–460.
28. Whittington RM, Robinson JS, Thompson JM. Fatal aspiration (Mendelson's syndrome) despite antacids and cricoid pressure. *Lancet* 1979;ii:228.
29. Madden AP. A knot for anesthesia. *Anaesthesia* 1992;47:822–823.

Airway Management, edited by
L.H. Hanowell, M.D. and R.J. Waldron, M.D.,
Lippincott-Raven Publishers, Philadelphia © 1996.

CHAPTER 6

Intubating Equipment

David A. White

INTRODUCTION

In any endeavor, using the proper tools often determines the success of one's efforts. When the goal of a physician's efforts, such as securing an airway, potentially affects whether a patient lives or dies, then the physician has no choice but to have the proper equipment and know how to use it. This chapter reviews the intubation equipment commonly used today. It describes what equipment is available, and what equipment should be used based on patient age and size and planned route of intubation.

Intubating equipment can be grouped into several categories, according to function. These include the following:

1. Equipment to maintain oxygenation and ventilation during the process of intubation
2. Equipment to provide access to the glottic opening in order to achieve intubation and placement of endotracheal tubes
3. Equipment that aids continued ventilation and oxygenation when intubation fails

The various categories of intubation equipment are reviewed here in approximately the order set forth above. Table 1 is a complete listing of the equipment that should be available for routine intubation. Success and safety necessitate immediate availability of proper equipment for all common contingencies.

D. A. White: Department of Anesthesiology, University of California, Davis School of Medicine and Medical Center, Sacramento, California 95817.

VENTILATION EQUIPMENT

During the process of intubation, it is vital to maintain oxygenation and ventilation. An individual maintaining spontaneous ventilation during the course of intubation requires only oxygenation and a patent airway. Appropriate equipment for delivering oxygen includes a fitted mask (Fig. 1), nasal oxygen tubing, or "blow-by" oxygen delivered in proximity to the mouth or nose by appropriate tubing. A pressurized oxygen source is also needed. A patent airway can be obtained through anterior displacement of the jaw by the care provider, a plastic airway placed within the oropharynx (Fig. 2), or a nasal airway placed via the nares into the posterior pharynx; each method lifts the tongue, thereby opening the airway. Placement of an oral or nasal airway is not well tolerated in the awake patient without topical anesthesia.

When the patient is not spontaneously ventilating during intubation, equipment must be at hand to provide ventilation. This equipment must include a tight-fitting mask and a manual resuscitator of the self-expanding type in order to assure ventilation when no external power source is available (Fig. 1). Ventilation systems that depend on external power sources, such as compressed gases or electromechanical devices, are also appropriate. The manual resuscitator is an open system using non-rebreathing valves suitable for short-term

TABLE 1. *Equipment that should be available for safe, routine endotracheal intubation*

All intubations
- 1. Ventilation equipment
  - Manual resuscitator, self-expanding
  - Tight-fitting mask
  - Oral airways
  - Oxygen source
- 2. Suction equipment
  - Tubing of adequate length, Yankauer-type suction tool, suction catheters
- 3. Miscellaneous
  - Syringe to inflate cuff
  - Tape or tie for securing endotracheal tube

Oral intubation
- 4. Blades
  - Macintosh (curved)
  - Miller (straight)
- 5. Handles, two available
- 6. Endotracheal tubes, size range appropriate for patient
- 7. Stylet for endotracheal tube

Nasal intubation: as above, plus
- 8. Topical anesthetics
  - Lidocaine 2% or 4% topical, benzocaine, or cocaine
- 9. Topical vasoconstrictors
  - Phenylephrine, cocaine

Optional
- 10. Gum elastic bougie or oxygenating tube changer
- 11. Laryngeal mask airway, appropriate sizes
- 12. Equipment for emergency cricothyroidotomy
  - Appropriate catheters, syringe to aspirate air and check for position in trachea; jet ventilation equipment

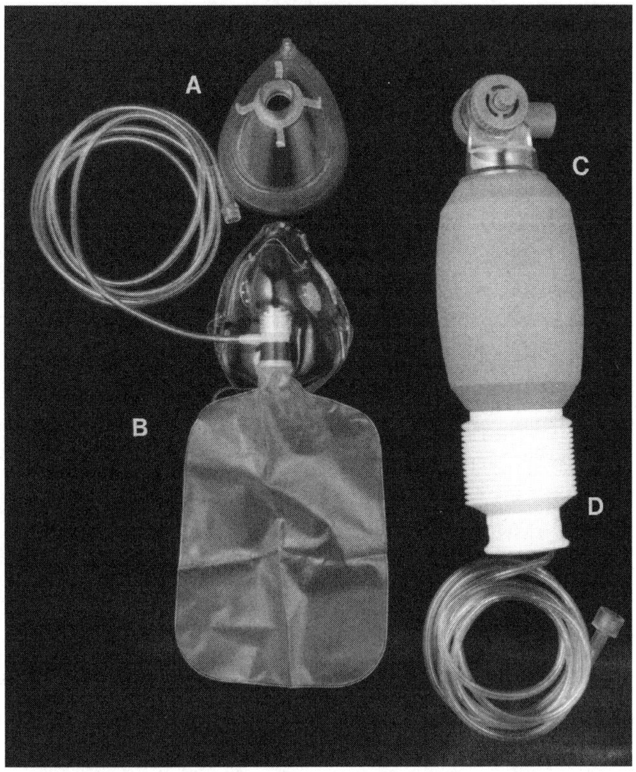

FIG. 1. Ventilation equipment. Fitted disposable mask (**A**). Non-rebreather mask for increased inspired O_2 in spontaneously ventilating patient (**B**). Pediatric-size self-expanding manual resuscitator (**C**). Oxygen reservoir of manual resuscitator (**D**).

ventilation. When fitted with oxygen reservoir systems, they are capable of providing 100% inspired oxygen. The oxygen reservoir of the manual resuscitator is seen in Fig. 1 as the large corrugated tube below the self-expanding bag. When the reservoir is extended, oxygen is stored in readiness for inflation of the bag during the next respiratory cycle, ensuring that oxygen enters the resuscitation bag undiluted by room air. Other manual ventilation systems may use a thin plastic bag as the reservoir for the oxygen. To provide 100% oxygen, the reservoir bag must have a volume greater than the resuscitator volume, with oxygen flow rates greater than the minute ventilation of the patient. Basic ventilation equipment is critical to providing a safe intubation environment.

INTUBATION EQUIPMENT

The major types of intubation equipment are subdivided according to their component parts. Equipment design may be categorized as conventional or specialized.

Laryngoscopes

Laryngoscopes, the primary tool for airway visualization, have evolved little over the last 30 or more years (1). Simplicity and sturdiness are their hallmark. Figure 3 shows examples of conventional adult and pediatric laryngoscope handle and blade assemblies.

Handles

Conventional Handle Designs

Laryngoscope handles are predominantly made of a corrosion-proof metal, sealed against leakage of water. Like most frequently used equipment that must be reliable, they have been kept simple and maintenance-free. Handles are manufactured in two sizes, adult and pediatric, although there are variations based on battery size. They most commonly use non-rechargeable dry cell batteries, because of the dry cell's greater energy storage and minimal need for maintenance. Handle-blade combinations may be either of standard construction,

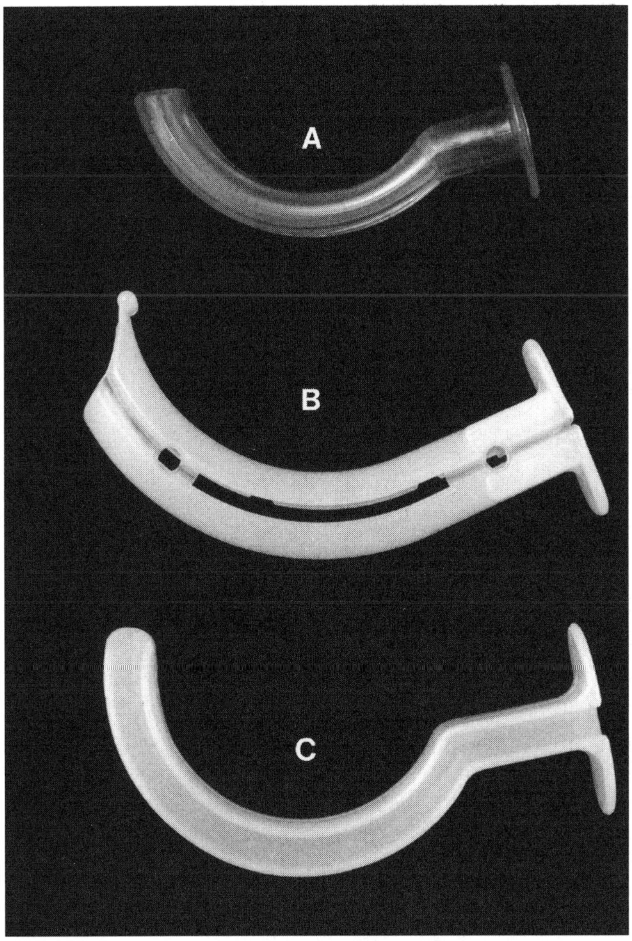

FIG. 2. Oral airways of three types. Guedel airway (**A**). Split "fiberoptic intubating" airway (**B**). Berman airway (**C**).

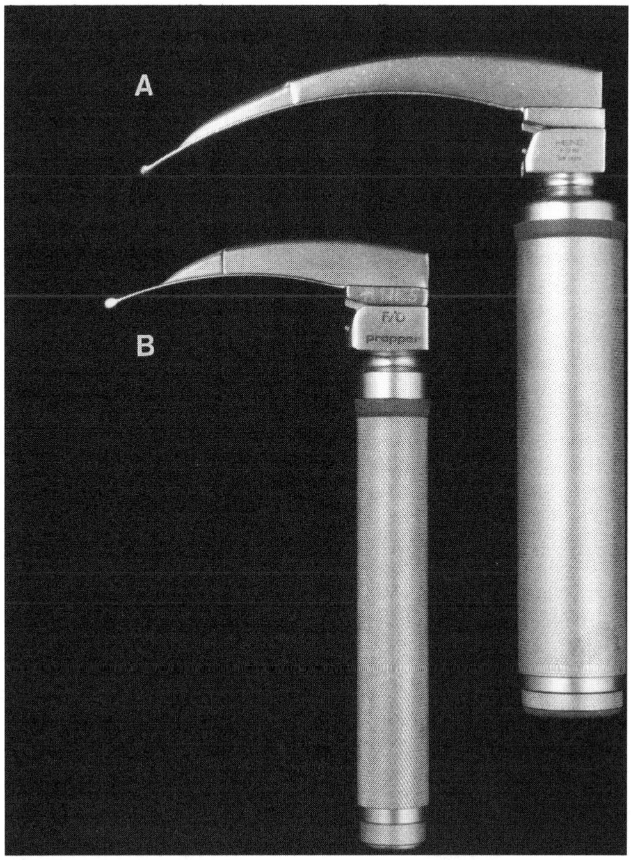

FIG. 3. Conventional laryngoscopes in adult **(A)** and pediatric **(B)** sizes.

with the blades containing the bulb near their tip, or fiberoptic, with the bulb remotely placed on the handle and the light transmitted to the blade tip via fiberoptics. The fiberoptic bundle encased within the blade transmits the light from the handle to the tip of the blade, obviating the need to have the bulb on the blade itself. The fiberoptic bundles incorporated within the laryngoscope blades are relatively inexpensive, since they do not need to be flexible or transmit an image. They are, however, susceptible to fiber fracture from repeated shocks, such as being dropped on hard surfaces. This design increases the reliability of the light source, since corrosion of the contact between the bulb and the socket acquired during frequent immersion for cleaning is eliminated. Cleaning has been further improved by eliminating the cracks and crevices present where the light bulb attaches to the blade.

Specialty Handle Designs

In an attempt to provide a bright, reliable light source, laryngoscope handles have been designed that have a remote light source. A long, flexible fiberoptic bundle transmits high-intensity light from a remote light source to the laryngoscope blade, which then conducts the light via an incorporated fiberoptic bundle. The remote light source gives the advantage of bright, cool, and presumably low-maintenance light. The disadvantages are its lack of mobility, expense, and the presence of another cable, which can become tangled with intravenous lines. This remote light source is not commonly used in the operating room environment.

Certain clinical situations make placement of the laryngoscope blade into the oropharynx difficult. This occurs in obese or parturient patients with short necks; in such cases, the patient's chest blocks the caudad rotation of the handle necessary for the proper placement of the blade into the oral opening. Modification of the laryngoscope handle to increase the angle between blade and handle (Fig. 4) can obviate this problem. A modified handle or a snap-on bracket placed on the handle that accepts a standard blade can be used. Although effective, modified handles are not commonly used. In most cases, the obstruction to intubation is no more than a nuisance and can be circumvented by experimenting with rotating the handle

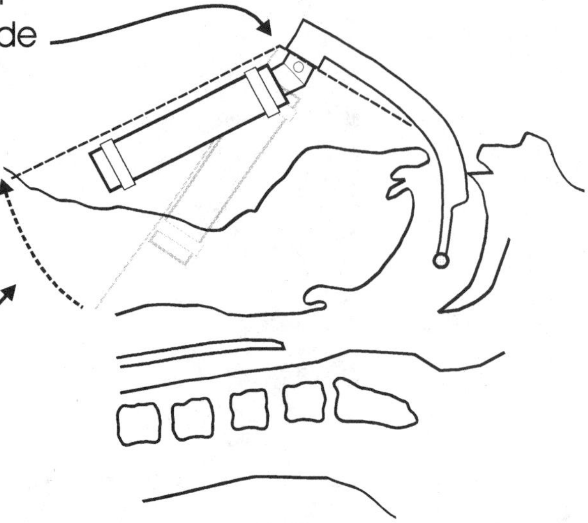

FIG. 4. Modification of laryngoscope to increase the angle between the handle and blade. This prevents interference by the chest when the blade is advanced into the oropharynx.

to the side, or removing the blade from the handle, and replacing it after the blade is placed into the mouth.

Blades

Conventional Blade Designs

Laryngoscope blades have been designed and redesigned over the years. The blades are configured to obtain the best view of the glottic opening with the least potential damage to the airway and associated structures. As expected, no single blade size or shape can attain these goals in all people. In recent years, several studies have been undertaken to evaluate the anatomic factors and associated blade shapes that may aid in visualization of the glottic opening (2,3). Despite this research, there does not appear to be an optimal design. Current supply catalogs show more than 12 different laryngoscope blade shapes, each of which may suit an individual's training and bias rather than provide clear scientific advantages. Despite the supply of various blades, few blades besides the Miller and Macintosh are in common

TABLE 2. *Commonly used laryngoscopic blades*

			Blade manufacturer, length (mm)[a]		
Blade type	Size	Age group	American Profile	Welsh-Allen	Sun-Lite
Macintosh	0	Neonate	80	—	—
	1	1–3 y	87	63	92
	2	3–6 y	108	82	108
	3	Adult	130	101	124
	4	Adult	158	135	158
Miller	0	Neonate	75	53	75
	1	1–3 y	102	79	102
	2	3–6 y	155	132	155
	3	Adult	195	172	195
	4	Adult	205	182	205

[a]From distributor information.

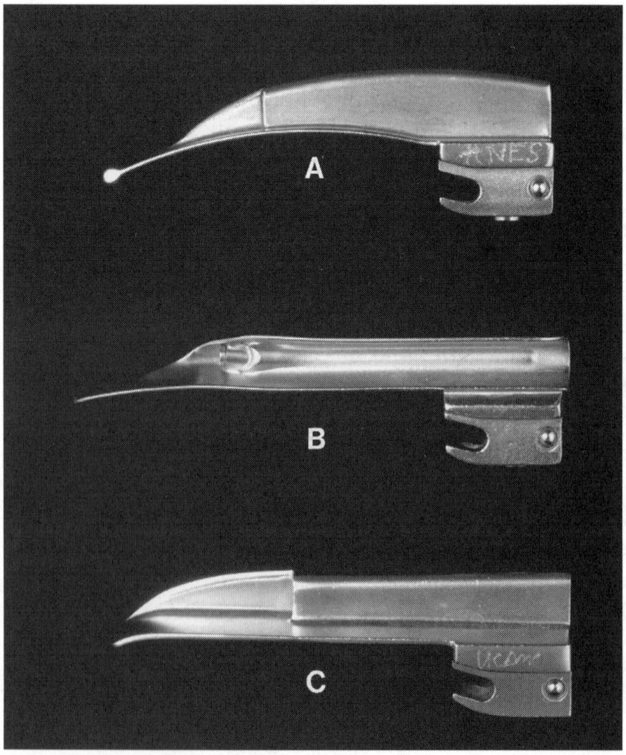

FIG. 5. Three laryngoscope blades. Curved Macintosh blade (**A**). Straight Miller (**B**) and Heine (**C**) blades.

use. Table 2 shows the sizes, appropriate age groups, and lengths available for the Miller and Macintosh blades. Note the nonstandardization of blade length with designated size. A blade designation does not necessarily mean it has the same "feel" across manufacturers. Three different blade configurations, both curved and straight, can be seen in Fig. 5.

Specialty Blade Designs

As intubation aids such as fiberoptic laryngoscopes and specialty equipment such as the Bullard scope become more readily available, the need for specialized laryngoscope blades has diminished. Alternative blade designs have included the incorporation of an oxygen delivery port into the blade to conduct oxygen toward the glottic opening. Prisms or mirrors have been placed midway down a curved blade to allow for indirect visualization of the glottic opening. These blades may allow for visualization, but the subsequent maneuvering of the tube into the larynx may not be improved with indirect visualization. Discussion of intubation equipment beyond the traditional laryngoscope is found in subsequent chapters.

Proper Use of the Laryngoscope Blade

In order to visualize the glottic opening, the laryngosope blade must be placed correctly and forces generated against the proper anatomic structures. The laryngoscope blade must be able to raise the epiglottis, either directly or indirectly, by upward movement of the hyoid bone to allow a direct line of view toward the glottic opening (3). The Miller blade, although commonly considered straight, has a curved tip, and it is perhaps the most commonly used of the straight blades. Straight blades are designed for the blade tip to be placed underneath the epiglottis, allowing direct upward displacement of the epiglottis and adjoining tissues (Fig. 6). Curved blades, such as the Macintosh, are designed for the blade tip to be placed in the vallecula, behind the epiglottis, to obtain optimal visualization (Fig. 7). Proper visualization requires displacement and compression of tissues of the tongue and supraglottic tissues to provide an unobstructed line of sight. The inability to compress or displace the soft tissues adequately interferes with proper blade tip placement and displacement of the tissues. This occurs with an anterior larynx, large tongue (each requiring greater tissue displacement), or receding chin (no place to move the tissues), or when redundant tissues block proper viewing. This may necessitate changing to a straight blade from a curved blade or vice versa to improve visualization, depending on individual anatomy. As is apparent in the figures, the hyoid bone is situated just beyond the anterior wall of the vallecula, providing a firm structure to transmit the forces from the tip of the blade into proper movement of the supraglottic structures and larynx for optimal visualization. Placement of the blade tip adjacent to the hyoid bone (above or below the epiglottis) is critical to proper movement and visualization of the supraglottic tissues.

The best blade for any individual patient is difficult to determine prior to laryngoscopy; therefore, the safest approach to a successful intubation is to have a selection of blades available, including straight and curved blades

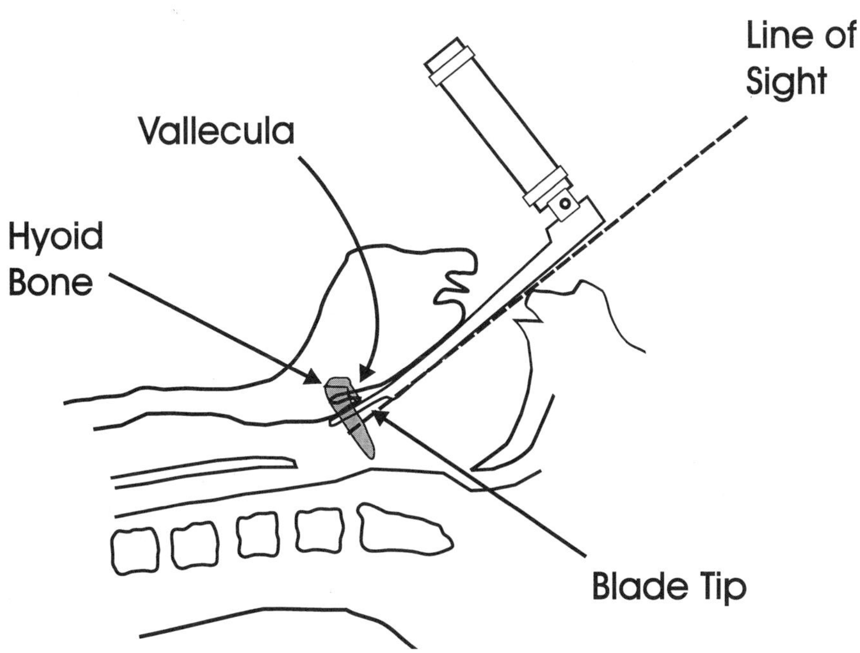

FIG. 6. Proper placement of the Miller (straight) blade under the epiglottis forces the glottic opening and larynx anteriorly. The hyoid bone is shown in relation to the blade tip.

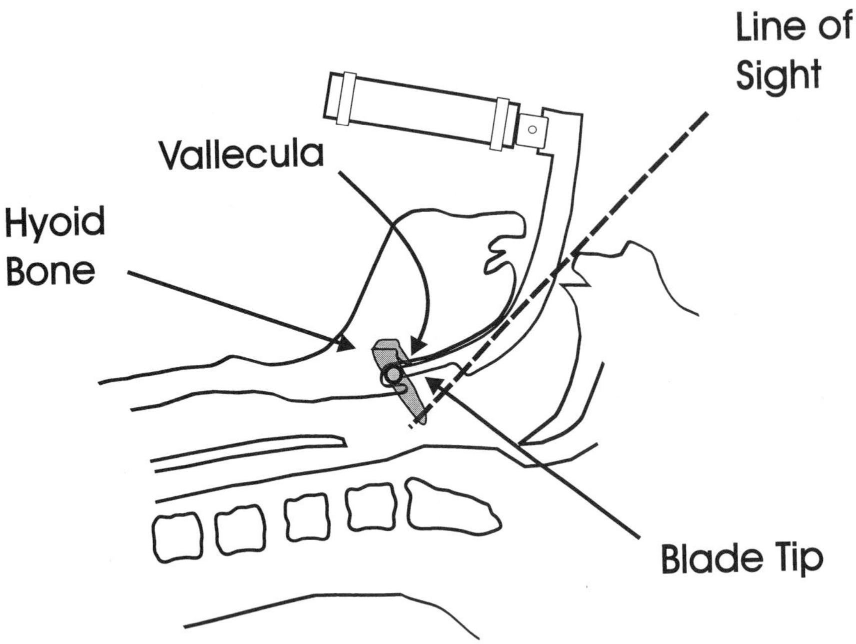

FIG. 7. Proper placement of the Macintosh blade into the vallecula forces the glottic opening and larynx anteriorly. The hyoid bone is shown in relation to the blade tip.

and multiple sizes of each type. Although visualization of the glottic opening is the primary aim of laryngoscopy, this does not guarantee intubation. Often, because of the shape of the laryngoscope blade and oral dimensions, the endotracheal tube cannot be maneuvered toward the glottic opening, which then necessitates a change in laryngoscope blade or alternative intubation technique.

Endotracheal Tubes

Endotracheal tubes have benefitted from the progress in materials technology over the years. With the need for flexibility, early endotracheal tubes were limited to available rubber compounds. Although useful, they were stiff, susceptible to kinking, and expensive, therefore not readily disposable. In addition to being flexible and resistant to kinking, endotracheal tubes must be nonirritating to tissues. With the development of modern plastics, the modern, inexpensive endotracheal tube with these desirable characteristics has evolved. With the availability of special materials and manufacturing techniques, specialty designs have been developed to allow greater flexibility without kinking. Newer tubes also have the advantage of relatively thin walls to improve patient safety and comfort.

Polyvinyl chloride (PVC) plastic is the most common material used for endotracheal tube construction because it has most of these properties. PVC plastic has been extensively tested and meets the Z-79 standards (4). The standard endotracheal tube is formed in a gentle curve, to mimic that of the bend from the oral or nasal pharynx into the glottic opening. In addition to conforming to the shape of the airway, the primary purpose of this gentle curve is to aid in placing the endotracheal tube tip near the glottic opening during intubation. The distal end of the tube may have one or two elongated holes, referred to as the "Murphy eye," to allow ventilation of both main bronchi when the tube is partially within a main bronchus. Small pediatric tubes (less than size 6.0) do not have a Murphy eye, as the small hole size leads to obstruction by secretions.

The endotracheal tube cuffs are designed to seal the tube against leaks during positive-pressure ventilation, with the additional advantage of preventing soiling of the airway from secretions entering the trachea from above the cuff.

Endotracheal tubes are supplied with inside diameters ranging from 2.0 mm to 10 mm, with 0.5-mm increments between tube sizes. It is important to realize that the reported sizes of endotracheal tubes are based on the internal diameter. The outer diameter, which is the dimension that determines whether a tube properly fits the glottic opening, larynx, and trachea, is determined by adding wall thickness of the endotracheal tube to its internal diameter. The wall thickness is optimized based on the needed tube rigidity and tube material. As the endotracheal tube becomes smaller, the wall thickness accounts for a greater portion of the outer diameter for a given inner diameter. As a result, there can be a small variation in necessary tube size (internal diameter) based on the tube's design or construction material for any given patient size. Because of the variation in body size with age and the poor predictors of appropriate tube size according to age, a selection of sizes should be available (Table 3).

Deciding what is the appropriate endotracheal tube for a patient requires taking a number of considerations into account, including patient age and size and surgical pro-

TABLE 3. *Endotracheal tube sizes*

Age	Size (ID), mm	Overall length, cm[a]	Placement depth, cm[b]	Extra-oral distance, cm
Premature	2.5[c]	12	10	2
Neonate	3.0[c]	14	10	4
1–6 mo	3.5[c]	16	10–11	5
6–12 mo	4.0[c]	18	12	6
2 y	4.5[c]	20	13	7
4 y	5.0[c]	22	14	8
6 y	5.5[c]	25	15	10
8 y	6.0[c]	26	16	10
10 y	6.5	26	17	9
12 y	7.0	28	18	10
Adult	7.5	29	18–24	4
Adult	8.0	30	18–24	6
Adult	8.5	31	18–24	7
Adult	9.0	32	18–24	8
Adult	9.5	32	18–24	8
Adult	10.0	32	18–24	8

[a]Length indicated on tube.
[b]Based on mean distance to carina.
[c]Uncuffed tubes.

cedure. All these factors are important to determine the proper endotracheal tube selection. Several guides to selection based on age have been employed. The following formula is commonly used for pediatric patients:

$$\text{Internal Diameter} = (\text{Age} - 16)/4$$

For adults, a size 8.0 for men and 7.5 for women is appropriate for the "average" person. Beyond age and size, the urgency of intubation, airway anatomy, the patient's medical condition, and planned duration of intubation should be considered when selecting the endotracheal tube size. As a general rule, the largest endotracheal tube should be chosen that can be passed through the glottic opening without applying excessive pressure on the airway structures. This minimizes resistance to airflow; it also permits better access to the airway, whether for suctioning secretions or for performing fiberoptic bronchoscopy for diagnostic or therapeutic intervention. However, for emergent intubation, a smaller endotracheal tube provides the advantage of easier placement through the glottic opening during a difficult intubation. This is especially true in the situation in which the glottic opening is obstructed or edematous. When prolonged intubation may be necessary, a low-pressure cuff is optimal to minimize tissue trauma. When high ventilation pressures are anticipated, a high-pressure cuff may be necessary.

Pediatric patients below the age of 8 years are generally intubated with uncuffed endotracheal tubes. The subglottic region of the airway is the narrowest point of the airway and is limited from expanding by the circumferential cricoid cartilage. Therefore, an overly large tube causes pressure on the airway mucosa, leading to ischemic damage and potential postoperative consequences. The lack of a cuff allows for evaluation of a gas leak around the tube, ensuring that there is no circumferential pressure on the tracheal mucosa. Additionally, the relatively increased outside diameter compared to the inner diameter in the smaller endotracheal tubes makes it advantageous to avoid the additional tube diameter incurred by a cuff, allowing for passage of the tube with the largest possible internal diameter in small children and infants.

Specialty Endotracheal Tubes

Preformed Endotracheal Tubes

Although the standard endotracheal tube is designed for both oral and nasal intubations, there are occasions when an endotracheal tube of a different shape is beneficial. Tube manufacturers have developed "preformed" tubes for nasal and oral intubation. These tubes have a fixed curvature that allows the tube connector to be placed away from the surgical field (Fig. 8). They are helpful during surgery of the head and neck, when alternative placement of the endotracheal connection aids in

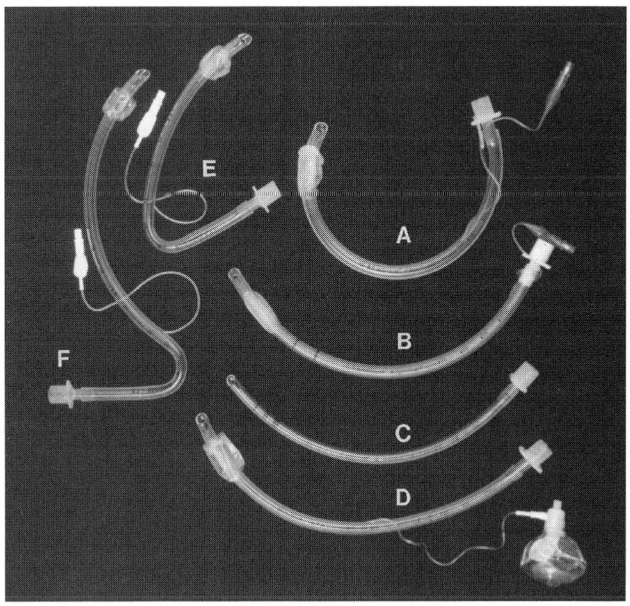

FIG. 8. Six endotracheal tubes are pictured. The four stacked endotracheal tubes include a "pull-tube" with pull ring to increase tube curvature (**A**). Note its marked curve created by a pull ring at proximal end of the tube. The reinforced endotracheal tube (**B**) is strengthened against kinking by a wire embedded within the wall of the tube. An uncuffed endotracheal tube (**C**) is commonly used in pediatric cases. A low-pressure endotracheal tube (**D**) is cuffed. The preformed endotracheal tubes are for oral intubation (**E**) and nasal intubation (**F**).

TABLE 4. *Preformed endotracheal tubes*

Tube size	Oral tube, length at lip (cm)	Nasal tube, length at nares (cm)
3.0	10.5	—
3.5	12	—
4.0	13	—
4.5	15	—
5.0	16.5	—
5.5	17	—
6.0	18	26
6.5	19	27
7.0	20	28
7.5	21	29
8.0	22	30
8.5	23	—
9.0	24	—

TABLE 5. *Length of the airway*

	Eagle (5)		Schellinger (6)	
Distance measured, cm	Female	Male	Female	Male
(1) Mean length from nose to vocal cords	18	20	—	—
(2) Mean length from teeth to vocal cords	12	13	—	—
(3) Mean distance from vocal cords to carina	12	13	—	—
(4) Distance from nose to carina	30[a]	33[a]	28	32
(5) Distance from teeth to carina	24[a]	26[a]	25	28

[a]Distance calculated from (1) or (2) plus (3).

access to the surgical site. As a result of the fixed curvature with preformed endotracheal tubes, the distance at which the tube tip is positioned above the carina depends on the distance from the preformed bend to the tube tip, which subsequently depends on the tube size selected (Table 4). Table 5 is a compilation of data from Eagle (5) and Schellinger (6). It shows the approximate distance from the nasal opening or teeth to the carina in male and female adults. In "average adults," the distance from the tube tip to the carina is approximately 3 to 4 cm (Tables 4 and 5). The preformed tube lengths and associated diameters are, by necessity, constructed for the average person. As the ideal tube length varies with a patient's height, in an unusually short or tall person the tube tip can be placed either too close to the carina or within the larynx when the tube is fixed at its predetermined bend. This problem must be accounted for when using preformed tubes, with the selection of a larger tube for the tall person, and a smaller tube for the short patient.

Tubes for Measuring End-tidal CO_2

Neonatal anesthesia provides many challenges. One challenge is accurate measurement of end-tidal CO_2. The small tidal volumes of neonates results in the expired alveolar gases being mixed with gases within the ventilation circuit, causing artificially low readings. A modified endotracheal tube is manufactured with a small-volume sampling port incorporated in its wall; this allows for transport of undiluted alveolar gases from the tip of the endotracheal tube to the gas monitor for more accurate measurements. This modification has been used most commonly during neonatal anesthesia.

Tubes Providing Topical Anesthesia to the Trachea

Sheridan-Kendall Catheter Corporation (Argyle, New York) makes an endotracheal tube (LTMA) with an injection port incorporated to allow for the placement of topical anesthetics above and below the endotracheal tube cuff. This provides mucosal anesthesia, minimizing the irritation to the airway caused by the endotracheal tube. It is intended for use in those patients in whom coughing or bucking at the termination of anesthesia would be deleterious. This approach to cough suppression during emergence, in conjunction with low-dose narcotics, allows 30% of patients emerging from anesthesia to have no cough, and decreases the severity of coughing in others (7).

Equipment for Nasal Intubation

Nasal intubation requires a change in technique, yet most of the necessary equipment is the same as for oral intubation. Alteration in technique includes steps necessary to guide the nasotracheal tube into the glottic opening, where direct manipulation of the proximal tube is no longer effective, and optimizing the nasal passage to minimize bleeding and patient discomfort. Forceps to guide the endotracheal tubes into the glottic opening should be available to assist with nasal intubation (Fig. 9). When a "blind" technique is planned, listening to the patient's breathing through the endotracheal tube aids in placement through the glottic opening. Whistles placed on the endotracheal tube connector have been marketed to aid in the identification of gas movement within the endotracheal tube, and therefore increase the likelihood of placement through the glottic opening. Nasal bleeding can be reduced by applying vasoconstrictive agents to the nasal mucosa. Additionally, it is important to obtain topical anesthesia of the nasopharyngeal and glottic mucosa for awake intubation. Often, vasoconstriction and topicalization can be obtained concurrently by combining pharmacologic agents. Flexible nasal airways (Fig. 9) are useful in spreading the topical anesthetic and

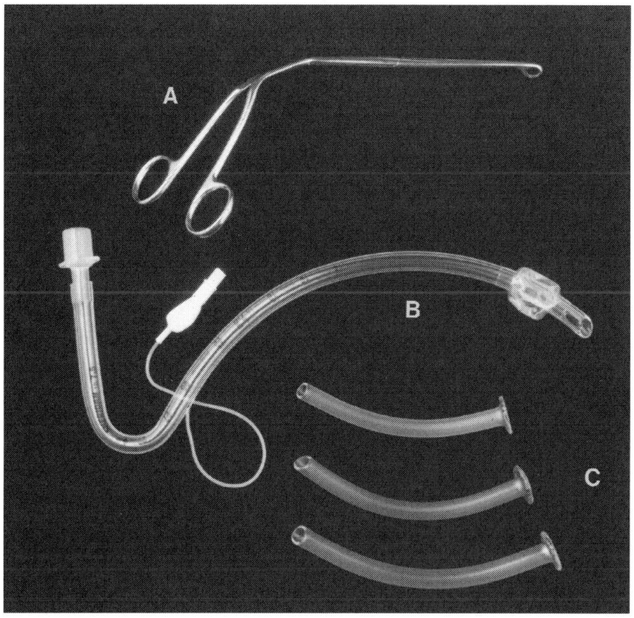

FIG. 9. Equipment necessary for nasal intubation. The Magill forceps are utilized to pick up the endotracheal tube tip and place it within the glottic opening (**A**). Nasal preformed endotracheal tube (**B**). Three sizes of flexible nasal airways (**C**).

vasoconstrictor within the nasal passage and indicating whether a nasal passage of adequate size is available. A preformed nasal endotracheal tube is often used in head and neck surgery (Fig. 9).

Equipment for Difficult or Failed Intubation

Endotracheal Tube Introducers and Changers

When endotracheal tubes must be placed or replaced in patients in whom airway visualization is anticipated or known to be difficult, endotracheal tube introducers or changers improve the likelihood of success with less tissue trauma. These facilitators of intubation are essentially malleable stylets that can be placed through the glottic opening under either complete or partial direct vision, or through an existing endotracheal tube without visualization. Once placed, these devices allow for the passage of an endotracheal tube "blindly" through the glottic opening. This avoids tissue trauma and the need for medications that might otherwise be necessary. During direct visualization of the glottic opening, these devices may be easier to manipulate into the airway than the bulkier endotracheal tube, especially in the confines of a small oropharynx.

Modified tube changers have a central channel, allowing for passage of oxygen into the pharynx or trachea during an endotracheal tube change. This can be life-saving in patients with severe lung disease and poor oxygenation, in whom hypoxemia follows only a few seconds of apnea. Extreme care must be taken to avoid wedging the tip of the tube changer into a small airway, where oxygen under pressure can rupture the airway during oxygenation through a tube changer.

Additional techniques for intubation are discussed in other chapters.

SUCTION EQUIPMENT

Maintenance of a clear, unobstructed airway is crucial to successful intubation. Suction of secretions, blood, or gastric contents is paramount to this goal. For any elective intubation, suction equipment must be available, including a flexible suction catheter useful for oral and tracheal suctioning, and a rigid Yankauer-type suction for oral suctioning. The flexible catheter also has the advantage of providing access to the pharynx when the mouth cannot be fully opened (Fig. 10). A suction pressure of at least negative 40 cm of water is needed for adequate suctioning of thick secretions. For emergency intubation, the airway is more likely to be soiled by such material, yet suction equipment may not always be available (espe-

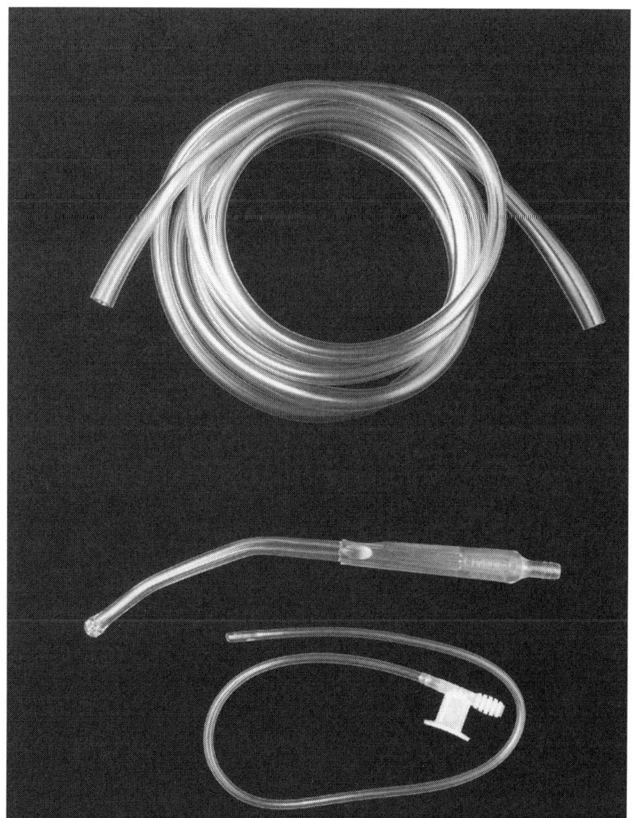

FIG. 10. Examples of suction equipment (flexible and rigid) required for elective intubation.

cially at remote sites where wall suction or electrical power is not available). In such situations, one does the best with what is available.

REFERENCES

1. Dorsch JA, Dorsch SE. Laryngoscopes. In: Anonymous, ed. *Understanding Anesthesia Equipment. Construction, Care and Complications*, 2nd ed. Baltimore: Williams & Wilkins; 1984:338–352.
2. Watanabe S, Suga A, Asakura N, et al. Determination of the distance between the laryngoscope blade and the upper incisors during direct laryngoscopy: comparisons of a curved, an angulated straight, and two straight blades. *Anesth Analg* 1994;79:638.
3. Marks RR, Hancock R, Charters P. An analysis of laryngoscope blade shape and design: new criteria for laryngoscope evaluation. *Can J Anaesth* 1993;40:262.
4. Watson WF. Development of the PVC endotracheal tube. *Biomaterials* 1980;1:41.
5. Eagle CC. The relationship between a person's height and appropriate endotracheal tube length. *Anaesth Intensive Care* 1992;20:156.
6. Schellinger, RR. The length of the airway to the bifurcation of the trachea. *Anesthesiology* 1964;25:169.
7. Gonzalez RM, Bjerke RJ, Drobychi T, et al. Prevention of endotracheal tube-induced coughing during emergence from general anesthesia. *Anesth Analg* 1994;79:792.

Airway Management, edited by
L.H. Hanowell, M.D. and R.J. Waldron, M.D.,
Lippincott-Raven Publishers, Philadelphia © 1996.

CHAPTER 7

Aspiration Prophylaxis and Rapid Sequence Intubation

Rajesh V. Patel and Ronald L. Katz

HISTORY

Hippocrates in 400 B.C. warned, "For drinking to provoke cough or for swallowing to be forced is bad," a reference to the risks of aspiration. Anacreon, a Greek poet, died after inhaling a grape seed in 475 B.C. An English poet Humphrey Gilbert aspirated a piece of mutton and died (1). John Hunter, while testifying at a murder trial in 1781, provided the first scientific observation of aspiration. Awareness of aspiration had been present for many years and continued over years with many illustrations. During the 1800s, more reports of aspiration associated with states of altered consciousness or pharyngeal dysfunction appeared.

Sir James Y. Simpson in 1848 argued that the first anesthetic death was not attributable to chloroform but to aspiration of brandy used to resuscitate the patient (2). A fifteen-year-old girl, while undergoing chloroform anesthesia via napkin, had an epileptic seizure. The physician administered brandy with water. When he saw the improvement, he gave more brandy. She rattled in her throat and died. Simpson maintained in his argument that the patient could have been saved "by simply removing the chloroform napkin from the face."

In the 1920s, Winternitz et al. described histologic changes of the lung with hydrochloric (HCL) acid. In 1937, Amberson described the first obstetric anesthetic aspiration. In 1946, Curtis Mendelson reported that aspiration occurred in 66/44,000 anesthetics, with an overall mortality rate of 3% for patients undergoing general anesthesia for vaginal deliveries (3). This report described the animal experiments to compare with the course of events in the clinical setting so well that even after 50 years, aspiration syndrome is known as *Mendelson's syndrome* (dyspnea, cyanosis, and tachycardia). Mendelson also demonstrated in rabbits that HCL acid, when instilled into the lungs, caused "cyanosis and

R. V. Patel and R. L. Katz: Department of Anesthesiology, University of Southern California School of Medicine; and Los Angeles County/University of Southern California Medical Center, Los Angeles, California 90033.

TABLE 1. *Incidence of subclinical regurgitation and aspiration*

Study (ref)	Regurgitation (n)	Comment
Turndorf et al. (4)	14.5% (152)	Upper abdominal surgery worst risk
Blitt et al. (5)	7.8% (900)	8.6% of episodes progressed to aspiration (0.67% of total)
Kofke et al. (6)	0% (20)	Small study, pH monitoring
Carlsson and Islander (7)	20% (138)	Many were emergency cases, many were done head down

TABLE 2. *Overall morbidity and mortality due to aspiration*

Study (ref)	Morbidity and mortality
Olsson et al. (10)	Incidence 1:2131 Mortality 0.2:10,000 anesthetics 47% developed pneumonitis 17% required mechanical ventilation
Gibbs (11)	8 of 324 (2.5%) anesthesia-related deaths due to aspiration
Pottecher et al. (12)	9 of 119 (7.6%) anesthesia-related deaths due to aspiration, 8 of 9 in recovery room
Nimmo (13)	25% of all maternal deaths, 19% of all anesthesia-related deaths in Great Britain

laboured respirations immediately with pink froth exuding from the respiratory passages in the terminal stages." The lung injury reported was similar to that caused by inhalation of the gastric contents.

INCIDENCE

The exact incidence of pulmonary aspiration is difficult to determine because clinically insignificant aspirations are difficult to diagnose, and those that are diagnosed are not always reported. Also, because the complication is infrequent, incidence cannot be ascertained from one institution alone. Mortality from different studies ranges from 1% to 20%. Turndorf et al. (4) in 1974 reported the incidence of regurgitation as 22/152 (14.5%). In this study, the incidence was significantly higher in the patients undergoing upper abdominal surgeries. Blitt et al. (5) in 1979 reported an incidence of 70/900 (7.8%) for silent regurgitation. Kofke and co-workers (6) found 0% incidence of gastropharyngeal reflux in 20 subjects undergoing mask general anesthesia with continuous hypopharyngeal pH monitoring. Carlsson and Islander (7) reported a 20% incidence of silent reflux in 138 women undergoing gynecologic surgery (Table 1). In this report, premedication consisted of morphine and scopolamine (which may decrease barrier pressures); nearly one-third were emergencies, and over half the surgeries were performed with head of the bed lowered. As we have seen, incidence varies widely among studies.

MORBIDITY AND MORTALITY

Morbidity consists of a multitude of complications like cyanosis, pneumonia, bronchospasm, sepsis, lung abscess, and end organ dysfunction. The average hospital stay after aspiration is 21 days, most of which is spent in the ICU (8,9). The mortality after aspiration ranges from 3% to 70% (3,8,9). Olsson et al. (10) provide newer and more accurate data (10). They reported an overall incidence of aspiration of 83/185,358 patients (1/2131). The mortality due to aspiration was 0.2/10,000. Almost half of patients who aspirated developed aspiration pneumonitis confirmed by chest x-ray, and 17% of patients who aspirated required mechanical ventilation. Gibbs (11) reported that 8 of 324 anesthesia-related deaths were due to aspiration. Pottecher et al. (12) reviewed 119 anesthesia-related cardiac arrests in a population of almost 200,000. Nine arrests were due to aspiration; of those, eight episodes were in the recovery room, indicating that vigilance and efforts at prevention should not end when anesthesia and surgery end. In 1982, aspiration was cited by Nimmo (13) as the cause of 25% of maternal deaths and 19% of all deaths attributed to anesthesia in Great Britain (Table 2). After reviewing all these reports, it is clear that a serious threat of aspiration during anesthesia does exist, and proper precautions to prevent this event are very important.

GASTRIC PHYSIOLOGY

The stomach is a muscular bag with very little tone. It aids in propulsion of food after it is mixed with digestive juices. The capacity is usually 1000–1500 ml. The pyloric portion has stronger peristaltic waves as compared to the fundal region. The peristaltic waves occur every 20 sec and exert 50–60 cm H_2O pressure. In an adult, gastric juice secretion is a continuous process: 1 ml/min in a nondigestive phase and 3–4 ml/min in a digestive phase (14). Swallowing of saliva is estimated at 1 ml/kg/hr (13,15).

The time required to empty the stomach varies according to the physiologic status of the patient. Pain, anxiety, narcotics, and labor all cause delayed gastric emptying (16,17). Liquids pass through the sphincter faster than do solids. Hormonal influence from gastrin and motilin also affects gastric motility; both increase lower esophageal tone. Gastrin also stimulates gastric secretion. Disease states delay gastric emptying, e.g., diabetes, hypothyroidism, peptic ulcer disease, and electrolyte disturbances (18). Hyperosmolar foods and lipids move through the stomach at a much slower rate than do proteins and carbohydrates. Because of the differences in gastric emptying times for clear liquids and solids, the recommendation of identical duration of preoperative fasting does not seem logical. It is also difficult to judge the level of anxiety in a patient preoperatively. There are data from gynecologic patients showing that when benzodiazepines versus placebo were given preoperatively, gastric fluid volume and gastric fluid pH were similar in both groups (19). The data from H_2 blockers suggesting that they retard gastric emptying are controversial (20).

PHYSIOLOGY OF REGURGITATION AND VOMITING

Regurgitation

Regurgitation is described as the passive flow of stomach contents past the lower esophageal sphincter (LES) when intragastric pressure exceeds LES pressure. Stomach contents can then enter the larynx if it is not protected. Regurgitation is referred to as *silent* if no immediate signs of aspiration are obvious or if no aspirate is recovered from the trachea.

As we know, the LES plays a very important role in prevention of gastric contents flow to the pharynx. Multiple mechanisms are described:

1. The circular smooth muscles in the anatomic LES. The length of the sphincter itself also plays an important role, because length increases with age.
2. Physiology of the sphincter, i.e., the tone of the muscle.
3. Pinch cork effect by crura of the diaphragm around the lower end of esophagus (21,22).
4. Angle formed between the esophagus and stomach.
5. Mucosal valve formation. This prevents fluid regurgitation but allows easy passage of food from esophagus to the stomach.
6. Mechanical factors.
7. Distance from gastroesophageal junction to pharynx. This is also important because gastric contents have a longer distance to travel in adults than in children. The distance between pharynx and gastroesophageal junction are: newborn, 11 cm; 3 years, 15 cm; 10 years, 17 cm; adult, 27 cm.

Lower esophageal sphincter control has two components: neuronal and hormonal. The neuronal component consists of a cholinergic reflex. Whenever there is an increase in intragastric pressure, there is an increase in lower esophageal tone, which would prevent regurgitation (23). There is a limit to this safety mechanism: Any rise in intragastric pressure above 25 cm H_2O is not matched by the neuronal mechanism to increase the sphincter tone. Smith et al. (24) described increases in intragastric pressure following fasciculations after succinylcholine administration (25). There are some interesting pressures to note. The normal intraabdominal pressure at rest is 10 cm H_2O. Normal LES pressure is 20 cm H_2O. The maximum increase in LES tone through reflex mechanism to prevent regurgitation is 25 cm H_2O. Cough increases intragastric pressure up to 60 cm H_2O. Properly applied crico-esophageal compression can withstand 100 cm H_2O of intragastric pressure.

The hormonal component of LES is controlled by gastrin and motilin. Both increase the lower esophageal sphincter tone (18,26). Prostaglandin E_2 and alkaline pH of stomach contents also increase the LES tone. Thus, the prophylactic use of antacids and H_2 blockers may help increase LES pressure. The factors that alter LES tone are shown in Table 3.

The intramuscular anticholinergics have very little effect on LES tone, but intravenous administration of anticholinergics causes prompt decrease in LES tone, which almost coincides with the increase in heart rate. All the beta adrenergic agonists and alpha adrenergic antagonists decrease LES tone. The agents commonly used for induction, including thiopentone, narcotics, and deep halothane (Fluothane) mask induction, all cause a decrease in LES tone. Isoflurane (Forane) does not decrease tone as much as do halothane and enflurane. A

TABLE 3. *Factors that alter LES tone*

Factors decreasing LES tone
Pregnancy
Obesity
Hiatal hernia
Drugs
• Anticholinergics
• Ganglion blocking agents
• Antidepressant medications
• β-adrenergic agonists
• α-adrenergic antagonists
• Sodium thiopentone
• Nitrous oxide
• Opioid analgesics
• Inhalation agents
Caffeine
Ethanol
Smoking
Factors that increase LES tone
Metoclopramide
Antacids
Cholinergic drugs
Muscle relaxants
• Succinylcholine
• Pancuronium
• Vecuronium
NM reversal agents
• Edrophonium
• Neostigmine
• α-adrenergic stimulants

LES, lower esophageal sphincter; NM, neuromuscular.

positive history of caffeine, alcohol, and smoking should alert anesthesia personnel to the increased risk of regurgitation and aspiration.

Succinylcholine in adults increases intragastric pressure, due to fasciculation of abdominal muscles. The fasciculations are seen much less in patients below the age of seven. Thus, succinylcholine may not increase intraabdominal pressure in children as much as it does in adults. Moreover, because LES is reflexly increased whenever intragastric pressure is increased up to 25 cm H_2O, this reflex would balance the increased intragastric pressure. Succinylcholine, thus, still appears to be the best agent to use in a patient suspected to have a full stomach, due to its fast onset of action. Although pancuronium has vagolytic effect, it increases LES tone.

Vomiting

Vomiting is described as active propulsion of stomach contents past a relaxed LES when simultaneous contraction of diaphragm and abdominal muscles squeeze the stomach. The vomiting center is located in the chemoreceptor trigger zone of the medulla. Figure 1 diagrams the zone's control. The motor responses travel through the fifth, seventh, ninth, and tenth nerves to the gastrointestinal tract and through spinal nerves to the abdominal muscles and diaphragm. The sequence of events in vomiting are as follows:

1. The soft palate moves upward to protect the nares.
2. The palatopharyngeal folds move medially to form a sagittal slit, permitting well-chewed food to pass easily but retarding passage of larger objects.
3. The epiglottis moves to cover the opening of the larynx, and the vocal cords become firmly approximated.
4. The larynx itself moves upward and forward, causing the esophagus to open widely (27).

HIGH-RISK GROUPS

In the area of high-risk groups, we should answer two questions:

1. Who is at risk of aspiration (Table 4)?
2. Who is at risk of aspiration pneumonitis, should aspiration occur?

Trauma Patients

The sentence to remember in this situation is **"stomach in trauma patient is full until proven otherwise."** The diagnosis of empty stomach can be made only in retrospect in trauma patients. From prior studies, it is well known that quality and quantity of food affects gastric emptying time. Pain, anxiety, and narcotics—which usually accompany trauma situations—also affect gastric emptying time. The more important NPO interval is the time between the last meal and accident—not the interval between last meal and induction of anesthesia. The usual policy of NPO refers to an interval of 6–8 hours between the last meal and an accident. H_2 blockers are not effective in this situation, because they do not influence existing acid in the stomach. If immediate surgery is required in a trauma patient, time since the last meal is irrelevant.

Pregnancy

Pregnancy tops the list for patients at risk for aspiration and deserves special consideration. Mechanical factors

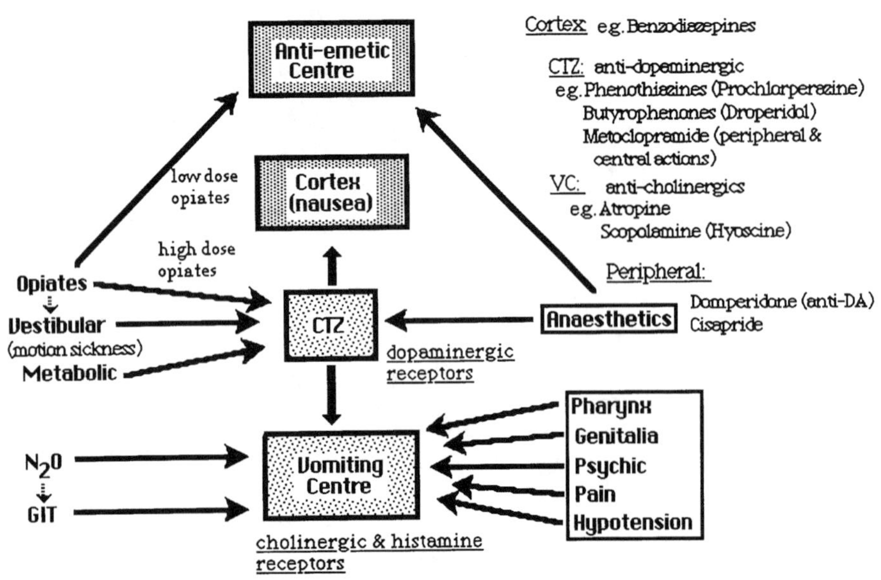

Figure 1. Diagramatic representation of "vomiting" pathways and sites of actions of antiemetic medications. CTZ, chemoreceptor trigger zone; VC, vomiting centre; GIT, gastrointestional track.

TABLE 4. *Predisposing factors to gastric aspiration*

Reduced level of consciousness
General anesthesia
Ethanol abuse
Deep sedation
Electrolyte abnormality (Na^+, Ca^{++})
Seizures
Hypoxia
Difficulty in swallowing
Elderly
Tracheostomies
Esophageal pathology (scleroderma)
GE junction pathology (hiatal hernia)
Fasting patients who are:
Obese
Diabetic
Pregnant
Decreased LES competence
Delayed gastric emptying
Increased gastric acid secretion
Increased intraabdominal pressure
Maternal stress
Distortion of gastric anatomy
Pediatric population
Delayed gastric emptying
Pain
Anxiety
Narcotics
Anticholinergics
Pregnancy
Diabetes
Particulate antacids/solid foods
Peptic ulcer disease
Myxedema
Reduced airway defenses
Prematurity (extremes of age)
NG tubes
Tracheostomy
Uncuffed endotracheal tubes
CPR

GE, gastroesophageal; NG, nasogastric tube; LES, lower esophageal sphincter.

distort the gastroesophageal junction because of the rising fundus of the uterus and cause heartburn (28,29). The hormones gastrin and motilin are important also. Gastrin is produced in the placenta, which increases acidity of the gastric content (30). Motilin, which speeds gastric emptying, is depressed during pregnancy (31). The rise in progesterone in early pregnancy may be related to decreased LES tone. Simpson et al. (32) found that gastric emptying was delayed in patients whose pregnancies were between 12 and 14 weeks gestation, but not in pregnancies of less than 11 weeks gestation (32). When the criteria of pH < 2.5 and gastric volume 25 ml were used, Wyner and Cohen (33) found 35% of patients for elective abortion to be at risk of aspiration (34). This risk also continues in the immediate postpartum period. James et al. (35) found that 40% to 73% of postpartum patients had more than 25 ml of low-pH gastric fluid, even 45 hours postdelivery.

In patients undergoing an elective Caesarean section (C-section), the time since the last meal bears some correlation with gastric volume; however, Roberts and Shirley (36) showed that 7 of 24 patients were still at risk of aspiration after an 8-hour fast. Patients who ate after labor began, weighed > 160 lb, had narcotics during labor, and who subsequently had a C-section had significantly higher gastric volumes (37).

ICU Patients

ICU patients who are intubated or have tracheostomies have 15% to 77% risk of aspiration (38). The intubated patient can be at increased risk due to asymmetry of cuff inflation, dilatation of the trachea with positive-pressure mechanical ventilation, and channeling of liquids down vertical cuff folds. The larynx is tethered to the skin in patients with tracheostomies. This prevents normal elevation necessary for glottic closure. There is also desensitization of the larynx that occurs with decreased air flow, leading to an attenuation of protective laryngeal reflexes (38). There is now increased awareness of keeping gastric pH higher in intubated and tracheostomized ICU patients. Pediatric patients are usually intubated with uncuffed tubes, and risk of aspiration is increased several fold, as compared to patients with cuffed ET tubes (23).

Prolonged Use of Endotracheal (ET) Tubes

Endotracheal tubes are available as low-volume/high-pressure cuffs (180–250 mm Hg) and high-volume/low-pressure cuffs (15–30 mm Hg). Mucosal ischemia occurs when more than 32 mm Hg pressure is continuously applied to the tracheal mucosa. Ideally, the cuff pressure should be maintained below 32 mm Hg at all times to avoid mucosal injury. Thus, high-volume/low-pressure cuffs appear more appropriate for prolonged periods of intubation. Nitrous oxide over a prolonged period can diffuse into the ET tube cuff and increase pressure in the cuff. In long operative cases, the cuff pressure should be adjusted frequently to avoid mucosal injury. Anterior mucosal ulcer (within 3–5 days) is the most common tracheal injury due to ET cuffs. The other rare complications are sloughing of the tracheal rings, posterior erosion into the esophagus, and anterior erosion into an innominate artery. Thick-wall cuffs (0.25 mm) are avoided because they form large folds through which aspiration might occur. Thin-wall (0.1 mm) cuffs are ideal for the ET tube.

Other Patients at Risk

The patient is currently thought to be at risk when: (a) gastric fluid pH is less than 2.5 and (b) gastric volume is more than 25 ml (0.4 ml/kg).

These data come not from human studies but from unpublished monkey studies where 25 ml gastric juice with pH < 2.5 was instilled directly into the lung (36). Serious lung injury was noted with the above experiment. Should 25 ml residual gastric content in man be a risk factor for lung injury? Even though the stomach may have 25 ml gastric juice, it is highly unlikely that all 25 ml will regurgitate and enter the trachea. With increasing use of measures to raise pH of the gastric juice prior to surgery, the more transient symptoms of even high volumes of gastric aspirate may be better tolerated by patients than will permanent, severe lung injury (39). Thus, increasing the gastric volume by the addition of 30 cc of sodium citrate should not be of concern if any risk of aspiration is suspected. Kennedy et al. (40) concluded that pH was the more critical factor in determining degree of lung injury. If we follow this strict criteria of pH < 2.5 and gastric residual volume > 25 ml, a significant number of patients, including pregnant, emergency, postpartum, obese, pediatric, and outpatients, is at risk of aspiration.

FASTING/NPO RECOMMENDATIONS

Many studies have challenged the conventional prolonged fasting during the preoperative period (41–43). Most of these studies have concluded that gastric contents present at the time of induction of anesthesia have a poor correlation with the time of last fluid intake. These studies were not done with solid food. Liberalization of fluid intake in our guidelines should be stressed after reviewing some literature here.

Shevde and Trivedi (44) looked at the effects of clear liquids (240 ml of water, black coffee, and pulp-free orange juice) on gastric fluid pH and volume in 30 adult volunteers (44). After overnight fasting, a salem sump nasogastric (NG) tube was inserted, and gastric contents were removed for measurement of baseline gastric fluid volume and pH. Gastric contents were then measured every 30 min and reinserted through the NG tube into the stomach until gastric fluid of < 25 ml was recovered. All volunteers had a gastric fluid volume of > 25 ml and a slight decrease in gastric fluid pH within 2 hours of ingestion of the test fluid. Read and Vaughn (45) evaluated the unlimited use of clear fluids until 2 hours preoperatively on 53 adult patients scheduled for surgery (45). Among all the patients, the average amount of fluid volume consumed preoperatively was 500 ml. These patients were compared with a group that fasted after midnight. After induction, neither group had significant difference in recovered gastric fluid volume and pH. In fact, the patients who were allowed unlimited use of clear liquids until 2 hours preoperatively were less anxious than were patients in the control group. This might reflect better absorption of oral benzodiazepines. Data from the studies done on pediatric cardiac patients showed less irritability in children who were allowed clear liquids preoperatively until 2 hours prior to induction (46). Based on these data, allowing children to drink clear liquids (water, soda, apple juice, and pulp-free orange juice) until 2 hours before anesthesia is justified.

TYPE OF GASTRIC ASPIRATE AND PATHOGENESIS

We have already discussed the fact that acidic materials cause more damage to the lung tissues. Pulmonary damage increases proportionately as pH is decreased below 2.5 (47,48). There are lung changes recently described by Kennedy et al. (40) in two stages. In stage I, almost immediately there is exudation of fluid into the alveoli, causing immediate hypoxemia. In stage II, after 4 hours, changes are seen secondary to the inflammatory process, where there is infiltration of red and white blood cells into the interstitial spaces (40). The lung architecture remains intact, unlike that following aspiration of food particles (49–51). Alveolar edema destroys surfactant and causes atelectasis. Reflex bronchospasm may occur. Hypovolemia and hypotension occur from loss of fluids into the lungs, causing pulmonary edema. Pulmonary hypertension occurs secondary to hypoxic pulmonary vasoconstriction, along with widening of arterial alveolar oxygen gradient. Aspiration of large particles of food may obstruct the airway, causing asphyxia if not removed immediately. Aspiration from grossly contaminated oral cavities can cause serious consequences. Aspiration of fecal material in a patient with intestinal obstruction may be fatal. Thus, it is usually wise to intubate the trachea awake in a patient with distal intestinal obstruction.

PREVENTION OF ASPIRATION

Table 5 shows broad principles that can be applied to prevent aspiration. Does every patient deserve prophylactic treatment for aspiration (Table 6)? There is no clear answer. We have to answer this in our clinical practice after evaluating patients individually for risk factors. Any suspicion of risk for aspiration should be considered seriously and prophylaxed. Before availability of drugs to decrease volume and increase pH of gastric juice, there were attempts made to induce vomiting with apomorphine or to remove stomach contents with NGs before induction of general anesthesia (52). The most common methods used today for aspiration prophylaxis are: emptying the stomach via an NG, decreasing gastric emptying time, neutralizing existing acid, and reducing acid production of gastric mucosa.

TABLE 5. *Prevention of aspiration*

NPO
Regional anesthesia
Awake intubation
Endotracheal intubation
Rapid sequence induction
Cricoid pressure
Nasogastric suction
Extubation with protective reflexes
Pharmacologic preparation
Metoclopramide
Liquid antacids (clear)
H_2 receptor antagonists

Drug Therapy

Metoclopramide

Metoclopramide is a central dopamine antagonist. It decreases gastric volume by increasing motility of the gastrointestinal tract, relaxing the pyloric sphincter, and emptying stomach contents in an anterograde fashion. Metoclopramide increases LES tone. Its effectiveness in reducing gastric volume preoperatively is controversial (53,54). Capen et al. (55) found a combination of metoclopramide and cimetidine (Tagamet) more effective in reducing both volume and acidity of gastric contents than when used individually (55). Manchikanti et al. (56) showed no advantage by combining metoclopramide and cimetidine. The action of metoclopramide may be antagonized by simultaneous administration of anticholinergics. Thus, use of glycopyrrolate may reduce the gastric-emptying effect of metoclopramide. Metoclopramide may exacerbate Parkinson's disease in elderly patients. Cisapride (Propulsid) has an anterograde gastric emptying property, but has not yet demonstrated its efficacy in routine anesthesia practice.

Antacids

Antacids neutralize existing acids. They are available as particulate, e.g., Gelusil,™ Mylanta,™ and clear (nonparticulate, e.g., Bicitra™). Antacids have an immediate onset of action. When mixed well with gastric contents, they can be 100% effective in raising pH above 2.5, if given in correct quantities. Particulate antacids do not mix well with gastric contents. If particulate antacid is aspirated, it causes a clinical course less severe than does acid aspiration, but late in the course, granulomatous changes occur. These changes are characterized by predominance of lymphocytes, macrophages, and granuloma formation, followed by fibrosis. In our clinical practice, we use soluble antacids like 0.3 molar solution of sodium citrate. Two tablets of Alka Seltzer Gold™ in 1 oz of water gives 0.3 molar sodium citrate after complete effervescence. In an emergency, even 50 ml of sodium bicarbonate IV preparation (8.4%) can be given by mouth. The commercially available Bicitra™ contains a mixture of sodium citrate and citric acid (the final concentration is 0.3 molar solution). When clear antacids were given preoperatively in 27 patients and gastric juice pH was measured after induction of anesthesia at different intervals, only 3 of 27 had pH less than 2.5 within 60 min duration of PO antacids. But when more than 60 min had elapsed after the antacid dose, 30 of 47 had a pH less than 2.5. We would recommend that antacid be given 10 min prior to the induction of anesthesia and be repeated if more than 60 min elapses from the last dose.

TABLE 6. *Who should receive prophylactic therapy?*

↑Intragastric pressure
Gastric pH < 2.5
Gastric volume > 25 ml
Preoperative risk factors
Delayed gastric emptying
Upper abdominal surgery
Emergency surgery

H_2 Blockers

H_2 blockers also reduce gastric acid secretion. Cimetidine, ranitidine (Zantac), and famotidine (Pepcid) are the three most commonly used H_2 blockers. All three are effective in reducing acid secretion. They differ in their duration of action and side effect profile. H_2 blockers are usually given the night before and on the morning of surgery. It is still justified to give H_2 blockers immediately before anesthesia or early during surgery, because decreased gastric acid secretion will be beneficial during extubation. Cimetidine has been known to cause dizziness and an altered state of consciousness, especially in elderly patients. Very rarely, cimetidine causes bradycardia and hypotension if given as a rapid intravenous bolus. Cimetidine is known to cause drug interactions by inhibiting cytochrome P-450 (mixed function oxidase system), interfering with gastrointestinal absorption, altering plasma protein binding, competing for renal excretion, and decreasing liver blood flow. The important drugs to remember for interaction with cimetidine are coumadin, diazepam, theophylline, propranolol, phenytoin (Dilantin), and lidocaine. Ranitidine is said to have lesser drug interactions. It also inhibits cytochrome P-450 system. Ranitidine is 4–10 times more potent and has a longer duration of action than does cimetidine (Table 7). It is not associated with confusion in the elderly. Famotidine has actions similar to other H_2 blockers. It has less cytochrome P-450 suppression. A one-time dose of 40 mg at night or IV 20 mg 45 min prior to induction is recom-

TABLE 7. *H_2 Receptor antagonists*

	Cimetidine (Tagamet)	Ranitidine (Zantac)
ADULT	PO 300 mg HS/300 mg 2 hr preop IV 300 mg HS/300 mg 45 min preop	PO 150 mg HS/150 mg 2 hr preop IV 50 mg/HS/ 50 mg 45 min preop
PEDS	PO 5–10 mg/kg HS/5–10 mg/kg 2 hr preop IV 5–10 mg/kg HS/5–10 mg/kg 45 min preop Rectal 40 mg/kg	PO 0.5–1 mg/kg HS/0.5–1 mg/kg 2 hr preop IV 0.25–0.5 mg/kg HS/0.25–0.5 mg/kg 2 hr preop
	Duration 4–6 hr	Duration 8–12 hr

mended. Nizatidine also is a new H_2 blocker, but its safety profile in routine anesthesia use is not established. It also has a weak suppression of cytochrome P-450 system.

Others

Anticholinergics like atropine and glycopyrrolate can reduce gastric acid secretion and help maintain pH above 2.5.

Misoprostol (Cytotec) is a synthetic prostaglandin E analog. It has mucosal protective properties. It decreases gastric acid secretion and is used for prophylaxis of ulcers secondary to NSAID therapy. Its safety and efficacy is not demonstrated in children. Misoprostol is contraindicated in pregnancy because it can induce premature labor. Misoprostol does not decrease cytochrome P-450 enzyme.

Anesthetic Technique Considerations

Regional anesthesia is preferable if it can be done safely in the patient at risk of aspiration. If general anesthesia is elected, rapid sequence induction becomes the choice in these patients with a normal airway examination. If any doubt exists about difficulty in intubation due to airway abnormality, it is always wise to intubate the patient awake. Many people (including the authors) believe that awake intubation is the safest technique, but others disagree.

RAPID SEQUENCE INTUBATION

Patient Position

There are a number of controversies about rapid sequence intubation (RSI). Should the induction be done in reverse Trendelenburg position? Passive regurgitation can be prevented by head up or semi-sitting position. Snow and Nunn (57) recommended that 20° to 40° head up tilt can decrease passive regurgitation. If the patient is hemodynamically stable, the operating table should be positioned with a 40° head up tilt. Thus the patient's larynx is elevated approximately 19 cm above the gastroesophageal junction. For oral contamination to occur, the gastric contents must overcome a barrier pressure and gravitational effects of 19 cm H_2O pressure (58). Some clinicians argue that the head down position is better because if there is regurgitation or vomiting, this position decreases the likelihood of pulmonary aspiration, should the oropharynx be filled with gastric contents. We prefer the head up position.

Cricoid Pressure

Sellick (59) described application of cricoid pressure in 1961, with neck and head extended to prevent passive regurgitation. It is very important not to apply pressure on the thyroid because it would make intubation difficult. The cricoid is a complete ring, and the purpose is to compress the esophagus between the anterior vertebral body and cricoid ring, causing an effective seal. Properly applied cricoid pressure can withstand a rise in intragastric pressure up to 100 cm H_2O, which is usually seen during coughing (59). Cricoid pressure should not be applied very early, because it can cause tracheal irritation, cough, and vomiting. Salem et al. (60) described an advantage of moving the cricoid cartilage cephalad to facilitate difficult intubations by improving visualization. Some have suggested that cricoid pressure be released with an act of active vomiting to avoid esophageal rupture. This is a theoretical possibility. However, in our opinion, maintaining cricoid pressure to prevent aspiration seems a better choice. Sellick (61) advised that as soon as the ET is inserted, the cuff should be inflated immediately, and only then should cricoid pressure be released. Some clinicians like to use one hand to support the neck while applying cricoid pressure. This would improve esophageal compression because if the neck is not supported it acts as a bridge between the shoulder blades and a pillow. Once the patient's muscles relax, single-handed cricoid pressure may not remain the most effective method of esophageal compression. Contraindications to cricoid pressure are esophageal foreign body, esophageal diverticula, and retropharyngeal abscess.

Nasogastric Tubes

Should the NG tube be left in place while providing cricoid pressure during RSI? Salem et al. in 1985 (62) evaluated the effectiveness of the Sellick maneuver in the presence of an NG tube. The experiment was done in cadavers. When NG tubes were clamped and 100 cm of intragastric pressure was created, there was no egress of gastric contents into the oral cavity. Thus, the NG need not be taken out during rapid sequence intubation, but should be suctioned before induction of anesthesia. If the patient was on low intermittent suction for many hours preoperatively, we can expect a fair degree of emptiness of the stomach.

Emptying of the stomach is not guaranteed if suction to the NG tube was applied preoperatively on the operating room table, after the NG tube was clamped for hours on the ward. An NG tube with a sump action is much more effective than a single lumen soft PVC catheter to empty the stomach. Some clinicians routinely empty the stomach after induction of anesthesia in any patient. A single lumen soft catheter is inexpensive and less traumatic, so it has become the choice among most clinicians. Since the NG tube passed orally or nasally is very effective in gastric emptying, it should be the choice in any patient suspected to have full stomach.

Performance of RSI

The process of RSI is a series of events with physiologic and pharmacologic importance. The goal is to secure the airway with an ET with the minimum duration after airway reflexes are lost. The consideration is given to:

1. Lungs full of oxygen, which would give enough time to intubate without positive pressure ventilation or hypoxia.
2. Rapid loss of consciousness via short-acting intravenous induction agents with minimal change in hemodynamics.
3. Rapid relaxation of muscles to help open the airway and intubate without coughing or bucking.
4. Properly applied cricoid pressure to prevent gastric contents entering the pharynx before intubation is complete.
5. Continued cricoid pressure until confirmation of the ET tube in the trachea.

The induction process would start with preoxygenation or denitrogenation. The patient may breathe 100% oxygen via face mask at normal depth for 3–5 minutes. Similar denitrogenation can be achieved by three to five vital capacity breaths with 100% oxygen.

The use of a nondepolarizing neuromuscular blocker to prevent fasciculation and thereby decrease intragastric pressure may be recommended, but some feel this is unnecessary. Pregnant patients fasciculate much less, especially preeclamptics on magnesium therapy. If the induction is delayed for any reason after a small defasciculant dose, then a feeling of weakness followed by anxiety in the patient will occur.

In most nonfull stomach cases we use preoperative sedation and give more on the operating room table, which decreases the amount of total induction dose required. It is not advisable to use sedation in patients suspected to have a full stomach, so a larger dose of induction agent may be necessary for complete loss of consciousness. Thiopental (Pentothal) is the most commonly used agent. It causes myocardial depression and venous dilatation (39,49). If the patient is hypovolemic, thiopental would cause hypotension and reflex tachycardia. Therefore, in mildly hypovolemic patients, ketamine might be more preferable. Ketamine has sympathomimetic effects, which raises blood pressure and heart rate. In the presence of severe hypovolemia where the sympathetic nervous system is already maximally stimulated, the sympathetic stimulatory effect of ketamine will not be obtained, and the direct myocardial depression effect will prevail. The dose of induction of ketamine should be reduced from 1–2 mg/kg to 0.25–0.5 mg/kg in such patients. If the patient has a depressed myocardium, some people believe that a safer agent for induction is etomidate in the dose of 0.1–0.3 mg/kg. The drawbacks of this drug are pain at the intravenous induction site, myoclonus, and 4 hours of adrenal cortical suppression after a single bolus dose (63,64).

Cricoesophageal compression may be applied by an assistant as soon as the patient loses consciousness and continued until the ET tube is confirmed to be present in trachea. It is very important that the person assigned to apply cricoid pressure does not release pressure while helping to pick up a stylet or manipulating the intravenous site. It is at this time that aspiration might occur. Should the first intubation attempt be unsuccessful, cricoid pressure must be continued. If hypoxia occurs, then a change in plan with gentle breaths and continued cricoid pressure will be beneficial until intubation is successful. Attempts at intubation should be done with some change each time, e.g., change in laryngoscopic blades, head position, and intubating personnel, if available. Traumatic intubation attempts should be avoided at all times. Usually, restricting intubation attempts to 3–4 times for a given person avoids excessive trauma and the soft tissue swelling that might make later indirect approaches to intubation more difficult. At this moment, if the patient starts moving and attempts to have spontaneous diaphragmatic movements, it would be appropriate to wake the patient and proceed with awake intubation. Continuing anesthesia with further paralysis at this time may be more detrimental to the patient, especially if ventilation attempts with cricoid pressures were not adequate.

ACID ASPIRATION SYNDROME

Clinical Features

The onset of the clinical syndrome may be acute or delayed, depending upon the amount of regurgitant aspirated into the trachea. The immediate clinical signs are cyanosis, diffuse rales, wheezing, tachypnea, and tachycardia. Symptoms include hypoxia in intubated patients, dyspnea and cough in nonintubated patients. Serious complications include pneumonitis, lung abscess, gastrointestinal hemorrhage, renal failure, pulmonary embolus, and myocardial infarction. The morbidity associated with gastric aspiration usually resulted in an average hospital stay of 21 days (65). Hospital costs associated with intensive monitoring, aggressive drug therapy, and prolonged length of stay can be significant. Most additional hospital days are spent in the ICU at a cost of $2000–$3000 per day or more.

There is no typical characteristic x-ray pattern that is a hallmark of aspiration. Not uncommonly, the initial chest x-ray after acute aspiration does not indicate the severity of the insult (34). The common changes seen on x-ray are infiltrates in the central location with radial distribution or involvement of lower lobes, usually the right side. The x-ray changes, when they do occur, do not disappear quickly and should be followed up for development of ARDS and/or pneumonia. There are some clinicians who assume that all patients who demonstrate signs and symptoms of ARDS during anesthesia or in the recovery period have aspirated stomach contents, even if regurgitation was not witnessed and tracheal suction does not reveal gastric material.

Treatment

Treatment of the patient who has suffered pulmonary aspiration is supportive. If the volume of liquid aspirate is large enough, acute respiratory symptoms will be present, regardless of pH (66). The changes produced by neutral pH liquid clears faster than do those produced by acidic pH (66). After aspiration, the aspirate reaches the alveolar region in 12–18 sec and completes the damage. Aspirated material is buffered within minutes (66,67). Some clinicians recommend that gastric fluid aspirate suctioned from the trachea be tested for pH with litmus paper. This is probably not necessary because pH is buffered immediately and treatment is not based on pH of the aspirate. For these reasons, it is not advisable to lavage with neutral or alkaline solutions because this would spread aspirate to the other areas of the lung, which are still good for oxygen exchange (66). Equal amount of acid with pH 1.6 if mixed with normal saline as lavage fluid will raise pH to only 1.8. This small change will probably not help limit further damage. Lavage would help to remove inspissated secretions or particulate material obstructing the airway. A bronchoscopic suction with 5–10 ml normal saline would help remove particulate matter.

The damage incurred by aspirate provides an excellent ground for bacteria to grow. If the aspiration occurred in an outpatient setting, the common pathogens suspected are bacteroids, Fusobacterium, and Peptostreptococcus. They are all penicillin-sensitive. If aspiration occurred in a patient who was hospitalized more than 48 hours, the gastric content normally gets colonized with gram-negative bacteria and staphylococcus aureus. The use of prophylactic antibiotics is usually discouraged to avoid emergence of antibiotic-resistant bacteria. The antibiotic use should be delayed until bacteria are identified and sensitivity determined (8,66). In cases of lower intestinal obstruction with fecal aspiration, where mortality is very high, antibiotics may be started early in the process. Complete coverage with high-dose crystalline penicillin and clindamycin or metronidazole is recommended for fecal aspiration.

In 1961, high-dose steroid therapy was recommended to alter the inflammatory process of chemical burn. The rationale for its use was that it reduced inflammation, stabilized lysosome membranes, protected type II pneumocytes, and prevented aggregation of leukocytes and platelets. The experimental studies done in early years related corticosteroid therapy to the pH of the aspirate. Steroids were beneficial in reducing water contents of the lung when given within 72 hours of injury if the pH of aspirate was between 1.5 and 2.5. When pH was less than 1.5, there was extensive damage, and steroids were not effective. When pH was greater than 2.5, the response to steroids was the same as with water aspiration.

However, more recent studies have shown that steroids do not affect outcome and can promote bacterial overgrowth, possibly interfering with immune mechanism and the healing process (66,68,69).

Supplemental oxygen can be given during spontaneous breathing as long as the patient can maintain PaO_2 compatible with life. A continuous positive airway pressure (CPAP) mask can be placed to improve oxygenation. If the patient needs more than 12 mm Hg CPAP to maintain oxygenation, then he or she should be intubated. Because > 12 mm Hg pressure of CPAP mask opens the gastroesophageal sphincter, there is an increased possibility of regurgitation. Positive end expiratory pressure (PEEP) should be continued even after intubation and should not be completely withdrawn until alveoli are capable of maintaining stability. A CVP line may be placed for a patient who has aspirated highly acidic material with extensive damage, because a substantial amount of fluids may be lost into the lungs.

A Swan-Ganz/PA catheter can be placed if the patient is hemodynamically unstable. The PA catheter would measure left atrial pressure and cardiac output to determine cardiac decompensation secondary to pump failure or ineffective circulatory volume. To optimize renal function, perform the usual differential diagnosis of oliguria before considering furosemide (Lasix). The most common cause of oliguria is hypovolemia. If treated appropriately, renal insufficiency will be prevented.

REFERENCES

1. Gardner AM. Aspiration of food and vomit. *GJ Med* 1958;27:227.
2. Simpson JY. Remarks on the alleged case of death from the action of chloroform. *Lancet* 1848;1:75.
3. Mendelson CL. The aspiration of stomach contents into the lungs during obstetric anesthesia. *Am J Obstet Gynecol* 1946;52:191.
4. Turndorf H, Rodis ID, Clark TS. "Silent" regurgitation during anesthesia. *Anesth Analg* 1974;53:700.
5. Blitt CD, Gutman HL, Cohen DD. "Silent" regurgitation and aspiration during general anesthesia. *Anesth Analg* 1979;49:707.
6. Kofke WA, Fasano M, Keamy MF, Darr JA. Continuous hypopharyngeal pH monitoring via mask. *Anesthesiology* 1987;67:434–436.
7. Carlsson C, Islander G. Silent gastropharyngeal regurgitation during anesthesia. *Anesth Analg* 1981;60:655–657.
8. LeFrock JL, Clark TS, Davies B. Aspiration pneumonia. A ten year review. *Am Surg* 1979;45:305.
9. Landay MJ, Christensen EE, Bynum LJ. Pulmonary manifestation of acute aspiration of gastric contents. *Am J Roentgenol* 1978;131:587.
10. Olsson GL, Hallen B, Hambraens-Jonzon K. Aspiration during anesthesia, a computer aided study of 185,358 anesthetics. *Acta Anaesthesiol Scand* 1966;30:84.
11. Gibbs JM. The anesthetic mortality assessment committee. *NZ Med J* 1986;99:55–59.
12. Pottecher T, Tiret L, Desmonts JM, Hatton F, Bilaine J. Cardiac arrest related to anesthesia. *Eur J Anaesthesiol* 1984;1:305–318.
13. Nimmo WS. Aspiration of gastric contents. *Br J Hosp Med* 1985;34:176–179.
14. Dubois A. Gastric emptying of liquids should not be studied independently from gastric secretion. In: Chey WY, ed. *Functional Disorders of the Digestive Tract*. New York: Raven Press, 1983;151.
15. Minami H, McCallum RW. The physiology and pathophysiology of gastric emptying in humans. *Gastroenterology* 1984;86:1592–1610.
16. Davison JS, Davison MC, Hay DM. Gastric emptying time in late pregnancy and labour. *Br J Obstet Gynaecol* 1970;77:37.
17. Holdsworth JD. Relationship between stomach contents and analgesia in labour. *Br J Anaesth* 1978;50:1145.
18. Mamel JJ. Gastric emptying disorders. In: Nord HJ, Brady PG, eds. *Critical Care Gastroenterology*. New York: Churchill Livingstone, 1982;113.
19. Harrik PE, Soreide E, Hofstad B, Steen PA. Does preoperative anxiety influence gastric fluid volume and acidity. *Anesth Analg* 1992;75:91–94.
20. Dobrilla G, de Pretis G, Comberlato M, Amplatz S. H_2-antagonists and motility of the upper gastrointestinal tract in man. *Hepatogastroenterology* 1988;35:30.
21. Marchand P. A study of the forces productive of gastro-oesophageal regurgitation and herniation through the diaphragmatic hiatus. *Thorax* 1957;12:189.
22. Botha GSM. Mucosal folds at the cardia as a component of the gastro-oesophageal closing mechanism. *Br J Surg* 1958;45:569.
23. Browning DH, Graves SA. Incidence of aspiration with endotracheal tube in children. *J Pediatr* 1983;102:582–534.
24. Smith G, Dalling R, Williams TIR. Gastroesophageal pressure gradient changes produced by induction of anesthesia and suxamethonium. *Br J Anaesth* 1978;50:1137.
25. Miller RD, Way WL. Inhibition of succinylcholine induced increased intragastric pressure by nondepolarizing muscle relaxants and lidocaine. *Anesthesiology* 1971;34:185.
26. You CH, Lee KY, Chey WY. Plasma motilin level and interdigestive motor complex in normal and abnormal states in man. In: Chey WY, ed. *Functional Disorders of the Digestive Tract*. New York: Raven Press, 1983;23.
27. Guyton AC. *Textbook of Medical Physiology*, 6th ed. Philadelphia: WB Saunders, 1981;784.
28. Greenan J. The cardio-oesophageal junction. *Br J Anaesth* 1961;33:432.
29. Williams NH. Variable significance of heartburn. *Am J Obstet Gynecol* 1941;42:814.
30. Attia RR, Ebeid AM, Fischer JE, et al. Maternal fetal and placental gastrin concentrations. *Anaesthesia* 1982;37:18.
31. Christofides ND, Ghatei MA, Bloom SR, et al. Decreased plasma motilin concentrations in pregnancy. *BMJ* 1982;285:1453.
32. Simpson KH, Stakes AF, Miller M. Pregnancy delays paracetamol absorption and gastric emptying in patients undergoing surgery. *Br J Anaesth* 1988;60:24.
33. Wyner J, Cohen SE. Gastric volume in early pregnancy: effect of metoclopramide. *Anesthesiology* 1982;57:209–212.
34. Landay MJ, Christensen EE, Bynum LJ. Pulmonary manifestations of acute aspiration of gastric contents. *Am J Roentgenol* 1978;131:587–592.
35. James CF, Gibbs CP, Banner T. Postpartum perioperative risk of aspiration pneumonia. *Anesthesiology* 1984;61:756.
36. Roberts RB, Shirley MA. Reducing risk of acid aspiration during Cesarean section. *Anesth Analg* 1974;53:859–868.
37. Holdsworth JD. Relationship between stomach contents and analgesia in labour. *Br J Anaesth* 1978;50:1145–1147.
38. Elpern EH, Jacobs ER, Bone RC. Incidence of aspiration in tracheally intubated adults. *Heart Lung* 1987;16:527–531.
39. James CF, Modell JH, Gibbs CP. Pulmonary aspiration: effects of volume and pH in rat. *Anesth Analg* 1984;63:665.
40. Kennedy TPM, Johnson KJ, Kunkel RG. Acute acid aspiration lung injury in he rat: biphasic pathogenesis. *Anesth Analg* 1989;69:87.
41. Cote CJ. NPO after midnight for children. *Anesthesiology* 1990;72:589–592.
42. Miller M, Wishart HY, Nimmo WS. Gastric contents at induction of anesthesia: is a 4 hour fast necessary? *Br J Anaesth* 1983;55:1185–1188.
43. Maltby JR, Sudherland AD, Sale JP, Shaffer EA. Is a five hour fast justified prior to elective surgery? *Anesth Analg* 1986;65:1112–1116.
44. Shevde K, Trivedi N. Effect of clear liquids on gastric volume and pH in healthy volunteers. *Anesth Analg* 1991;72:528–531.
45. Read MS, Vaughn RS. Allowing preoperative patients to drink. *Acta Anaesthesiol Scand* 1991;35:591–595.
46. Nicolson SC, Dorsey AT, Schreiner MS. Shortened preanesthetic fasting interval in pediatric cardiac surgical patients. *Anesth Analg* 1992;74:694–697.
47. Teabeaut JR II. Aspiration of gastric contents: an experimental study. *Am J Pathol* 1952;28:51.
48. Taylor G, Pryse-Davies J. The prophylactic use of antacids in the prevention of the acid pulmonary-aspiration syndrome (Mendelson's syndrome). *Lancet* 1966;1:288.
49. Schwartz DJ, Wynne JW, Gibbs CP. The pulmonary consequences of aspiration of gastric contents at pH values greater than 2.5. *Am Rev Respir Dis* 1980;121:119.
50. Jones JG, Grossman RF, Berry M. Alveolar capillary membrane permeability correlation with functional, radiographic and postmortem changes after fluid aspiration. *Am Rev Respir Dis* 1979;120:399.
51. Wynne JW, Reynolds JC, Hood CI. Steroid therapy for pneumonitis induced in rabbits by aspiration of foodstuff. *Anesthesiology* 1979:51:11.
52. Holdsworth JD, Furness RMB, Roulston RF. A comparison of apomorphine and stomach tubes for emptying the stomach before general anesthesia in obstetrics. *Br J Anaesth* 1974;46:526–529.
53. Howard FA, Sharp DS. Effect of metoclopramide on gastric emptying during labour. *BMJ* 1973;1:446.
54. Cohen SE, Jasson J, Talafre ML. Does metoclopramide decrease gastric volume in Caesarean section patients? *Anesthesiology* 1984;61:604.
55. Capan LM, Rosenberg AD, Carni A. Effect of cimetidine and meto-

clopramide combination on gastric acidity: effectiveness at the time of induction of anesthesia. *Can J Anaesth* 1981;j 28:29.
56. Manchikanti L, Colliver JA, Marrero T. Ranitidine and metoclopramide for prophylaxis of aspiration pneumonitis in elective surgery. *Anesth Analg* 1984;63:903.
57. Snow RG, Nunn JF. Induction of anesthesia in the foot down position for patients with full stomach. *Br J Anaesth* 1959;31:493–497.
58. Salem MR. Anesthetic management of patients with full stomach. *Anesth Analg* 1970;49:47.
59. Sellick BA. Cricoid pressure to control regurgitation of stomach contents during induction of anesthesia. *Lancet* 1961;2:404.
60. Salem MR, Heyman JH, Livschultz v, Mehdi M. Cephalad displacement of the larynx facilitates tracheal intubation. *Anesthesiology* 1987;67:3.
61. Sellick BA. Rupture of the esophagus during cricoid pressure. *Anaesthesia* 1982;37:213.
62. Salem MR, Joseph NJ, Hayman HJ. Cricoid compression is effective in obliterating the esophageal lumen in the presence of nasogastric tube. *Anesthesiology* 1985;63:443–446.
63. Gooding JM, Corssen G. Effect of etomidate on the cardiovascular system. *Anesth Analg* 1977;56:717.
64. Kettler D, Sonntag H, Donath U. Cardiovascular hemodynamics by etomidate. *Anaesthetist* 1974;23:116.
65. Arms RA. Morbidity and mortality in pulmonary aspiration. *Chest* 1974;65:136.
66. Wynne JW, Modell JH. respiratory aspiration of stomach contents. *Ann Intern Med* 1977;87:466–474.
67. Hamelberg W, Bosomworth PP. Aspiration pneumonitis, an experimental study and clinical observations. *Anesth Analg* 1964;43:669–676.
68. Wynne JW, Raynolds TC, Hood CI. Steroid therapy for pneumonitis induced in rabbits by aspiration of food stuff. *Anesthesiology* 1979; 51:11–19.
69. Downs JB, Chapman RL, Modell JH. An evaluation of steroid therapy in aspiration pneumonitis. *Anesthesiology* 1974;40:129–135.
70. Linda JF, Warrian WG, Wankling WJ. Responses of the gastroesophageal junctional zone to increases in abdominal pressure. *Can J Surg* 1966;9:32.

Airway Management, edited by
L.H. Hanowell, M.D. and R.J. Waldron, M.D.,
Lippincott-Raven Publishers, Philadelphia © 1996.

CHAPTER 8

Application of the ASA Difficult Airway Algorithm

William C. Wilson

INTRODUCTION

Maintenance of adequate gas exchange is the fundamental responsibility of the anesthesiologist. Failure to maintain a patent airway for more than a few minutes can lead to brain injury or death and constitutes the single most common cause of anesthesia-related morbidity and mortality (1). The ASA (American Society of Anesthesiologists) difficult airway algorithm was developed by a task force of academic clinicians with the goal of reducing airway-related catastrophes (2).

Prior to discussing the ASA difficult airway algorithm in detail, the "difficult airway" will be defined and described. Next, an overview of the algorithm will be pursued, and finally, each of the critical decision-tree components will be amplified and discussed in greater detail.

DEFINING THE DIFFICULT AIRWAY

Several outstanding reviews of the anesthetic implications of the difficult airway exist (3,4). However, all of these reviews suffer from a wide disparity in the operational definition of difficult airway. Benumof has recently reviewed the difficult airway and the ASA difficult airway algorithm (5). The review by Benumof is recommended because it is current and has direct applicability to patients in the operating room and intensive care unit and to posttraumatic patients.

It must be recognized that airway difficulty can occur during mask ventilation or during endotracheal intubation. The two are not synonymous, and indeed, some patients who may be difficult to mask ventilate (for example, those with mandibular fractures) may actually be quite easy to intubate. Maintenance of gas exchange utilizing mask ventilation can range from zero degree of difficulty to infinite (Fig. 1). Zero degree of difficulty during ventilation with a face mask means that the patient breathes spontaneously and maintains a patent airway without any external adjunctive intervention. There is a continuum of increasing difficulty in maintaining airway patency, beginning with mask ventilation, as increasingly more aggressive airway manipulations are required to achieve gas exchange. Not only does Figure 1 serve as a conceptual framework for the definition of airway difficulty with mask ventilation, it also serves as a reminder of the progressive steps that

W. C. Wilson: Department of Critical Care Medicine and Cardiothoracic Anesthesiology, University of California, San Diego Medical Center, San Diego, California 92103.

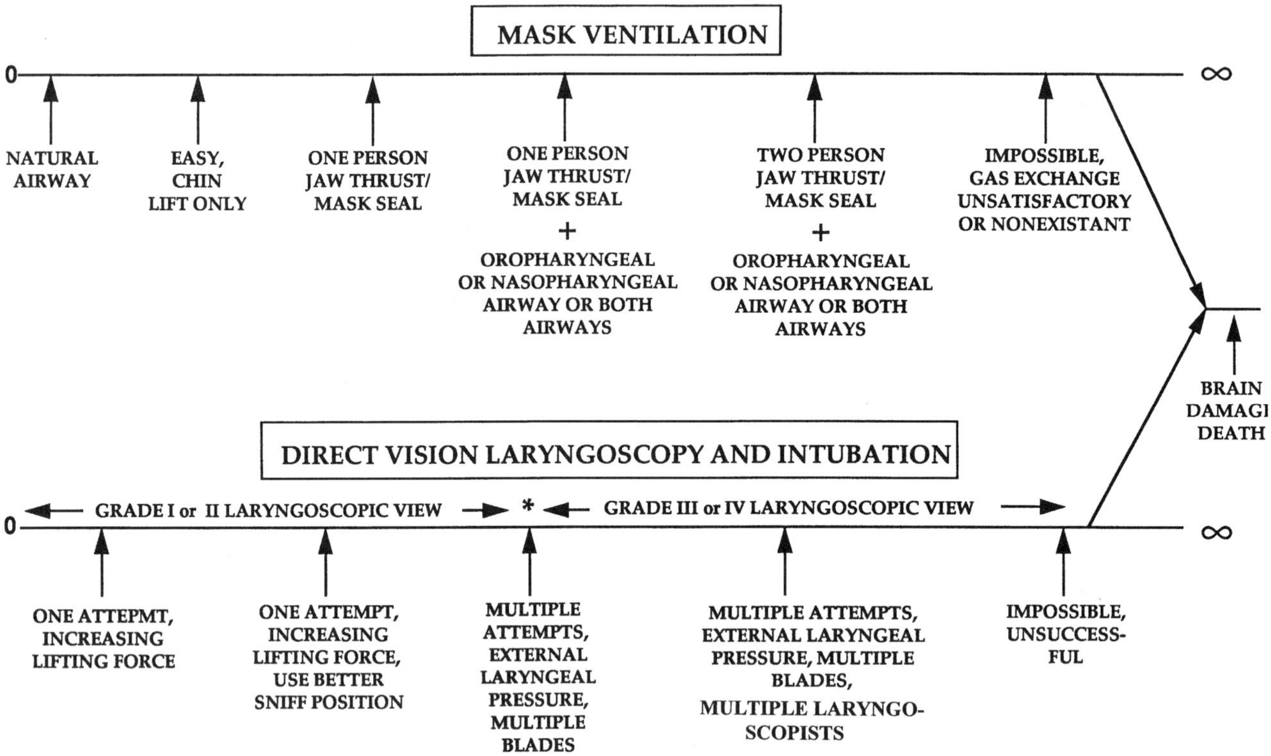

FIG. 1. Definition of a difficult airway. The airway refers to either the natural airway with mask ventilation or endotracheal intubation using rigid, direct-vision laryngoscopy. The degree of difficulty for both mask ventilation (*top*) and direct-vision laryngoscopy (*bottom*) ranges from easy (zero degree of difficulty) to difficult/impossible (infinite degree of difficulty). The amount of difficulty can vary in the same patient with different anesthesiologists using various techniques and having unequal experience. The grade of laryngoscopic view refers to Fig. 2. Modified from Benumof (5).

can be utilized to improve mask ventilation and gas exchange. These steps begin with 1) *chin lift*, proceed to 2) *chin lift with jaw thrust*, advance further to 3) *use of adjunctive airway devices* (oropharyngeal and nasopharyngeal airways), and continue further with all the aforementioned interventions plus 4) *assistance of another person* (one person maintaining a tight mask fit and two-handed jaw thrust, the other person squeezing the gas reservoir bag). If these maneuvers are unsuccessful, the consequence may be the inability to maintain gas exchange.

Difficulty of intubation using direct laryngoscopy also proceeds along a similar continuum from easy to very difficult/impossible (Fig. 1). Difficult intubation can be defined as multiple attempts to intubate with multiple maneuvers that include external laryngeal pressure, use of multiple laryngoscope blades, and attempts by multiple endoscopists.

The best definition of difficult intubation for documentation in the medical record (to inform future care providers of a previous difficult intubation) or for research purposes involves the grading of laryngoscopic views (Fig. 2). Grade I is visualization of the entire laryngeal aperture; grade IV is visualization of only the soft palate; grades II and III are intermediate views (3).

Difficult intubation correlates well with a grade III or IV laryngoscopic view in the vast majority of patients (3,6). However, there are some relatively uncommon situations that provide exceptions to this rule. First, the skill of the endoscopist in manipulating the patient's endotracheal tube and choosing the proper laryngoscope blade may have a significant effect on the grade visualized. Second, a grade III laryngoscopic view has been described differently by different investigators (3,6). Third, the blade used for laryngoscopy affects the grade applied. For example, a long floppy epiglottis may yield a high-grade view (III or IV) when one blade is used, but a relatively low-grade view (I or II) with another blade. Finally, pathologic conditions such as laryngeal webs or tumors may dissociate the laryngoscopic view from the actual difficulty of tracheal intubation. Despite these considerations, the laryngoscopic grading system of Cormack and Lehane is used by most authors to define laryngoscopic views during endotracheal intubation (3).

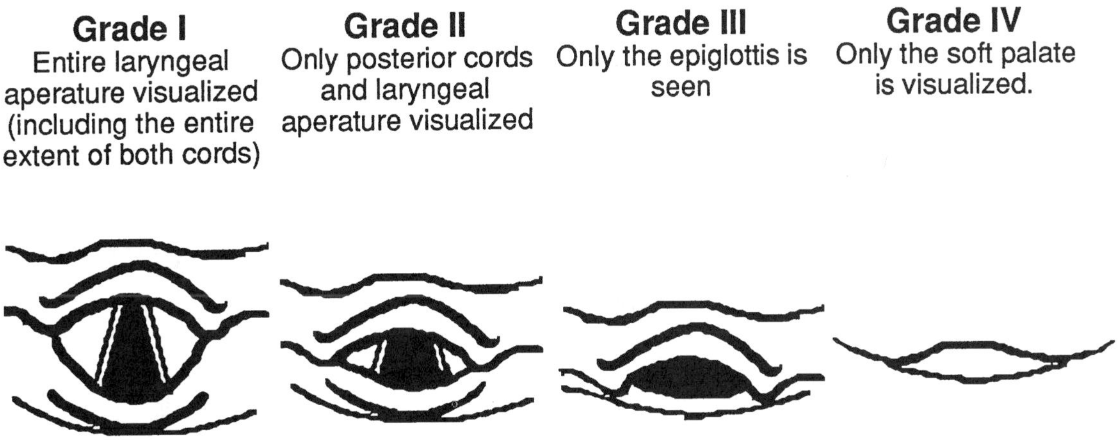

FIG. 2. The four grades of laryngoscopic view. The grading of laryngoscopic view is based on the anatomic features visualized during direct laryngoscopy. Modified from Cormak and Lehane (3).

OVERVIEW OF THE ASA DIFFICULT AIRWAY ALGORITHM

Application of the ASA difficult airway algorithm assumes that a fully trained and board-certified anesthesiologist is attempting to maintain airway patency at all times.

The ASA difficult airway algorithm (Fig. 3) begins with *recognition* of airway difficulty. When confronted with buckteeth, micrognathia, a massive fungating neck abscess, and respiratory stridor, the physician can clearly tell that the patient will be a difficult intubation. However, there may be more subtle anatomic or pathologic causes of airway difficulty that can go unrecognized with a hasty preoperative evaluation. Missed signs of a difficult airway can be minimized if one looks carefully for pathologic or anatomic abnormalities. Once the patient is recognized to have a difficult airway, the clinician should plan to *secure the airway awake.*

Awake Limb of the ASA Difficult Airway Algorithm

The ASA difficult airway algorithm does not endorse any particular awake technique. However, it does emphasize that the patient must be *properly prepared.* If the awake intubation technique fails, the physician must determine whether alternative maneuvers will improve the likelihood of success, and these should be undertaken (more choices are available if the patient is still spontaneously ventilating). Once the patient's trachea is intubated, having successfully utilized an awake technique, one must *confirm endotracheal tube position* with determination of end-tidal carbon dioxide or other tests. If subsequent *extubation* of the trachea is to be performed and the circumstances that caused the difficult airway are still present, a jet stylet should be inserted through the endotracheal tube and the endotracheal tube removed over the stylet. The stylet provides a ready means of ventilation and oxygenation, pending replacement of the endotracheal tube over the stylet, if the patient does not have a sufficient airway.

If awake intubation techniques lead to failure of intubation despite manipulations that might improve intubating conditions, then a tracheostomy or a cricothyroidotomy must be considered. If proper equipment or personnel are not available, one should consider stopping, maintaining spontaneous ventilation, allowing the patient to recover from topicalization (topical local anesthesia) or sedative medications, and resuming management later with a better plan (other equipment and/or personnel). If at any time during attempts at awake intubation the patient cannot be ventilated by face mask and intubation is unsuccessful, transtracheal jet ventilation or a surgical airway must be considered.

Anesthetized Limb of the ASA Difficult Airway Algorithm

If the patient is anesthetized with an unrecognized difficult airway, or if the patient is noted to have possible airway difficulty but is uncooperative or unstable, then the physician moves down the anesthetized limb of the difficult airway algorithm. *Preparation* with tools necessary for intubation and proper patient positioning are critical in order to improve chances of a successful intubation. Once the patient is anesthetized or rendered apneic or presents comatose and the trachea cannot be intubated, one should *call for help* and *ensure mask ventilation.*

Provided that mask ventilation is adequate, one may proceed to any number of techniques that would allow for

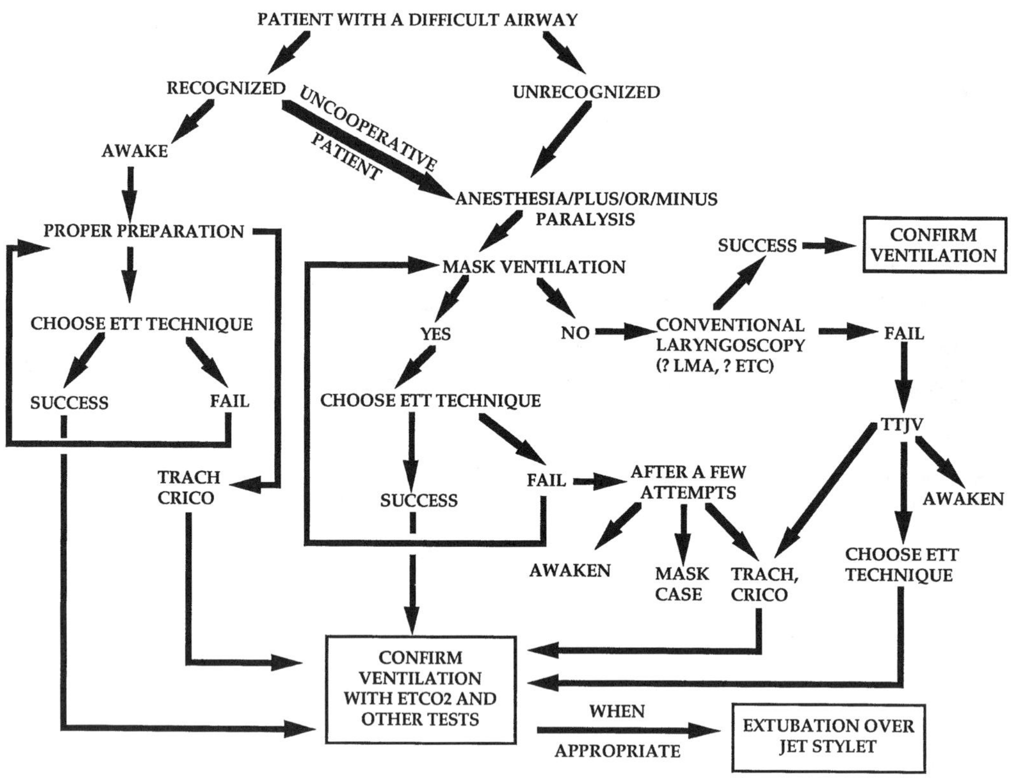

FIG. 3. The ASA difficult airway algorithm. This provides airway management guidelines that emphasize maintaining airway patency at all times, recognizing airway difficulty, utilizing awake techniques to secure the airway when airway difficulty is anticipated, confirming ventilation following attainment of a secure airway, and extubating the trachea in patients with a known difficult airway over a jet stylet. Modified from Benumof (5).

endotracheal intubations (some allow for continuous ventilation during airway manipulations and others require an interruption of mask ventilation).

Positive-pressure ventilation can be *continuously maintained* while a definitive airway is obtained using an anesthesia mask with self-sealing diaphragm and an oral airway intubating device. A fiberoptic bronchoscope can be preloaded with an endotracheal tube. The fiberoptic bronchoscope can be passed through the self-sealing diaphragm of the airway intubating mask, and then through an oral intubating airway and into the trachea while ventilation is maintained the entire time.

Alternatively, other devices and techniques that require a *cessation of mask ventilation* (at least temporarily) can be employed, such as new laryngoscopy/retraction blades with illuminating stylets, retrograde techniques, and light wands.

Once the trachea is intubated, *correct position of the endotracheal tube must be confirmed* with end-tidal carbon dioxide measurement or other techniques. It should be remembered that a difficult intubation is likely to be a difficult extubation. In such cases, it may be prudent to perform extubation of the trachea using a jet stylet if the condition(s) that caused intubation difficulties still persists.

However, if the patient's trachea still cannot be intubated using these techniques or if ventilation cannot be maintained, the use of *three recently introduced airway-manipulation devices* should be considered:

1. The laryngeal mask
2. The esophageal-tracheal Combitube
3. Transtracheal jet ventilation apparatus

Transtracheal jet ventilation (TTJV) should be considered in any patient at any time if other manipulations are failing and gas exchange is not being maintained (Chapters 13, 14, and 17).

Finally, if *transtracheal jet ventilation* is unsuccessful, then one should proceed to an emergency cricothyroidotomy. If TTJV is successful, then one may proceed to other intubation techniques, such as fiberoptic bronchoscopy or retrograde intubation, while maintaining gas exchange through the TTJV catheter. No matter what technique has been used to introduce an endotracheal tube into the trachea, confirmation of correct placement with end-tidal carbon dioxide or other tests must be performed.

MAJOR DECISION-TREE COMPONENTS OF THE ASA DIFFICULT AIRWAY ALGORITHM

Several critical decision-tree elements are present in the ASA difficult airway algorithm, including the following:

Recognition of the difficult airway
Preparation of the patient for airway manipulations
Awake techniques
Techniques for the anesthetized patient with a difficult airway
Techniques for the patient who cannot be ventilated or intubated
Verification of endotracheal tube position
Extubation or tube change for the patient with a known difficult airway

Recognition of the Difficult Airway

Prior to attempting endotracheal intubation, the clinician should assess the patient's airway from the viewpoint of technical ease of ventilation/intubation.

Pathologic Causes of the Difficult Airway (Typically Apparent)

Several *pathologic* causes of airway difficulty are known to cause *difficulty with mask ventilation*, e.g., mandibular fractures, thick beard, massive jaw, lack of teeth, and large tongue (macroglossia). None of these situations, except for macroglossia, are associated with *difficulty of intubation*. Indeed, mandibular fractures not involving the temporomandibular joint can actually make intubation easier. Pathologic factors associated with difficult intubation include congenital facial and upper airway deformities, maxillary facial airway trauma, and the requirement for cervical spine immobility. Most of the *pathologic* causes of airway difficulty are readily apparent and thus are typically recognized prior to induction of anesthesia. However, *anatomic* variations in patients without other *obvious* risk factors may be subtle. Patients who present with unrecognized anatomically challenging airways and then become anesthetized comprise a significant group of anesthesia-related airway catastrophes (brain damage and death).

TABLE 1. *Predictors of difficult intubation*

Obesity (> 110 kg)
Buckteeth
Large tongue
Decreased jaw movement
Decreased head extension or neck flexion
Receding mandible or anterior larynx

Anatomic Characteristics That Impair Direct Laryngoscopy

These characteristics, listed in Table 1, include obesity (weight over 110 kg); short, stout neck; buckteeth; large tongue; decreased jaw movement; decreased head and neck movement; and receding mandible. In the fully extended adult neck, if the distance between the mandible and the upper border of thyroid cartilage is less than 6.0 cm, visualization of the vocal cords is predictably difficult (7).

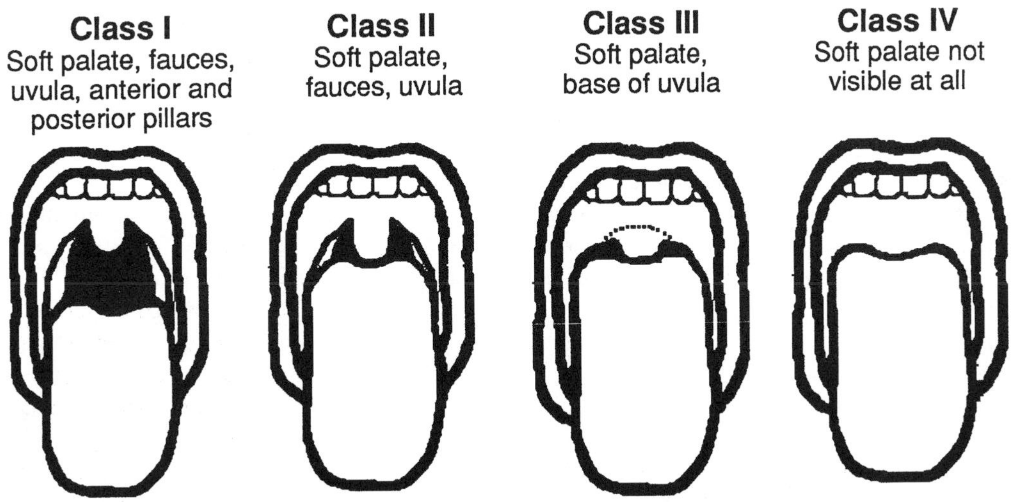

FIG. 4. Mallampati classification. Classification of the upper airway based on anatomic features seen with the mouth open, directly relating tongue to pharyngeal size. Modified from Mallampati et al. (8).

Three Easily Performed, Risk-Free Airway-Evaluation Tests

In the last 10 years, numerous investigators have invested their efforts to determine anatomic characteristics that correlate with difficult intubation. Recently, three airway-assessment methods have emerged as highly predictive indicators of intubation difficulty.

1. Relative tongue-pharyngeal size (Mallampati class). The size of the tongue in relation to the size of the oral cavity is an important factor (Fig. 4) (8). Lewis et al. (9) have recently demonstrated that the Mallampati classification is more predictive and easier to perform if the patient assumes the sitting position, holds the head in full extension, protrudes the tongue, and phonates.
2. Mandibular space. The space anterior to the larynx (hyomental or thyromental distance) is another factor. A hyomental distance greater than 6 cm suggests that direct laryngoscopy will be relatively easy (10).
3. Atlanto-occipital joint extension. Thirty-five degrees of extension are normally possible at the atlanto-occipital joint. Bellhouse and Dore (11) have demonstrated that atlanto-occipital joint extension can be easily measured clinically and is highly predictive of ease of intubation.

When these three tests are used in the same patient, the predictive power becomes quite substantial. In cases of trauma (with suspected cervical spine injury), the spine cannot be moved. Such patients are analogous to those with little or no atlanto-occipital extension. Luckily, mandibular space measurement and Mallampati classification are very strong predictors of intubation ease. When combined with a low Mallampati classification, a hyomental distance greater than 6 cm becomes a strong predictor of easy intubation (12,13).

Proper Preparation

Requirements for Safe Airway Management

Regardless of the anticipated level of airway difficulty, the following are always necessary for safe intubation: 1) oxygen, 2) positive-pressure bag-mask ventilation capability and airway equipment, 3) suction, 4) functioning intravenous line, 5) vasopressors, 6) patient preparation and positioning, 7) an alternate plan, and 8) availability of extra help (see Chapter 27).

Awake Technique Preparation

If a blind nasal or fiberoptic intubation is planned, the patient should be psychologically prepared, and the clinician must ensure that the nasopharynx and oropharynx are properly anesthetized with topically applied local agents.

Positioning for General Anesthesia and Rigid Direct Laryngoscopy

The sniffing position (forward flexion of the neck on chest and atlanto-occipital extension) is the optimal position for direct laryngoscopy and endotracheal intubation. This aligns the oropharyngeal, laryngeal, and tracheal axes.

Awake Techniques

Whenever there is concern that the patient has a difficult airway, the airway should be secured awake. After deciding to intubate the trachea using an awake technique, the anesthesiologist must select a technique with which he or she is familiar and that is clinically appropriate. Numerous techniques are available, including the following:

1. Direct laryngoscopy after administration of topical anesthesia
2. Flexible fiberoptic (bronchoscopic) intubation using either a nasal or oral route
3. Retrograde intubation, light wands, or combinations of the fiberoptic, retrograde, and direct laryngoscopic techniques

These techniques are described in much greater detail in other chapters of this textbook (Chapters 15–18).

The technique chosen is not as important as the anesthesiologist's experience and judgment regarding suitability, given the patient's difficult airway circumstances. Indeed, the ASA algorithm does not endorse any particular airway technique. Regardless of the technique chosen, the patient must be mentally and physically prepared for an awake technique, and the physician must ensure that oxygen saturation is maintained throughout the procedure.

Techniques for the Anesthetized Patient with a Difficult Airway (Recognized or Not)

Conditions Associated with an Anesthetized Patient with a Difficult Airway

There are three situations in which an anesthesiologist is confronted with the need to intubate the trachea of an unconscious or anesthetized patient with a difficult airway. The first occurs when the anesthesiologist has failed to recognize airway difficulty in preoperative evaluation prior to induction of anesthesia. The second is patient unconsciousness prior to assessment by an anesthesiologist (trauma, drug overdose, or coma of medical etiology). The last is hemodynamic instability (e.g., following trauma or other catastrophe) or patient refusal to cooperate with an awake intubation (a child, a mentally retarded adult, a combative patient). All these conditions are handled by the anesthetized limb of the ASA difficult airway algorithm. In the last situation (uncooperative patient), preoperative assessment should have identified factors that might make intubation of the trachea difficult, and the anesthesiologist should consider using a technique that *maintains spontaneous ventilation* despite the need for anesthesia.

Four Steps to Improve Success at Intubation with Rigid Direct Laryngoscopy

When confronted with the anesthetized patient whose airway is difficult, one proceeds down the anesthetized limb of the ASA algorithm as described above. Additionally, the anesthesiologist should take four steps, as suggested by Benumof (14), to optimize or improve laryngoscopic view.

Step 1: Proper sniff position should be ensured. Proper sniff position is best appreciated from the lateral view of the patient and sometimes requires more than elevating the head, especially in a very obese patient. Elevating and supporting the shoulders will optimize positioning of the very obese patient. This maneuver creates room for extension of the head, in addition to elevating the head.

Step 2: Optimal external laryngeal pressure should be used to improve laryngoscopic view. Optimal external laryngeal pressure is not analogous to cricoid pressure. (The cricoid cartilage is 2 to 3 cm caudad to the larynx.) Optimal external laryngeal pressure should be determined by having the laryngoscopist move the larynx with the right hand while holding the laryngoscope in the left hand. The optimal position may be forward, backward, up, down, left, or right from the initial position. Once optimal position is determined, the laryngoscopist should have a helper reproduce the proper pressure under guidance of the laryngoscopist. Then the laryngoscopist can perform intubation.

Step 3: The choice of muscle relaxant may be important. If it is feasible to wake the patient and no muscle relaxant has been given (not possible in the comatose or severely traumatized patient), then no muscle relaxant should be given. The airway should be maintained, and the patient should be allowed to emerge from anesthesia so that an alternate plan for airway management can be developed. If succinylcholine has been given and ventilation can be maintained, awakening the patient is still a viable option. However, in situations in which one must proceed and awakening the patient is not an option, then a nondepolarizing neuromuscular blocker such as vecuronium should be considered to optimize relaxation of tongue and jaw muscles.

Step 4: Finally, changing blades may occasionally be helpful. The Macintosh blade is useful for patients with large, floppy tongues, whereas a straight Miller blade may be superior when laryngoscopy shows a long, floppy, and posteriorly directed epiglottis. The Miller blade may also be helpful for intubation of the patient with a receding chin or anterior larynx (defined as a hyomental distance of less than 6 cm).

Most importantly, one should ensure to as great a degree as possible that the first attempt at laryngoscopy is the best attempt when confronted by the anesthetized patient with a difficult airway.

Techniques for the Patient Who Cannot Be Ventilated or Intubated

In some cases, it may be impossible either to ventilate the lungs by mask or to intubate the trachea *despite* the use of multiple awake or anesthetized laryngoscopic techniques. Under these circumstances, the anesthesiologist must proceed to an alternate form of airway manipulation, such as a surgical airway. Otherwise, brain injury and death rapidly ensue.

Three Quick, Low-Risk, Emergency Airway Techniques

Recently, three alternative ventilation methods have been described that can be instituted blindly and quickly and that appear to have a low risk-to-benefit ratio. These are the esophageal-tracheal Combitube (ETC), laryngeal mask airway (LMA), and transtracheal jet ventilation (TTJV). When confronted with the patient who cannot be ventilated or intubated, the physician should consider these alternative ventilation methods. Once ventilation is established with one of these methods, other, more time-consuming techniques can be performed. These include the use of a wire for retrograde intubation or a fiberoptic bronchoscope for oral or nasotracheal intubation.

Precautions (Supraglottic Solutions Should Not Be Used for Subglottic Airway Problems)

One must also bear in mind that if the reason for failure to ventilate is a laryngeal or sublaryngeal problem (i.e., laryngeal fracture), then the LMA and ETC are contraindicated, as they are both supralaryngeal airway solutions. TTJV is an extremely effective means of providing oxygen in these settings, and can provide adequate ventilation for 30 to 40 minutes (15).

Confirmation of Correct Endotracheal Tube Placement

Verification of endotracheal tube position and confirmation of ventilation must occur following intubation in the operating room, or immediately after the previously intubated patient arrives from the field.

The Importance of Recognition

Esophageal intubation is a problem of recognition, not of prevention. Indeed, unrecognized esophageal intubation has been identified as a significant contributor to cardiac arrests attributed solely to anesthesia (16). Thus, immediately after the trachea is intubated, the position of the endotracheal tube must be verified.

Few esophageal intubation detection techniques are error-free. Birmingham et al. (17) have elucidated the sources of error with most clinical esophageal intubation detection maneuvers, including chest movement, chest and epigastric auscultation, balloting the balloon in the suprasternal notch, tube condensation, and reservoir bag compliance.

Direct Confirmation

Direct vision of the endotracheal tube passing through the cords is considered "the gold standard." The only foolproof techniques for confirming tracheal position are seeing the tube pass through the cords, or looking through the endotracheal tube into the trachea with a fiberoptic bronchoscope and visualizing the tracheal rings.

Other Techniques

Two indirect methods of determining endotracheal tube position are useful for patients with unconfirmed endotracheal position: end-tidal carbon dioxide measurement and the esophageal detector device.

End-tidal Carbon Dioxide Measurement

Carbon dioxide detection devices are effective in determining endotracheal vs. esophageal intubation. However, in circumstances of cardiopulmonary arrest with little or no cardiac output, very little carbon dioxide will be detected. Similarly, patients with carbon dioxide in their stomach from sodium bicarbonate or soft drinks can give a false-positive test (18). Provided the patient has a blood pressure, the presence of carbon dioxide is a useful test. Additionally, carbon dioxide detection devices are now available in hand-sized colorimetric versions; these are accurate and can be used to detect esophageal intubation. These devices can also quantify the efficacy of cardiopulmonary resuscitation in the emergency room and other locations where an infrared carbon dioxide analyzer may not be present (19).

The Esophageal Detector Device

Recently, an esophageal detector (comprised of an Ellicks evacuator applied to the supposedly "tracheal" tube) has proved to be highly sensitive and specific for esophageal detection (20). If the tube is in the esophagus, the deflated bulb fails to expand completely because suction created by bulb expansion collapses the esophageal walls, obstructing the tube. On the other hand, a tracheally placed tube allows air to flow out of the lungs and reinflate the bulb. (This device is illustrated in Chapter 21.)

Indication of Esophageal Intubation by Delayed Oxygen-Hemoglobin Desaturation

The problem of esophageal intubation is further compounded by the fact that following pre-oxygenation, the patient may not manifest oxygen-hemoglobin desaturation (a decline in percent saturation detected by pulse oximetry) for as long as 10 minutes after intubation. Thus, any cyanosis or desaturation that occurs in this time frame should be considered an indication of esophageal intubation until proved otherwise by immediate verification of endotracheal tube position.

Extubation or Endotracheal Tube Change of the Difficult Airway

Extubation of the trachea or tube change in the patient with a difficult airway should be considered a high-risk endeavor.

Indications

Indications for *extubation* of the patient with a known difficult airway include: (1) that the patient has been weaned from mechanical ventilation, (2) the patient is awake, (3) the patient can protect his or her airway (intact gag response), and (4) pathologic airway problems have resolved.

There are four main reasons for an endotracheal tube change:

1. The tube is malfunctioning (is obstructed, or has an air leak from a ruptured cuff).
2. A larger tube is needed (especially during weaning).
3. A change from a single-lumen tube to a double-lumen tube is required secondary to a major pulmonary vascular or airway injury following trauma.
4. Replacement of a double-lumen tube with a single-lumen tube is required at the end of an anesthetic case.

The techniques described below are applicable to endotracheal tube changes in any ventilator-dependent patient in the operating room or the intensive care unit.

Technique for Extubation

Step 1: Place patient on 100% oxygen.

Step 2: Suction the oropharyngeal and nasopharyngeal area as well as the endotracheal tube.

Step 3: Deflate the balloon cuff of the endotracheal tube, occlude the endotracheal tube, and determine if the patient can exhale air out of the lungs and trachea around the obstructed endotracheal tube. If no air flows out, it is unlikely that the patient is ready for tracheal extubation. The patient's endotracheal tube should be reconnected to the ventilator and the source of airway obstruction determined using a fiberoptic bronchoscope. If there is a large audible air flow out of the trachea alongside the obstructed endotracheal tube, there is a high likelihood that periglottic swelling will not be a deterrent to extubation, and one can advance to step 4.

Step 4: Place a jet stylet (a fiberoptic bronchoscope is preferably used) through the endotracheal tube, deflate the balloon cuff, and remove the endotracheal tube over the translaryngeal jet stylet.

Step 5: If no difficulty with ventilation is encountered with the jet stylet still through the cords, then the jet stylet may be removed. However, if ventilation becomes labored, reinsert the endotracheal tube into the trachea over the jet stylet.

Step 6: Once the tube is replaced through the cords, verification of endotracheal tube position should be performed.

Technique for Endotracheal Tube Change in the Ventilator-Dependent Patient Without Expected Airway Difficulty

These reintubations can be challenging because of the presence of airway edema and hypoxemia.

Step 1: The patient is placed on 100% oxygen.

Step 2: A nondepolarizing neuromuscular blocker is administered, neuromuscular blockade is documented with a twitch monitor, and adequate anesthesia is ensured.

Step 3: The oropharynx and the endotracheal tube are thoroughly suctioned.

Step 4: Direct laryngoscopy is performed with the original endotracheal tube in place. If the glottis is easily visualized and cords and surrounding structures are normal in appearance, the original endotracheal tube is removed, and a styleted replacement endotracheal tube is passed through the cords under direct vision.

Step 5: If direct laryngoscopy fails to present an adequate view of the glottis, or if there is significant periglottic swelling (and the tube absolutely must be changed), the endotracheal tube should be changed over a jet stylet endotracheal tube changer as described by Bedger and Chang (21) and outlined below.

Technique for Endotracheal Tube Change in the Ventilator-Dependent Patient with Known Difficult Airway

Patients with known difficult airways (swollen glottis, cervical spine injury) should have tracheal extubation over a jet stylet (preferably a fiberoptic bronchoscope). Ventilator-dependent patients who require a tube change pose a special challenge; all such cases warrant a tube change over a jet stylet.

Steps 1–3: As above (technique for tube change in ventilator-dependent patient without expected airway difficulty).

Step 4: A fiberoptic elbow adapter with self-sealing diaphragm is placed between the ventilator circuit and the existing endotracheal tube.

Step 5: A tube exchanger of appropriate size is placed through the self-sealing diaphragm of the fiberoptic elbow adapter and down through the existing endotracheal tube to the carina. Apparatus for possible jet ventilation and appropriate connectors should be immediately available (at the bedside) when this technique is performed. (Several varieties of tube exchangers are available. These are essentially stylets that permit jet ventilation.)

Step 6: The existing endotracheal tube is removed over the tube changer, and the replacement tube is then inserted over the tube changer. The endotracheal tube may occasionally hang up at the cords (be difficult to pass through the vocal cords) with this maneuver. However, rotation of the endotracheal tube at the cords usually overcomes this problem. If difficulty placing the new tube persists, ventilation can be performed using the jet stylet by the method described by Goskowicz et al. (22).

Step 7: Next, the fiberoptic elbow with self-sealing diaphragm is slid over the tube changer and placed on the replacement endotracheal tube, allowing for the assessment of end-tidal carbon dioxide samples. Once the replacement tube is documented to be in the trachea by this means, the tube exchanger is withdrawn from the replacement tube and out of the self-sealing diaphragm.

Step 8: Final verification using a fiberoptic bronchoscope should always be encouraged, especially after placement of a double-lumen endotracheal tube.

SUMMARY

After assessment of the airway and evaluation of the patient's underlying pathologic condition, the physician must devise a plan for intubation. The plan for securing the airway must minimize the risks of airway loss, aspiration, and hemodynamic compromise. The clinician must reorganize the priority list as the patient's condition changes. If there is any concern that the patient's airway will be difficult, an awake technique with spontaneous ventilation should be chosen. Alternative plans must be thought out beforehand and be physically ready to go. Finally, tracheal extubation of a patient with a difficult airway over a jet stylet (preferably a fiberoptic bronchoscope) allows for a controlled and reversible withdrawal from the airway (because ventilation and reintubation are possible at any time).

REFERENCES

1. Caplan RA, Posner KL, Ward RJ, et al. Adverse respiratory events in anesthesia: a closed claim analysis. *Anesthesiology* 1990;72:828.
2. Meeting of American Society of Anesthesiologists Difficult Airway Task Force Members (J Benumof, M Bishop, C Blitt, R Caplan, F Cheney, T Davidson, D Gaba, E Pierce) on November 2, 1990, in San Francisco.
3. Cormack RS, Lehane J. Difficult tracheal intubation in obstetrics. *Anaesthesia* 1984;39:1105.
4. McIntyre JRW. The difficult intubation. *Can J Anaesth* 1987;34:204.
5. Benumof JL. Management of the difficult airway. *Anesthesiology* 1991;75:1087.
6. Samsoon GLT, Young JRB. Difficult tracheal intubation: a retrospective study. *Anaesthesia* 1987;42:487.
7. Wilson ME, Spiegelhalter D, Robertson JA, et al. Predicting difficult intubation. *Br J Anaesth* 1988;61:211.
8. Mallampati SR, Gatt SP, Gugino LD, et al. A clinical sign to predict difficult tracheal intubation: a prospective study. *Can J Anaesth* 1985; 32:429.
9. Lewis M, Keramati S, Benumof JL, et al. What is the best way to determine oropharyngeal classification and mandibular space length to predict difficult laryngoscopy? *Anesthesiology* 1994;81:69.
10. Finucane BT, Santora AH. Evaluation of the airway prior to intubation. *Principles of Airway Management.* Philadelphia: FA Norris; 1988:69.
11. Bellhouse CP, Dore C. Criteria for estimating likelihood of difficult intubation with the Macintosh laryngoscope. *Anaesth Intensive Care* 1988;16:329.
12. Frerk CM. Predicting difficult intubation. *Anaesthesia* 1991;46:1005.
13. Rose KD, Cohen MM. The airway: problems and predictions in 18,500 patients. *Can J Anaesth* 1994;41:372.
14. Benumof JL. Difficult laryngoscopy: obtaining the best view. *Can J Anaesth* 1994;41:361.
15. Benumof JL, Scheller MS. The importance of transtracheal jet ventilation in the management of the difficult airway. *Anesthesiology* 1989;71:769.
16. Keenan RL, Boyan CP. Cardiac arrest due to anesthesia: a study of incidence and causes. *JAMA* 1985;253:2373.
17. Birmingham PK, Cheney FW, Ward RJ. Esophageal intubation. *Anesth Analg* 1986;65:886.
18. Sum Ping ST, Mehta MP, Symreng T. Reliability of capnography in identifying esophageal intubation with carbonated beverage or antacid in the stomach. *Anesth Analg* 1992;74:333.
19. Ornato JP, Shipley JB, Racht EM, et al. Multicenter study of a portable hand held colorometeric end-tidal carbon dioxide detection device. *Ann Emerg Med* 1992;21:518.
20. Williams KN, Nunn JF. The esophageal detector device. *Anaesthesia* 1989;44:412.
21. Bedger RC, Chang JL. A jet stylet catheter for difficult airway management. *Anesthesiology* 1987;66:221.
22. Goskowicz R, Gaughn S, Benumof JL, Ozaki GT. It is not necessary to remove a jet stylet in order to determine tracheal tube location. *J Clin Anesth* 1992;4:42.

PART III

Pharmacology

Airway Management, edited by
L.H. Hanowell, M.D. and R.J. Waldron, M.D.,
Lippincott-Raven Publishers, Philadelphia © 1996.

CHAPTER 9

Nonopiate Intravenous Anesthetic Agents

Jonathan L. Howes, Richard J. Waldron, and Dennis L. Fung

INTRODUCTION

Anesthesia dates back to ancient times when civilizations such as the Egyptians and the Incas used opium poppies, coca leaves, and mandrake roots—or even went to the extremes of bleeding their patients, almost to unconsciousness—before operating. Dioscorides, a Greek philosopher, is reported to have first used the term *anesthesia* to describe the effects of the mandrake root. Other definitions, dating from the eighteenth century, describe a "defect of sensation" and a "privation of the senses." The sleeplike state that enables painless surgery to be performed was described by Oliver Wendell Holmes in 1846.

The origins of intravenous anesthesia began after the development of the hypodermic needle in 1855 by Alexander Wood. Agents that were initially used included chloral hydrate in 1872, intravenous chloroform and ether in 1909, and morphine and scopolamine in 1916. Barbiturates, originally synthesized in 1903 by Fischer and von Mering, gained popularity as induction agents. Development continued with hexobarbital in 1927 and with thiopentone in 1934, resulting in barbiturates becoming the most commonly used agents for the induction of anesthesia. Methohexitone, first used in 1957, is the only other barbiturate currently used for anesthetic induction. The benzodiazepines were introduced in subsequent years and have found widespread applications in anesthesia, in particular, diazepam (1959) and midazo-

J.L. Howes: Sir Humphry Davy Department of Anaesthesia, Bristol Royal Infirmary, Bristol, United Kingdom BS2 8HW.
R. J. Waldron: Department of Anaesthetic Services, Royal Hobart Hospital; and University of Tasmania, Hobart, Tasmania, Australia, 7001.
D. L. Fung: Department of Anesthesiology, University of California, Davis School of Medicine, Sacramento, California 95817.

lam (1976). Ketamine and etomidate were introduced in 1970 and 1972, respectively, and the most recent nonopiate intravenous anesthetic agent to be released was propofol in 1989 (in its current formulation). A number of new agents are currently being investigated for use as induction agents, including the steroid pregnanalone and older agents such as propanidid (originally withdrawn due to the unacceptable incidence of allergic reactions to the solvent Cremphor-EL). These may be released as new formulations in intralipid.

There are many drugs which may be described as "general anesthetic" agents, including barbiturates, opiates, alcohol, and even local anesthetic agents. The following chapter describes the clinical pharmacology of the more commonly used nonopiate intravenous anesthetic agents, including the benzodiazepines (often referred to as *co-induction agents*) and the antagonist flumazenil. Each section will follow a similar format, consisting of a description of the basic pharmacokinetics (absorption, distribution, metabolism, and excretion of the drug), pharmacodynamics (i.e., the effect of the drug on the body), doses used, routes of administration, and the major complications and side effects associated with their use. For quick reference of indications, dosages, and precautions with these drugs, see Appendix B.

Intravenous anesthetic induction agents should be used only by those trained in anesthesia and where facilities for maintenance of a patent airway, artificial ventilation, oxygenation, and other resuscitative measures are immediately available. Hypotension and apnea may follow the use of these agents, particularly with rapid administration. The concomitant use of other sedative/hypnotic agents or medical conditions altering the normal pharmacokinetics and pharmacodynamics dramatically affect the dosage of these drugs. As with all anesthetic agents, caution should be exercised when used in patients with cardiac, respiratory, renal, or hepatic impairment; or in hypovolemic and debilitated patients.

THIOPENTONE (THIOPENTAL)

Description

Thiopentone is an ultra-short-acting thiobarbiturate (Fig. 1), first used in 1934 in the US by Lundy and Waters. It was used during World War II on US servicemen at Pearl Harbor, where a 5% solution was used, compounding problems with overdosage.

It is formulated as a yellow, amorphous powder (500 mg in single-dose vials), together with 6% anhydrous sodium carbonate, producing a water-soluble, alkaline solution. It is also sealed under nitrogen to prevent precipitation of the insoluble free acid by atmospheric carbon dioxide. The resulting 2.5% clear, yellow solution has a pH of 10.6 and is incompatible with acidic solutions such as the opiates, catecholamines, and neuromuscular blocking agents (particularly succinylcholine). This alkalinity imparts a bacteriostatic effect. Thiopentone is not recommended for use if reconstituted for more than 48 hours, even if refrigerated (do not use a cloudy solution).

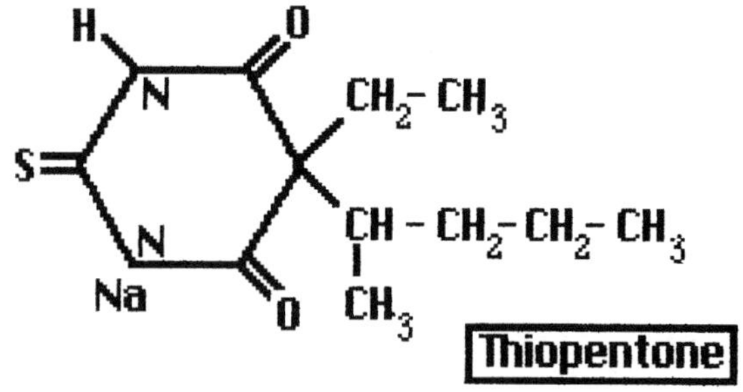

FIG. 1. Structural formula of thiopentone.

Mechanism of Action

The mechanism by which barbiturates induce anesthesia is incompletely understood, but is thought to be via the polysynaptic reticular activating system within the brainstem. Barbiturates inhibit these pathways both pre- and postsynaptically, suppressing excitatory neurotransmitters such as acetylcholine and augmenting transmission of inhibitory neurotransmitters such as γ-amino butyric acid (GABA). By acting at the level of the thalamus, barbiturates inhibit ascending conduction in the reticular formation, preventing impulses from reaching the cortex.

There is a close relationship between the structure and the pharmacodynamics of the barbiturates. They are all derived from barbituric acid (Fig. 2), and by substituting alkyl or aryl groups at the carbon 5 position, the hypnotic and sedative activity is increased. The addition of phenyl groups, at the carbon 5 or on one of the nitrogens of the ring, confers *anticonvulsant* properties (phenobarbitone); whereas, alkyl groups in excess of five carbons increase the *convulsant* properties (methohexitone). Substitution

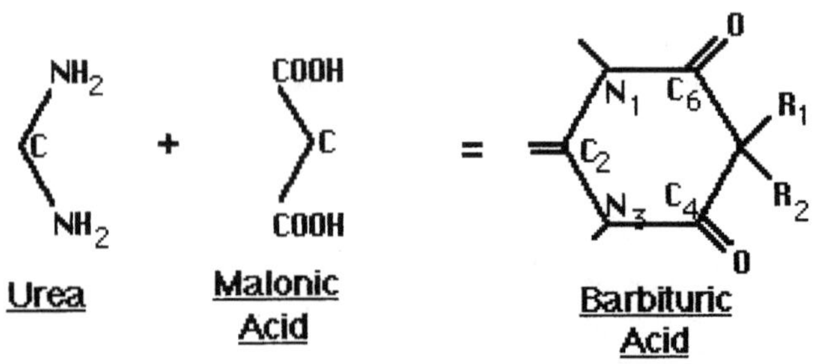

FIG. 2. Formation of barbituric acid (with positions marked).

of sulfur for oxygen at the carbon 2 position increases lipid solubility (thiobarbiturates).

Pharmacokinetics

Absorption

Thiopentone is generally given as an intravenous injection of the 2.5% solution, although rectal induction in children with a 5% or 10% solution is another well-described route. With a pH of 10–11 and a pKa of 7.6, approximately 60% of molecules are in the nonionized or diffusible form at normal body pH. In addition, it is extremely lipid-soluble; thus, with high cerebral blood flows, uptake by the brain is rapid and maximal within 30 sec, despite the high degree of protein binding (80%). Uptake of a given dose of thiopentone is, therefore, easily influenced by changes in pH, protein binding, and volume status. For example, in low albumin states, such as chronic liver disease or displacement by sulfonamides and NSAIDs, more "unbound" drug is available for uptake by the brain. Similarly, hypovolemia increases the relative concentration of a given dose, and acidosis increases the nonionized fraction, both of which may result in a relative overdose of thiopentone.

Distribution

The duration of action of thiopentone is determined by redistribution. Plasma levels of thiopentone decrease as it is taken up by less vascular tissues such as lean muscle, viscera, and finally, fat. It is this redistribution from the brain to other tissues that is responsible for the "offset" in action. Repeat doses, however, would slowly increase the muscle and fat content of thiopentone, resulting in a reduced concentration gradient and slower recovery. When these compartments become saturated, as with continuous infusions, duration of action becomes dependent on metabolism and elimination.

Metabolism

The principal site of metabolism is the liver; others include the brain and kidneys. The metabolic half-life is 6 hours; clearance is in the order of 1.6–4.3 ml/kg/min. Of the injected dose, 10% to 15% is metabolized each hour, primarily by hepatic oxidation to inactive, water-soluble metabolites and then renally excreted.

Excretion

Very little thiopentone is excreted unchanged by the kidney. High protein binding reduces glomerular filtration and high lipid solubility favors reabsorption by the renal tubules.

Pharmacodynamics

Cardiovascular System

Intravenous induction with thiopentone causes mild and transient hypotension associated with a slight elevation of heart rate. This is due to depression of the medullary vasomotor center and decreased sympathetic outflow, resulting in vasodilatation of the peripheral capacitance vessels, increased venous pooling, and a reduction in venous return. Thiopentone also has a direct myocardial depressant action and is mildly vagolytic, hence the tachycardia. However, unlike the inhalation anesthetic agents, thiopentone does not sensitize the myocardium to epinephrine or other sympathomimetic amines.

Under controlled conditions, cardiac output may be maintained by this rise in heart rate and through compensatory baroreceptor reflexes. As a result, systemic vascular resistance may actually increase by 10% to 20%. However, in the presence of hypovolemia, β-blockade, or congestive cardiac failure, the baroreceptor response is obtunded, resulting in profound hypotension. The myocardial depressant action of thiopentone is exposed under such conditions, the degree of hypotension being related to autonomic tone, preexisting disease, speed of injection, and volume status of the patient.

Respiratory System

Thiopentone acts directly on the medullary respiratory center, depressing the ventilatory response to hypoxia and hypercapnia. As with other induction agents, a period of apnea may follow intravenous induction, the degree of respiratory depression depending on dose, speed of administration, and concomitant drug therapy.

Laryngeal and pharyngeal reflexes are not completely depressed following induction. Laryngospasm may be triggered by airway instrumentation, pharyngeal secretions, or surgical stimulation if the patient is not satisfactorily anesthetized. Similarly, bronchospasm may be induced in asthmatics as a result of stimulation or release of histamine. This may make insertion of the laryngeal mask airway more difficult as compared with an agent such as propofol. Laryngeal and bronchial vagal reflexes may be suppressed with the prior administration of an antimuscarinic agent, e.g., atropine.

The neonatal blood–brain barrier is more permeable to a lipid-soluble agent such as thiopentone. Also, the neonatal respiratory center is particularly susceptible to the respiratory depressant effects of thiopentone.

Central Nervous System

The major actions of thiopentone on the central nervous system are rapid onset of sedation, hypnosis, anesthesia, reduction in cerebral metabolism and blood flow, and anticonvulsant activity.

Thiopentone reduces intracranial pressure (ICP) by inducing cerebral vasoconstriction (cerebrovascular resistance increases by up to 70%) and decreasing cerebral blood flow by as much as 50%. This reduction in ICP is less than the fall in mean arterial pressure (MAP); thus, cerebral perfusion pressure (CPP) is well maintained (CPP=MAP–ICP). In addition, the cerebral metabolic requirement for oxygen ($CMRO_2$) is reduced, but to a greater degree than is cerebral blood flow. Thus, the ratio of oxygen supply to demand is increased, provided cerebral perfusion pressure is well maintained. These beneficial effects are thought to protect the brain from hypoxic/ischemic events.

The degree of central nervous system depression is dependent on dose. Small doses may, however, cause paradoxical excitation and disorientation due to an antianalgesic effect. Though tolerance to, and dependence on, the sedative effects of barbiturates can develop rapidly, this is not likely to be a problem with thiopentone.

Liver

Barbiturates, in general, induce liver microsomal enzyme activity, increasing the metabolism of some drugs. Phenobarbitone is the most potent in this regard. They also stimulate the activity of an enzyme known as δ-aminolevulinic acid synthetase, a mitochondrial enzyme, which results in accelerated production of heme. This may precipitate acute intermittent, or variegata porphyria in susceptible individuals.

Renal

A reduction in renal blood flow and glomerular filtration rate occurs in proportion to the degree of hypotension and increased renal vascular resistance.

Eyes

Thiopentone reduces intraocular pressure (IOP). Typically, on induction of anesthesia, the pupils initially dilate and then constrict. Sensitivity to light remains until the patient is deep enough to permit a skin incision.

Musculoskeletal system

Reduced tone of skeletal muscle.

TABLE 1. *Dosages of thiopentone*

Induction of anesthesia	
Intravenous (healthy adult)	3–5 mg/kg slowly.
Rectal (children)	20–40 mg/kg (5–10% solution)
Convulsions/status epilepticus	
Intravenous	1–2 mg/kg IV increments

Pregnancy

Thiopentone readily crosses the placenta and reaches peak levels 2–3 min after an intravenous bolus. However, fetal plasma concentrations are substantially less than are maternal levels and produce little clinical effect. There is little or no effect on uterine tone; thiopentone is, therefore, of no value in external cephalic version.

Small amounts may appear in breast milk, following large doses, though this is not clinically significant.

Neonatal

Thiopentone's elimination half-life is prolonged, in the vicinity of 11–42 hours. The blood–brain barrier of the neonate is also more permeable to drugs; thus, the dose should be reduced.

Other

Thiopentone reduces the tone of the lower esophageal sphincter. Patients may also experience a taste of garlic after an intravenous dose, prior to onset of anesthesia.

Dosage and Administration

Thiopentone is administered intravenously, as a 2.5% solution (25 mg/ml), and rectally (Table 1). Intramuscular injections are contraindicated as this causes muscular necrosis. Dose is dependent on age, sex, weight, and physical status of the patient. Cloudy solutions or those older than 24 hours should be discarded.

Precautions and Side Effects

General

Thiopentone should be administered only by those qualified in the use of intravenous anesthetic agents, where equipment for resuscitation and tracheal intubation are available.

Specific contraindications include allergy to barbiturates, acute intermittent or variegata porphyria, and concurrent use of disulfiram (Antabuse).

Thiopentone should be used with care in the presence of coronary artery disease, constrictive pericarditis, congestive cardiac failure, hypovolemic states, mitral and aortic valve disease, and other causes of hypotension. Cardiovascular collapse may occur with rapid injection in these circumstances.

Laryngeal spasm, bronchospasm, respiratory obstruction, and apnea may occur, leading to difficulties with airway management. Thiopentone may exacerbate bronchospasm in the asthmatic patient due to release of histamine and, as such, is contraindicated for use in asthmatic patients, particularly status asthmaticus.

Patients should be warned of the possible adverse effects on driving and the performance of other skilled tasks. Psychomotor impairment following barbiturate anesthesia may last up to 24 hours or even longer, depending on the dose and drugs used.

Local

Urticaria

An urticarial, blotchy red rash may occur. This is usually transient and due to local histamine release.

Extravascular injection

This causes severe pain, erythema, and swelling and may lead to tissue sloughing and necrosis. The irritant effect can be treated with the injection of 2% procaine (Novocain) to relieve pain and reduce the venospasm. Hyaluronidase (Wydase) may help tissue dispersion.

Intraarterial injection

Intraarterial injection induces intense arterial spasm, producing a white hand, cyanosed fingers, and severe, burning pain. It may even cause sudden death. This is thought to be due to precipitation of thiopentone crystals and local release of norepinephrine, causing vasospasm and, later, hemolysis of red blood cells. However, no permanent complications have been recorded with 2.5% solutions.

Immediate treatment to prevent gangrene consists of injecting saline through the same needle, diluting the thiopentone. Intravenous papaverine (40–80 mg diluted) or procaine (5 ml of 2%) induces local vasodilatation and helps perfuse the limb. Stellate ganglion or brachial plexus block have similar effects, producing analgesia and vasodilatation. Heparinization should be commenced to preserve arterial patency. Selective intraarterial injection of urokinase has been used with good clinical effect (1).

METHOHEXITONE (METHOHEXITAL)

Description

Methohexitone was first described by Chernish in 1956 and used clinically by Stoelting in the US in 1957. It is a methylated oxybarbiturate, three times as potent as thiopentone, but with a shorter recovery time. It is formulated as a white crystalline powder and is mixed with anhydrous sodium carbonate. Methohexitone is readily soluble in water, producing a 1% solution that is stable for several weeks. The chemical structure for methohexitone is shown in Fig. 3.

The mechanism of action and many of the pharmacological effects are similar to those of thiopentone, in particular, the cardiovascular and respiratory depressant effects. However, methohexitone does have some advantages, in particular, earlier recovery and less accumulation with repeat doses.

Pharmacokinetics

Absorption

Methohexitone is administered as a 1% solution for intravenous induction. It has a pH of 11 and pKa of 7.9; thus, 75% is nonionized at physiologic pH. It is highly lipid soluble and has a rapid onset of action, despite high protein binding. Uptake of methohexitone is influenced by the same factors as with thiopentone.

Distribution

Recovery of consciousness is due to redistribution of the drug from the central nervous system to muscle and fat. Rapid redistribution, combined with a metabolic clearance rate four times higher than thiopentone, results in a shorter elimination half-life, which is reflected in the rapid clinical recovery.

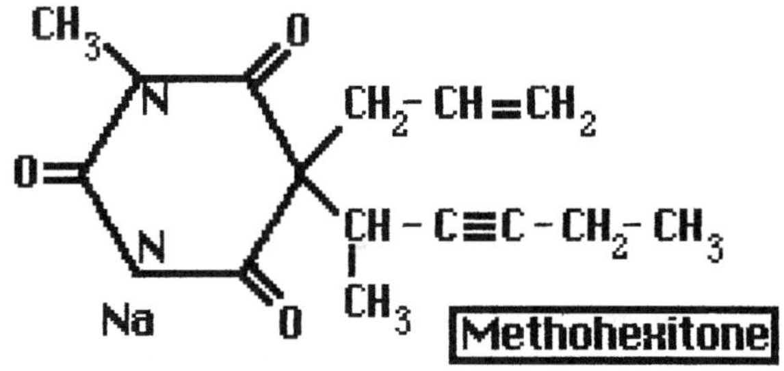

FIG. 3. Structural formula of methohexitone.

Metabolism and Excretion

Methohexitone is cleared by the liver three to four times more rapidly than is thiopentone. It is filtered by the kidney, but the high degree of protein binding limits the magnitude of filtration. Some is excreted in the feces.

Pharmacodynamics

Central Nervous System

Methohexitone, due to the methyl group on the first carbon and the long alkyl group at the fifth carbon position, is associated with more excitatory phenomena on induction. Although perhaps a disadvantage when compared with thiopentone, use is made of this property for induction of anesthesia in electroconvulsive therapy (ECT). Prolonged convulsions may be treated with diazepam or phenytoin (Dilantin). Methohexitone should be avoided in epileptic patients. The incidence of tremor and involuntary movements is dose-dependent and may be reduced with the use of opiate premedication.

Respiratory System

The respiratory system action is similar to that of thiopentone. Dose-dependent respiratory depression and transient apnea occur. There is a higher incidence of coughing, hiccup, and generalized muscle twitching following induction with methohexitone. As a result, laryngospasm may be precipitated, particularly following stimulation under light anesthesia. The incidence of coughing and the production of secretions can be reduced with anticholinergic medication.

Cardiovascular System

Transient hypotension and tachycardia may occur.

Pregnancy

The safe use of methohexitone in pregnancy has not been established with certainty; however, there is no evidence of teratogenicity at present. It does cross the placenta.

Dosage and Administration

Methohexitone may be administered intravenously as a 1% solution or rectally as a 10% solution (Table 2). Higher concentrations given intravenously are associated with a greater incidence of muscle movements and respiratory complications.

TABLE 2. *Recommended dosages for methohexitone*

Induction of anesthesia	
Intravenous (healthy adult)	1–2 mg/kg
Rectal (children)	25 mg/kg of a 10% solution
Sedation	
Intravenous	0.2–0.4 mg/kg

As with thiopentone, methohexitone does not mix with acidic solutions such as succinylcholine, atropine or d-tubocurarine.

Precautions and Side Effects

General

Methohexitone should be administered only by those qualified in the use of intravenous anesthetic agents, where equipment for resuscitation and tracheal intubation are available.

Muscle twitching and seizure-like movements may occur on induction. Methohexitone should be used with caution in patients with severe cardiovascular disease, hypertension, congestive cardiac failure, or valvular heart disease, and in those with asthma, particularly status asthmaticus and obstructive pulmonary disease. Erythema, urticaria, and rare cases of anaphylaxis have been reported.

Patients should be warned of the possible adverse effects on driving and the performance of other skilled tasks. Psychomotor impairment following barbiturate anesthesia may last up to 24 hours, depending on the dose and drugs used.

Local

Intraarterial Injection

As with thiopentone, intraarterial injection may lead to severe arterial spasm, thrombosis, necrosis, and, eventually, gangrene. The conscious patient may complain of severe pain in the arterial distribution, those who are anesthetized may develop blanching or blotchy cyanosis of the limb. The extent of injury is related to concentration and is, therefore, less likely with 1% solutions of methohexitone. Treatment is as for thiopentone.

PROPOFOL

Description

Propofol is an intravenous agent used for the induction and maintenance of anesthesia and for sedation of venti-

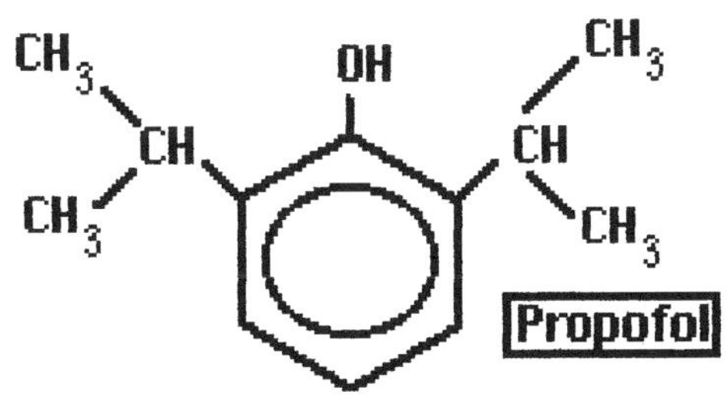

FIG. 4. Structural formula of propofol.

lated patients in intensive care. The structure is that of a phenol ring with two isopropyl groups attached at the 2 and 6 carbon positions (Fig. 4).

It is extremely lipid soluble and, thus, very water insoluble. This caused problems initially with the preparation of a suitable parenteral solution. Originally released in 1977, propofol was formulated in Cremphor EL (polyhydroxylated castor oil), which was associated with an unacceptably high incidence of allergic reactions.

The current formulation of propofol consists of 1% aqueous solution (10 mg/ml) as an oil-water emulsion containing 10% soybean oil, 1.2% egg phosphatide, and 2.25% glycerol. This solution is similar to intralipid 10% and has a calorific value of 1.1 kcal/ml. Consequently, it is not bacteriostatic, and strict aseptic techniques should be observed, particularly when preparing an intravenous infusion. Sepsis and death have been associated with contaminated propofol preparations; unused open ampules or syringes should be discarded. Although this preparation does not appear to stimulate the release of histamine, it can cause quite severe pain on injection.

Pharmacokinetics

Absorption and Distribution

Propofol is available for intravenous administration only. It has a rapid onset of action, followed by a rapid recovery due to a very short initial redistribution half-life. The extensive redistribution and metabolic clearance results in a more rapid recovery, with less "hangover" effect than following induction with other agents and is, therefore, ideally suited for day-case (ambulatory) anesthesia and for long-term sedation by infusion. These beneficial pharmacokinetic effects are also seen in obese patients following induction and maintenance with propofol (2).

Metabolism and Excretion

Extensive hepatic metabolism occurs to inactive glucuronide and sulfate conjugates, which are renally excreted. However, the clearance exceeds hepatic blood flow, suggesting additional extrahepatic metabolism. The pharmacokinetics of propofol do not seem to be altered by chronic renal failure or cirrhosis.

Pharmacodynamics

Central Nervous System

Propofol produces a dose-dependent depression of central nervous system function. Low doses produce drowsiness and sedation, while higher doses lead to unconsciousness and anesthesia. Propofol acts synergistically when used in combination with short-acting opiates such as fentanyl (3). There is some debate as to whether propofol has anticonvulsant properties. There are reports of successful treatment in status epilepticus (4). Nevertheless, it is associated with excitatory phenomenon, including involuntary movements, opisthotonus, and seizures, which may occur at induction or emergence.

A reduction in cerebral blood flow and intracranial pressure occurs. There may also be a dramatic reduction in cerebral perfusion pressure, resulting from a fall in mean arterial pressure exceeding the fall in intracranial pressure.

Other advantages are a reduction in intraocular pressure, and a lower incidence of headache, nausea, and vomiting in the recovery from propofol anesthesia. Boluses doses of 10–20 mg may be of benefit in postoperative nausea and vomiting. Propofol has been used successfully as an antiemetic in chemotherapy.

Cardiovascular System

Intravenous injection of propofol results in dose-dependent cardiovascular depression, with a fall in systolic and diastolic blood pressures. The compensatory tachycardia seen with other agents does not occur; indeed, bradycardia is more common and can be particularly profound when used in conjunction with suxamethonium (succinylcholine) or fentanyl.

Systemic vascular resistance, cardiac output, myocardial blood flow, and myocardial oxygen consumption may also be reduced. Propofol is a cardiac depressant and should be administered cautiously to patients with limited cardiac reserve or hypovolemia, where a fall in systemic vascular resistance or cardiac output may be disastrous. However, when propofol is used with caution, these patients seem to tolerate it surprisingly well. Administration by infusion retains the beneficial pharmacodynamic effects while attenuating the hypotensive response (5). This may relate to a reduction in myocardial oxygen consumption. Cardiac dysrhythmias are uncommon.

Respiratory

Propofol produces dose-dependent respiratory depression, initially inducing a reduction in tidal volume and increased respiratory rate, followed by apnea that may last 30–60 sec (or longer if used in conjunction with other respiratory depressant drugs).

Propofol appears to inhibit laryngeal reflexes to a far greater extent than do other induction agents, enabling patients to tolerate oropharyngeal and laryngeal mask airways. There is no effect on resting bronchomotor tone, and it is considered safe for use in asthmatics.

Pregnancy and Neonates

Propofol crosses the placental barrier and is excreted in breast milk.

Others

There is no impairment of renal or hepatic function in adults.

Dosage and Administration

Administration by slow intravenous injection avoids excessive hypotension, usually in boluses of 20–30 mg over 10 sec (Table 3). Intravenous infusions for total intravenous anesthesia (TIVA) should be titrated carefully against the cardiovascular response to the drug.

Dosage should be titrated against the response of the patient. Propofol is not recommended for intensive care sedation in children (see below), and (generally) is to be used for not more than 3 days for sedation in adults.

TABLE 3. *Recommended dosages for propofol*

Induction	
Healthy adult	2.0–2.5 mg/kg
Elderly or high risk patient	1.0–1.5 mg/kg
Children > 3 years	Up to 3–3.5 mg/kg
Maintenance	
Adults	4–12 mg/kg/hr
A typical regime would be:	2–3 mg/kg bolus followed by 10 mg/kg (1 ml/kg) for 10 min 8 mg/kg (0.8 ml/kg) for 10 min 6 mg/kg (0.6 ml/kg) thereafter (Or intermittent boluses of 25–50 mg)
Sedation	
Adults	1–4 mg/kg/hour
Children > 3 years	9–15 mg/kg/hour

Precautions and Side Effects

General

Contraindications include known allergy to propofol (an allergy to egg is not necessarily a contraindication, since allergies are normally to the yolk component, whereas the egg phosphatide comes from the egg white). Anaphylactoid reactions have been reported.

Excitatory phenomenon, involuntary movements, coughing, and hiccup may occur in up to 14% of patients. Caution must be exercised when given to those with cardiac or respiratory impairment, in hypovolemic or critically ill patients, and in those with raised intracranial pressure.

The manufacturers do not recommend the use of propofol in ECT, although it may have some beneficial effects. Propofol, as compared with methohexitone, reduces blood pressure and heart rate on induction and significantly reduces the increase in systolic blood pressure on stimulation. However, it also significantly reduces the clinical duration of the seizure (6). A considerable amount of controversy exists as to the relationship of seizure duration to the therapeutic effect of ECT.

A number of deaths have been associated with propofol used for sedating children in intensive care, resulting in neurological, cardiac, and renal effects; hyperlipemia; hepatomegaly; and metabolic acidosis (7).

Propofol appears to be safe in patients susceptible to malignant hyperthermia (8) and porphyria (9,10).

Local

Probably the most common and noticeable side effect is pain on injection, particularly when used in small veins on the back of the hand (28%). This can usually be overcome by adding 10 mg of lidocaine or by using a larger vein. Venous thrombosis is not a problem with the current formulation.

ETOMIDATE

Description

Etomidate is an intravenous induction agent that was first synthesized and studied by Janssen and co-workers in 1971. It is a carboxylated imidazole compound that is structurally unrelated to any other induction agent (Fig. 5). The result is a sedative-hypnotic compound that is characterized by rapid onset and offset of action with excellent cardiovascular stability. However, it is associ-

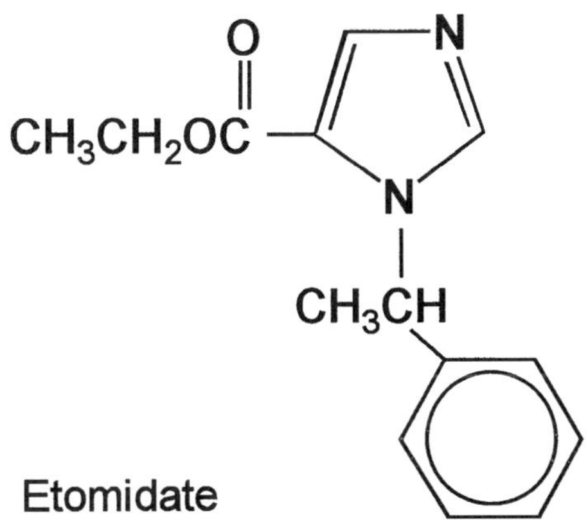

FIG. 5. Structural formula of etomidate.

ated with a high incidence of involuntary movements, pain on injection, nausea, and adrenocortical depression.

Etomidate is thought to act by depressing the reticular activating system, mimicking the inhibitory effects of GABA. It has a "disinhibitory" effect on parts of the extrapyramidal system, resulting in a high incidence of involuntary movements.

It is a white crystalline powder soluble in a wide range of solvents including water, ethanol, and propylene glycol. The imidazole ring confers water solubility in acidic solutions and lipid solubility at physiologic pH. Commercial preparations are presented as 10-ml ampules containing 2 mg/ml of the hydrochloride dissolved in water, with 35% propylene glycol.

Pharmacokinetics

Absorption and Distribution

Induction of anesthesia occurs rapidly after intravenous injection and may last 6–10 min following a single bolus. Etomidate is 76% plasma protein bound, primarily to albumin, but, despite this, is characterized by a rapid onset of action as a result of the high lipid solubility and greater proportion of nonionized drug at physiologic pH (pKa 4.2). Recovery from anesthesia occurs as a result of redistribution.

Only 2.5% of a bolus dose remains in the circulation 2 min after injection, and repeated doses are not cumulative.

Metabolism and Excretion

Etomidate's clearance is five times greater than that of thiopentone. It is rapidly hydrolyzed by hepatic microsomal enzymes and plasma esterases to an inactive carboxylic acid ester. The end products are primarily excreted in the urine, with some in the bile—less than 3% is excreted unchanged.

Pharmacodynamics

Central Nervous System

Etomidate induces rapid loss of consciousness. It decreases cerebral blood flow, cerebral oxygen consumption ($CMRO_2$), and, consequently, reduces intracranial pressure. Cerebral perfusion pressure is well maintained because of the minimal cardiovascular depressant effects. It is sedative and hypnotic but lacks any analgesic action.

Involuntary muscle movements, occasionally severe, are not uncommon following induction. As a result, etomidate should be used cautiously in patients with epilepsy. Opiates reduce the incidence of myotonic contractions; however, atropine premedication may potentiate them.

Cardiovascular System

Induction doses of etomidate result in minimal cardiovascular depression. A slight reduction in arterial blood pressure occurs following a fall in peripheral vascular resistance. Myocardial contractility and cardiac index are unchanged.

Respiratory System

Etomidate has minimal effects on the respiratory system unless used in conjunction with other central respiratory depressants. Any reductions in tidal volume are offset by increases in respiratory rate. About 10% of patients develop hiccup.

Endocrine System

One of the disadvantages of etomidate is that it suppresses adrenocortical function. This effect appears to result from enzymatic blockade (11-β-hydroxylase) of the adrenal steroidogenic pathway, reducing cortisol and aldosterone synthesis and lasting 6–8 hours after an induction dose. The clinical effect of this transient adrenal suppression is unknown, but infusions in critically ill patients are contraindicated as septic complications are likely to ensue (11). Etomidate is, therefore, restricted to induction of anesthesia, and should be used with caution in those with preexisting adrenal suppression.

Others

Thirty-three percent of patients complain of nausea and vomiting that is independent of premedication. Pain on injection is common, though less so when formulated in propylene glycol and may be reduced by using a large forearm vein or the prior injection of lidocaine.

TABLE 4. *Recommended dosages for etomidate*

Induction	
Healthy adult	0.1–0.4 mg/kg

Dosage and Administration

Intravenous induction in the healthy adult is 0.1–0.4 mg/kg (Table 4).

Precautions and Side Effects

Allergy

Although etomidate is thought not to stimulate the release of histamine, hypersensitivity reactions have been described, including urticaria and anaphylaxis (12).

Porphyria

Etomidate is thought not to be safe in acute porphyria as it is porphyrinogenic in animals (13).

KETAMINE

Description

Ketamine is an intravenous anesthetic agent that produces a state of "dissociative anesthesia." It is not strictly an induction agent in the true sense of the word, as the time to onset of anesthesia exceeds one arm–brain circulation time.

The mode of action of ketamine differs from other intravenous anesthetic agents in that it functionally "dissociates" the thalamus from the limbic cortex. As a result, sensory impulses passing from the reticular activating system via the thalamus to the cerebral cortex are prevented from reaching conscious awareness (the limbic system). The patient appears to be awake (breathing, swallowing, eyes open) but does not respond to stimulation.

Ketamine exerts a number of other effects on the central nervous system, including inhibition of polysynaptic reflexes within the spinal cord and inhibition of excitatory neurotransmitters in other parts of the brain. In subanesthetic doses it is a potent analgesic; the mechanism of action is unclear but may be related to an interaction with opioid receptors and antagonism of N-methyl-d-aspartate (NMDA) receptors.

Structurally, ketamine is an arylcyclohexylamine (Fig. 6), an analog of phencyclidine (PCP or "angel dust") with similar psychotomimetic effects, hence the abuse potential as a recreational drug ("Special-K"). Formulated as a

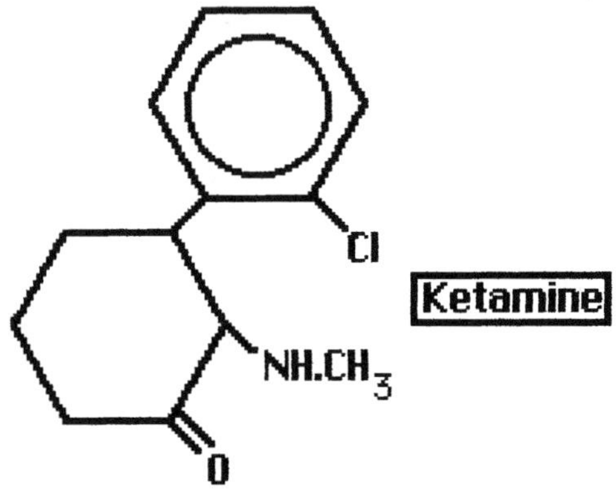

FIG. 6. Structural formula of ketamine.

white crystalline powder containing 0.01% benzethonium chloride as a preservative, it is readily soluble in water, producing an acidic solution of pH 3.5. This formulation will precipitate when in contact with basic preparations such as barbiturates and diazepam. The asymmetric carbon atom results in a racemic solution, containing both (+) and (–) isomers. The (+) isomer produces more intense analgesia with a more rapid recovery and is less likely to cause emergence reactions that are associated with the (–) isomer.

Pharmacokinetics

Absorption and Distribution

Ketamine can be administered by intravenous or intramuscular injection. It is more lipid soluble than is thiopentone, though less protein bound and equally ionized at physiologic pH. Combined with the increases in cerebral blood flow and cardiac output, this leads to a rapid brain uptake and loss of consciousness in 30–60 sec. Subsequent redistribution to peripheral compartments results in recovery after 10–15 min. When given intramuscularly, surgical anesthesia is normally reached in 3–5 min, with peak plasma levels after 10–15 min and a duration of up to half an hour.

Metabolism and Excretion

Metabolism is a complex process that takes place primarily in the liver, producing about 8–16 active metabolites, some of which may be responsible for the emergence phenomena, others of which have residual anesthetic activity. Remarkably, ketamine has a hepatic extraction ratio of 0.9 and a clearance of 18 ml/kg/min, which accounts for the relatively short elimination half-life of 2 hours.

The principal metabolites, resulting from hydroxylation and N-demethylation, are then conjugated with glucuronic acid and excreted in the urine.

Pharmacodynamics

Central Nervous System

The most important effects are increases in cerebral blood flow and intracranial pressure. Potent cerebral vasodilatation and increases in cerebral blood flow by up to 60% occurs, even in the presence of normocapnia. However, unlike other agents, cerebral oxygen consumption is not reduced. Thus, ketamine is probably best avoided in neurosurgical anesthesia and in patients with head injuries. Although not directly epileptogenic, ketamine anesthesia is associated with increases in muscle tone that may at times resemble seizure activity.

The dissociative anesthesia produced is associated with a high incidence of emergence reactions, particularly during recovery. These include vivid, unpleasant dreams, hallucinations, confusion, and irrational behavior. These side effects may be reduced or prevented by using benzodiazepine premedication and by keeping verbal, tactile, and visual stimuli to a minimum during recovery.

Other central nervous system effects include anterograde amnesia and intense analgesia. The analgesia tends to outlast the period of anesthesia and occurs at subanesthetic doses. Lacrimation, diplopia, nystagmus, and increases in intraocular pressure have also been described, as well as a relatively high incidence of nausea and vomiting.

Cardiovascular System

Intravenous administration of ketamine increases mean arterial pressure, pulmonary arterial pressure, central venous pressure, heart rate, and cardiac output, though hypotension and dysrhythmias have been described. There is some controversy concerning the mechanism by which ketamine produces these effects. There is undoubtedly a marked increase in circulating catecholamine levels; however, it is unclear whether this is due to central sympathetic stimulation or to inhibition of catecholamine reuptake.

The positive inotropic effects of ketamine are valuable in the poor-risk, hypovolemic patient, though caution should be exercised when administering to patients with valvular or ischemic heart disease.

Respiratory System

Ketamine differs significantly from most other induction agents in that the response to hypoxia and hypercapnia is maintained, and the pharyngeal and laryngeal reflexes remain intact. It is also a bronchodilator. These properties, as well as analgesia, make ketamine well suited as a sedative for short surgical procedures. Following large intravenous doses, however, respiratory depression and apnea may still occur.

The profound bronchodilation produced by ketamine makes it a useful agent for induction in those with asthma and obstructive airway disease, and, as such, it has been used for the emergency intubation and treatment of status asthmaticus (14). Continuous intravenous infusions of ketamine have been used successfully in pediatric patients where conventional bronchodilator therapy has failed (15). An antisialogogue should be given simultaneously, as ketamine stimulates profuse salivation.

The preservation of the upper airway reflexes during ketamine anesthesia may make aspiration less likely but can also precipitate coughing and laryngospasm as a result of the accumulation of secretions or following instrumentation of the airway.

Pregnancy

Ketamine crosses the placenta and has the potential to produce neonatal respiratory depression; however, when used as an adjunct or at light planes of anesthesia, there is little clinical effect.

Others

Ketamine does not release histamine and rarely causes allergic reactions, though transient rashes and pain at the site of injection may occur.

Dosage and Administration

Following intravenous or intramuscular injection (Table 5) a state of dissociative anesthesia (catalepsy, amnesia, and analgesia) is produced and may persist into the recovery period. Atropine or another suitable antimus-

TABLE 5. *Recommended dosages for ketamine*

Induction of surgical anesthesia	
Intravenous	1–2 mg/kg (Onset 30 sec, lasts 5–15 min)
Intramuscular	5–10 mg/kg (Onset 3–4 min, lasts 15–30 min)
Analgesia	
Intravenous	0.2–0.75 mg/kg
Epidural/intramuscular	30 mg bolus*

*From Naguib et al. (32).

carinic (antisialogog, e.g., glycopyrrolate) should be administered prior to induction. A benzodiazepine such as diazepam or midazolam given prior to and during ketamine anesthesia may help to reduce the incidence of emergence phenomenon.

The dose, like all other induction agents, should be modified according to ASA grade, age, and physical status. For example, in cases of severe trauma and low blood pressure, doses of 10–20 mg may be all that is required for anesthesia.

Precautions and Side Effects

Ketamine should be used with caution in patients with a history of the following:

Cerebrovascular accidents and raised intracranial pressure.
Valvular and ischemic heart disease.
Uncontrolled hypertension, cardiac failure, or pulmonary hypertension.
Recent penetrating eye injury.

The cardiovascular depressant effects of ketamine are unmasked by beta blockers and other sympathetic antagonists, including verapamil, halothane (Fluothane), and, to a lesser extent, other volatile agents.

Disadvantages of the use of ketamine include slow onset and recovery with associated emergence sequelae, increased muscle tone and jerky movements following induction, cardiovascular stimulation, postoperative nausea and vomiting, and increase in cerebral blood flow and intracranial pressure.

Ketamine has been used safely in patients with myopathies and acute intermittent porphyria. Although rare, malignant hyperthermia has been reported.

BENZODIAZEPINES

The benzodiazepines are a group of drugs with sedative, hypnotic, anticonvulsant, amnestic, and tranquilizing properties. Diazepam also acts as a muscle relaxant, the mechanism of action being different from that of neuromuscular blocking agents. There are numerous benzodiazepines in clinical use; however, diazepam and midazolam are most commonly used in anesthesia as "co-induction" agents. They have a common structure that includes a seven-member diazepine ring and a benzene ring (1,4-benzodiazepine nucleus). Substitutions at various points on these rings affects the potency and biotransformation. The chemical structure of diazepam is shown in Fig. 7.

Mechanism of Action

Over recent years, the understanding of the mechanism of action has been described in more detail. Gamma-aminobutyric acid, the major inhibitory neurotransmitter in the cerebral cortex, acts by binding to specific receptors within the brain, increasing the membrane conductance of chloride ions. This results in hyperpolarization of the cell membrane, inhibiting neuronal transmission. The GABA receptor protein complex incorporates the chloride ion channel and three separate binding sites. One binds GABA, one the benzodiazepines, and the third binds barbiturates and ethanol. Benzodiazepines have a synergistic action at these cortical receptors, augmenting GABA-minergic neurotransmission, producing sedative and anticonvulsant properties (16).

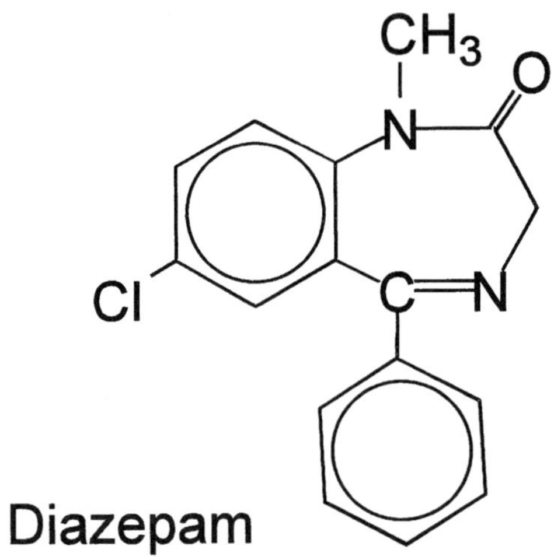

FIG. 7. Structural formula of diazepam.

Specific benzodiazepine "receptors" or, more specifically, high-affinity binding sites, have been identified within the cerebral cortex, hypothalamus, cerebellum, and medulla. Isolation of these binding sites has resulted in the development of selective benzodiazepine antagonists such as flumazenil.

Diazepam

Description

Diazepam is a long-acting benzodiazepine (see Fig. 7) available for oral and parenteral administration. It is widely used as a co-induction agent in anesthesia, as a premedicant, to produce sedation and amnesia for short surgical procedures, and as an anticonvulsant, particularly in status epilepticus or febrile convulsions. Diazepam is also used in the management of severe, disabling anxiety disorders associated with alcohol withdrawal states; insomnia; and in control of muscle spasm resulting from spasticity, cerebral palsy, and tetanus.

As can be seen from its chemical structure, it is poorly water soluble. Parenteral preparations contain various organic solvents, including propylene glycol (40%), ethyl alcohol (10%), and sodium benzoate (5%), which as a result are associated with a high incidence of thrombophlebitis. An alternative formulation, Diazemuls, uses a lipid emulsion solvent similar to intralipid.

Pharmacokinetics

Absorption and Distribution

Diazepam is rapidly and completely absorbed from the gastrointestinal tract; peak plasma levels are usually achieved after an hour. Intramuscular injections result in lower peak plasma concentrations and are not recommended. Diazepam is highly lipid soluble and, after intravenous administration, rapidly crosses the blood–brain barrier. Redistribution is fairly rapid and, as with most induction agents, is responsible for the decrease in effect. Diazepam has a biphasic half-life, an initial rapid distribution phase of up to 3 hours, followed by a more prolonged terminal elimination phase lasting 1 or 2 days. The effects may be further prolonged by the principal active metabolite, desmethyldiazepam, which has a half-life of 2–5 days.

Metabolism and Elimination

Extensive hepatic metabolism occurs, primarily by oxidation, to water-soluble glucuronide metabolites. In addition to desmethyldiazepam, other active metabolites include oxazepam and temazepam (Fig. 8); up to 70% of these metabolites are then excreted either free or conjugated in the urine. Enterohepatic circulation may result in a secondary peak in plasma concentrations some 6–12 hours later. This, together with the active metabolites, may account for the prolonged sedative effects seen with diazepam.

The plasma half-life of diazepam and its metabolites are prolonged in the elderly, in neonates, in patients with liver disease, and in those taking cimetidine (Tagamet), which inhibits the liver microsomal enzymes necessary for hepatic oxidation.

Pharmacodynamics

Cardiovascular System

Diazepam has been used as an induction agent in patients with cardiovascular disease, due to its relative cardiovascular stability, particularly when compared with barbiturate anesthetics. Intravenous administration results in a slight fall in arterial pressure, cardiac output, and peripheral vascular resistance, with a small transient increase in heart rate. This relative hemodynamic stability makes diazepam a useful induction agent in those with valvular or ischemic heart disease. However, as is often the case, diazepam is used as a co-induction agent with an opiate such as fentanyl. In this situation there is an additive, negative inotropic effect resulting in a greater reduction in blood pressure, cardiac output, and peripheral vascular resistance.

Respiratory System

Respiratory depression is of little clinical importance after oral or low-dose intravenous administration in normal individuals. However, when administered in combination with an opiate, or if larger doses are used, apnea may result.

Central Nervous System

Diazepam, given intravenously, is rapidly anxiolytic, has amnestic and sedative effects, and will result in unconsciousness. However, the onset is slower than that of the barbiturates, and the dose required varies greatly,

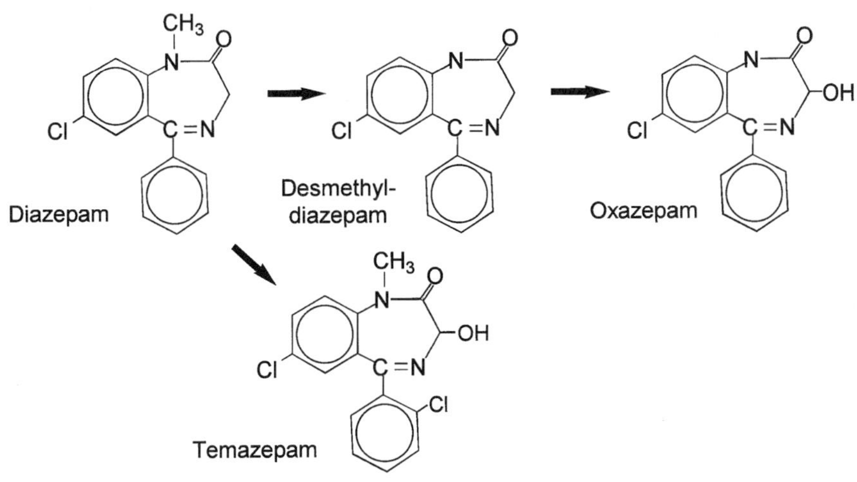

FIG. 8. Metabolism of diazepam. Note the active metabolites, des-methyl diazepam, oxazepam, and temazepam.

requiring individual titration. When used for sedation, marked anterograde, but not retrograde, amnesia occurs, a useful premedicant property. Diazepam has no direct analgesic action.

A reduction in cerebral oxygen consumption, cerebral blood flow, and intracranial pressure follow the use of diazepam, though to a lesser extent than with thiopentone. The GABA-minergic properties result in strong anticonvulsant activity. Diazepam can be used to stop or prevent generalized seizures in epileptics or those induced by local anesthetics.

The muscle relaxant properties are mediated at the brainstem and spinal cord level, probably via several mechanisms involving inhibitory interneurones.

Pregnancy and the Neonate

The use of diazepam in the first trimester has been implicated as a cause of various congenital malformations; however, no clear relationship has been established (17). Administration of benzodiazepines later in pregnancy is associated with neonatal drowsiness and respiratory depression, as well as the features of the floppy infant syndrome such as hypotonia, hypothermia, and suckling difficulties (18). These effects may last several days due to immaturity of neonatal hepatic metabolism. Withdrawal symptoms may occur in the infants of mothers who have been on long-term benzodiazepines. Competition with bilirubin for plasma protein binding and conjugation pathways may result in hyperbilirubinemia (19).

Diazepam is also transferred into breast milk at concentrations approximately 10% of maternal levels. If large doses are used, breast feeding should be stopped. Diazepam is not indicated in the management of severe hypertension in pregnancy; however, it may be used to prevent or control convulsions in preeclampsia, provided the adverse effects on the fetus are appreciated (19).

TABLE 6. *Recommended dosages for diazepam*

Premedication/sedation	
Adults—intravenous	0.05–0.2 mg/kg (max 20 mg)
Adults—oral	0.2–0.5 mg/kg (max 20 mg)
Children—oral	0.1–0.2 mg/kg (max 4 doses)
Induction	
Adults—intravenous	0.3–0.6 mg/kg
Children—intravenous	0.1 mg/kg
Anticonvulsant	
Adults—intravenous	5–10 mg initially (max 30 mg)
Children > 5 years —intravenous	1 mg slowly (max 10 mg)
Children > 30 days —intravenous	0.2–0.3 mg/kg slowly (max 5 mg)
Muscle spasm	
Adults—intravenous	5–10 mg initially
Acute anxiety states/alcohol withdrawal	
Adults—oral	2–10 mg 8 hourly

Dosage and Administration

Oral and intravenous routes are preferred (Table 6). Intramuscular injections are not only painful, but can result in the formation of sterile abscesses, and absorption is unpredictable. A rectal solution of diazepam is useful for the control of convulsions in children. Elderly patients may be particularly sensitive to the sedative effects of benzodiazepines. Up to half the adult dose is recommended, and particular care is needed when the intravenous route is used.

To reduce thrombophlebitis, a large vein should be used or, alternatively, administration through a running drip, though a cloudy precipitate usually forms. Problems may arise when infusions are set up as in excess of 50% may be adsorbed onto the walls of polyvinyl chloride administration sets. In view of the risks of tolerance and dependence, diazepam should always be given in the lowest dose needed to control symptoms; however, for short-term use this is not usually a problem.

Complications and Side Effects

Central Nervous System

Drowsiness, sedation, and ataxia as a result of CNS depression are the most frequently seen side effects of diazepam use. Other side effects include vertigo, confusion, dysarthria, muscle weakness, visual disturbances, amnesia, and paradoxical excitation and disinhibition. Rebound anxiety and insomnia may result from tolerance or may be part of the withdrawal syndrome following chronic use.

Overdose can produce CNS depression and unconsciousness, particularly when taken in combination with other CNS depressants, alcohol, antihistamines, general anesthetics, antidepressants, and opiates. High doses may be taken for the euphoriant effects or for suicidal overdose.

Cardiovascular

Pain and thrombophlebitis may occur with some formulations. Higher doses, especially when used in combination with other cardiovascular depressants, may result in marked hypotension.

Respiratory

Diazepam should be avoided in patients with preexisting CNS depression, acute respiratory problems, or sleep apnea and used with caution in patients with chronic respiratory disease. Care must be exercised in the elderly and in those with renal or hepatic impairment, as relatively small doses may result in respiratory depression and unconsciousness.

Hypersensitivity and Local Reactions

Anaphylaxis and other hypersensitivity reactions are rare with diazepam. Reactions have been reported with early formulations in Cremphor EL. Accidental intraarterial injection has been associated with ischemia and gangrene.

Midazolam

Description

Midazolam is a short-acting, water-soluble benzodiazepine used as a premedicant, a sedative for minor surgical procedures, and for the co-induction of anesthesia. It is also used for sedation in intensive care. Midazolam is available for parenteral, oral, or rectal administration, though the parenteral route is most often used.

The structure of midazolam is unusual in that it contains an imidazole ring. This ring contributes to the water solubility characteristics by exhibiting a pH-dependent ring-opening phenomenon (Fig. 9). At high pH—greater than 4.0—the ring remains closed and enhances lipid solubility; however, at low pH—less than 4.0—the ring opens and becomes water soluble. The intravenous formulation of midazolam is buffered to a pH of 3.5, enhancing water solubility; therefore, it does not require a solvent. As a result, the incidence of injection pain and thrombophlebitis is low. Once it enters the body, at physiological pH of 7.4, the ring closes and midazolam becomes extremely lipid-soluble.

Pharmacokinetics

Absorption and Distribution

Midazolam is the most lipid-soluble benzodiazepine available and rapidly crosses the blood–brain barrier after intravenous administration. When used as an induction agent, anesthesia occurs in 2–3 min. Synergism is exhibited when coadministered with an opiate such as fentanyl (21) or when used in combination with propofol (22), necessitating a marked reduction in the expected dose.

In contrast to diazepam, intramuscular injections are rapidly absorbed and free from pain and local irritation. Onset of sedation occurs within 15 min, with peak levels achieved in 30–60 min, the overall bioavailability being in excess of 90%. Oral midazolam is rapidly absorbed from the gastrointestinal tract; however, it undergoes significant first-pass metabolism, resulting in a bioavailability of 50%. It is sometimes given intranasally (as premedication) for this reason.

Metabolism and Elimination

Midazolam is hydroxylated in the liver to the principal metabolite, 1-hydroxymidazolam. This is less active than midazolam and is excreted in the urine as glucuronide conjugates. Less than 0.03% of the original dose is excreted unchanged. The relatively large volume of distribution (0.8–1.8 L/kg), short elimination half-life (1–2.8 hours), and high clearance (0.24–0.73 L/hour/kg) results in a short duration of action and rapid recovery. Midazolam is, therefore, not likely to accumulate following intravenous infusions and is used in this respect for sedation in intensive care. Nevertheless, the elimination half-life has been found to be increased by up to sixfold in some intensive-care patients and in the elderly, sedated long-term with midazolam. Infusions should, therefore, be tailored to the therapeutic effect required.

Enzyme-inhibiting drugs such as erythromycin may reduce the clearance of midazolam, resulting in raised

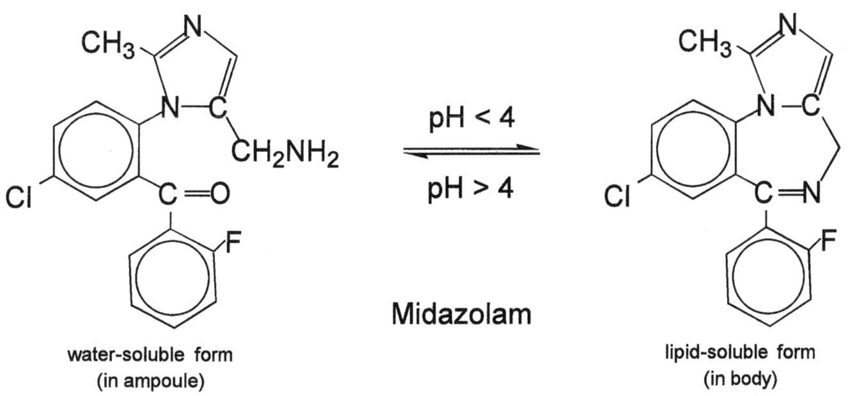

FIG. 9. Structural formula of midazolam. Note the pH-dependent changes in the structure.

plasma levels and unexpected CNS depression. Midazolam does not suppress adrenal steroidogenesis, as does etomidate, a similar imidazole-based induction agent.

Pharmacodynamics

The pharmacodynamics of midazolam are essentially very similar to diazepam—in particular, the anxiolytic, sedative, anticonvulsant, muscle relaxant, and amnestic properties. An outline of the fundamental differences is presented below.

Central Nervous System

In common with diazepam, cerebral metabolic rate, oxygen consumption, and blood flow are reduced with midazolam; however, cerebral perfusion pressure (mean arterial pressure less intracranial pressure) may be decreased. This is due to a fall in blood pressure greater than the fall in intracranial pressure. If used with caution, this effect is of little clinical significance, and midazolam may be safely used to induce anesthesia in neurosurgical patients.

Cardiovascular System

Midazolam may cause a greater fall in blood pressure and peripheral vascular resistance than does diazepam and produces an increase in heart rate due to preservation of the baroreceptor response. It does not abolish the hemodynamic response to laryngoscopy and intubation.

Respiratory System

A number of fatalities have been reported due to respiratory depression with the use of midazolam, in both the UK and US. This effect is probably comparable to diazepam; however, the onset is far quicker. Midazolam has no effect on pulmonary compliance or bronchomotor tone.

Pregnancy and the Neonate

Midazolam is not recommended for obstetric use as it crosses the placenta and may result in neonatal CNS depression. Though the concentrations (and half-life) of midazolam and its hydroxy-metabolite, found in breast milk, are small and likely to be of little clinical significance, it is not recommended for nursing mothers (23).

Dosage and Administration

Midazolam is most often administered intravenously, but can also be given orally and rectally (see Table 7).

TABLE 7. *Recommended dosages for midazolam*

Sedation/premedication	
Adults—intravenous	0.02–0.05 mg/kg (Normally 2–7 mg in healthy adults. Bolus in 1–2 mg increments to desired effect)
Adults—intramuscular	0.02–0.08 mg/kg
Children—rectal*	0.5 mg/kg
Children—intranasal	0.1 mg/kg (onset around 10 min)
Intravenous infusions (in ICU)	0.03–0.2 mg/kg/hour IV
Induction	
Adults—intravenous	0.15–0.35 mg/kg
Children > 7 years —intravenous	0.15 mg/kg
Insomnia	
Adults—oral	7.5–15 mg (at night)

*From Beebe et al. (33).

Recently, intranasal (24,25), sublingual (26), and intrathecal (27) routes of administration have been described.

Midazolam should be administered slowly, according to effect, and reduced in the elderly, debilitated patients and in those with hepatic or renal impairment. Full cardiovascular monitoring and facilities for resuscitation must be available.

Precautions and Side Effects

Central Nervous System

Many of the side effects are common to all benzodiazepines. The critically ill and those with hepatic or renal impairment are particularly prone to the central sedative effects of benzodiazepines. Discontinuing midazolam after prolonged use may result in withdrawal symptoms. There are also reports of agitation, tonic/clonic movements, muscle tremor, and hyperactivity occurring with therapeutic sedative doses.

Cardiovascular

Particular care is needed when midazolam is administered to those with impaired cardiovascular function or hypovolemia. Patients with cardiac failure have a reduced clearance rate and may, therefore, suffer from prolonged sedation.

Respiratory

The most significant side effect is probably respiratory depression and apnea. Patients with compromised respiratory function—particularly, chronic obstructive pulmonary disease, sleep apnea, or those who have received other central nervous system depressants—are unusually sensitive. Hiccup and coughing may occur following intravenous midazolam, precipitating laryngospasm.

The availability of the antagonist flumazenil should not encourage a more relaxed attitude to the use of intravenous midazolam for sedation.

Local

Pain, tenderness, and thrombophlebitis have been reported, but are rare.

Flumazenil

Description

Flumazenil, a specific benzodiazepine antagonist, reverses most of the sedative effects of benzodiazepines by competitive inhibition at central benzodiazepine receptors. An imidazobenzodiazepine structurally related to midazolam (Fig. 10), it is presented as a clear aqueous solution for intravenous injection, each 5-ml ampule containing 0.5 mg. The hypnotic and sedative effects are reversed within a few minutes, even after large doses of benzodiazepines. However, because of its short duration of action, these effects may slowly return, necessitating further doses or an intravenous infusion. It is well tolerated and has few side effects.

Flumazenil is indicated for the reversal of benzodiazepine-induced effects following anesthesia and sedation, and to diagnose and treat known or suspected cases of benzodiazepine overdose. Patients who may benefit from its use include those at increased risk of postoperative complications and those in whom a postoperative neurological assessment is required. Flumazenil may be of benefit in weaning patients off ventilation in the intensive care unit, when benzodiazepines have been used for sedation, although for long-term patients this is not recommended, due to the risk of precipitating withdrawal symptoms.

Beneficial responses have also been observed when administered during the early stages of hepatic encephalopathy (28,29). This is not a universal phenomenon and is not as yet an indication for its use.

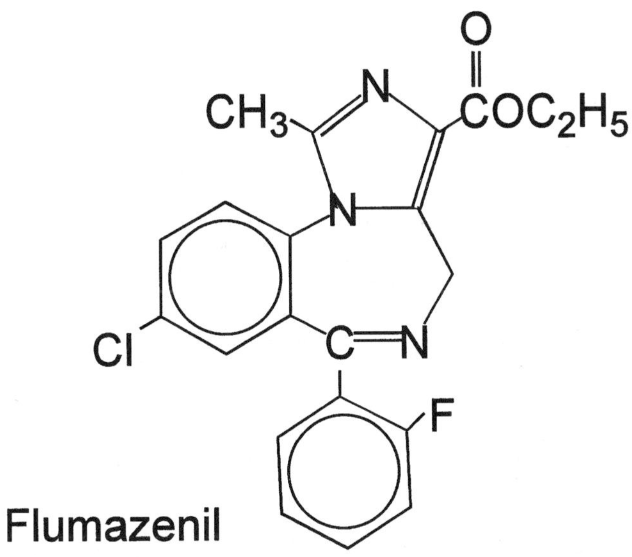

FIG. 10. Structural formula for flumazenil.

Pharmacokinetics

Flumazenil is a weak lipophilic base, 50% bound to plasma proteins, that rapidly crosses the blood–brain barrier following intravenous administration, leading to an onset of action within minutes. The rapid and extensive hepatic metabolism and elimination half-life of 53 min are reflected in the short duration of action (1–3 hours). The products of metabolism, principally the carboxylic acid, are inactive as either agonists or antagonists, and are renally excreted in the free and conjugate forms.

Pharmacodynamics

Central Nervous System

Flumazenil antagonizes the anxiolytic, sedative, muscle relaxant, anticonvulsant, and amnestic properties of the benzodiazepines. It is specific for the benzodiazepine receptor and does not reverse the effects of barbiturates, alcohol, or opiates. In high doses, it has a weak agonist-like effect, but none at normal therapeutic doses.

The reversal of benzodiazepine effects may precipitate withdrawal symptoms or convulsions in those with benzodiazepine dependency or in those who have been on long-term benzodiazepine treatment.

Cardiorespiratory

Flumazenil has minimal cardiorespiratory effects, and those seen are due to a reversal of the central depressant effects of the benzodiazepines, i.e., transient increases in blood pressure and heart rate and reversal of the respiratory depression.

Pregnancy and Children

No evidence of teratogenicity. Few data are available in children.

TABLE 8. *Recommended dosages for flumazenil*

Reversal of therapeutic doses of benzodiazepines	
Initially	0.2 mg IV slowly
If no response after 60 sec further	0.1-mg increments (max 1 mg with usual dose being 0.3–0.6 mg)
Reversal of benzodiazepine overdose	
Initially	0.3 mg IV slowly
If no response after 60 sec further	0.2-mg increments (max 2 mg)

Dosage and Administration

See Table 8 for dosage recommendations. If drowsiness recurs, an infusion of 0.1–0.4 mg/hr can be used, titrated according to the response required. The benefits of the use of flumazenil in reversing sedation should be balanced against the risks of precipitating withdrawal symptoms.

Precautions and Side Effects

Side effects, although rare, include nausea, vomiting, flushing, anxiety, and headache. Flumazenil is not recommended in epileptics who have received benzodiazepines, as convulsions may be precipitated. Extreme caution is needed when administered to those with known or suspected benzodiazepine dependency. If withdrawal symptoms occur, midazolam or diazepam should be administered.

In cases of mixed overdose, benzodiazepines may have a protective effect from the psychotropic and cardiovascular effects of other drugs. In particular, the presence of autonomic, neurologic, or cardiovascular symptoms arising from an overdose of tricyclic antidepressants is a contraindication to its use (30,31).

Although flumazenil may reverse the obvious effects of sedation, higher cognitive functions may remain impaired. Patients should not, therefore, operate dangerous machinery or drive for 24 hours after administration. There is the additional risk of resedation, particularly when antagonizing longer-acting agents such as diazepam.

REFERENCES

1. Vangerven M, Delrue G, Brugman E, Cosaert P. A new therapeutic approach to accidental intra-arterial injection of thiopentone. *Br J Anaesth* 1989;62:98–100.
2. Servin F, Farinotti R, Haberer JP, Desmonts JM. Propofol infusion for maintenance of anesthesia in morbidly obese patients receiving nitrous oxide. A clinical and pharmacokinetic study. *Anesthesiology* 1993;78(4):657–665.
3. Ben-Shlomo I, Finger J, Bar-Av E, Perl AZ, Etchin A, Tverskoy M. Propofol and fentanyl act additively for induction of anaesthesia. *Anaesthesia* 1993;48(2):111–113.
4. Wood PR, Browne GP, Pugh S. Propofol infusion for the treatment of status epilepticus. *Lancet* 1988;1(8583):480–481.
5. Hullander RM, Leivers D, Wingler K. A comparison of propofol and etomidate for cardioversion. *Anesth Analg* 1993;77:690–694.
6. Rampton AJ, Griffin RM, Stuart CS, Durcan JJ, Huddy NC, Abott MA. Comparison of methohexital and propofol for electroconvulsive therapy: effects on hemodynamic responses and seizure duration. *Anesthesiology* 1989;70:412–417.
7. Parke TJ, Stevens JE, Rice AS, Greenaway CL, Bray RJ, Smith PJ, Waldmann CS, Verghese C. Metabolic acidosis and fatal myocardial failure after propofol infusion in children: five case reports. *BMJ* 1992;305:613–616.
8. Harrison GG. Propofol in malignant hyperthermia. *Lancet* 1991;337:503.
9. Meissner PN, Harrison GG, Hift RJ. Propofol as an IV anaesthetic induction agent in variegate porphyria. *Br J Anaesth* 1991;66:60–65.
10. Tidmarsh MA, Baigent DF. Propofol in acute intermittent porphyria. *Br J Anaesth* 1992;68(2):230.
11. Ledingham IM, Watt I. Influence of sedation on mortality in critically ill multiple trauma patients. *Lancet* 1983;1:1270.
12. Watkins J. Etomidate: an 'immunologically safe' anaesthetic agent. *Anaesthesia* 1983;38:Suppl 34–38.
13. Moore MR, McColl KEL. *Porphyria: Drug Lists*. Glasgow: Porphyria Research Unit, University of Glasgow, 1991.
14. L'Hommedieu CS, Arens JJ. The use of ketamine for the emergency intubation of patients with status asthmaticus. *Ann Emerg Med* 1987; 16:568–571.
15. Rock MJ, Reyes de la Rocha SL, L'Hommedieu CS, Truemper E. Use of ketamine in asthmatic children to treat respiratory failure refractory to conventional therapy. *Crit Care Med* 1986;14:514–516.
16. Snyder SH. Drug and neurotransmitter receptors. New perspectives with clinical relevance. *JAMA* 1989;261:3126–3129.
17. Laegreid L, Olegard R, Conradi N, Hagberg G, Wahlstrom J, Abrahamsson L. Congenital malformations and maternal consumption of benzodiazepines: a case-control study. *Dev Med Child Neurol* 1990; 32:432–441.
18. Cree JE, Meyer J, Hailey DM. Diazepam in labour: its metabolism and effect on the clinical condition and thermogenesis of the newborn. *BMJ* 1973;4:251–255.
19. Notarianni LJ. Plasma protein binding of drugs in pregnancy and in neonates. *Clin Pharmacokinet* 1990;18:20–36.
20. Chamberlain G. ABC of antenatal care. Raised blood pressure in pregnancy. *BMJ* 1991;302:1454–1458.
21. Ben-Shlomo I, abd-el-Khalim H, Ezry J, Zohar S, Tverskoy M. Midazolam acts synergistically with fentanyl for induction of anaesthesia. *Br J Anaesth* 1990;64:45–47
22. Short TG, Chui PT. Propofol and midazolam act synergistically in combination. *Br J Anaesth* 1991;67:539–545.
23. Matheson I, Lunde PK, Bredesen JE. Midazolam and nitrazepam in the maternity ward: milk concentrations and clinical effects. *Br J Clin Pharmacol* 1990;30:787–793.
24. Walberg EJ, Wills RJ, Eckhert J. Plasma concentrations of midazolam in children following intranasal administration. *Anesthesiology* 1991;74:233–235.
25. Rey E, Delaunay L, Pons G, Murat I, Richard MO, Saint-Maurice C, Olive G. Pharmacokinetics of midazolam in children: comparative study of intranasal and intravenous administration. *Eur J Clin Pharmacol* 1991;41:355–357.
26. Wong L, McQuenn KD. Midazolam routes of administration. *DICP* 1991;25:476–477.
27. Cripps TP, Goodchild CS. Intrathecal midazolam and stress response to upper abdominal surgery. *Clin J Pain* 1988;4:125–128.
28. Grimm G, Ferenci P, Katzenschlager R, Madl C, Schneeweiss B, Laggner AN, Lenz K, Gangl A. Improvement of hepatic encephalopathy treated with flumazenil. *Lancet* 1988;2:1392–1394.
29. Mullen KD. Benzodiazepine compounds and hepatic encephalopathy. *N Engl J Med* 1991;325:509–511.
30. Burr W, Sandham P, Judd A. Death after flumazenil. *BMJ* 1989;298:1713.
31. Marchant B, Wray R, Leach A, Nama M. Flumazenil causing convulsions and ventricular tachycardia. *BMJ* 1989;299:860.
32. Naguib M, Adu-Gyamfi Y, Absood GH, Farag H, Gyasi HK. Epidural ketamine for postoperative analgesia. *Can Anaesth Soc J* 1986;33:16–21.
33. Beebe DS, Belani KG, Chang PN, Hesse PS, Schuh JS, Liao JC, Palahniuk RJ. Effectiveness of preoperative sedation with rectal midazolam, ketamine, or their combination in young children. *Anesth Analg* 1992;75:880–884.

Airway Management, edited by
L.H. Hanowell, M.D. and R.J. Waldron, M.D.,
Lippincott-Raven Publishers, Philadelphia © 1996.

CHAPTER 10

Inhalational Anesthetic Agents

Wendy J. Falloon, Richard J. Waldron, Dennis L. Fung

INTRODUCTION

The introduction of the inhalational agents heralded the beginning of modern anesthesia and surgery. The first successful demonstration of anesthesia was performed at the Massachusetts General Hospital in 1846 by W.G. Morton, a dentist and second-year medical student, using ether. Within a year of this demonstration, ether was being used for surgical anesthesia around the world.

Despite recent developments with intravenous agents, inhalational agents (also known as *volatiles*) remain the most commonly used agents for maintenance of surgical anesthesia. Inhalational (gaseous) induction of anesthesia is also useful in children (where intravenous access may be difficult) and in patients with either incomplete obstruction of the upper airways or suspected difficulty in airway management.

Due to their mode of administration, certain considerations specific to the inhalational agents must be understood before the individual drugs are discussed. Two of the most important concepts are:

W.J. Falloon: Special Anaesthetist, Hobart, Tasmania, Australia 7000.

R.J. Waldron: Department of Anaesthetic Services, Royal Hobart Hospital; and University of Tasmania, Hobart, Tasmania, Australia 7001.

D.L. Fung: Department of Anesthesiology, University of California, Davis School of Medicine, Sacramento, California 95817.

1. Minimum alveolar concentration (MAC)
2. Uptake and distribution of inhalational agents

MINIMUM ALVEOLAR CONCENTRATION

Minimum alveolar concentration (MAC) is the concentration of an anesthetic gas or vapor that inhibits movement in response to a surgical stimulus in 50% of a population at one atmosphere (1). The concept that the alveolar concentration of an inhalational agent reflects its partial pressure at the site of anesthetic action (see Uptake and Distribution of Inhalational Anesthetic Agents) has made MAC an extremely useful index of anesthetic potency, allowing comparisons to be made between inhalational agents. If inhalational agents are combined, their total anesthetic effect is determined by simple addition of their MAC fractions.

Another measure of potency is the AD_{95} (anesthetic dose), which is the alveolar concentration of an inhalational agent required to inhibit movement in response to surgery in 95% of patients. This is approximately 1.5 MAC. The AD_{95} may be a more useful estimate of actual anesthetic requirement than is MAC, but MAC is used more commonly.

Minimum alveolar concentration is altered by many factors (2,3). For example, MAC requirements are maximum at 3–4 months of age and declines thereafter. Elderly patients have a significantly decreased requirement for inhalational anesthetic agents. Many drugs

TABLE 1. *Factors affecting minimum alveolar concentration*

Decreases MAC	No effect	Increases MAC
Elderly/neonates	Gender	Age 3–4 months
Concurrent drug administration	Anemia	Alcohol abuse
Hypothermia	Hypertension	Hyperthermia
Hypercarbia	Hypocarbia	Hypernatremia
Severe hypoxia		Amphetamine use
Hypotension		
Pregnancy		

MAC, minimum alveolar concentration.

TABLE 2. *Summary of factors affecting uptake of inhalational anesthetic agents*

Anesthetic machine to alveolus	• Inspired concentration • Second gas effect • Alveolar ventilation/fresh gas flow
Alveolus to pulmonary capillary	• Blood:gas solubility • Cardiac output • Alveolar/mixed venous pressure gradient
Pulmonary capillary to brain	• Tissue blood flow • Arterial/tissue pressure gradient

reduce the amount of volatile agent required to maintain anesthesia, including opioids, benzodiazepines, local anesthetic agents, and nitrous oxide. Other factors that may alter MAC (or have no effect) are listed in Table 1.

UPTAKE AND DISTRIBUTION OF INHALATIONAL ANESTHETIC AGENTS

The objective of inhalational anesthesia is to achieve an optimal partial pressure of anesthetic agent in the brain (see Figure 1 for chemical structures). Delivery of inhaled anesthetic agents to their site of action occurs as a result of the presence of a series of partial pressure gradients from the anesthetic machine to the brain. This gradient causes a greater movement of agent into the body than out until equilibrium is reached, that is:

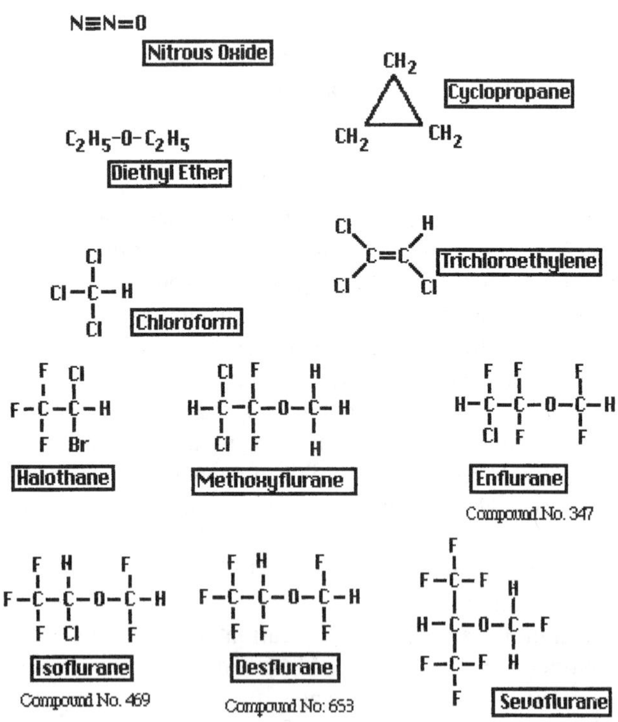

FIG. 1. Chemical formulas of inhalational anesthetic agents.

$$P_i \leftrightarrow P_A \leftrightarrow P_a \leftrightarrow P_{br}$$

where P_i is inspired partial pressure of inhalational agent; P_A is alveolar partial pressure of inhalational agent; P_a is arterial partial pressure of inhalational agent; and P_{br} is brain tissue partial pressure of inhalational agent.

At equilibrium, the alveolar partial pressure of anesthetic agent will determine arterial and, therefore, brain partial pressure, as indicated by the above equation. Alveolar partial pressure depends on the delivery of anesthetic agent to the alveolus and its removal (uptake) into the body. The balance of these factors, therefore, ultimately determines brain partial pressure.

The main variables that alter the rate of delivery, uptake, and distribution of inhalational anesthetic agents in the body are listed in Table 2. Most of these variables will not operate independently, and factors affecting one may alter another.

Anesthetic Machine to Alveolus

Inspired Concentration (Ci)

The higher the inspired concentration of inhalational agent, the more rapidly alveolar concentration (and, therefore, brain partial pressure) will reach an anesthetic level (4). This occurs because, at higher inspired concentrations, a greater mass of agent is delivered to the alveolus per unit volume of fresh gas flow (FGF).

This "concentra*tion* effect" is modified by the time taken for the concentration dialed at the vaporizer to be achieved at the patient/circuit interface. This time ("washin") is prolonged by:

1. Decreased FGF.
2. Increased volume of anesthetic circuitry.
3. Increased solubility of anesthetic agent in rubber and soda lime.
4. Use of a rebreathing circuit.

Second Gas Effect

This effect occurs when two inhalational agents are delivered together, most noticeably with the use of nitrous oxide in high concentration (5,6). The rapid transfer of large volumes of N_2O from the alveolus to pulmonary capillary (due to the presence of a large concentration gradient) results in (a) an increase in the concentration of the remaining anesthetic vapor (e.g., halothane)—the concentra*ting* effect; and (b) an increase in alveolar ventilation as the space previously occupied by N_2O is passively filled by fresh gas. The result is a more rapid rise in alveolar and, therefore, brain concentration of inhalational agent.

Alveolar Ventilation

In practice, alveolar ventilation can be approximated by the fresh gas flow. Increasing FGF will, therefore, increase the amount of anesthetic agent delivered to the alveolus and, therefore, the rate of rise of alveolar concentration (7). This effect is maximal with the more soluble agents but scarcely affects N_2O.

When a patient under anesthesia is breathing spontaneously, ventilation is depressed in a dose-dependent fashion by inhalational agents. This acts as a negative feedback system, limiting the rise of alveolar concentration above a level that might dangerously depress respiration and the cardiovascular system.

Alveolus to Pulmonary Capillary

Solubility

The greater the solubility of an anesthetic agent in blood, the more rapidly it passes from the alveolus to the pulmonary capillary and is removed by the pulmonary circulation. This results in a slower rise in alveolar partial pressure and a delay in the development of adequate brain partial pressures. Solubility is measured as the blood:gas partition coefficient (8). For example, isoflurane has a blood:gas coefficient of 1.2, i.e., the blood concentration of isoflurane will be 1.2 times greater than its gaseous concentration, although at equilibrium their partial pressures will be equal.

Methoxyflurane and ether are both highly soluble agents (blood:gas coefficients >10), and inhalational induction of anesthesia is, therefore, slow in comparison with the moderately soluble agents (halothane, enflurane, and isoflurane). The most rapid rise in alveolar partial pressure occurs with the least soluble agents such as cyclopropane, N_2O, sevoflurane, and desflurane (blood: gas coefficients < 1). Desflurane is not recommended for inhalational inductions, however, as it has a very pungent odor and provokes airway irritability.

Cardiac Output

An increase in cardiac output (and pulmonary capillary blood flow) will result in a more rapid removal of anesthetic agent from the alveolus and will, therefore, delay the achievement of the required alveolar concentration of agent (9). Children have relatively high cardiac outputs and will, therefore, take longer to achieve the optimal concentration than will the elderly, who have relatively low cardiac outputs.

Alveolar to Mixed Venous Anesthetic Partial Pressure Gradient

Transfer of anesthetic agent across the alveolar–capillary membrane occurs as simple diffusion down a concentration gradient and is, therefore, limited by the size of this gradient, i.e., the relative alveolar to mixed venous agent partial pressure. It is also affected by membrane thickness (not likely to be clinically significant) and the solubility coefficient of the agent.

Pulmonary Capillary to Tissues

Tissue Solubility

Unlike blood:gas coefficients that vary widely, tissue:blood coefficients (i.e., tissue solubilities) in lean tissues range from < 1 to 4 (10). In other words, the affinity of all anesthetic agents for lean tissues is roughly equal. Tissue:blood coefficients for fat, however, are significantly greater than 1, ranging from 2.3 for N_2O to 62 for halothane. This means that almost all of the agent carried by blood flowing through fat will be transferred to it, but as fat blood flow is so low, its anesthetic partial pressure will rise very slowly (see next section).

Tissue Blood Flow

Tissue blood flow (TBF) affects tissue uptake of inhalational agents. Highly perfused tissues such as brain will have more agent delivered per unit of time than will those with poor perfusion and will, therefore, equilibrate more rapidly. Tissues can be grouped on the basis of their perfusion (and tissue solubility) and, therefore, on the time taken to reach equilibrium (11).

The vessel-rich group (VRG) consists of the brain, heart, splanchnic bed (including liver), kidneys, and endocrine organs. These organs weigh less than 10% of the total body weight but receive 75% of the cardiac output (75 ml/100g/min). Equilibration is 90% complete by 10 min, with actual times varying with the tissue solubility of the individual agent. Uptake after 10 min is determined by the muscle group.

The muscle group (MG) is made up of lean muscle and skin, comprising 50% of total body weight but receiving only 20% of cardiac output. It has a much lower perfusion than does the VRG (3 ml/100g/min). Equilibration occurs after 1–4 hours of anesthesia.

The fat group (FG) is the only remaining depot for agent uptake after muscle equilibration is complete. In a patient of average proportions, it comprises 20% of body weight and has a blood flow of 300 ml/min. On a weight-for-weight basis, this is similar to the perfusion of resting muscle; however, fat differs from muscle in its high affinity for anesthetic agents, which prolongs the period over which it will continue to absorb anesthetic. Equilibration will not occur during a normal anesthetic with enflurane, for example, although it may occur with N_2O (5–6 hours), due to its lower fat:blood coefficient.

The vessel-poor group (VPG) contains ligament, tendon, bone, and cartilage. It makes up 20% of body mass, but its lack of significant blood flow prevents its participation in the anesthetic uptake process.

Arterial to Tissue Partial Pressure Gradient

Transfer of anesthetic agent from the arterial system to the tissues occurs by simple diffusion down a concentration gradient. At equilibrium, the same amount of agent is transferred from the tissue back to the circulation as is transferred into the tissue, i.e., effective uptake will cease. The time taken to equilibrate is altered by tissue solubility and blood flow, as discussed earlier.

FACTORS AFFECTING RECOVERY FROM ANESTHESIA

In general, the factors influencing the uptake and distribution of anesthetic agents also affect recovery; i.e., alveolar ventilation, solubility, cardiac output, and the venous–alveolar partial pressure difference. Of these, the most important is solubility, recovery being rapid for the less soluble drugs such as desflurane (12).

It is important to note, however, that recovery differs from induction in two important respects.

1. The inspired concentration of agent cannot be reduced below zero. In other words, the reverse of the concentration effect does not apply.
2. It may take hours for muscle and fat to equilibrate. Fat continues to take up halothane for several hours after the vaporizer has been turned off and will, therefore, be released from the body for a long period of time, resulting in "hangover" effects.

Diffusion Hypoxia

The concentration effect and the second gas effect occur during induction of anesthesia, due to the uptake of large volumes of nitrous oxide. During recovery, the concentration gradient is reversed, and large amounts of nitrous oxide will move rapidly from the blood into the alveoli. The inspired air also has a high concentration of nitrogen (~78%). This produces the effect known as *diffusion hypoxia* (13), in which inspired ambient oxygen (F_I=21%) will be diluted by N_2O and nitrogen. Dilution of alveolar CO_2 may also result, reducing respiratory drive and increasing the likelihood of arterial hypoxemia (14). This problem is very simply overcome by supplying the patient with enriched oxygen mixtures during recovery from anesthesia.

Agent Loss Via Other Routes

As well as their normal route of excretion via the lungs, inhalational agents are removed from the body via the skin and through biodegradation. Transcutaneous loss is minimal (15), although with a 70% alveolar concentration of N_2O, 5–10 ml/hour will pass through the skin. As well, N_2O passes into closed gas spaces that may be compliant (bowel, pneumothorax, pneumoperitoneum) or noncompliant (middle ear, skull,), which may be of clinical significance.

Metabolism of inhalational agents can be significant, with 20% to 50% of halothane and up to 75% of methoxyflurane being degraded in the body. Agents such as enflurane, isoflurane, and desflurane are minimally metabolized (16).

OLDER INHALATIONAL AGENTS

Historical Perspectives

Ether

The beginning of modern anesthesia came about in 1846 with the first successful public demonstration of ether anesthesia by Morton, on Mr. Gilbert Abbott, for removal of a vascular malformation below the mandible (17). Ether, while having the considerable disadvantages of explosivity in oxygen or N_2O, excessive salivation, postoperative nausea and vomiting, and slow induction and recovery, remains one of the safest anesthetics in relatively unskilled hands. In 1858, John Snow commented in his writings *On Chloroform and Other Anaesthetics*, "I hold it therefore to be almost impossible that a death from this agent can occur in the hands of a medical man who is applying it with ordinary intelligence and attention." Ether is still used today in many third-world countries because of its low cost of production and ease of use.

Chloroform

Chloroform was introduced into clinical practice and popularized by James Simpson in 1847. Within a short time it had become more popular than ether, but its first recorded casualty, a young girl having a minor procedure, occurred in less than 2 months. Its disadvantages include hypotension, delayed liver damage, and sudden cardiac arrest.

Trichloroethylene

This agent was introduced into clinical practice by Christopher Langton Hewer in London, who published case reports in 1941. Its advantages include good analgesia, nonflammability, little cardiorespiratory depression, and low cost. Its less attractive characteristics, however, are tachypnea, dysrhythmias, nausea and vomiting, lack of muscle relaxation, and the production of a neurotoxic breakdown product in the presence of soda lime.

Methoxyflurane

Methoxyflurane was first used in clinical anesthesia by Artusio and Van Poznak in 1960. It is a good analgesic, and induction is slow due to its high solubility. Its major disadvantage is the production of high levels of free F^- ions, which may result in a high output renal failure.

HALOTHANE

The introduction of halothane into clinical anesthetic practice marked the beginning of a new era in anesthesia. For the first time, anesthetists had available an agent that was noncombustible, low in toxicity (in comparison to previously available agents), and allowed relatively rapid induction and emergence (18). It was synthesized in the laboratories of Imperial Chemical Industries (ICI) near Manchester by C.W. Suckling in 1951 (19) and was first used in clinical practice in 1956 by Johnstone of Manchester (20).

Physical Properties

Carbon-fluorine compounds were developed to reduce flammability, and the presence of the trifluorocarbon confers molecular stability (21). Halothane is subject to decomposition when exposed to light, so it is stored in amber bottles with 0.01% thymol to stabilize the halothane. Thymol slowly accumulates, particularly in older model vaporizers, and can cause turnstiles or temperature compensation devices to malfunction. The physicochemical properties of halothane are listed in Table 3.

Pharmacokinetics

Uptake and Elimination

With its intermediate solubility (blood:gas coefficient 2.3), gaseous induction of halothane is not particularly rapid. However, it remains the agent of choice for this technique in most situations, due to its comparatively pleasant odor and low MAC, although sevoflurane has proven to be useful also for inhalational inductions.

Biotransformation

Halothane biotransformation during anesthesia affects at least 20% of the inhaled agent (22) and occurs via two principle pathways:

1. Oxidative pathway, in which the principal metabolite is trifluoroacetic acid, which has no known toxic effects. Bromide and chloride are other by-products. High bromide levels (also produced by the reductive pathway) may contribute to postoperative somnolence and confusion.
2. Reductive pathway, releasing volatile metabolites Br^- and F^-, which occurs only with halothane of the inhalational agents. Halothane degradation in soda-lime releases CF_2CBrCl into the gas mixture. Reductive metabolites have been implicated in the etiology of so-called halothane hepatitis.

Hepatotoxicity

The major disadvantage of the use of halothane is its association with hepatic dysfunction (23). Predisposing

TABLE 3. *Comparison of physicochemical properties*

Property	Halothane	Enflurane	Isoflurane	Desflurane	Sevoflurane	Nitrous oxide
Molecular weight (Da)	197.4	184.5	184.5	168	200.1	44
Boiling point (°C)	50.2	56.5	48.5	23.5	58.5	–89
Vapor pressure at 20°C (mm Hg)	243	172	238	664	160	—
Blood:gas partition coefficient	2.3	1.9	1.4	0.42	0.6–0.7	0.47
MAC in O_2 (%)	0.75	1.58	1.28	6–9	~2.0	105–110
MAC in 70% N_2O (%)	0.29	0.57	0.56	—	~1.0	—
Metabolism (%)	~20%	~2%	~0.2%	~0.02%	2–3%	—
Ozone depletion	Marked	Yes	Yes	Minimal	Minimal	Yes

MAC, minimum alveolar concentration.

factors include female sex, obesity, atopy, previous exposure to halothane, hypoxemia or reduced hepatic perfusion, preexisting hepatic disease, age, and enzyme induction (24). Two distinct forms have been observed. The most common manifestation, occurring in up to 20% of exposed patients, occurs 2–5 days following exposure, with fever, nausea, and vomiting, often followed by jaundice. Fortunately the more severe form, leading to hepatic failure, is very rare.

Massive hepatic necrosis was first reported in 1958 following halothane administration, though widespread attention was not drawn to the problem until 1963. The US National Halothane Study was published in 1966. It comprised a review of 850,000 halothane anesthetics given between 1959 and 1962. The frequency of severe damage was estimated as 1:6,000–1:35,000. There is no diagnostic laboratory test to confirm halothane hepatitis.

A large number of mechanisms have been proposed for the etiology of halothane hepatotoxicity, including a hypersensitivity reaction, the production of an antigenic metabolite-protein hapten, liver hypoxia, production of damaging reactive metabolites via the reductive pathway, and the unmasking of a previously asymptomatic viral hepatitis. Of these, two major mechanisms have attracted the most support and research (a) biotransformation of halothane to toxic intermediates; and (b) allergy or sensitization to halothane or a metabolite-protein hapten. This mechanism is supported by the common presence of a rash, eosinophilia, and autoantibodies.

Pharmacodynamics

Central Nervous System

Administration of halothane results in depression of the reticular activating system, cardiovascular and respiratory centers, and cerebral metabolism ($CMRO_2$). Paralysis of the respiratory center precedes vasomotor depression; therefore, apnea will occur before cardiovascular collapse, preventing the further inhalation of halothane. This can be seen particularly during inhalational induction in premature and very small neonates.

Halothane is a potent cerebral vasodilator, resulting in an increased cerebral blood flow (CBF), which causes an increase in intracranial pressure (ICP) (25). Therefore, halothane is not recommended for use in neurosurgery, following head injury, or in the presence of raised ICP. It is not as analgesic as methoxyflurane in low dose and is thought to be less emetic than other inhaled anesthetic agents.

Cardiovascular System

In addition to depression of the central vasomotor center, halothane produces a dose-related direct myocardial depression. Cardiac output falls initially but tends to return toward normal as the heart rate rises, compensating for the fall in stroke volume (26). Arterial hypotension is common and is due to a combination of peripheral vasodilation, myocardial depression, depression of the vasomotor center, sympathetic ganglion blockade, and inhibition of the baroreceptor reflex (preventing reflex vasoconstriction and tachycardia in response to a fall in blood pressure).

Halothane sensitizes the myocardium to exogenous and endogenous catecholamines, thus increasing the risk of dysrhythmias during anesthesia (27). If halothane cannot be avoided, it is recommended that the epinephrine dose be limited to 10 ml of 1:100,000 for short procedures or to 30 ml of the same concentration per hour of halothane anesthesia (adults). Epinephrine doses in children are reduced in proportion to their weights.

Dysrhythmias may also be due to a combination of direct inhibition of the conducting system by halothane, hypercapnia, hypoxemia, and light anesthesia (27). Rhythm disturbances that may be seen during halothane anesthesia include (a) ventricular extrasystoles, ventricular tachycardia, and even ventricular fibrillation due to increased myocardial excitability; and (b) bradycardias, the most common being nodal rhythm, which may be associated with hypotension.

Respiratory system

Respiratory depression is a significant side effect of all of the volatile anesthetic agents. Depression of the respiratory center by halothane results in decreased tidal volume and minute volume. Both the central chemoreceptors responsible for increasing ventilation in response to hypercapnia and the peripheral chemoreceptors responsible for increasing ventilation in response to hypoxemia are depressed. Respiratory rate is often increased. The pattern of spontaneous ventilation under halothane anesthesia is, therefore, rapid and shallow (28).

Other effects of halothane include a decrease in bronchomotor tone, resulting in bronchodilation. Halothane has been used successfully in patients with status asthmaticus when other pharmacological therapies have failed. It decreases salivary and bronchial secretions, as well as producing early depression of pharyngeal and laryngeal reflexes. This makes halothane a good agent for inhalational induction, particularly in the presence of upper airway obstruction.

Renal System

Halothane causes a reversible decrease in glomerular filtration rate (GFR) and renal blood flow (RBF). It has no direct effect on the renal parenchyma (29).

Muscle

As with all inhalational agents, halothane potentiates nondepolarizing neuromuscular blockade (30). Halothane-induced "shakes" are not uncommon, particularly after prolonged anesthesia, and are aggravated by hypothermia but can occur in normothermic patients. Shivering is also seen after the use of other anesthetic agents (isoflurane, enflurane, etc). This shivering can result in dramatic increases in oxygen consumption and may be dangerous in patients with ischemic heart disease.

Reproductive System

Halothane causes uterine muscle relaxation (via the β receptor) with inspired concentrations above 0.5%. It may also contribute to uterine atony and postpartum hemorrhage.

Liver

By virtue of its effects on blood pressure, the administration of halothane decreases hepatic blood flow by 25% to 30% (31). The association of halothane with postoperative hepatic dysfunction has already been discussed.

ENFLURANE

Enflurane, a fluorinated methyl ethyl ether, was developed in the US by Ross Terrell (32) in 1963 (agent 347 of over 700). The first clinical accounts of its use appeared in 1966. It has been widely and, for the most part, safely used around the world. However, with the cost reduction of isoflurane in the last few years, enflurane is believed by most to have been superseded.

Physical Properties

Enflurane is a clear, colorless, nonflammable, volatile agent that is more stable than halothane (it does not require the addition of a preservative) but less potent (MAC 1.6). Its lower blood:gas coefficient (1.9) is offset by its less acceptable odor, reducing its suitability for inhalational induction. It is stable when used with soda lime. The important physicochemical properties of enflurane are listed in Table 3.

Pharmacokinetics

Uptake and elimination of enflurane are governed by its physical properties and by the factors discussed earlier. It is excreted mostly unchanged by the lungs, but 2% to 3% is metabolized in the body to nonvolatile fluorinated metabolites. Of concern is the release of fluoride ions (F^-), which are excreted by the kidney and are potentially nephrotoxic above 50 μmol/L. This may occur after prolonged enflurane anesthesia (33) or in the presence of enzyme-inducing drugs (34).

Enflurane has been implicated as a cause of postoperative liver damage (35), though this link is not definite. A postulated mechanism is that of cross-sensitization with halothane.

Pharmacodynamics

Central Nervous System

Overall, enflurane results in cerebral depression but causes seizure activity on EEG. Tonic-clonic facial muscle twitching may be observed during administration of high concentrations, especially in association with hypocapnia (36). Although seizure activity has not been shown to be provoked in epileptics, it is not recommended for use in these patients.

Other central nervous system effects include cerebral vasodilation with increased cerebral blood flow and variable effects on ICP, depending on the $PaCO_2$ and inspired concentration.

Cardiovascular System

Enflurane produces dose-dependent myocardial depression, probably greater than that of halothane. Levels above 1.5 MAC may cause marked cardiovascular depression. Therefore, it has a narrow safety margin between the dose required for adequate anesthesia and the level at which dangerous side-effects may occur. Arterial hypotension is primarily due to its negative inotropic effect, although a decrease in systemic vascular resistance does also occur (37).

Enflurane does sensitize the myocardium to catecholamines but has a lower incidence of epinephrine-associated dysrhythmias than does halothane.

Respiratory System

Enflurane causes a more marked depression of ventilation than do other inhalational agents at similar MAC levels of anesthesia (38). Tidal volume is decreased but respiratory rate is unchanged or slightly increased. The ventilatory response to $PaCO_2$ and PaO_2 is depressed. It is relatively nonirritant to the respiratory tract and produces bronchodilation.

Renal System

Enflurane anesthesia produces a reduced renal blood flow, glomerular filtration rate, and, subsequently, urine output as a result of its cardiovascular effects. The formation of F^- is associated with renal damage (as discussed earlier); enflurane is, therefore, contraindicated in patients with renal failure.

Liver

Evidence of slight hepatic dysfunction has been reported following enflurane anesthesia. More significant liver damage has also been reported (see earlier).

Muscle

Enflurane potentiates neuromuscular blockade (39). This effect is not reversed by neostigmine.

Reproductive System

Although enflurane causes uterine muscle relaxation, the response to oxytocin is preserved if inspired concentrations are less than 2.5%. It has been used in obstetrics in low concentrations (0.5–0.8%) without causing significant fetal depression.

ISOFLURANE

Isoflurane is a methyl ethyl ether and was the 469th compound synthesized by Terrell in 1965. It is an isomer of enflurane. It was first used in clinical anesthesia in 1971.

Physical Properties

Isoflurane is a clear, colorless, nonflammable liquid that is extremely stable. The absence of a fluoride atom on the a-carbon results in almost no fluoride ion being produced by metabolism. Its physical characteristics (boiling point and saturated vapor pressure) are very similar to those of halothane (see Table 3) Theoretically, the same vaporizer could be used for both.

Pharmacokinetics

Isoflurane anesthesia is characterized by rapid induction and emergence in comparison to earlier agents, reflecting its physicochemical characteristics (i.e., low blood:gas coefficient). The presence of significant airway irritability may result in a slower-than-expected induction.

Isoflurane is extremely resistant to degradation, in and out of the body. Metabolism has been estimated at 0.2%, resulting in a minor increase in urinary F^- excretion. This is insufficient to cause any renal toxicity. Trifluoroacetic acid is also formed via oxidative pathways and appears to be nontoxic.

Pharmacodynamics

Central Nervous System

Isoflurane, like all the inhalational agents, produces dose-related central nervous system depression. No increase in cerebral blood flow is observed at 1.1 MAC or less, if $PaCO_2$ remains constant (40). At higher MAC levels, cerebral blood flow and intracranial pressure will increase (less than with halothane or enflurane), although this can be effectively abolished by hypocarbia. It is, therefore, the inhalational agent of choice for neurosurgery, although its role has recently been undermined by the increasing popularity of propofol total intravenous anesthesia in this context.

Isoflurane does not increase EEG activity like enflurane; in fact, at 2.0 MAC the EEG becomes isoelectric.

Cardiovascular System

Isoflurane appears to be less depressant to the myocardium than are halothane or enflurane. Cardiac output is maintained in humans by an increase in heart rate (41). Heart rate and cardiac output are further increased during spontaneous ventilation as a result of the rise in $PaCO_2$. Arterial blood pressure drops more than with halothane or enflurane, due primarily to a profound decrease in peripheral vascular resistance, although direct myocardial depression also occurs (40).

In patients with normal coronary arteries, studies have demonstrated a reduction in coronary vascular resistance, resulting in improved global coronary perfusion (42). However, it has been suggested that in patients with critical coronary stenoses, isoflurane may increase blood flow to normal myocardium at the expense of a potentially ischemic area, the so-called coronary steal phenomenon. This issue has not been resolved, although a subgroup of patients with total occlusion of one or more major coronary arteries and significant stenosis of the vessel supplying collateral circulation are felt to be at increased risk (43). Dysrhythmias are relatively uncommon, and there is little sensitization of the myocardium to catecholamines.

Respiratory System

Isoflurane is a respiratory depressant, intermediate in potency between halothane and enflurane, resulting in a decreased tidal volume and, uniquely, a decrease in respiratory rate (44). It is relatively irritant to airways, causing coughing, breath-holding, and even laryngospasm, making inhalational induction difficult (considered by some to be contraindicated in this instance). However, it is a bronchodilator and has been used successfully in status asthmaticus. In fact, it may be a better agent to use than halothane, as it causes less sensitization to circulating catecholamines.

Renal System

Isoflurane decreases renal blood flow, glomerular flow rate, and urine output during anesthesia. It is not nephrotoxic.

Liver

Isoflurane reduces hepatic portal vein blood flow in animals, but hepatic arterial flow is increased, suggesting preservation of hepatic oxygenation during isoflurane anesthesia to a greater extent than with halothane (39). There is no evidence of isoflurane-induced hepatotoxicity in humans.

Muscle

Isoflurane directly depresses skeletal muscle contractility and potentiates the effects of nondepolarizing neuromuscular blocking agents. Its effect is greater than that of halothane or enflurane.

DESFLURANE

Desflurane was the 653rd compound of approximately 700 synthesized by Terrell between 1959 and 1966. It is a fluorinated methyl ether structurally similar to isoflurane, differing only in the substitution of fluorine for chlorine on the a-carbon. Initially desflurane (I-653) was not considered to be commercially viable, for the following reasons:

1. Production required a potentially explosive reaction.
2. Desflurane had a vapor pressure close to 1 atmosphere, requiring an alternative vaporization system.
3. Its potency was low (MAC ~6%).

However, increased emphasis on outpatient anesthesia and the probability that desflurane would be rapidly taken up and excreted (suggested by its structure) led to a search for a safer method of synthesis and commencement of further pharmacokinetic investigations and animal studies in 1981. The first clinical trials in human volunteers were undertaken in London in 1988 (18). It is in use in routine clinical anesthesia in the US.

Physical Properties

Desflurane is nonflammable and nonexplosive in clinical concentrations and is more stable in the presence of soda lime than are any of the presently used volatile agents (45). Some of its physicochemical properties are very different from the more traditional agents (see Table 3). In particular, its molecular weight (168) and boiling point (22.8°C) are significantly lower than those of other agents, requiring the development of new vaporizer technology. Desflurane vaporizers (Ohmeda Tec 6) are electrically powered, more bulky than standard Tec vaporizers, and much more expensive, as is the vapor itself.

It also differs from other agents (other than sevoflurane) in that it has a very low solubility, with a blood:gas coefficient less than that of nitrous oxide (0.42) (46). Desflurane MAC is 6% to 7.2%, varying considerably with age (47).

Pharmacokinetics

Uptake and Elimination

As a result of its low solubility, alveolar concentration of desflurane rises rapidly toward the inspired concentration on induction and falls rapidly during elimination (48). Its pungency and airway irritability limit the usefulness of inhalational induction.

Recovery is extremely rapid, being 2–4 times as fast as recovery from isoflurane. Emergence, unlike that with halothane, enflurane, or halothane, is not markedly prolonged by duration of anesthesia.

Metabolism and Excretion

Desflurane resists biodegradation in animals and humans more than any of the other available inhalational agents and appears, therefore, to be devoid of toxicity. Degradation is apparently one-tenth that of isoflurane, and excretion of trifluoroacetic acid is 100 times less than after exposure to low average doses of isoflurane (49,50).

Pharmacodynamics

Central Nervous System

The cerebral effects of desflurane parallel those of isoflurane, producing a dose-dependent central nervous system depression, with EEG suppression and periods of electrical silence at 1.7 MAC. Desflurane does increase cerebral blood flow and intracranial pressure in a fashion similar to that of isoflurane, i.e., the effect is minimal at less than 1 MAC. Normal cerebrovascular responsiveness to $PaCO_2$ is maintained (51).

Cardiovascular System

Overall, the observed circulatory effects of desflurane again parallel those of isoflurane. Early studies in healthy volunteers demonstrated that desflurane causes a fall in arterial blood pressure, primarily due to a fall in systemic vascular resistance. Cardiac output does not alter significantly. Heart rate is increased at deeper levels of anesthesia (1.66 MAC) (52). These findings have been reproduced during clinical anesthesia in surgical patients. Desflurane does not appear to predispose to dysrhythmias.

Desflurane does not increase coronary blood flow or cause coronary steal in the chronically instrumented animal model.

Respiratory System

Concentrations of desflurane up to 6% do not appear to produce airway irritation (18); however, higher concentrations required for inhalational induction cause coughing, breath-holding, salivation, and laryngospasm (47). This irritation is worse than that caused by isoflurane and is more pronounced in children. It is not recommended for use as an induction agent, particularly in children.

Respiratory depression occurs, as evidenced by a decreased tidal volume and increased $PaCO_2$, demonstrating a depressed ventilatory response to CO_2. Respiratory rate is increased, but minute ventilation falls. This depression, which is dose-dependent and slightly more marked than that of isoflurane, is lessened by the addition of nitrous oxide.

Renal System

Desflurane has little or no effect on renal blood flow. There has been no evidence of renal injury in clinical trials or in enzyme-induced rats.

Liver

There has been no demonstrable hepatic injury following desflurane anesthesia, a finding consistent with its minimal biodegradation, small alteration in cardiac output, and rapid elimination from the body.

SEVOFLURANE

Sevoflurane is a halogenated methyl isopropyl ether that was synthesized in 1969 by Regan and further investigated by Wallin and Napoli in Illinois. The reaction of sevoflurane with soda lime was reported by Wallin et al. in 1975, and the potential toxicity of "compound A" played a major part in the decision not to pursue its development at that time, although the introduction of enflurane and isoflurane probably contributed (53).

It is currently used almost exclusively in Japan, where it has apparently replaced halothane as the agent of choice for inhalational induction in children. As of April 1993, sevoflurane had been administered to 800,000 patients in Japan, with no reports of associated renal or hepatic toxicity (54). It is now used clinically in the U.K. and the U.S., and is more widely available.

Physical Properties

Sevoflurane is a potent, nonexplosive, and nonflammable agent that degrades when in contact with soda lime, as well as being absorbed by it. This produces concerns related to (a) potential toxicity of breakdown products; and (b) cost implications of the loss of agent into the circuit.

It is potent relative to desflurane (MAC 2.0–2.5) and has a similarly low blood:gas coefficient (0.6), although its higher brain solubility is the cause of a slightly longer emergence time. Its boiling point and vapor pressure are such that conventional vaporizer techniques can be employed. Its physicochemical properties are listed in Table 3.

Stability of Sevoflurane

Sevoflurane degrades in soda lime at a rate of 6.5% per hour at 22°C. This rate increases by 1.6% per hour for each degree rise in temperature, and is 57.4% at 54°C (55). Degradation is increased in dry soda lime (56) and in the presence of baralyme, although this effect is probably less marked than was originally thought (57). Among the breakdown products are:

$$CF_2 = C(CF_3)\text{-}O\text{-}CH_2F \text{ (compound A)}$$

and

$$CH_3OCF_2CH(CF_3)OCH_2F \text{ (compound B)}$$

Toxicity in animals appears to be low for compound B. Compound A has the highest levels following sevoflurane anesthesia. It has a lethal concentration (LC_{50}) in rats of >1000 ppm after 1 hour and >340 ppm after 3 hours. Quantitative studies in humans have produced mean levels of 8–20 ppm after prolonged exposure. One patient had a peak level of 60 ppm. None of the patients so far studied has developed clinical or biochemical evidence of organ toxicity.

Pharmacokinetics

As suggested by its physicochemical parameters, sevoflurane has been demonstrated to produce more rapid induction than does enflurane (58) and more rapid emergence than does isoflurane. Recovery of response to command was ~7.5 min versus ~19 min for isoflurane in comparable groups of patients. Emergence time does not correlate with duration or dose of sevoflurane anesthesia.

The extent of biotransformation is similar to that of enflurane, releasing similar levels of F^- (22 mmol/L), but its low solubility and rapid elimination confine this to the period of exposure. Toxic effects on the kidneys, liver, and hemopoietic system have not been demonstrated.

Pharmacodynamics

Central Nervous System

Sevoflurane produces "anesthesia of excellent quality." (59) There are no epileptiform changes seen on EEG. Sevoflurane at 0.5–2.0 MAC appears to be a less potent cerebral vasodilator than is isoflurane in rats (60).

Cardiovascular System

Sevoflurane produces a dose-dependent decrease in heart rate, mean arterial pressure, pulmonary artery pressures, systemic vascular resistance, and cardiac index in animal studies. In humans it decreases blood pressure, with little change in heart rate (57). Depression of cardiac output is similar to that seen with isoflurane. Sevoflurane does sensitize the myocardium to catecholamines to a slightly lesser extent than does enflurane. There is no alteration of regional coronary blood flow.

Respiratory System

Respiratory function is depressed by sevoflurane, with decreased tidal volume and little change in respiratory rate. $PaCO_2$ is elevated during spontaneous ventilation.

NITROUS OXIDE

Nitrous oxide was first prepared in 1772 by Joseph Priestly, its anesthetic properties suggested by Sir Humphrey Davy in 1799. Colton popularized its use in dental anesthesia in 1867, and it became available in cylinders in 1868 (17). It remains in wide use throughout the world.

Physical Properties

Nitrous oxide is a colorless, nonirritant, slightly sweet-smelling gas. It supports combustion but is not flammable. Because it has a critical temperature of 36.5°C (above this temperature it cannot exist in liquid form), it is stored in pressurized cylinders (standardized blue in color) as a liquid in equilibrium with its vapor. The cylinder pressure remains constant until only N_2O vapor remains, when it falls rapidly.

It has a MAC of 105% and cannot, therefore, be used as sole anesthetic agent. It is a good analgesic, producing relatively little cardiorespiratory depression and is, therefore, frequently used with oxygen as a carrier gas for the more potent agents. Its physicochemical properties are listed in Table 3.

Nitrous oxide is produced by heating ammonium nitrate to 240–270°C. Impurities include nitric oxide (NO) and nitrogen dioxide (NO_2), which are toxic (producing laryngospasm, pulmonary edema, and chemical pneumonitis) and must be removed before clinical use.

Pharmacokinetics

Nitrous oxide has a low blood:gas solubility coefficient and, therefore, a rapid onset and offset of action. Its presence in high inspired concentrations results in the second gas effect (see earlier) and may produce diffusion hypoxia (see earlier).

Nitrous oxide is excreted predominantly unchanged, although an estimated 0.004% of an absorbed dose undergoes reductive metabolism to N_2 in the gut. Anaerobic bacteria such as Pseudomonas are responsible for this.

Pharmacodynamics

Central Nervous System

Nitrous oxide is a central nervous system depressant and a good analgesic. It does increase cerebral blood flow and intracranial pressure, although this is less significant than that of the other agents. Cerebral vasoconstriction will still occur in response to arterial CO_2 tension.

Cardiovascular System

Nitrous oxide is a direct myocardial depressant, resulting in a decrease in cardiac output, heart rate, and contractility without altering blood pressure, due to an increase in systemic vascular resistance (probably a sympathomimetic effect). This depression is not as marked as that of the more potent inhalational agents. As a result, the use of N_2O-volatile mixtures will result in less cardiovascular depression than will the use of equivalent MAC quantities of volatile. In contrast, the administration of N_2O with opioids results in significant circulatory depression characterized by decreased cardiac output, although the effects vary in different surgical groups.

Respiratory System

Nitrous oxide has little effect on the respiratory system. It does not alter the ventilatory response to CO_2 or bronchomotor tone. It may slightly decrease tidal volume and increase respiratory rate.

Musculoskeletal System

Nitrous oxide may increase muscle tone.

Reproductive System

Nitrous oxide does not change uterine tone or contractility during labor and delivery. It does produce teratogenic effects when administered to experimental animals in early pregnancy. There is currently no definitive evidence that brief exposure to anesthetic concentrations or longer exposure to subanesthetic doses of N_2O have adverse fetal effects.

Hematologic System

Nitrous oxide reacts with vitamin B_{12}, oxidizing Cob(I)alamin to Cob(III)alamin, thus inhibiting methionine synthetase, interfering with DNA synthesis and folate metabolism. Leukopenia, thrombocytopenia, megaloblastic anemia, and subacute combined degeneration of the spinal cord have all been described following N_2O exposure. In healthy patients, an estimated minimum 5 hours' exposure is required before bone marrow suppression is demonstrable. Bone marrow aplasia and fatal agranulocytosis have followed prolonged administration of nitrous oxide in the treatment of poliomyelitis and tetanus.

Other Effects of Nitrous Oxide

Air Space Expansion

Nitrous oxide has a blood:gas coefficient (0.47), 35 times higher than that of nitrogen (0.013). It will, therefore, move more rapidly into air spaces, causing rapid expansion—for example, in the middle ear, bowel, pneumothoraces, air emboli, and endotracheal tube cuffs.

Greenhouse Effect

Nitrous oxide has the same molecular weight as has CO_2 and does trap thermal radiation reflected from the earth's surface. The consensus of opinion is that nitrous oxide does contribute (<5%) to the total greenhouse effect. Of the nitrous oxide in the atmosphere, approximately one-third results from human activities, of which 1% is attributable to anesthesia.

REFERENCES

1. Eger EI II, Saidman LJ, Brandstater B. Minimum alveolar anesthetic concentration: a standard of anesthetic potency. *Anesthesiology* 1965; 26:756.
2. Quasha AL, Eger EI II, Tinker JH. Determination and applications of MAC. *Anesthesiology* 1980;53:315.
3. Stanski DR. Monitoring depth of anesthesia. In: Miller RD, ed. *Anesthesia*, 2nd ed. New York: Churchill Livingstone, 1990;1:1012.
4. Eger EI II. The effect of inspired concentration on rise of alveolar concentration. *Anesthesiology* 1963;24:153.
5. Epstein RM, Rackow H, Salanitre E, Wolf GL. Influence of the concentration effect on the uptake of anesthetic mixtures: the second gas effect. *Anesthesiology* 1964;25:364.
6. Tunstall ME, Hawksworth GM. Halothane uptake and nitrous oxide concentration. *Anaesthesia* 1981;36:177
7. Yamamura H, Wakasugi B, Okuma Y, Maki K. The effects of ventilation on the absorption and elimination of inhalational anesthetics. *Anaesthesia* 1963;18:427.
8. Eger EI II, Larson CP. Anesthetic solubility in blood and tissues: values and significance. *Br J Anaesth* 1964;36:140.
9. Munson ES, Eger EI II, Bowers DL. Effects of anesthetic depressed ventilation and cardiac output on anesthetic uptake. *Anesthesiology* 1971;35:401.
10. Yasuda N, Targ AG, Eger EI II. Solubility of I-653, sevoflurane, isoflurane and halothane in human tissues. *Anesthesiology* 1988;69A: 615.
11. Eger EI II (ed). MAC, *Anesthetic Uptake and Action*. Baltimore: Williams and Wilkins, 1974.
12. Eger EI II, Johnson BH. Rates of awakening from anesthesia with I-653, halothane, isoflurane and sevoflurane: a test of the effect of anesthetic concentration and duration in rats. *Anesth Analg* 1987;66:977.
13. Fink BR. Diffusion anoxia. *Anesthesiology* 1981;54:3.
14. Rackow H, Salanitre E, Frumin MH. Dilution of alveolar gases during nitrous oxide excretion in man. *J Appl Physiol* 1961;16:723.
15. Stoelting RK, Eger EI II. Percutaneous loss of nitrous oxide, cyclopropane, ether and halothane in man. *Anesthesiology* 1972;36:278.
16. Carpenter RL, Eger EI II, Johnson BH. The extent of metabolism of inhaled anesthetics in humans. *Anesthesiology* 1986;65:201.
17. Atkinson RS, Rushman GB, Davies NJH. In: *Lee's Synopsis of Anaesthesia*, 11th ed. Oxford: Butterworth-Heinemann Ltd., 1990:87.
18. Jones RM, Cashman JN, Mant TGK. Clinical impressions and cardiorespiratory effects of a new fluorinated inhalation anesthetic, desflurane (I-163) in volunteers. *Br J Anaesth* 1990;64:11.
19. Suckling CW. Some chemical and physical factors in the development of fluothane. Br J Anaesth 1957;29:466.
20. Johnstone M. The human cardiovascular response to fluothane anesthesia. *Br J Anaesth* 1956;28:392.
21. Bryce-Smith R, O'Brien HD. Fluothane: a non-explosive anesthetic agent. *Br Med J* 1956;2:969.
22. Rehder K, Forbes J, Alter H, Hessler O, Stier Q. Halothane biotransformation in man. A quantitative study. *Anesthesiology* 1967:28:711.
23. Elliott RH, Strunin L. Hepatotoxicity of volatile anesthetics. *Br J Anaesth* 1993:70:339.
24. Wood M. Inhalational anesthetic agents. In: Wood M, Wodd AJJ, eds. *Drugs and Anesthesia: Pharmacology for Anesthesiologists*, 2nd ed. Baltimore: Williams & Wilkins, 1990:248.
25. McDowell DG. Effects of clinical concentrations of halothane on the blood flow and oxygen uptake of the cerebral cortex. *Br J Anaesth* 1967;39:186.
26. Bahlman SH, Eger EI II, Halsey MJ, Stevens WC, Shakespeare TF, Smith NT, Cromwell TH, Fourcade H. The cardiovascular effects of halothane in man during spontaneous ventilation. *Anesthesiology* 1972;36:494.
27. Atlee JL, Bosnjak ZJ. Mechanisms for cardiac dysrhythmias during anesthesia. *Anesthesiology* 1990;72:347.
28. Munson ES, Larson CP, Badad AA, Regan MJ, Buechel DR, Eger EI II. The effects of halothane, fluroxene and cyclopropane on ventilation: a comparative study in man. *Anesthesiology* 1966;27:716.
29. Mazze RI, Schwartz FD, Slocum HC, et al. Renal function during anesthesia and surgery I. The effects of halothane anesthesia. *Anesthesiology* 1963;24:279.
30. Waud BE. Decrease in dose requirements of d-tubocurarine by volatile anesthetics. *Anesthesiology* 1979;51:298.

31. Gelman S, Fowler KC, Smith LR. Liver circulation and function during isoflurane and halothane anesthesia. *Anesthesiology* 1984;61:726.
32. Terrell RC. Physical and chemical properties of anesthetic agents (with and appendix on the manufacture of isoflurane). *Br J Anaesth* 1984;56:3S.
33. Mazze RI, Calverley RK, Smith NT. Inorganic fluoride nephrotoxicity: prolonged enflurane and halothane anesthesia in volunteers. *Anesthesiology* 1977;46:265.
34. Mazze RI, Woodruff RE, Heerdt MD. Isoniazid induced defluorination in humans. *Anesthesiology* 1982;57:5.
35. Lewis JH, Zimmerman HJ, Ishak KG, Mullack FG. Enflurane hepatotoxicity. A clinicopathologic study of 24 cases. *Ann Intern Med* 1983;98:984.
36. Neigh JL, Garman JK, Harp JR. The electroencephalographic pattern during anesthesia with enflurane. Effects of depth of anesthesia, $PaCO_2$ and nitrous oxide. *Anesthesiology* 1971;35:482.
37. Calverley RK, Smith NT, Prys-Roberts C, EgerEI II, Jones CW. Cardiovascular effects of enflurane anesthesia during controlled ventilation in man. *Anaesth Analg* 1978;57:619.
38. Jones RM. Clinical comparisons of inhalational anesthetic agents. *Br J Anaesth* 1984;56:57.
39. Rupp SM, Miller RD, Gencarelli PJ. Vecuronium induced neuromuscular blockade during enflurane, isoflurane and halothane anesthesia in humans. *Anesthesiology* 1984;60:102.
40. Eger EI II. The pharmacology of isoflurane. *Br J Anaesth* 1984;56:71S.
41. Stevens WC, Cromwell TH, Halsey MJ, Eger EI II, Shakespeare TF, Bahlman SH. The cardiovascular effects of a new inhalation anesthetic, forane, in human volunteers at constant carbon dioxide tension. *Anesthesiology* 1971;35:8.
42. Gelman S, Fowler KC, Smith LR. Regional blood flow during isoflurane and halothane anesthesia. *Anesth Analg* 1984;63:557.
43. Priebe HJ. Coronary circulation and factors affecting coronary 'steal.' *Eur J Anaesthesiol* 1991;8:177.
44. Fourcade, Stevens, Larson. Cromwell, et al. The ventilatory effects of Forane, a new inhaled anesthetic. *Anesthesiology* 1971;35:8.
45. Eger EI II. Stability of I-653 in soda lime. *Anesth Analg* 1987;66:983.
46. Eger EI II. Partition coefficients of I-653 in human blood, saline and olive oil. *Anesth Analg* 1987;66:971.
47. Rampil IJ, Lockhart SH, Zwass MS, et al. Clinical characteristics of desflurane in surgical patients: minimum alveolar concentration. *Anesthesiology* 1991;71:429.
48. Yasuda N, Lochart SH, Eger EI II, Weiskopf RB, Johnson BH, Freire BA, Fassoulaki A. Kinetics of desflurane, isoflurane and halothane in humans. *Anesthesiology* 1991;74:489.
49. Sutton TS, Koblin DD, Weiskopf RB, et al. Fluoride metabolites following exposure of volunteers to desflurane. *Anesth Analg* 1990;71: S398.
50. Jones RM,Koblin DD, Cashman JN, Eger EI II, Johnson BH, Damask MC. Biotransformation and hepatorenal function in volunteers after exposure to desflurane (I-653). *Br J Anaesth* 1990;64:482.
51. Eger EI II. In: *Desflurane, a Compendium and Reference*. Anaquest, 1993.
52. Weiskopf RB, Calahan MK, Eger EI II, et al. Cardiovascular actions of desflurane in normocarbic volunteers. *Anesth Analg* 1991;73:143.
53. Mazze RI. The safety of sevoflurane in humans. *Anesthesiology* 1992; 77:1062.
54. Bito H, Ikeda K. Closed-circuit anesthesia with sevoflurane in humans. Effects on renal and hepatic function and concentrations of breakdown products with soda lime in the circuit. *Anesthesiology* 1994;80:71.
55. Strum DP, Johnson, Eger EI. Stability of sevoflurane in soda lime. *Anesthesiology* 1987;67:779.
56. Strum DP, Eger EI. The degradation, absorption, and solubility of volatile anesthetics in soda lime depend on water content. *Anesth Analg* 1994;78:340.
57. Frink EJ, Malan TP, Morgan SE, Brown EA, Malcolmson M, Brown BR. Quantification of the degradation products of sevoflurane in two CO_2 absorbents during low-flow anesthesia in surgical patients. *Anesthesiology* 1992;77:1064.
58. Saito S, Goto F, Kadoi Y, Takahashi T, Fujita T, Mogi K. Comparative clinical study of induction and emergence time in sevoflurane and enflurane anesthesia. *Acta Anaesthesiol Scand* 1989;33:389.
59. Holaday DA, Smith FR. Clinical characteristics and biotransformation of sevoflurane in healthy human volunteers. *Anesthesiology* 1981;54:100.
60. Lu GP, Gibson JA, Frost EA, Goldiner PL. Cerebral vasodilating effect of sevoflurane versus isoflurane. *Anesthesiology* 1981;73: A625.

Airway Management, edited by
L.H. Hanowell, M.D. and R.J. Waldron, M.D.,
Lippincott-Raven Publishers, Philadelphia © 1996.

CHAPTER 11

Neuromuscular Blockade

Christopher S. Butler, Richard J. Waldron, and Dennis L. Fung

INTRODUCTION

Neuromuscular blocking (NMB) agents have an important role in safe airway management for both elective and emergency patients (1). The existence of these agents was first described in 1596 by Sir Walter Raleigh when he described South American arrow poison in his book *Discovery of the Large, Rich, and Beautiful Empire of Guinea*. The first use of d-tubocurarine to produce muscle relaxation during surgery was by Harold Griffith and Enid Johnson in Montreal, Canada in 1942.

This chapter will concentrate first on the physiology of the neuromuscular junction (NMJ), as well as describing clinical monitoring and factors affecting the degree of blockade. The individual agents will then be discussed separately, followed by applications in certain clinical situations. In general, indications for the use of NMB agents include:

1. Providing optimal conditions for direct laryngoscopy and endotracheal intubation.
2. Facilitation of intermittent positive pressure ventilation (IPPV) and control of carbon dioxide levels (e.g., raised intracranial pressure).
3. Reduced requirements for sedative/anesthetic agents (e.g., trauma, operative obstetrics, neonatal anesthesia).
4. Optimization of surgical exposure (e.g., abdominal surgery, thoracic surgery).

CONCEPTS OF NEUROMUSCULAR TRANSMISSION

Prejunctional Events

Acetylcholine Synthesis and Release

Figure 1 shows the junction between a motor nerve ending and its corresponding motor end-plate (a thickened area of muscle membrane). This is a specialized func-

C. S. Butler: Department of Anaesthesia and Intensive Care, Townsville General Hospital, Townsville, Queensland, Australia 4810.
R. J. Waldron: Department of Anaesthetic Services, Royal Hobart Hospital, and University of Tasmania, Hobart, Tasmania, Australia 7001.
D. L. Fung: Department of Anesthesiology, University of California, Davis Medical Center, Sacramento, California 95817.

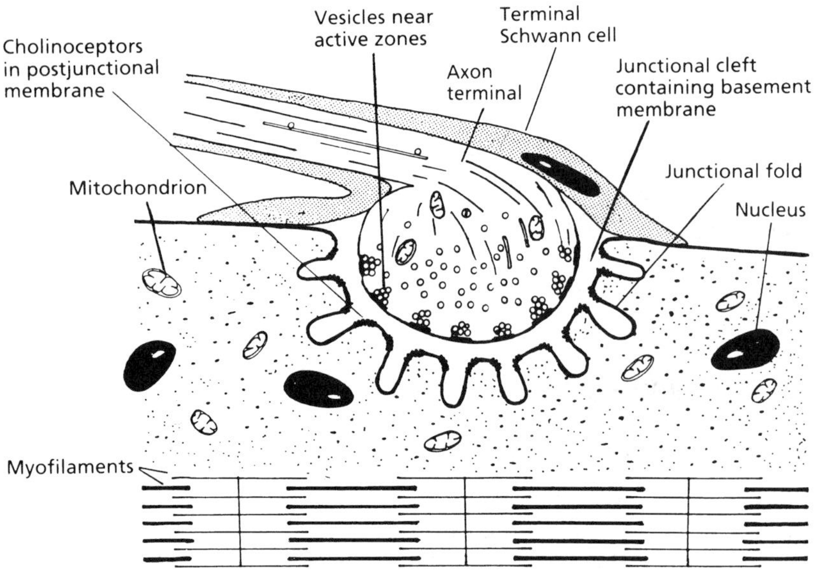

FIG. 1. Diagrammatic representation of the neuromuscular junction (NMJ) between a myelinated motor nerve ending and a muscle fiber. The presynaptic (axon) terminal shows vesicles containing acetylcholine gathered together near "active zones." Postjunctional receptors are located on the "shoulders" of folds in the postjunctional membrane—see text for details. From: Bowman WC. *Pharmacology of neuromuscular function, 2nd edition.* Oxford: Butterworth-Heinemann; 1990, with permission.

tional unit called the *neuromuscular junction* (NMJ). As a motor nerve approaches this end-plate region of a muscle fiber, it sheds its myelin sheath and divides into a number of prejunctional nerve endings or "terminals." The neurotransmitter at all NMJs in the body is acetylcholine (Ach), which is synthesized (and stored) in the prejunctional area of the NMJ according to the following chemical reaction:

Choline → Acetyl CoA → Acetylcholine
(enzyme is **choline acetyl transferase**)

Choline is 50% derived from the diet and 50% recycled from breakdown at the NMJ. It is actively transported into the nerve endings by a carrier mechanism (this mechanism is blocked by hemicholinium).

Eighty percent of the Ach is stored in the vesicles of nerve endings (each vesicle containing 10,000 molecules of Ach), and there are approximately 300,000 vesicles in each nerve ending. A typical nerve impulse arrives at a nerve ending and releases about 300 of these synaptic vesicles. These vesicles are synthesized in the cell body and transported via the microtubular system. They may be used repeatedly in the terminal. During stimulation, the synthesis of vesicles rises. Each vesicle (a quantum) results in the opening of channels on the postjunctional membrane (PJM) for Na^+ entry.

Following stimulation, the wall of the vesicle fuses with the nerve membrane at "active zones" in the terminal. There are about 1000 active zones in each terminal. Each active zone is aligned opposite the shoulders of a junctional fold of PJM, where the Ach receptors are found in the greatest density (see Fig. 1).

Acetylcholine Release

Ach release requires a Ca^{++} influx; it will not occur in its absence. The "active zones" contain Ca^{++} channels also. A wave of depolarization activates adenylate cyclase, which converts adenosine triphosphate (ATP) to cyclic adenosine monophosphate (cAMP), in turn activating a protein kinase that phosphorylates proteins that control several functions. One of these functions is the regulation of Ca^{++} entry and transmitter release. Ca^{++} causes vesicles to move up to the edges of the "active zones" and fuse with the membrane. The inward Ca^{++} current is normally stopped by the flow of K^+ at the end of the action potential.

Synaptic Cleft Transmission

The synaptic cleft lies between the nerve ending and the PJM and is about 50 nm wide. It is filled with so-called basement membrane, which is a collagen material rich in carbohydrates and containing most of the junctional acetylcholinesterase. It is the access point to the NMJ for NMB agents to exert their effect.

There is abundant acetylcholinesterase in the cleft that destroys up to 66% of the released Ach even before it reaches PJM, and all the Ach is hydrolyzed in a millisecond. One acetylcholinesterase hydrolytic site removes 1,000,000 molecules of Ach in 1 sec.

Postjunctional Events

Postjunctional Receptor

These receptor complexes are organized into discrete clusters, each of which is 0.1 microns in diameter and contains a few hundred receptors. They are usually found on the "shoulders" of the junctional curves. Ach receptors of the PJM are of nicotinic (N) type.

The receptor channel is different from the typical Na^+ channel of a nerve axon (Fig. 2) (2). The two alpha sub-

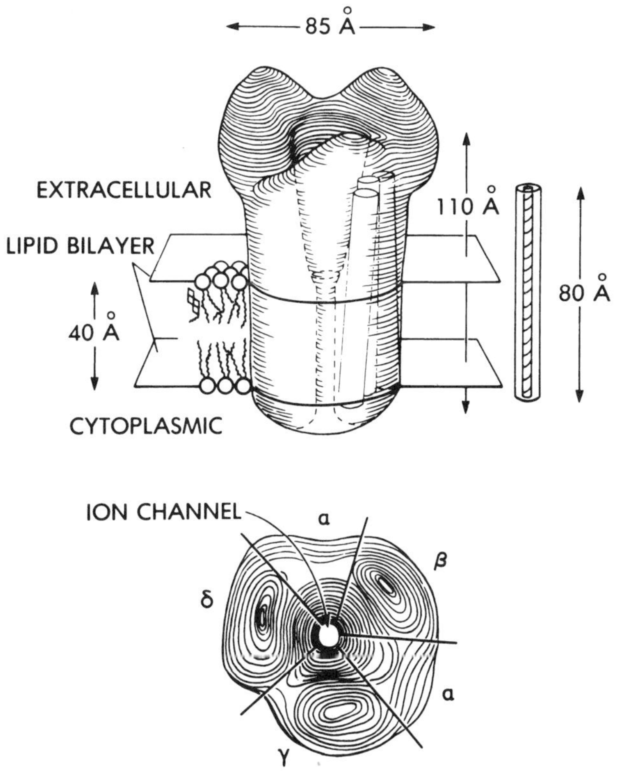

FIG. 2. Diagrammatic representation of the acetylcholine receptor showing subunits. The alpha subunits are critical for receptor activation by acetylcholine (see text for details). From: Kistler J, Stroud RM, Klymkowski MW, et al. Structure and function of an acetylcholine receptor. *Biophys J* 1982; 37:371–383, with permission.

units (MW 40,000 daltons) contain the N receptors, and both must be occupied to open the channel. The other subunits are beta, delta, and epsilon and are larger than the alphas. In fetal muscle, there is a gamma subunit which replaces the adult epsilon subunit.

Occupation of the receptor sites on the two alpha subunits induces a conformational change in the protein of the receptor complex, which results in opening the channel. The opened channel allows small cations like Na^+, K^+, Ca^{++} to move along their concentration gradients. Na^+ is initially the most important ion as it induces postjunctional depolarization, sometimes called the *motor endplate potential* (mepp).

The number of receptors present is far in excess of that necessary for neuromuscular transmission. This gives a so-called margin of safety. Because of this margin of safety, it is believed that about 75% of these receptors must be blocked before paralysis commences (3). The other aspect of margin of safety is that 5 times the amount of Ach necessary for the critical membrane potential is released as a result of prejunctional events.

Postjunctional Membrane and Depolarization

The PJM is part of and continuous with the cell membrane of the muscle fiber. It differs from the normal muscle cell membrane in that it is 1000 times more sensitive to Ach. This sensitivity to Ach makes it the area from which a postjunctional depolarization will commence, leading to contraction of the muscle fiber.

Initially, there is a small collapse of the transmembrane polarization, the mepp. When the mepp reaches 30 mV, the adjacent muscle membrane is stimulated and a muscle action potential (AP) occurs. The mepp and AP are complete in about 8 msec, by which time the muscle is starting to contract.

Extrajunctional Receptors

Extrajunctional receptors are thought to play prominence in the abnormal sensitivity of muscle in denervated situations, e.g., spinal cord trauma, burns (4). These receptors are regulated in normally innervated muscle so that they are usually low in number (i.e., neural activity suppresses their formation), and have a short half-life. They are more sensitive to agonists [like succinylcholine (Sch)], while being poorly responsive to antagonists (like nondepolarizing NMB agents). These extrajunctional receptors appear over the entire PJM rather than being confined to the NMJ. They are thought to be responsible for the increased K^+ release seen with Sch when given to patients with spinal cord trauma and burns.

MONITORING THE NEUROMUSCULAR JUNCTION

Monitoring the degree of neuromuscular blockade provides useful information as regards timing of intubation and extubation. Other reasons for monitoring include:

1. Clinical assessment of neuromuscular blockade ("relaxation") during anesthesia (particularly when using infusions) and degree of recovery before extubation (Table 1).
2. Adjustment of dosage of NMB agent.
3. Assessment of unexpected, prolonged neuromuscular blockade. Use of a monitor may assist in the detection of Phase II blockade.

TABLE 1. *Clinical criteria of recovery from neuromuscular blockade*

The awake patient responding to command is able to:
Open the eyes widely
Cough effectively
Sustain tongue protrusion, hand grip, head lift for 5 sec
Produce a vital capacity of at least 15–20 ml/kg
Generate an inspiratory force of at least 20–25 cm H_2O negative pressure
The patient who is asleep and unable to respond to command:
Normal tidal volume (approximately 500 ml or 10 ml/kg)
Inspiratory force of at least 25 cm H_2O negative pressure
Sustained response to tetanic stimulation for 5 sec

4. Early recognition of patients with abnormal plasma cholinesterase, particularly when a rapid sequence intubation has been performed.

Types of Neuromuscular Blockade

The importance of differentiating between different types of neuromuscular blockade, although mainly historical, is related to: (a) the action of depolarizing and nondepolarizing NMB agents and (b) assessing the cause of prolonged neuromuscular blockade.

Distinguishing between these types requires an understanding of neuromuscular monitoring, which will be briefly dealt with later in this chapter (Fig. 3). There are three types of neuromuscular blockade (depolarizing, nondepolarizing, and Phase II) that are described, and their features are as follows:

Depolarizing Neuromuscular Blockade (Noncompetitive)

This type of block is best typified by that produced by Sch. The characteristic features are outlined in Table 2.

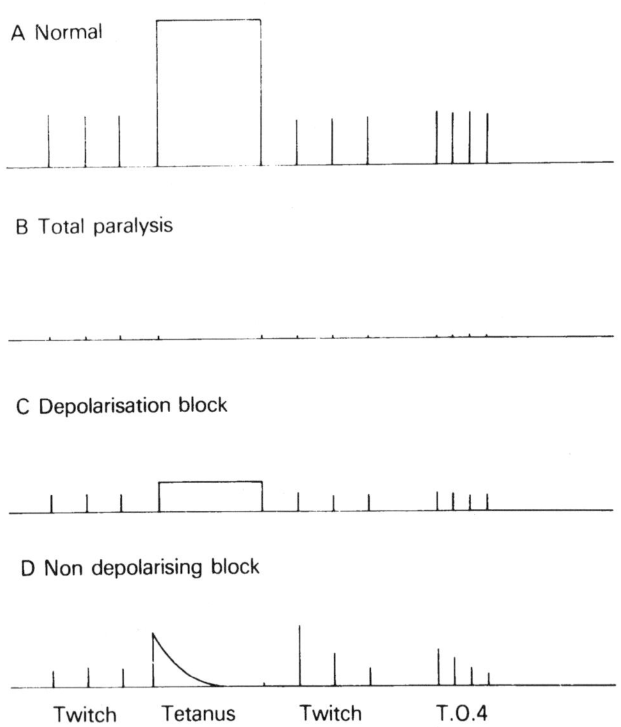

FIG. 3. Illustration of the different types of neuromuscular blockade (single twitch, tetanus, and train-of-four) using neuromuscular function monitoring (see text for details). This figure illustrates the effects of single twitch, tetanus, and train-of-four assessed by a force transducer recording the contraction of the abductor pollicis muscle. From: Smith G, Aitkenhead AR. *Textbook of anaesthesia 1985.* London: Churchill Livingstone; 1985:175, with permission.

TABLE 2. *Characteristics of depolarizing neuromuscular blockade*

Muscle fasciculation (preceding onset of paralysis)
Absence of:
Fade (at slow and fast stimulation rates)
Post-tetanic potentiation
Potentiation by anticholinesterases and other depolarizing NMB agents.
Antagonism by nondepolarizing NMB agents.

NMB, neuromuscular blocking.

It is often complete in clinical anesthesia; nerve stimulation or added cholinergics may prolong the block. Note that although removal of Sch molecules in the NMJ is rapid, transmission to the adjacent muscle membrane is blocked for a period of minutes. This is a form of accommodation where the adjacent muscle membrane becomes totally resistant to stimulation.

Nondepolarizing Neuromuscular Blockade (Competitive)

This type of block is produced by nondepolarizing NMB agents and is by far the most common form of clinical neuromuscular blockade. The characteristic features are outlined in Table 3.

Note that it is not a complete block, i.e., it can be overcome by increasing the concentration of Ach. Muscle groups vary in sensitivity in the same species, e.g., muscular activity of the diaphragm returns before that of the protective airway muscles (5).

Phase II (Dual) Blockade

This phenomenon is usually due to large, repeated doses of Sch, typically up to dosages of 300–400 mg. It was commonly seen with infusions of Sch used for surgery of short duration requiring neuromuscular blockade, e.g., rigid bronchoscopy. Importantly, it may occur at relatively normal dosage levels in the following conditions:

TABLE 3. *Clinical characteristics of nondepolarizing neuromuscular blockade*

Absence of fasciculation.
Fade following slow (twitch) or fast (tetanic) rates of stimulation and train-of-four (TO4).
Post-tetanic potentiation.
Antagonism by anticholinesterases, depolarizing NMB agents.
Potentiation by nondepolarizers.

Neonates
Myasthenia gravis
Patients with atypical cholinesterase enzyme

The mechanism of this so-called dual block is unknown. The NMJ is initially depolarized, but then slowly recovers its membrane potential. The blockade is refractory to reversal by cholinesterase inhibitors, and recovery is unpredictable. With the advent of newer, short-acting nondepolarizing NMB agents, this phenomenon will become less common.

Types of Stimulus

Evoked responses do not require the cooperation of the individual and are, therefore, suitable for use in the anesthetized/unconscious patient. The resulting activation of the muscle fibers can be measured either mechanically (tension) or electrically (EMG). The hand muscles are used most commonly, especially the adductor pollicis of the thumb (Fig. 4). Other sites include the feet and the face. Because the anatomic position of the adductor pollicis is remote from the point of stimulation of the ulnar nerve, the probability of direct muscle stimulation is diminished. The stimulating electrodes are applied either as surface or as percutaneous needle electrodes along the ulnar nerve, with the negative electrode overlying the nerve and the positive electrode placed about 1 cm proximally. Ideally, evoked potentials should be commenced soon after induction and prior to injection of an NMB agent. The following is a brief outline of some of the more commonly used forms of evoked potentials in the monitoring of neuromuscular blockade.

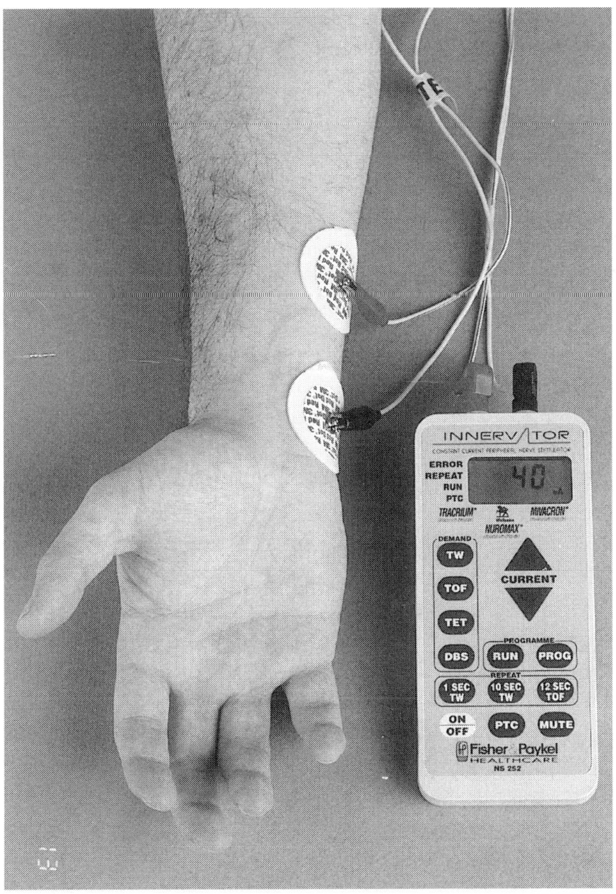

FIG. 4. Photograph of a typical nerve stimulator with electrodes placed over the ulnar nerve. Movement of the adductor pollicis is assessed.

Single Twitch

The term *single twitch* refers to a supramaximal stimulus lasting 0.2 msec. The control height of the twitch must be determined prior to administration of NMB agent. A supramaximal stimulus means all fibers are involved, and a duration of 0.2 msec prevents repetitive firing. A 95% twitch suppression corresponds to good intubating conditions and adequate surgical relaxation. However, it is not a sensitive indicator of onset or recovery from blockade as 75% of receptors must be occupied for twitch height to decrease. Difficulty is also encountered in assessing how much twitch suppression has occurred.

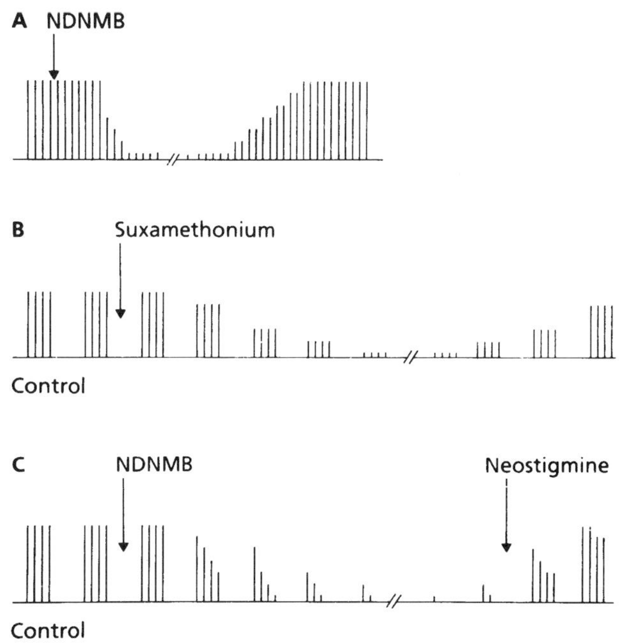

FIG. 5. Typical train-of-four (TO4) response to depolarizing (suxamethonium/succinylcholine) and nondepolarizing neuromuscular blocking agents (NDNMB). Twitch response **(A)**, TO4 monitoring of depolarizing neuromuscular block **(B)**, and nondepolarizing neuromuscular block **(C)**. NDNMB, nondepolarizing neuromuscular blocking agent. From: Nimmo WS, Rowbotham DJ, Smith G. *Anaesthesia, 2nd edition.* London: Blackwell Scientific Publications; 1989:415, with permission.

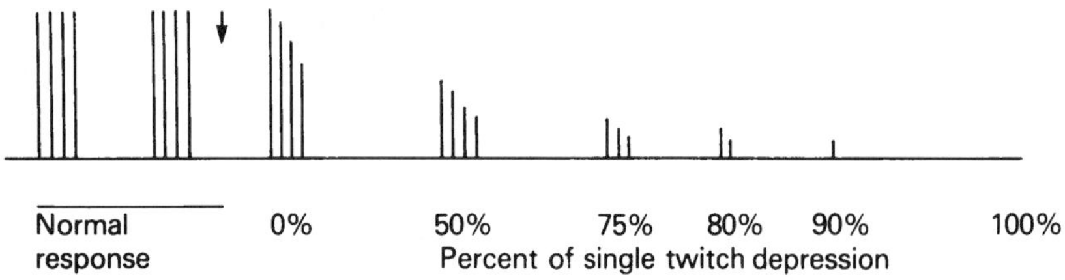

FIG. 6. TO4 stimulation observed with a transducer and recorder permitting assessment of TO4 count and TO4 ratio. The TO4 ratio is the ratio of the height of the fourth to the first twitch. A ratio greater than 70% indicates adequate transmission following use of nondepolarizing neuromuscular blockers. The TO4 is more sensitive than single twitches: a TO4 count of two corresponds to 80% blockade of a single twitch response. From: Smith G, Aitkenhead AR. *Textbook of anaesthesia 1985.* London: Churchill Livingstone; 1985: 176, with permission.

Tetanic Stimulus

Tetanic stimulus detects whether response is sustained or fades during the stimulus. Stimulus frequency ranges from 50 to 200 Hz. With a depolarizing block, the peak tension is diminished but sustained; whereas, with a nondepolarizing or Phase II block, the peak height is reduced and fades. A tetanic stimulus of 50 Hz for 5 sec correlates with maximal voluntary effort, but frequent tetanic stimulation can induce muscle recovery.

Post-tetanic Single Twitch/Post-tetanic Count (PTC)

This is the resumption of single twitch stimulation 6–10 sec after a tetanic stimulus, essentially causing posttetanic potentiation (PTP). A nondepolarizing or Phase II block will give a PTC, whereas a depolarizing block will not. A PTC is used when there is no response to a TO4 stimulus (see next section). In general, a PTC of >6 precedes the return of TO4 by 10–15 min, and a PTC of 20 corresponds to the return of the first twitch of a TO4 stimulus.

Train-of-Four (TO4)

Train-of-Four is the delivery of 4 supramaximal stimuli at 2 Hz repeated at intervals no less than 10 sec apart. The number of twitches to a TO4 stimulus can indicate the degree of nondepolarizing neuromuscular blockade (Table 4) (Fig. 5).

With a TO4 ratio of 0.75 (Fig. 6), a single twitch has returned to its control height and tetanus at 50 Hz for 5 sec is fully sustained. This correlates with adequate clinical recovery.

TABLE 4. *Correlates of train-of-four (TO4) stimuli to the degree of neuromuscular blockade*

Disappearance of fourth response	→	75% depression of a single twitch
Disappearance of third response	→	80% depression of a single twitch
Disappearance of second response	→	90% depression of a single twitch
Disappearance of first response	→	100% depression of a single twitch

Double Burst Stimulation

Double burst stimulation usually consists of two trains of three impulses (each impulse lasting 0.2 msec) (Fig. 7A) at 50 Hz, separated by 750 msec, which is used to evaluate recovery from neuromuscular blockade. The first "burst" is then compared with the second by either visual or tactile

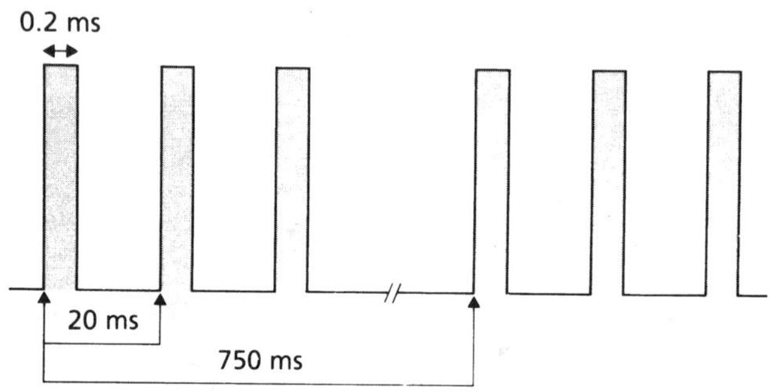

FIG. 7A. Double burst stimulation (DBS). Diagram shows three tetanic stimuli given at 20 msec intervals, repeated 750 msec later. DBS is used to assess recovery from competitive neuromuscular blockade and is regarded as more sensitive than TO4. From: Nimmo WS, Rowbotham DJ, Smith G. *Anaesthesia, 2nd edition.* London: Blackwell Scientific Publications; 1989:417, with permission.

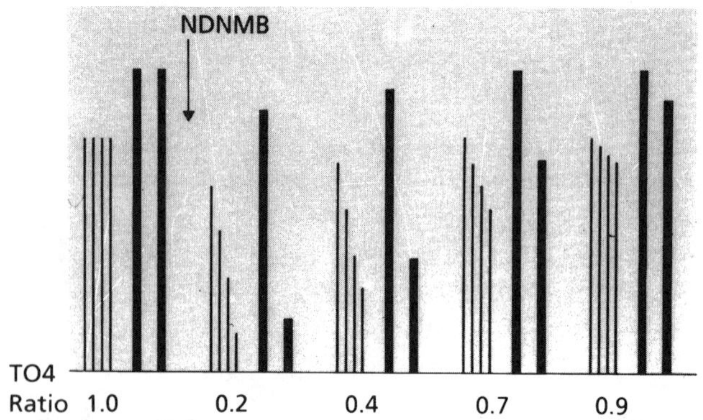

FIG. 7B. Double burst stimulation compared with TO4. Note the exaggerated "fade" of a DBS stimulus after a dose of nondepolarizing muscle relaxant, compared with a smaller "fade" with TO4. From: Nimmo WS, Rowbotham DJ, Smith G. *Anaesthesia, 2nd edition.* London: Blackwell Scientific Publications; 1989:417, with permission.

means. The absence of fade between the two suggests that any residual neuromuscular blockade is clinically insignificant. Double burst stimulation is a more sensitive test of recovery than is TO4 (Fig. 7B) and can be tolerated by the awake patient.

FACTORS AFFECTING NEUROMUSCULAR BLOCKADE

There are many factors and conditions that will affect the dynamics of neuromuscular blockade in patients (Table 5). Although many of these factors will not affect the onset of NMB agents, their importance lies in their prolongation of paralysis, affecting the patient's ability to maintain the airway after extubation. There are also some important conditions, however, that a practicing clinician should be aware of that may increase the difficulty of managing a patient's airway.

Volatile Anesthetics and Other Drugs

The volatile anesthetic agents produce a dose-dependent enhancement of the magnitude and duration of NMB due to nondepolarizing NMB agents. In general, isoflurane and enflurane have a more pronounced effect than does halothane. There are many drugs that patients may be taking for medical conditions that affect the duration of neuromuscular blockade. Some of the agents that have known interaction with NMB agents are shown in Table 5.

Muscle Group Variation

Different muscle groups within the body vary in their sensitivity to NMB agents, affecting the onset, duration, and intensity of blockade. The practical significance of this occurs in: (a) monitoring neuromuscular blockade; and (b) protecting the patient's airway, particularly on emergence from anesthesia.

In general, the muscles involved in airway protection are more sensitive to NMBs than are the diaphragm, limb muscles, and muscles of the face. Thus, even though monitoring of the adductor pollicis or orbicularis may indicate return of adequate function, the function of the protective airway muscles may still be deficient.

Muscle Diseases

In myasthenia gravis, the patient is sensitive to nondepolarizers but resistant to depolarizers. However, in myasthenia due to the Eaton-Lambert syndrome, the patient is very sensitive to nondepolarizers and depolarizers. Myotonia congenita is a condition where Sch is likely to cause generalized rigidity and should be avoided. Although these patients respond normally to nondepolarizing NMB, myotonia is not relieved by these agents, as it is a disease of the muscle membrane. Anticholinesterase drugs can also exacerbate myotonias. Other neural disease (e.g., lower motor neurone lesions, syringomyelia) are also very sensitive to nondepolarizing NMB agents.

Electrolyte Disturbances

The presence of low extracellular concentrations of K^+ and Ca^{++}, and high concentration of Mg^{++} increases sensitivity to nondepolarizing NMB agents.

Hypothermia

The prolongation of neuromuscular blockade may reflect the decrease in metabolism/excretion from the liver and kidney.

Disease States

In general, the severely diseased patient is more susceptible to NMB agents. In renal failure, avoid agents

TABLE 5. *Drugs affecting the duration of action of neuromuscular blocking agents*

Drug	Effect	Mechanism
Ca^{++} channel blockers	↑ Duration	Blockade of calcium flux
Antibiotics	↑ Duration	Antibiotics, in general, may exert effects at the prejunctional membrane similar to magnesium. There may also be a stabilization of the postjunctional membrane.
Neomycin, aminoglycosides	↑ Duration	Inhibit Ach release from presynaptic membrane
Tetracyclines	↑ Duration	Chelate calcium
Penicillins and cephalosporins	No effect	
Anticholinesterases	↑ Duration	Reduce the rate of hydrolysis of Ach
Local anesthetics, e.g., procaine, lidocaine	↑ Duration	Interfere with prejunctional release of Ach; stabilize postjunctional membrane
Magnesium	↑ Duration	Decrease release of Ach and reduces sensitivity of the postjunctional membrane
Frusemide (Furosemide)	↑ Duration	Probable prejunctional mechanism
Lithium	↑ Duration	Interfere with sodium flux

Ach, acetylcholine.

TABLE 6. *Mode of elimination of some of the neuromuscular blocking agents*

Drug	Renal	Biliary	Metabolic
Mivacurium	—	—	100%
Rocuronium	30%	70%	—
Atracurium	<10%	—	>90%
Vecuronium	>25%	20%	50–60%
Pancuronium	30–80%	10%	15–40%
Pipecuronium	~80%	~20%	—
Doxacurium	~80%	~20%	—
Gallamine	100%	—	—
Alcuronium	70–90%	10–30%	—
Tubocurarine	40–60%	40–60%	—

(e.g., pancuronium, gallamine, metocurine, decamethonium, pipecuronium, doxacurium) that rely principally on renal excretion (Table 6). Although most NMB agents are excreted unchanged by the kidney, liver disease will impact on some agents dramatically. Succinylcholine and mivacurium are both metabolized by plasma (pseudo) cholinesterase, which is produced by the liver. Also note that 15% to 40% of pancuronium is metabolized by the liver.

Age

Neonates are regarded as being sensitive to nondepolarizing NMB agents. The receptor at the NMJ is more sensitive to NMB agents, but this is offset by an increase in the volume of distribution. Similarly, elderly patients are sensitive, but for a different reason. With increasing age, there is a decrease in lean body mass, so that a relatively lower dosage of NMB agents is required to produce the same degree of blockade.

Burns

A threefold increase in dose and a fivefold increase in plasma concentrations of d-tubocurarine are required to produce the same degree of NMB (6). It is speculated that there is a proliferation of extrajunctional NMJ receptors that are responsive to Ach. As such, there is an apparent resistance to d-tubocurarine and other nondepolarizing NMB agents in the presence of a burn injury, due to a change in the pharmacodynamics and not pharmacokinetics.

SUCCINYLCHOLINE

Description

Succinylcholine is a depolarizing NMB agent that produces a sustained opening of the receptor channels. It was first used in 1906 but not recognized as an NMB agent until 1949. The structure of Sch is two molecules of Ach joined together (Fig. 8).

It acts by attaching to each of the alpha subunits of the postjunctional N receptor and mimics the action of Ach. Succinylcholine also has prejunctional effects, but these are minor compared to the postjunctional actions. It is unstable at room temperature and should be kept refrigerated.

Pharmacokinetics

Absorption and Distribution

Succinylcholine is generally given intravenously but can be used intramuscularly. About 90% of dose is destroyed in the blood before it reaches its site of action. As it is highly ionized, it is largely confined to the extracellular fluid and does not cross the blood–brain barrier (BBB). Succinylcholine is rapidly hydrolyzed in the plasma, and there are no significant levels in the circulation after 3 min (7).

Metabolism and Excretion

Succinylcholine is metabolized by plasma (pseudo) cholinesterase to succinyl-monocholine (which is 2% to 10% as active as the dicholine). About 5% of Sch is

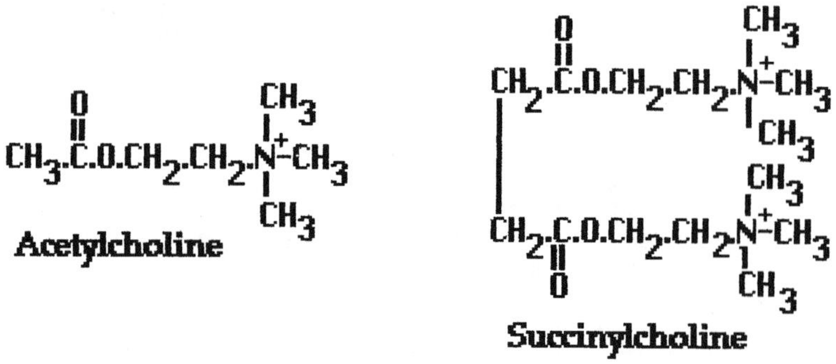

FIG. 8. Diagram of the succinylcholine molecule. It is composed of two molecules of acetylcholine (shown).

slowly hydrolyzed by alkaline tissue fluid. This is normally unimportant in clinical use unless there is pseudocholinesterase abnormality. Two percent of the administered dose of Sch is excreted unchanged by the kidney.

Pharmacodynamics

Central Nervous System

There is controversy surrounding the effects of Sch on cerebral blood flow (CBF) and, subsequently, on intracranial pressure (ICP). Traditionally, Sch has been thought to increase ICP (in the vicinity of 4–6 mm Hg). However, most clinicians still advocate the use of Sch in the head-injured patient for the purpose of airway control and subsequent hyperventilation. Recently, Kovarik et al. (8) have published a study of ten patients with neurological injuries who received Sch, demonstrating little change in ICP and cortical electrical activity.

Cardiovascular System

The muscle fasciculations may increase venous return and, subsequently, increase cardiac output. Bradycardia and AV nodal blocks may occur due to an agonist action on myocardial muscarinic receptors (particularly with repeat doses and in pediatric anesthesia).

Respiratory System

Apart from rapid paralysis of protective airway muscles and the muscles of respiration, there may be some increase in bronchial secretions.

Musculoskeletal System

The cause of fasciculations is not known. Muscle pain associated with the use of Sch may be a result of asynchronous contraction of muscle fibers. Patients who complain of postanesthetic muscle pains find it commonly affects the neck, back, and abdomen.

Gastrointestinal System

There is an inconsistent increase of intragastric pressure. Prevention of skeletal muscle fasciculations by prior administration of a nonparalyzing dose of a nondepolarizing NMB agent prevents increases in intragastric pressure by subsequent administration of Sch. The risk of increased intragastric pressure (the lower gastroesophageal sphincter can open at pressures above 28 cm H_2O) is the passage of gastric fluid into the esophagus, pharynx, and subsequently into the lungs.

Eyes

There is an increase in intraocular pressure. The mechanism is not clearly defined but presumably involves contraction of tonic myofibrils or transient dilation of the choroidal blood vessels. This increase occurs 2–4 min after Sch administration and is transient, lasting only 5–10 min.

Uterus and Placenta

There is no change in intrauterine pressure and Sch does not reach the fetal circulation (high levels of plasma cholinesterase are present in the placenta).

Dosage and Administration

Succinylcholine can be given intravenously at 1–1.5 mg/kg or intramuscularly (in emergency situations where intravenous access has not been achieved) at 4 mg/kg.

Precautions and Side Effects

Immediate, Life-Threatening

The use of Sch can result in immediate mortality if certain patient conditions exist. Examples of this are allergy to Sch, history of malignant hyperthermia, patients with known or suspected difficult airways (cannot intubate, cannot ventilate), and patients at risk of hyperkalemic cardiac arrest. Careful evaluation of a patient is always an essential step prior to pharmacological assistance in airway control.

Normally, Sch will increase the plasma concentration of K^+ by 0.5 mmol/L, which is not usually of any clinical significance. Certain patients are at risk of exaggerated increases of K^+ however, which may lead to hyperkalemic cardiac arrest. These include those with burns, denervation leading to skeletal muscle atrophy, upper motor neurone lesions, and severe intraabdominal infections. Pretreatment with a nonparalyzing dose of nondepolarizing NMB agents does not affect the magnitude of the K^+ release (although it tends to modify the other adverse effects). With burn patients, this potential for excessive K^+ leak develops within 2 days and may persist up to 2 years.

Abnormal Muscle Response to Sch

The action of Sch may be abnormal in certain patients. The best example of this is myotonia congenita (particularly the percussion form). In these people, Sch results in contraction, rather than relaxation, making control of the airway difficult. In myasthenia gravis, a muscle disorder where there are decreased numbers of NMJ receptors (usually due to antibodies), patients may have resistance to the action of Sch.

There may also be abnormally prolonged duration of Sch paralysis. This is due generally to inadequate function of the enzyme pseudo-cholinesterase. There are inherited forms (so-called Sux apnea), where abnormal forms of the enzyme are present in normal concentrations but fail to hydrolyze Sch at the normal rate. Paralysis may last for several hours and should be managed with positive-pressure ventilation and sedation until spontaneous resolution occurs. The enzyme may be at low levels as a result of decreased production (liver disease) or drug interactions (e.g., insecticides, ester local anesthetics, ecothiopate).

Repeat Doses of Sch

Careful consideration should be given to repeated administration of Sch. The propensity to bradycardias and Phase II blockade are well documented. Concurrent administration of atropine will avert life-threatening bradycardias.

Pressure Effects of Sch

The main areas of concern are gastric, intracranial, and intraocular pressures. In general, the use of Sch is not contraindicated in airway emergencies in patients with suspected alteration in these pressures. Cricoid pressure (Sellick's maneuver) should always be applied in intubating patients with a potentially full stomach.

Myalgia

Although a relatively minor side effect, myalgia can be distressing to the patient. The severity of the myalgias is not related to the magnitude of the fasciculations. They are thought to be less common if preceded by a small dose of nondepolarizing NMB, with the exception of pancuronium (9). Myoglobinuria may suggest skeletal muscle damage associated with Sch-induced fasciculations.

In summary, despite the many problems associated with its use, Sch has the most rapid onset and offset of any NMB agent currently available. As such, it is still the NMB agent of choice for emergency airway control and rapid sequence intubation (RSI) in most situations.

MIVACURIUM

Description

Mivacurium is a benzylisoquinolinium-type nondepolarizing relaxant, structurally related to atracurium but possessing a shorter duration of action (Fig. 9) (Table 7). It differs significantly, however, from atracurium in its metabolic pathway.

It is in three stereoisomers; trans-trans (57.4%), cis-trans (36.2%), and cis-cis (6.4%). The cis-cis form is pharmacologically inactive (10).

Pharmacokinetics

Absorption and Distribution

Mivacurium is administered intravenously and, like other NMBs, has a small volume of distribution (V_d = 0.1–0.2 L/kg) (Table 7).

Metabolism and Excretion

The half-life of mivacurium is about 17 min, the clinical duration of a normal intubating dose (0.2–0.25 mg/kg) being around 15 min. Clearance is higher than in other nondepolarizing relaxants, at 50–100 ml/kg/min.

It is metabolized by plasma cholinesterase at 70% to 80% of the rate seen with Sch, producing pharmacologically inactive metabolites. The block may be prolonged

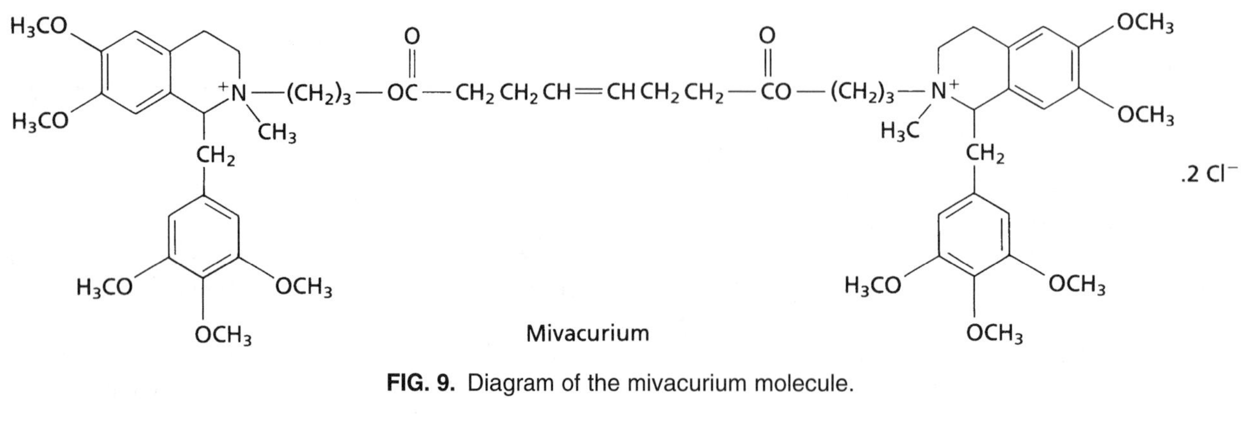

FIG. 9. Diagram of the mivacurium molecule.

TABLE 7. *Pharmacokinetic data for the intermediate acting neuromuscular blocking drugs*

	Rocuronium	Mivacurium	Vecuronium	Atracurium
ED_{95} (mg/kg)	0.3	0.07	0.04–0.07	0.15–0.30
Onset to maximal twitch depression (min)	1.5–3	2–4	3–5	3–5
Time to 25% recovery of twitch height (min)	42		20–35	20–35
Recovery Index (25–75% of control) (min)	15	2–8	15–25	15–25
Continuous infusion (mcg/kg/min)	5–12	4–8	1	6.2
Volume of Distribution (L/kg)	0.21	0.11	0.27	0.20
Clearance (ml/kg/min)	2.9	70	5.2	5.5
Active metabolites		No	Slight	No
Degradation dependent on:				
Body temperature		No	Yes	Yes
Blood pH		No	No	Yes
Renal function	Yes	No	Yes	No
Hepatic function	Yes	No	Yes	No
Plasma cholinesterase	No	Yes	No	No

in liver disease (11) and in patients with atypical cholinesterase (12). Unlike Sch, the use of neostigmine may assist in the reversal of prolonged block that is associated with atypical cholinesterase.

Pharmacodynamics

Neuromuscular Junction

Mivacurium produces a nondepolarizing block of shorter duration than atracurium and vecuronium. However, onset to acceptable intubating conditions appears to be similar to these agents at 1.5–2 min (13).

Cardiovascular System

It produces a dose- and rate-dependent release of histamine in a fashion similar to atracurium. Hypotension and facial flushing have been reported at higher doses. There are no reports of effects on autonomic ganglia or cardiac muscarinic receptors.

Dosage and Administration

The normal intubating dose is 0.2–0.25 mg/kg, and infusion rates vary significantly between 4 and 8 mcg/kg/min. It is recommended that neuromuscular monitoring be employed when infusions are in use. There is no evidence of accumulation with prolonged infusions at this stage.

Implications for Patient Management

It will obviously be useful for patients who require short-term airway control, e.g., short surgical procedures less than 15–20 min. It may permit one to avoid the use of reversal agents in certain patient groups, e.g., bowel anastomosis, patients with ischemic heart disease or a history of postoperative nausea and vomiting.

Its most disappointing aspect is that it does not provide a suitable alternative to Sch for urgent airway control. Although it is pharmacologically similar to atracurium, its different metabolic pathway must be remembered, particularly in patients with liver disease or atypical cholinesterase.

ROCURONIUM (ORG 9426)

Description

Rocuronium is a monoquaternary amino-steroid nondepolarizing neuromuscular blocking agent (Fig. 10). It has been recently commercially released in the US (1994). It has an intermediate duration of action similar to vecuronium, but its main attribute is its rapid onset of action with good intubating conditions. Its potency is around one-sixth to one-eighth that of vecuronium. It appears that drugs with a relatively low potency may have a faster onset time to adequate conditions for intubation, an important consideration when looking at potential replacements for Sch (14,15).

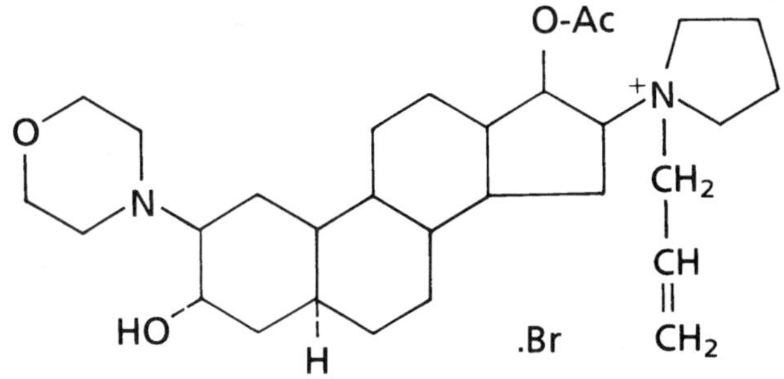

FIG. 10. Diagram of the rocuronium molecule.

Pharmacokinetics

Absorption and Distribution

Like all NMBs, rocuronium is given intravenously and has a low volume of distribution (V_d = 0.21 L/kg) (Table 7). This is increased in patients with hepatic cirrhosis (16).

Metabolism and Excretion

Rocuronium does not appear to undergo significant metabolism in the body and has an elimination half-life between 70 and 90 min. Originally, it was thought that all of the dose was taken up by the liver and biliary excretion was unchanged, with a clearance of 2.9 ml/kg/min. There are now data supporting elimination unchanged by the kidney of up to 30% to 40% of the dose administered (17).

Pharmacodynamics

Musculoskeletal System

Rocuronium causes a rapid onset of a nondepolarizing block with good intubating conditions within 60 sec. However, the clinical duration of action is still similar to vecuronium.

Cardiovascular System

Most studies of the cardiovascular stability of rocuronium support the contention that there is little change in blood pressure or heart rate. There is no effect on the autonomic ganglia or cardiac muscarinic receptors. Likewise, there is no histamine release of significance.

Dosage and Administration

The intubating dose (ED_{95}) is 0.6–0.8 mg/kg with a clinical duration of action of 20–30 min. Infusion rates of 8–12 mcg/kg/min are required to maintain 90% twitch depression. Note that there may be accumulation with prolonged infusions, as with vecuronium.

Implications for Patient Management

The main feature of rocuronium is the decreased time to adequate intubation conditions as compared with the other nondepolarizing NMB agents (18) and the current concern with hyperkalemic cardiac arrest associated with the use of Sch. However, in the difficult airway scenario, it does not have the rapid offset of action that Sch offers.

VECURONIUM

Description

Vecuronium is an intermediate duration, nondepolarizing NMB drug first introduced into clinical practice in 1980 (19). It is currently regarded as the gold standard for cardiovascular stability among the NMB agents.

Structurally, it is a monoquaternary analog of pancuronium (Fig. 11). The absence of this quaternary methyl group in the A ring of the steroid nucleus reduces the vagolytic activity by 20-fold. This modification also increases its lipid solubility (but its V_d is still the same as pancuronium). It is unstable in solution and is supplied as a powder to be dissolved in sterile water.

Pharmacokinetics

Absorption and Distribution

Vecuronium is administered intravenously. The extensive hepatic uptake of vecuronium may contribute to the rapid decline in plasma levels and its relatively short duration of action (Table 7).

The onset of action may be enhanced by giving a "priming" or subparalyzing dose (e.g., 0.01 mg/kg) followed in 3–6 min by the remaining intubating dose (0.1 mg/kg). This technique is useful when administration of Sch is contraindicated.

Metabolism and Excretion

Metabolism and excretion occurs mainly via the liver, 15% to 30% of an administered dose appearing in the urine as unchanged drug and metabolites in the first 24 hours. Because of its lipid solubility, it enters the hepatocyte readily, where it undergoes deacetylation to 3-hydroxyvecuronium, 17-hydroxyvecuronium, and 3,17-

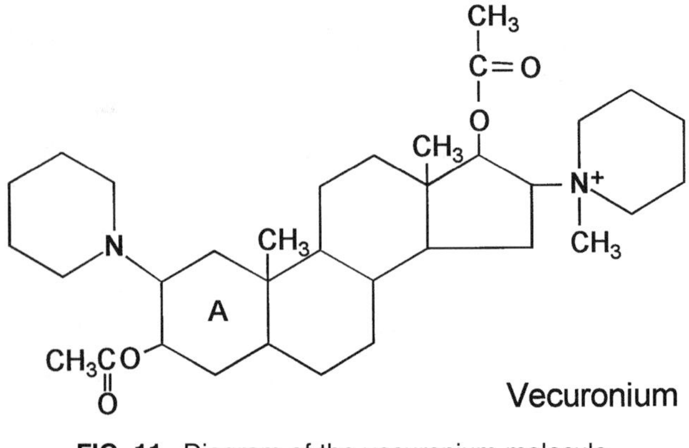

FIG. 11. Diagram of the vecuronium molecule.

dihydroxyvecuronium. Even though the elimination half-life is about 50 min as compared with 22 min for atracurium, the two drugs have a similar duration of clinical action of 30 min. Its excretion is slightly prolonged by renal failure (20).

Pharmacodynamics

Cardiovascular System

Vecuronium has little or no effect on heart rate or blood pressure, when compared with other NMB agents (21). Although it does not alter plasma histamine levels, it may actually inhibit the degradation of histamine (22).

Others

At the time of publishing, this agent appears to have little impact on other organ systems.

Dosage and Administration

Vecuronium is given intravenously at a usual intubating dose of 0.1 mg/kg. It may be given by infusion at 0.9 mcg/kg/min. Note that it may be cumulative over long infusion times.

Implications for Patient Management

Vecuronium is a reliable, very cardiovascularly stable NMB agent with few side effects. It is probably the agent of choice in trauma patients with unstable blood pressure or in those suffering from ischemic heart disease. It can be used in double the normal intubating dosage for rapid sequence inductions in patients with contraindications for the use of Sch.

ATRACURIUM

Description

Atracurium is a bisquaternary ammonium structure (Fig. 12). The iodized salt, besylate, provides water solubility, and commercial preparations adjusted to a pH of 3.25–3.65 minimize *in vitro* degradation. However, the potency of atracurium stored at room temperature declines about 5% every 30 days (23).

It has gained widespread use for neuromuscular blockade as a result of its unique process of degradation. This process is called *Hofmann degradation*, which is a physicochemical process that is temperature- and pH-dependent, not involving enzymes. It is also subjected to enzymatic degradation in the plasma, probably by a carboxylesterase enzyme.

Pharmacokinetics

Absorption and Distribution

Atracurium is administered intravenously only and has only a small V_d (150–180 ml/kg) (Table 7).

Metabolism and Excretion

There are two routes of metabolism:

1. *Hofmann Elimination*, which is a purely chemical process resulting in the loss of positive charges by molecular fragmentation to laudanosine (a tertiary amine) and a monoquaternary acrylate. It is a nonbiologic process that does not require renal, hepatic, or enzymatic function. It occurs at physiologic pH and temperature, and a decrease in pH or temperature will slow Hofmann degradation.

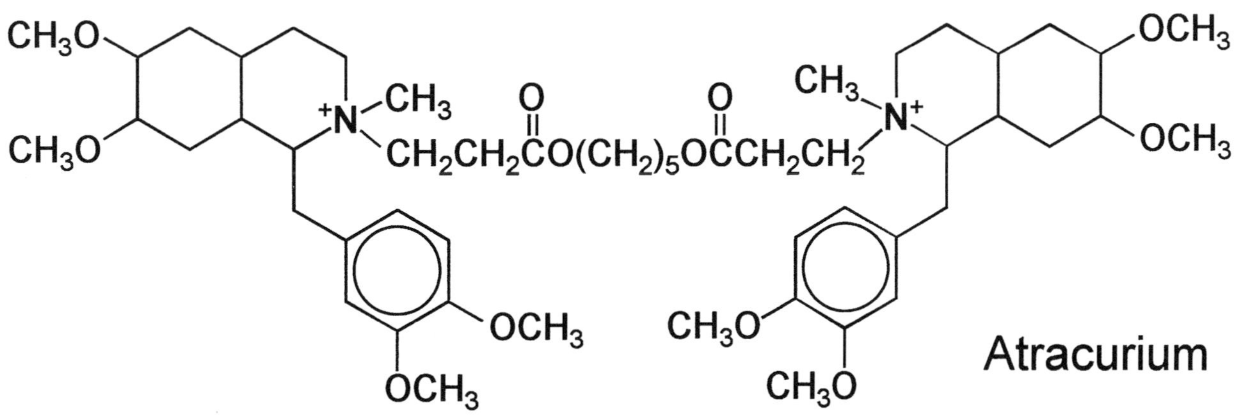

FIG. 12. Diagram of the atracurium molecule.

2. *Ester hydrolysis* does occur and there may be other pathways involved also. Laudanosine is also a metabolite of ester hydrolysis. This ester hydrolysis occurs by nonspecific esterases that are unrelated to plasma cholinesterase. There is no prolonged blockade of atracurium in patients with atypical plasma cholinesterase.

Laudanosine has a half-life of 2–4 hours and is excreted unchanged by the kidney. It is inactive at the NMJ. However, it freely crosses the BBB (peak CSF concentrations in 3–10 min) and has CNS-stimulating properties. In doses of 1–2.5 mg/kg to dogs breathing subanesthetic doses of halothane, there is evidence of arousal in the EEG in the absence of changes to CBF, $CMRO_2$, or ICP (24). Much higher blood levels are needed for seizures, but a 30% increase in anesthetic requirement (MAC) and arousal pattern on EEG is commonly found. As such, there is the possibility of awareness in the lightly anesthetized patient.

Pharmacodynamics

Cardiovascular System

Atracurium has been associated with histamine release that is dose- and rate-dependent. The histamine usually causes cutaneous manifestations only, and cardiovascular changes rarely correlate (25). It is estimated that the plasma histamine levels must double before cardiovascular changes manifest. Atracurium does not evoke sufficient histamine release until 3 times the ED_{95} is administered. There is no histamine release with 3.5 times the ED_{95} dose of vecuronium.

Respiratory System

The release of histamine modifies the use of this drug in patients with atopic dispositions, particularly asthmatics.

Dosage and Administration

The normal intubating dose of atracurium is 0.5 mg/kg. As it is noncumulative, it is ideal for infusion at rates of 0.3–0.5 mg/kg/hour.

Clinical Implications

Atracurium is used routinely in anesthetic practice for intubation. It is a reliable form of nondepolarizing NMB in patients with hepatic or renal failure. However, due to its histamine release, it is not as stable cardiovascularly as other agents (e.g., vecuronium). Caution should be exercised with the administration to asthmatic patients.

PANCURONIUM

Description

Pancuronium is an aminosteroid-based molecule (Fig. 13) that has fragments very similar to acetylcholine, which accounts for its high NMB activity, action on cardiac muscarinic receptors, and plasma cholinesterase inhibiting action.

Pharmacokinetics

Absorption and Distribution

It is 90% plasma protein bound and, like other NMB agents, it has a small V_d (0.26 L/kg). Aging is associated with a decreased rate of decline in the plasma concentration. This reflects declining renal function in the elderly.

Metabolism and Excretion

About 15% to 40% is deacylated in the liver into 3-OH, 17-OH or 3,17-OH derivatives. The 3-OH form is the major metabolite, and the most potent (having 50% of the NMB activity of the parent compound). Its duration of action and pharmacokinetics are similar to that of its parent compound. Despite this, an estimated 80% of a single dose of pancuronium is eliminated unchanged in the urine.

Pharmacodynamics

Central Nervous System

There is a decreased requirement of halothane by 25% when pancuronium is administered to patients.

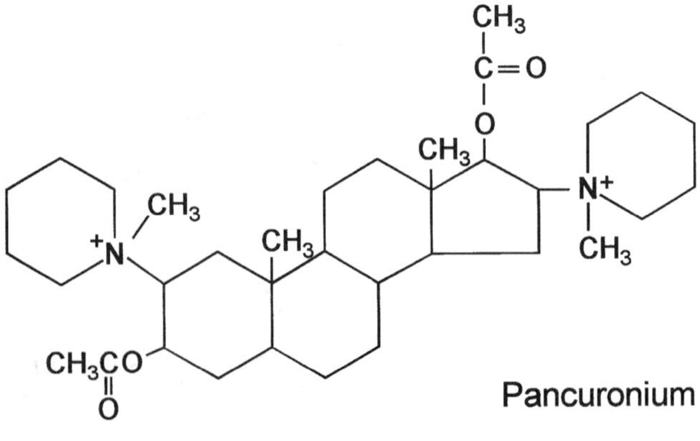

FIG. 13. Diagram of the pancuronium molecule.

Cardiovascular System

Pancuronium produces a modest 10% to 15% increase in heart rate, mean arterial pressure, and cardiac output. These effects are attributed to selective cardiac vagal blockade (i.e., atropine-like effect) and activation of the sympathetic nervous system.

The increased heart rate is due to blockade of muscarinic receptors at the S-A node. The magnitude of the increase in heart rate is more dependent on the preexisting rate (an inverse relationship) than on the dose administered. Marked increases are more likely to occur in patients with altered AV conduction of cardiac impulses, as characteristic of AF. The increase in blood pressure is a reflection of the changes in heart rate, with no change in peripheral resistance. There are no demonstrated direct inotropic effects.

Autonomic Nervous System

There is both release of norepinephrine from adrenergic nerve endings and blockade of re-uptake back into postganglionic nerve endings that have been proposed as the mechanisms of SNS activation. It may also interfere with activity of preganglionic muscarinic receptors that normally inhibit the release of NA. Nonetheless, there is an increase in the circulating levels of catecholamines in the plasma.

Dosage and Administration

The intubating dose is 0.1 mg/kg intravenously with a clinical duration of 30–40 min.

Clinical Implications

Pancuronium was perhaps the most commonly used long-acting nondepolarizing NMB agent until the advent of pipecuronium and doxacurium. Its main disadvantage is the tachycardia that may be detrimental to patients with a history of ischemic heart disease.

PIPECURONIUM

Description

Pipecuronium was introduced in the US in 1991 and is an aminosteroid nondepolarizing neuromuscular agent that is structurally related to pancuronium (Fig. 14). It has a longer duration of action than does pancuronium and, due to structural modifications, it does not have the vagolytic properties of pancuronium.

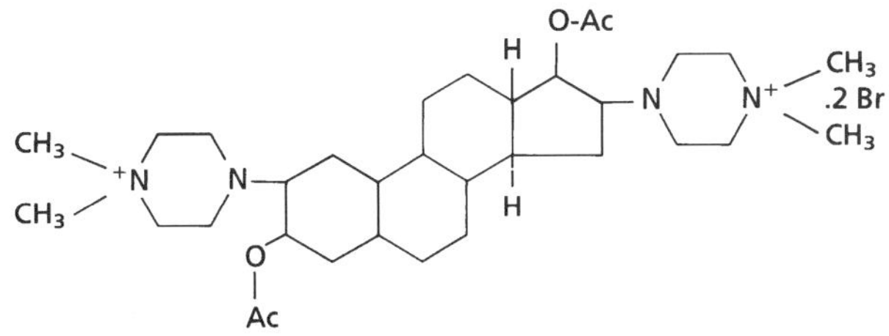

Pipecuronium bromide

FIG. 14. Diagram of the pipecuronium molecule.

Pharmacokinetics

Absorption and Distribution

Pipecuronium is administered intravenously.

Metabolism and Excretion

Elimination of pipecuronium is almost exclusively renal. The liver does provide a minor role but the kinetics of pipecuronium are not significantly affected by cirrhosis (26).

Pharmacodynamics

Cardiovascular System

There are minimal changes in heart rate and blood pressure. No histamine release occurs with intubating doses.

Neuromuscular Junction

Pipecuronium has slow onset (2–3 min) of adequate intubating conditions (like pancuronium) with the normal intubating dose. Concurrent use of isoflurane decreases maintenance dosage requirements by 30% (27)

Dosage and Administration

The normal intravenous intubating dose is 0.1 mg/kg with a clinical duration of action up to 120 min.

Clinical Implications

Pipecuronium provides an alternative, long-acting NMB agent to pancuronium.

DOXACURIUM

Description

Doxacurium is a benzylisoquinolone derivative first introduced in 1991. It is structurally related to atracurium (Fig. 15). It is a long-acting, nondepolarizing NMB agent devoid of cardiovascular side effects.

Pharmacokinetics

Absorption and Distribution

Doxacurium is administered intravenously at an intubating dose of 0.05–0.06 mg/kg. It has a small V_d of 0.22 L/kg.

Metabolism and Excretion

The half-life is 99 min (clearance 2.7 ml/min/kg). It is mainly excreted unchanged in the urine, with a small amount in the bile (28). There is no Hofmann degradation or ester hydrolysis.

There is no drug accumulation with repeated doses but duration is prolonged in renal failure (29). Duration is also increased in the elderly patient.

Pharmacodynamics

Cardiovascular System

Unlike atracurium, there is no histamine release. Doxacurium is regarded as cardiovascularly stable, although there may be a small drop in heart rate with large doses (30).

Neuromuscular Junction

It has a slow onset to adequate intubating conditions, similar to pancuronium (3–4 min) with normal intubating doses. The clinical duration of action of an intubating dose is 90–120 min (time to recovery of 25% of control single twitch). It also has a slow recovery index, so that the blockade it causes should always be reversed.

Dosage and Administration

Normal intubating dose is 0.05–0.06 mg/kg intravenously.

Clinical Implications

It is a long-acting agent with cardiovascular side effects but does not appear to offer a marked advantage over pancuronium (31). There is also no real advantage over infusions of the intermediate acting agents like vecuronium and atracurium. Its long onset time to intubating conditions precludes it from use in emergency airway conditions. It may be useful for long-term intermittent blockade in ICU or transfer situations where infusions are not practical.

CLINICAL IMPLICATIONS

In most anesthetic situations, it generally doesn't matter which NMB agent is used. However, certain situations require consideration of the side effects of each of the agents that may endanger the well-being of the patient. We will discuss some of the more common difficulties encountered.

The Patient with the Full Stomach and Sch Contraindicated

Most patients requiring urgent surgery and general anesthesia (typically trauma victims) need an RSI. Succinylcholine is the most suitable NMB agent for RSI due to its rapid onset and offset of action. At present, there is

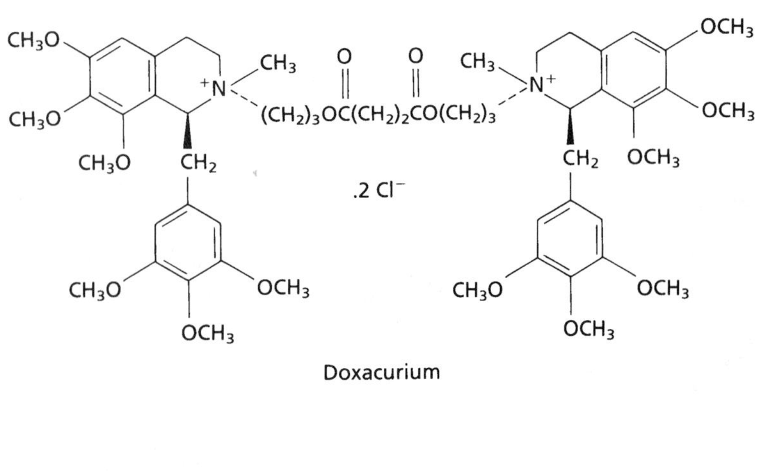

FIG. 15. Diagram of the doxacurium molecule.

no other agent that has these same characteristics. Urgent airway access is difficult in patients with a contraindication to Sch, e.g., allergy to Sch, myotonia, hyperkalemia, burns (more than 24–48 hours old), spinal cord injuries more than 24–48 hours old, penetrating eye injuries, and malignant hyperthermia.

The alternatives to the use of Sch include:

1. Awake intubation (nasotracheal, fiberoptic, tracheotomy).
2. Modified rapid sequence intubation using either double-dose vecuronium, a small priming dose of a nondepolarizing NMB, or a large dose of rocuronium.

The main determinants of which approach to use are: (a) the clinician's assessment of the difficulty expected in intubation; (b) the clinician's experience; and (c) available drugs.

In the situation where a difficult intubation is not anticipated (and Sch is contraindicated), a modified RSI is our technique of choice. We use double-dose vecuronium (0.2 mg/kg) and wait for 60–90 sec following routine preoxygenation. Rocuronium (1.0 mg/kg) may be a alternative if available.

If a difficult airway is anticipated, wherever possible, an awake procedure is preferable. The choice of technique depends upon the experience of the operator.

The Patient with Known Ischemic Heart Disease (IHD)

Most of the cardiovascular problems associated with intubation and extubation relate to direct laryngoscopy and airway stimulation (see the chapter regarding laryngoscopy and intubation). Drugs used for intubation/extubation may exaggerate this response. The patient with IHD obviously is at risk of ischemia with increased cardiac work, i.e., changes in rate and blood pressure.

With intubation, it is prudent to avoid drugs that may be associated with changes in heart rate, particularly pancuronium and gallamine (direct effect on autonomic ganglia). One should also be wary of the use of atracurium and alcuronium (due to hypotension from histamine release), which may result in a reflex tachycardia. Remember that Sch may cause significant bradycardia, particularly in elderly and pediatric patients, or in those receiving a second dose.

At extubation, the concern is with the use of anticholinergic drugs to antagonize the muscarinic effects of anticholinesterase agents (neostigmine, edrophonium). There is debate as to how patients should be managed. There are advocates for allowing neuromuscular function to recover spontaneously. Equally, there are those who will always "reverse" NMB agents. Our practice is to use an agent like glycopyrrolate, rather than atropine, to diminish the tachycardia in these patients.

Organ Failure

The main problem in patients with an organ system failure (liver, renal, etc.) is the altered pharmacokinetic profile of the NMB agent, generally resulting in altered duration of action. These agents are otherwise generally very safe for use in such patients; it is just that the reliability of reversal of neuromuscular blockade is in question. Where reliable reversal is required, atracurium is probably the agent of choice. See Table 3 for the mode of elimination of some of the more commonly used agents.

The exception to this is Sch. It should be avoided in patients with renal failure in the presence of known hyperkalemia.

Patients with Allergic Diathesis

Atracurium, alcuronium, mivacurium, and curare are all associated with elevation of plasma histamine levels. The problems with the elevation in plasma histamine levels include rash, tachycardia, hypotension, and bronchospasm. Generally, the changes in plasma histamine levels are not enough to alter patient well-being. However, we would avoid such agents in patients with known allergic predispositions, e.g., asthma. Vecuronium and pancuronium are generally regarded as safe in such patients but there is evidence that vecuronium will increase the severity of anaphylaxis due to its inhibition of N-methyl transferase.

REFERENCES

1. Ligier B, Buchman TG, Breslow MJ, Deutschman CS. The role of anesthetic induction agents and neuromuscular blockade in the endotracheal intubation of trauma victims. *Surgery, Gynecology and Obstetrics* Dec 1991;173(6):477–481.
2. Kistler J, Stroud RM, Klymkowski MW, Lalncette RA, Fairclough RH. Structure and function of an acetylcholine receptor. *Biophys J* 1982;37:371–383.
3. Waud BE, Waud DR. The relation between tetanic fade and receptor occlusion in the presence of competitive neuromuscular block. *Anesthesiology* 1971;35:456–464.
4. Azar I. The response of patients with neuromuscular disorders to muscle relaxants: a review. *Anesthesiology* 1984;61:173–187.
5. Pavlin EG, Holle RH, Schoene RB. Recovery of airway protection compared with ventilation in humans after paralysis with curare. *Anesthesiology* 1989;70:381–385.
6. Martyn JAJ, Szyfelbein SK, Ali HH, Matteo RS, Savarese JJ. Increased d-tubocurarine requirement following major thermal injury. *Anesthesiology* 1980;52:352–355.
7. Holst-Larsen H. The hydrolysis of suxamethonium in human blood. *Br J Anaesth* 1976;48:887–891.
8. Kovarik WD, Mayberg TS, Lam Am, Mathisen TL, Winn HR. Succinylcholine does not change intracranial pressure, cerebral blood flow velocity, or the electroencephalogram in patients with neurological injury. *Anesth Analg* 1994;78:469–473.
9. Brodsky JB, Brock-Utne JG, Samiels SI. Pancuronium pretreament and post-succinylcholine myalgias. *Anesthesiology* 1979;51:259–261.
10. Cook DR, Freeman JA, Lai AA, et al. Pharmacokinetics of mivacurium in normal patients and in those with hepatic or renal disease. *Br J Anaesth* 1992;69:580–585.
11. Devlin JC, Head-Rapson AG, Parker CJR, Hunter JM. Pharmacody-

namics of mivacurium chloride in patients with hepatic cirrhosis. *Br J Anaesth* 1993;71:227–231.
12. Goudsouzian NG, d'Hollander AA, Viby-Mogensen J. Prolonged neuromuscular block from mivacurium in two patients with cholinesterase deficiency. *Anesth Analg* 1993;77:183–185.
13. Goldberg ME, Larijani GE, Azad SS, et al. Comparison of tracheal intubating conditions and neuromuscular blocking profiles after intubating doses of mivacurium chloride or succinylcholine in surgical outpatients. *Anesth Analg* 1989;69:93–99.
14. Bowman WC, Rodgers IW, Houston J, et al. Structure: relationships among some desacetoxy analogues of vecuronium and pancuronium in the anesthetised cat. *Anesthesiology* 1988;69:57–66.
15. Kopman AF. Gallamine, pancuronium, and d-tubocurarine compared: is onset time related to drug potency? *Anesthesiology* 1989;70:915–920.
16. Khalil M, D'Honneur G, Duvaldestin P, Slavov V, De Hys C, Gomeni R. Pharmacokinetics and pharmacodynamics of rocuronium in patients with cirrhosis. *Anesthesiology* 1994;80:1242–1247.
17. Cooper RA, Maddineni VR, Mirakhur RK, et al. Time course of neuromuscular effects and pharmacokinetics of rocuronium bromide (org 9426) during isoflurane anesthesia in patients with and without renal failure. *Br J Anaesth* 1993;71:222–226.
18. Bartkowski RR, Witkoski TA, Azad S, et al. Rocuronium onset of action: a comparison with atracurium and vecuronium. *Anesth Analg* 1993;77:574–578.
19. Crul JF, Booij LHDJ. First clinical experiences with Org NC 45. *Br J Anaesth* 1980;52:49–51S.
20. Lynam DP, Cronnelly R, Castagnoli KP, Canfell PC, Caldwell J, Arden J, Miller RD. The pharmacodynamics and pharmacokinetics of vecuronium in patients anesthetized with isoflurane with normal renal function or with renal failure. *Anesthesiology* 1988;69:227–231.
21. Marshall RJ, McGrath JC, Miller RD, Docherty JR, Lamar JC. Comparison of the cardiovascular actions of org NC 45 with those produced by other non-depolarizing neuromuscular blocking agents in experimental animals. *Br J Anaesth* 1980;52:21–31S.
22. Futo J, Kupferberg JP, Moss J, Fahey MR, Cannon JE, Miller RD. Vecuronium inhibits histamine N-methyl transferase. *Anesthesiology* 1988;69:92–96.
23. Russell WJ, Meyer-Witting M. The stability of atracurium in clinical practice. *Anaesth Intensive Care* 1990;17:55–552.
24. Parker CJR, Jones JE, Hunter JM. Deposition of infusions of atracurium and its metabolite, laudanosine, in patients in renal and respiratory failure in an ITU. *Br J Anaesth* 1988;61:531–540.
25. Barnes PK, de Renzy-Martin N, Thomas VJE, Watkins J. Plasma histamine levels following atracurium. *Anesthesia* 1986;41:821–824.
26. D'Honneur G, Khalil M, Dominique C, Habere JP, Kleef UW, Duvaldstein P. Pharmacokinetics and pharmacodynamics of pipecuronium in patients with cirrhosis. *Anesth Analg* 1993;77:1203–1206.
27. Pittet J, Tassonyi E, Morel DR, Gemperie G, Richter M, Rouge J. Pipecuronium-induced neuromuscular blockade during nitrous oxide-fentanyl, isoflurane, and halothane anesthesia in adults and children. *Anesthesiology* 1989;71:210–213.
28. Savarese JJ, Wastila WB, Rudd D, Welch RE, Samara B. Pharmacodynamics and pharmacokinetics of doxacurium chloride (BW A938U): background and overview. *J Cardiovasc Anesth* 1990;4 (Supp 4):14–19.
29. Cook DR, Freeman JA, Lai AA, et al. Pharmacokinetics and pharmacodynamics of doxacurium in normal patients and in those with hepatic or renal failure. *Anesth Analg* 1991;72:145–150.
30. Emmott RS, Bracey BJ, Goldhill DR, Yate PM, Flynn PJ. Cardiovascular effects of doxacurium, pancuronium and vecuronium in anesthetized patients presenting for coronary artery bypass surgery. *Br J Anaesth* 1990;65:480–486.
31. Rathmell JP, Brooker RF, Prieplipp RC, Butterworth JF, Gravlee GP. Hemodynamic and pharmacodynamic comparison of doxacurium and pipecuronium with pancuronium during induction of cardiac anesthesia: does the benefit justify the cost? *Anesth Analg* 1993;76:513–519.

Airway Management, edited by
L.H. Hanowell, M.D. and R.J. Waldron, M.D.,
Lippincott-Raven Publishers, Philadelphia © 1996.

CHAPTER 12

Opiates and Airway Management

Jennifer Hall and Dennis L. Fung

INTRODUCTION

Opiates are seldom used as the sole pharmacologic agent in emergency airway management, but they are commonly administered as an adjunct. The use of opiates can contribute to the effectiveness of management, but it can also lead to complications. Understanding the pharmacokinetics and pharmacodynamics of opiates is critical to their logical application. Knowledge of kinetics enables appropriate drug and dosage selection, and knowledge of pharmacodynamics enables prediction of side effects and facilitates their management.

J. Hall and D. L. Fung: Department of Anesthesiology, University of California, Davis School of Medicine, Sacramento, California 95817.

Ideal Intubating Conditions and the Role of Opiates

For effective emergency airway management, a patient's airway must be secured rapidly with a minimum of adverse sequelae. A decision is made as to whether the patient will be awake for the procedure or anesthetized, with or without paralysis. If the patient is awake and breathing and has airway analgesia, then judicious use of sedation may minimize patient distress and improve patient cooperation. If the decision is to induce anesthesia, then ideally the patient will be unaware and the vocal cords will be open and still. In either scenario, it is important to avoid major hemodynamic or respiratory consequences of intubation, in particular, acute rises in heart rate and blood pressure, or coughing and bucking. Opiates have a role in controlling many of these conditions. After the airway has been secured, opiates can be used to improve tolerance of the endotracheal tube by blunting of airway reflexes and suppression of respiratory drive, thereby facilitating positive-pressure ventilation.

History of the Opiates

Traditionally, opiates such as morphine were used for their analgesic or euphoric properties. They were known to alter the conscious state without cardiac depression, but their dosage was limited by side effects, especially respiratory depression. Mechanical ventilation overcame this problem to some extent, but histamine release with vasodilation and hypotension limited the use of large doses. Fentanyl was synthesized in 1960 (1). Not only did it have a shorter duration and more potency than morphine, it also caused minimal histamine release. Also, this opiate maintained circulatory stability and inhibited the elevation in pulse and blood pressure that often accompany endotracheal intubation. Accordingly, fentanyl became popular as an induction agent for cardiac anesthesia. Unfortunately, in large doses it still produced prolonged respiratory depression and could precipitate truncal rigidity on induction, causing acute respiratory embarrassment. Also, cases of awareness were reported. Alfentanil and sufentanil were two of the drugs synthesized to try to overcome these characteristics, and together with fentanyl they can be useful opiates for the emergency situation.

Selection of Opiates

Use of opiates in emergency airway management requires a selection of drug, dose, and rate of administration, and consideration of potential adverse effects. Since time is a factor in successful emergency management, the onset and duration of effect are important selection criteria. With administration of equipotent doses, there are differences among the opiates. The short-acting opiates, such as fentanyl, sufentanil, and alfentanil, also have rapid onset. These short-acting opiates may be preferred if it is important to evaluate the patient's neurologic status serially. On the other hand, when continued control of ventilation is needed, a longer-acting opiate, such as morphine, may be more useful. If a long-acting opiate is used but the patient needs to be evaluated neurologically, the opiate effects can be reversed (sometimes only transiently) by administering naloxone. This is best done by titration, using small amounts, because of the risk of inducing hypertension, tachycardia, and pain.

PHARMACOKINETICS

Important pharmacokinetic characteristics in the emergency use of opiates are onset of action and duration of effect. These characteristics are difficult to define without an objective measure of opiate effect. Analgesia, respiratory depression, and EEG pattern have all been used to quantitate opiate effect (2,3). Studies using the EEG have been performed under general anesthesia. Since anesthesia may alter the pharmacokinetics and pharmacodynamics of opiates, the applicability of results from anesthetized patients to awake patients is uncertain. Further, the relation of EEG pattern to analgesic, cardiovascular, and respiratory effects is unclear. Nevertheless, the pharmacokinetic parameters that are of special interest for comparing onset and duration of single doses are the transfer rate from the central compartment to the effect compartment (Ke_0) (Fig. 1) and the distribution and elimination half-times ($t_{1/2}\alpha$ and $t_{1/2}\beta$). These and other pharmacokinetic values are listed in Table 1.

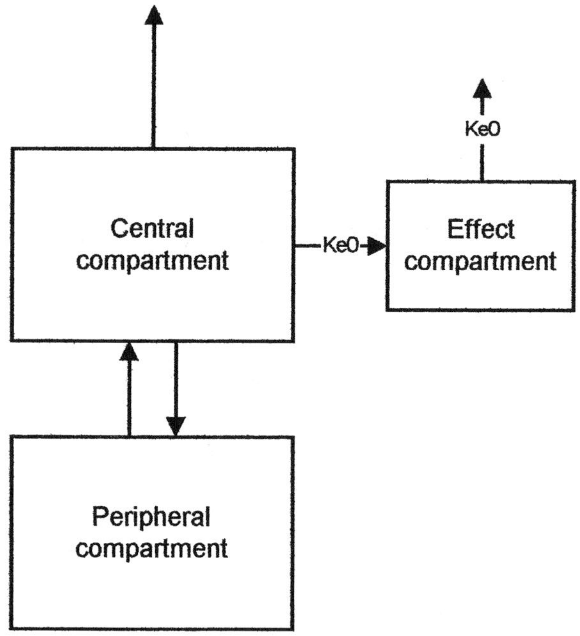

FIG. 1. Transfer rate from the central compartment to the effect compartment (Ke_0).

Onset of Opiate Effect

The onset of opiate effect depends on the ease with which opiate molecules move from the site of administration to the site of effect. Access to the site of effect is described pharmacokinetically by the parameter Ke_0, the transfer rate from the central compartment (which includes the intravascular volume and very highly perfused areas) to the site of action. Ke_0 is expressed in units of inverse time and is a parameter of pharmacokinetic-pharmacodynamic models. It is usually assumed for simplicity that there is one effect compartment containing all effect sites. A drug with a large Ke_0 value has greater access to the effect site than a drug with small Ke_0.

TABLE 1. *Pharmacokinetic values*

Opiate	Volume of distribution (steady state), L/kg	Clearance (elimination), mL/min	Half-time (β), h	Half-time (α), min	Peak time, min	Duration, h	Ke_0, min–1
Fentanyl	2–4	850	3–5	1–2	3–5	0.5–1	0.147
Sufentanil	2–4	850	3–5	1.2	3–5	0.5–1	0.227
Alfentanil	0.2–0.5	275	1–3	1–4	1.5–2	0.2–0.3	0.770
Meperidine	2–4	850	3–5	4–17	5–7	2–3	
Morphine	3	814	2.4–3.0	1–4	20–30	3–4	

Ke_0, transfer rate from central compartment to effect compartment.

Among the short-acting opiates, alfentanil has the largest Ke_0 value.

Duration of Opiate Effect

The duration of effect after a single opiate dose usually depends on the rate of redistribution from the highly perfused brain. Brain concentration of fentanyl follows plasma concentration closely unless hyperventilation or hypoventilation is imposed. After a single dose, the early decline in plasma concentration is described by $t_{1/2}\alpha$. (In some descriptions, two half-times are used to describe this early phase: $t_{1/2}\alpha$ and $t_{1/2}\pi$.) After repeated doses or infusion, the decline in plasma concentration is more likely to be described by $t_{1/2}\beta$. This shift in the observed plasma half-time is referred to as "context sensitivity." Unless an acute change in sensitivity (tolerance) occurs, a shift to the longer $t_{1/2}\beta$ with large, repeated doses or infusion should result in a longer duration. In situations in which $t_{1/2}\beta$ describes the decline in plasma and brain concentration, changes in clearance and volume of distribution have clinical significance. For example, the reduced clearance that accompanies liver cirrhosis causes an increase in $t_{1/2}\beta$ and an increase in duration. Onset and duration are also affected by the dose and rate of administration. A large dose produces a fast onset and a longer duration. Rapid administration causes a more rapid onset and a higher peak effect. A smaller dose given rapidly can achieve the same peak effect as a larger one given slowly.

Onset and Duration of Specific Opiates

Using the values from EEG studies in a computer simulation, it can be predicted that alfentanil will have the fastest onset, but sufentanil will have the most rapid recovery. However, in the first 90 minutes after bolus administration, there is little difference in rate of recovery among fentanyl, sufentanil, and alfentanil (4). Comparable studies for meperidine and morphine have not been performed. Clinical observation suggests that both meperidine and morphine exhibit slower onset and longer duration of effect.

Fentanyl has been useful because of its rapid onset (30 seconds) and short duration (30 minutes). These favorable characteristics can be explained by fentanyl's high lipid solubility. It readily crosses the blood-brain barrier for a rapid onset, and then it redistributes to other tissues, such as skeletal muscle and fat, for a short duration (5). Alfentanil and sufentanil have similar effect times.

OPIATE RECEPTORS AND ENDOGENOUS LIGANDS

Opiates exert many of their effects by interacting with specific receptors. These opiate receptors were first isolated in 1973, by Pert and Snyder (6). Later, naturally occurring opiates or endogenous ligands that bind to the receptors were identified and classified into three families using recombinant DNA techniques (7). Although originally described only in the central nervous system, receptors have also been identified more recently at peripheral nerve endings and on immune cells (8,9). Endogenous opiates seem to play a role in regulating many physiologic functions, including the stress response, food intake, fluid balance, and mood control. They interact extensively with other neurotransmitters, such as serotonin and adenosine (10,11). The spinal cord receptors and their role in pain modulation are the best studied; less is known about the supraspinal and peripheral receptors.

Opiate Receptors

Of the five types of opiate receptors described in animal studies, only three have been identified in humans. They are designated according to the agonist that was used experimentally to activate each of them, as described below.

Mu (μ) Receptors for Morphine

The μ receptors are now subdivided into μ_1 and μ_2 receptors. Many authors believe that the μ_1 receptors are responsible for supraspinal analgesia, whereas the μ_2

receptors are responsible for spinal analgesia. The supraspinal receptors may exert their effect by descending inhibition of spinal pathways. Brain stem μ_2 receptors appear responsible for respiratory depression (12). Activation of μ receptors also causes miosis, bradycardia, and hypothermia. In immune cells in vertebrate and invertebrate animals, μ_3 receptors have been described; they may have a role in modulation of immune function (9).

Delta (δ) Receptors for DADL (D-Alanine-D-Leucine) enkephalin

The δ receptors are subdivided into δ_1, δ_2, and δ_3 receptors. They may contribute to control of respiration, being located in strategic brain stem areas, but seem likely to have a lesser role than μ receptors. Other roles may include olfaction, motor integration, and analgesia (13).

Kappa (κ) Receptors for Ketocyclazocine

The κ receptors are subdivided into κ_1, κ_2, and κ_3 receptors. Stimulation of κ_1 receptors spinally appears to mediate spinal analgesia. Distribution and function of κ_2 receptors are unclear. However, κ_3 receptors mediate analgesia and are the most numerous of the supraspinal opiate receptors. They have been identified supraspinally in association with μ_1 receptors. The significance of their association with μ receptors is not yet certain.

Physiology of Opiate Receptors

Whereas there is some consensus regarding the location and function of μ receptors, there is less regarding the role of the κ and δ receptors (13,14). Activation of any of the three receptors (μ, δ, or κ) causes inhibitory effects. However, the mechanisms differ. Activation of μ and δ receptors results in opening of K^+ channels, via cAMP and a G-protein. There is consequent hyperpolarization and decreased firing of the neuron. At a nerve terminal, this hyperpolarization then leads to a secondary inhibition of Ca^{2+} influx, thereby preventing transmitter release. By contrast, κ-receptor activation directly leads to closure of Ca^{2+} channels, causing inhibition of transmission (10,15,16).

No true endogenous antagonists at the opiate receptor sites have been identified. Several agents from other neurologic pathways that modify pain transmission have been identified. For example, cholecystokinin has been implicated as part of an antagonist system (14). Excitatory amines (e.g., glutamate and aspartate) can act at N-methyl-D-aspartate receptors to reduce the effectiveness of opioids (17).

Whereas spinal cord receptors are involved in pain modulation, the opiate effects that facilitate intubation (i.e., conscious state changes, respiratory and circulatory effects) are probably mediated supraspinally. Truncal rigidity appears to be spinally mediated. Some side effects of opiates do not involve opiate receptors at all. Two examples of nonopiate-receptor effects are histamine release by morphine and the antimuscarinic activity of meperidine.

Endogenous Ligands

Although in humans there are three groups of opiate receptors and at least three distinct groups of naturally occurring peptides, any one group of peptides is not necessarily selective for a particular type of receptor (10). Details of the role of these endogenous opiates in physiologic pain control and regulation of autonomic function are incomplete. They have short half-lives and are difficult to study directly. The endogenous ligands fall into three groups: β-endorphins, enkephalins, and dynorphans.

β-Endorphins

Pro-opiomelanocortin is the precursor molecule for β-endorphins and contains sequences for β-LPH (lipotropin) and nonopiate hormones such as ACTH (corticotropin). The β-LPH sequence contains β-endorphin, which is found in the pituitary, hypothalamus, spinal cord, small intestine, plasma, and placenta.

Enkephalins

The precursor for enkephalins, pro-enkephalin, is found widely in the central nervous system and in the adrenal medulla, gastrointestinal tract, and plasma. Delta receptors have high sensitivity to enkephalins (14).

Dynorphans

Prodynorphan is the precursor for dynorphans and is found in high concentration in hypothalamus but also elsewhere in the central nervous system and peripheral tissues. The dynorphans appear to have a role in neurotransmission and its regulation. Dynorphans are now widely acknowledged as the endogenous ligand for κ receptors (15).

Structure-Activity Relationships

There is little consistency observed between structure and activity of opiate ligands (Fig. 2). This may stem from the heterogeneity of opiate receptors (18). However some trends exist for benzmorphans (e.g., morphine) and

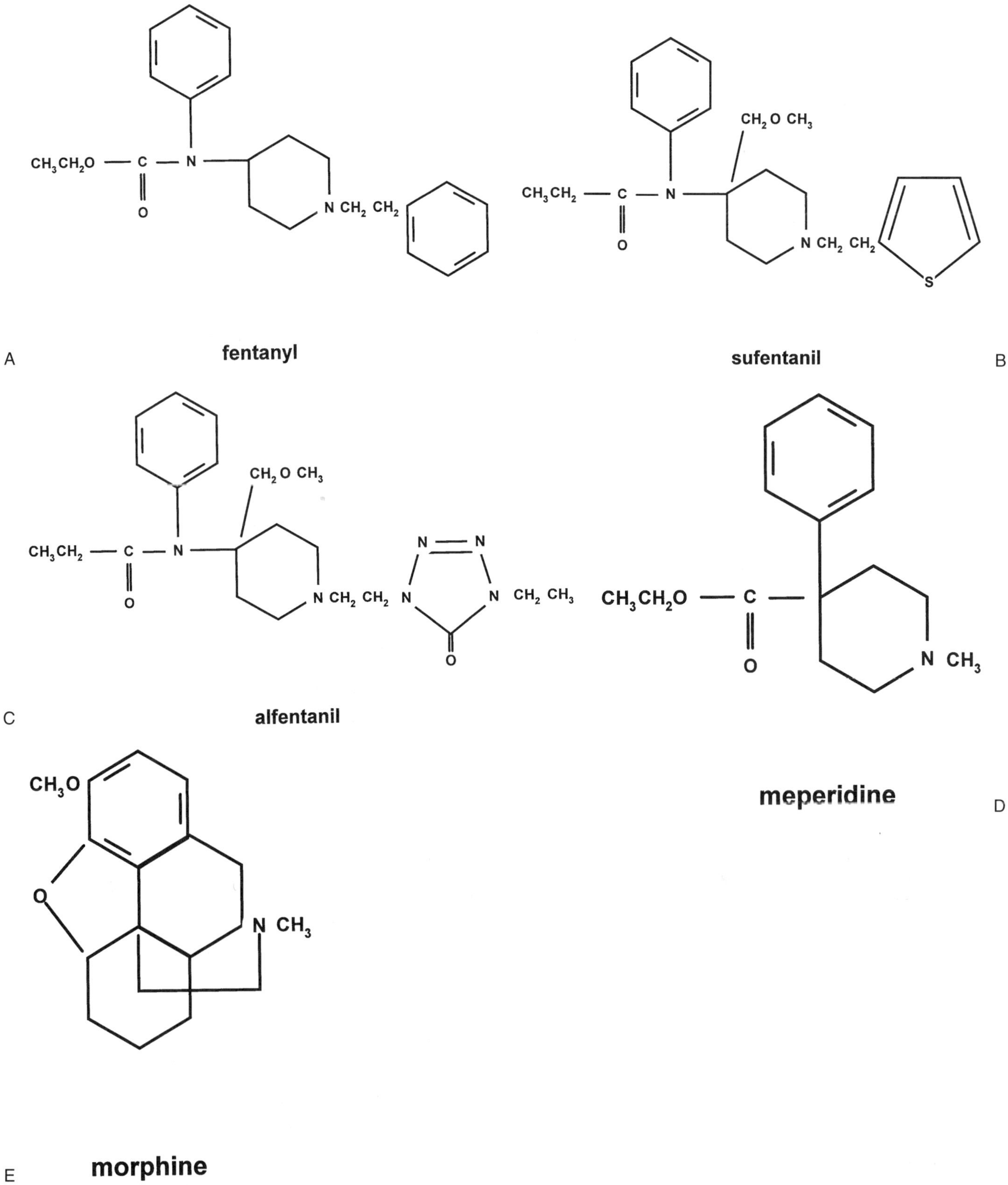

FIG. 2. A–E: Structure of opiate ligands.

their effect at μ receptors. For example, in the benzmorphan series, the levo-optical isomer is more active than the dextro-optical isomer. Substitution of a hydroxyl group at carbon atom 14 leads to antagonist activity.

The conformation of the phenoperidines (e.g., meperidine) differs from that of the benzmorphans such that the chain of the molecule is equatorial, not axial, with respect to the phenol ring (18). The synthetic agents (fentanyl, sufentanil, and alfentanil) are based on this phenoperidine structure. The effects of substitutions have been less predictable than with benzmorphans.

Now that μ, κ, and δ opioid receptors have been cloned, their active sites can be identified and structure-activity relationships may be better established (19,20, 21). For example, aspartate residues in the δ receptor appear to bind strongly to the positively charged nitrogen moiety in a δ agonist. It also appears that a receptor may have several active domains, such that drugs with diverse structures may interact with a given receptor at different domains (22).

PHARMACODYNAMICS OF SPECIFIC OPIATES

Specific Drugs and Their Actions

Just as there is variation in the pharmacokinetic profiles of the different opioid drugs, there is pharmacodynamic diversity, with differences in terms of affinity for receptors and degree of agonist activity at the receptor. Morphine is the prototype agonist at the μ receptor. Buprenorphine is an example of an opiate that binds tightly, but it is only a partial agonist at this receptor. Thus, it has a high affinity for the receptor and is hard to displace with another agonist or antagonist, but it is less potent than a full agonist in terms of its effects.

Of the opiate drugs used clinically, almost all possess μ-receptor activity. Naloxone is a pure antagonist that is relatively specific for the μ receptor. Fentanyl, alfentanil, and sufentanil can be described as pure μ agonists, with high affinity and potency. Sufentanil is 5 to 10 times as potent as fentanyl, which is, in turn, 5 to 10 times as potent as alfentanil. In other words, 10 μg/kg fentanyl is equivalent to 1 to 2 μg/kg sufentanil or 50 to 100 μg/kg alfentanil. The high potency of sufentanil is attributable to its high affinity for the μ receptor.

Hemodynamic Effects of Opiates

Endotracheal intubation is well described as a potent stimulus, producing elevated catecholamine levels, tachycardia, and high blood pressure (23,24). The possible consequences of these changes include myocardial ischemia, pulmonary edema, ventricular dysrhythmias, and cerebral hemorrhage (25). Fentanyl produces bradycardia, particularly in moderate to high doses. This is an effect of fentanyl on brain stem vagal centers (26). A recent study suggests that the afferent nerve fibers of the glossopharyngeal and vagus nerves have a high density of opiate receptors in the medulla (27). This inhibition of oropharyngeal reflex transmission may represent another mechanism by which opiates inhibit the response to laryngoscopy and intubation. Sufentanil and alfentanil similarly produce bradycardia.

Several papers have described the use of these drugs during induction of anesthesia in an effort to diminish the hemodynamic response to intubation (28–33). Cork et al. (31) used a thiopental (Pentothal) rapid-sequence induction technique with or without fentanyl 5 μg/kg and demonstrated less increase in rate and blood pressure in the fentanyl group. Kautto et al. (32) found that a fentanyl dose of 2 μg/kg limited blood pressure increase at laryngoscopy but that 6 μg/kg was more effective in preventing tachycardia during induction with thiopental. Moderate doses of fentanyl (5 μg/kg) have been shown to reduce the heart rate response to intubation, whereas higher doses (10 μg/kg) more reliably reduce both the rate and pressor response, but with an increased incidence of hypotension (33). Alfentanil 15 μg/kg blunted pressor and rate response to intubation (31). Many of these studies have been in patients undergoing coronary artery bypass grafting.

With minimal histamine release, the synthetic opioids, unlike morphine, do not cause dilation of capacitance vessels (34). Crosby et al. (34) found that sufentanil 10 μg/kg, but not fentanyl 50 μg/kg, caused a drop in systemic vascular resistance and mean arterial pressure when used as a bolus for induction. Similarly, sufentanil 15 μg/kg caused this blood pressure drop in patients being induced for elective coronary artery surgery, whereas fentanyl 75 μg/kg and alfentanil 125 μg/kg did not (35). In this particular study, it appeared that high doses of alfentanil may have caused anaerobic myocardial metabolism, based on lactate measurements.

Unfortunately, no threshold plasma level or dose of opiate has been found invariably to limit the hemodynamic response to laryngoscopy and intubation. Even at high doses, there is no guarantee of hemodynamic stability (35,36). Furthermore, it is hard to compare the drugs when equipotent doses cannot be well established.

Respiratory Effects

μ-Receptor agonists produce dose-dependent respiratory depression. This is probably the consequence of a direct effect on μ_2 receptors in the brain stem. There is suppression of the normal ventilatory response to CO_2 such that a higher level of plasma CO_2 is needed before a given level of ventilatory response is evoked. Also, the ventilatory response to hypoxia is suppressed. A patient with opiate-induced respiratory depression who is arousable may require instruction to breathe. However, the use of an opiate in a large dose or one with a longer half-life increases the likelihood of the need for prolonged mechanical ventilation. Interestingly, sufentanil appears to cause less respiratory depression at equianalgesic doses than does fentanyl, despite the fact that both agents are described as pure μ agonists. This may be caused by a greater affinity for μ_1 than μ_2 receptors (37).

Coughing or bucking of the patient on intubation is undesirable because it worsens the conditions for intubating. It may also worsen the patient's underlying condition. For instance, in a patient with a head injury and raised intracranial pressure, coughing could potentially markedly increase that pressure, or the movement might worsen a cervical cord injury. One study compared alfentanil doses in combination with lidocaine and propofol and evaluated the conditions produced (38). The use of 20 μg/kg alfentanil with propofol 2.5 μg/kg, but not the use of 10 μg/kg alfentanil with propofol, was associated with an easier direct laryngoscopy and less coughing after endotracheal tube placement. Interestingly, the use of intravenous lidocaine further improved the conditions with either of these regimens.

Central Nervous System Effects

Conscious State

None of the opiate agents alone can be relied on to produce total anesthesia (39). Large doses do not always blunt autonomic response to noxious stimuli (36), nor does the absence of an autonomic response during high-dose opiate anesthesia guarantee lack of patient awareness. Therefore, the supplementary use of an agent that produces hypnosis, such as a barbiturate or benzodiazepine, is advisable to prevent recall.

Confusion, acute psychosis, nightmares, and disturbed sleep patterns have been well described with opiates. Visual hallucinations also occur, in the presence of a clear sensorium. It seems that the critical neurons are located in the hypothalamus and temporal lobes, and that κ-receptor activation may be responsible. Acute mood changes such as sedation and euphoria are thought to be μ-receptor-mediated, as are chronic changes of decreased motivation (40).

Truncal Rigidity

Truncal rigidity has been reported with moderate- to high-dose fentanyl, alfentanil, and sufentanil, typically at induction of anesthesia for cardiac surgery. It is believed to be caused by inactivation of inhibitory supraspinal neurons, such that spinal reflexes are unopposed. Smith et al. (41) described this rigidity with upper limb flexion, lower limb extension, athetoid or myoclonic movements of the limbs, and vertical nystagmus in the presence of a normal EEG. This phenomenon was described in all nine patients receiving a bolus induction dose of 175 μg/kg alfentanil (41). Similarly, fentanyl, when used in an average dose of 28 μg/kg, produced chest wall rigidity in 22% of patients, while sufentanil at an average dose of 4.2 μg/kg produced rigidity in 28% of patients (42). The skeletal muscle rigidity can be sufficient to prevent effective positive-pressure ventilation of the lungs. The response is modified by the use of a muscle relaxant, such as pancuronium. Clearly, these high doses of opiate are appropriate for use in securing an airway only if there is certainty about the ability to intubate a patient and to use muscle relaxants to allow ventilation.

Seizure Activity

Apparent seizures have been described after administration of fentanyl (43,44), alfentanil (45), and sufentanil (46,47). This phenomenon is different from that seen with the metabolite normeperidine following the administration of meperidine to patients with impaired renal function, or to those taking anticonvulsant therapy. There has been controversy as to whether these represent true cortical seizures, subcortical seizures, or an exaggerated form of muscular rigidity with spinal disinhibition. EEG recordings have not shown any cortical seizure activity, and it is difficult to record subcortical activity with superficial electrodes. These myoclonic jerks appear to occur at lower doses than those producing truncal rigidity. One theory is that these movements represent subcortical seizure activity. Others have demonstrated EEG epileptiform activity in the uninvolved temporal lobe of patients with complex partial (temporal lobe) epilepsy, after administration of doses of fentanyl of 17 to 35 μg/kg (48). Limbic system seizure activity and associated neurologic lesions have also been demonstrated in rats given high-dose alfentanil (49). At present, it would seem prudent to avoid giving boluses of narcotic in high dosages to patients with epilepsy.

Tolerance and Dependence

A patient who is a chronic user of opiates will require higher doses to achieve any effect, whether that be analgesia or attenuation of response to intubation. Also, a patient with prolonged recent exposure to high-dose opiates will require an increased dose. This increased requirement is not the consequence of enzyme induction but of changes at a receptor level (11). Receptor desensitization occurs first, as the receptor uncouples from the

G-protein. This is followed by down-regulation, that is, a decrease in the number of receptors (11). Antagonists at the N-methyl-D-aspartate receptor have been demonstrated to prevent and reverse pharmacologic tolerance in animals after long-term morphine administration, that is, to maintain sensitivity to morphine (18). This effect may be mediated by nitric oxide (15). Rapid onset of tolerance has been described within hours with fentanyl administration in dogs (50), and with alfentanil in humans (51).

Nonopiate-Receptor-Mediated Effects

Nausea and Vomiting

Stimulation of the chemoreceptor trigger zone by opioids causes nausea and vomiting. This appears to be caused by activation of dopamine receptors and is opposed by dopamine antagonists, such as metoclopramide and droperidol. Other factors may contribute, however. Opiates delay gastric emptying. Nausea and vomiting occur more commonly with motion than when a patient is supine, suggesting a vestibular effect.

Drying of Secretions

The synthetic opioids do not appear to have the anticholinergic actions of meperidine, such as drying of oral and bronchial secretions. An antimuscarinic drug such as glycopyrrolate may be needed to improve conditions for fiberoptic intubation.

Bronchospasm

Unlike morphine, the synthetic opioids do not cause significant histamine release. Thus, the precipitation of bronchospasm is unlikely. Sufentanil does cause some histamine release, but in the clinical range of doses, this is minimal.

Pruritis

Opiate-induced pruritis may also be caused by histamine release, which is triggered by μ agonists. It is less common with the synthetic agents, and less common with intravenous rather than spinal or epidural administration. Intravenous fentanyl frequently causes patients to want to scratch the nose, without other sites of itch. Troublesome systemic itching can be managed with an antihistamine, such as hydroxyzine or diphenhydramine. Nalbuphine may also be helpful as a partial opiate antagonist, but increased drowsiness or decreased opiate effect may occur.

OPIATE ANTAGONISTS

Naloxone

Agents such as naloxone can be used to reverse the effects of opiate agonists, particularly respiratory depression. Naloxone is an antagonist at all three receptors, but with greatest affinity for the μ receptor. Problems with its use include pulmonary edema (52), especially if there has been preceding laryngospasm (53). Ventricular arrhythmias have also occurred with naloxone administration in patients with cardiac irritability (54). Sudden reversal of analgesia and sedation may result in patient self-extubation. Restraint of an intubated patient's hands in anticipation of this response is advisable. It is recommended that the drug be given as cautiously as possible (e.g., 40-μg increments in adults) to minimize the risk for these complications. A 400-μg ampule can be diluted to 10 mL and administered 1 mL at a time. Naloxone has a $t_{1/2}\alpha$ of only several minutes, a $t_{1/2}\beta$ of about 60 minutes (55), and clinically a short duration of 10 to 30 minutes, depending on dosage. Hence, when it is used to counteract the effects of opiates, there can be inadequate duration of effect, such that narcotization recurs in uncontrolled circumstances. Such patients need to be observed for several hours for evidence of "renarcotization," and a naloxone infusion should be commenced if necessary.

In an emergency prehospital setting, naloxone has been used in patients with a decreased level of consciousness and depressed respiration, to treat possible narcotic overdose. Preferably, this is done in conjunction with intubation, as the drug may have any of the above-mentioned side effects and may not improve the patient's level of consciousness if symptoms are not the consequence of a narcotic overdose (56).

Nalbuphine

Nalbuphine has been suggested as an alternative to naloxone in the treatment of acute respiratory depression. It is an antagonist at μ receptors but an agonist at κ_1 and κ_3 receptors (52). It is postulated that a less sudden reversal of opiate effect may reduce the potential for adverse effects.

Nalmefene

Nalmefene is an antagonist at both μ and κ receptors, like naloxone. However, it is more potent and has a longer half-life of 4 to 8 hours. It is currently under investigation for clinical use (57).

CLINICAL APPLICATIONS OF OPIATES

In light of the preceding discussion, doses should be individualized. Table 2 offers some suggested dose ranges as guidelines.

Pediatric Patients

There are serious limitations to the use of opiates in pediatric airway management. Pediatric patients are particularly at risk for complications from airway obstruction and hypoventilation. Any medication that impairs a child's ability to maintain an open airway or adequate ventilation, without also permitting immediate control of airway and ventilation, can lead to disaster. This is the case with opiates, because they can cause apnea, hypoventilation, and upper airway obstruction, but they do not always facilitate laryngoscopy or prevent laryngospasm. In addition, the rapid administration of opiates such as fentanyl can cause chest wall rigidity and inability to apply effective ventilation by mask.

Elderly Patients

Elderly patients may need emergency airway management for complications of chronic illnesses. Pneumonia, respiratory failure, congestive heart failure, and coma are indications that commonly arise in elderly patients. Sedation with opiates prior to "awake" laryngoscopy or fiberoptic procedures may lead to severe carbon dioxide retention or apnea with hypoxia. Airway and resuscitation equipment must be available. It is advisable to monitor with pulse oximetry, electrocardiography, and, if possible, capnography. Attenuation of hemodynamic response is a favorable effect of opiates in patients at risk for myocardial ischemia.

Obstetric Patients

Emergency airway management in obstetric patients frequently involves intubation for cesarean section. Other emergency obstetric situations that may require airway management are eclampsia and respiratory paralysis as a result of magnesium sulfate overdose.

In any decision to use opiates during childbirth, the ease with which opiates cross the placenta and the potential for impaired neonatal respiratory efforts must be considered. On the positive side is the fact that opiate-induced neonatal respiratory depression is readily reversed by naloxone. However, this should be avoided in the neonate of a mother who is a chronic opiate user, as the rapid reversal of opiate effect will produce a withdrawal syndrome (58). Intubation and ventilation are the preferred management of this neonate.

Alfentanil 10 μg/kg or fentanyl 2.5 μg/kg has been used at induction in pre-eclamptic patients. The great risk in these patients is an exaggerated increase in blood pressure and heart rate during laryngoscopy. The morbidity arises from cerebral hemorrhage or, less often, pulmonary edema. Both alfentanil and fentanyl obtund the pressor response to intubation (59). Ashton et al. (60) found that alfentanil 7.5 μg/kg when given in addition to magnesium 30 mg/kg was more effective than magnesium 40 mg/kg in controlling heart rate and pressure rises with intubation in pre-eclamptic women.

Dann et al. (61) investigated the effect of alfentanil 10 μg/kg on maternal hemodynamics and fetal status in healthy women undergoing cesarean section. For induction, sodium thiopental 3.5 mg/kg was administered alone or with alfentanil. The pressor response to intubation was attenuated in the alfentanil group without any neonatal depression based on Apgar scores. These neonates were delivered approximately 10 minutes after alfentanil administration. The high protein binding and low lipid solubility of alfentanil contribute to its short duration of action and make it a suitable opiate for this application.

Cardiac Patients

Opiates are frequently used in cardiac anesthesia. Their lack of association with myocardial depression and their preservation of arterial pressure are valuable in patients with limited cardiovascular reserve. For these reasons, opiates should also be useful in emergency airway management for cardiac patients. The main drawbacks are the risk of chest wall rigidity, and possibly the incomplete control of the cardiovascular response to laryngoscopy and intubation. Additional drugs such as labetalol, esmolol, and even nitroglycerin should be available or should be used prophylactically to avoid increasing myocardial oxygen requirements in patients with coronary artery disease. Conversely, drugs such as ephedrine and atropine should be available to manage bradycardia or hypotension resulting from use of opiates.

TABLE 2. *Suggested dose range (μg/kg) for opiate use in adults*

Opiate	As sole agent for induction	As adjunct during intubation	For awake airway manipulation
Fentanyl	20–100	3–10	1–5
Sufentanil	2–5	0.5–2	0.2–1.5
Alfentanil	50–100	7.5–50	5–20

Neurosurgical Patients

The hypoventilation and impairment of airway reflexes that can result from elevated intracranial pressure may necessitate endotracheal intubation, both to protect the airway from aspiration and also to facilitate hyperventilation. The use of an opiate allows better maintenance of mean arterial pressure than a typical induction agent might. However, the possible risk of seizure activity at moderately high doses must be considered. This could cause an increase in cerebral metabolic requirement for oxygen, increased cerebral blood flow, and a consequent increase in cerebral blood volume and intracranial pressure. Hanowell et al. (62) studied alfentanil given prior to endotracheal suctioning in head-injured patients. When doses of 15 or 30 μg/kg were given prior to suctioning, there was an increase in intracranial pressure and a decrease in cerebral perfusion pressure that were greater than with a saline control. The mechanism for these changes is not clear. It seems that opiates in low dose as an adjunct may be useful in patients with raised intracranial pressure, but that high doses should be avoided.

Trauma Patients

The most common indications for emergency airway management in trauma patients are injuries to the chest, head, or neck. If an immediate airway is needed, opiates have limited use. Scheduled drugs are locked and not readily available. Other problems are that opiates may impair airway protective reflexes and ventilation, and they may cause nausea. In less urgent circumstances, opiates might be useful for facilitating fiberoptic laryngoscopy, although the risks for nausea and hypoventilation should be considered. In some situations, opiates may be a useful adjunct, e.g., in a patient with the potential for significant myocardial ischemia in whom blood pressure changes or tachycardia pose significant risk.

Awake Patients

Opiates are frequently used alone or with benzodiazepines for sedation prior to awake fiberoptic laryngoscopy or blind nasal intubation. However, the emphasis should be on airway anesthesia with topical sprays or local neural blockade, while the sedation is intended for anxiolysis. Doses that render a patient unresponsive to laryngopharyngeal stimulation would also produce apnea and unresponsiveness. Particular care is required with a midazolam and fentanyl combination (63). While fentanyl blunts ventilatory responses to hypoxemia and elevated plasma CO_2, midazolam further blunts the response to hypoxemia. Neither fentanyl 2 μg/kg nor midazolam 0.05 mg/kg alone produced apnea in 12 healthy subjects, but the combination produced apnea in 6 of the 12 subjects (63). No subject receiving midazolam alone had an arterial oxygen saturation of less than 90%; however, 6 of 12 receiving fentanyl, and 11 of 12 receiving midazolam and fentanyl, had desaturation to this level. Thus, supplemental oxygen and oximetry are recommended. For long procedures with relative hypoventilation, end-tidal capnography or arterial CO_2 sampling is suggested.

SUMMARY

The usefulness of the newer synthetic agents fentanyl, sufentanil, and alfentanil in airway management is limited. They have rapid onset, maintain cardiovascular stability, and limit the hemodynamic response to laryngoscopy and intubation. However, their ability to produce apnea and truncal rigidity, as well as problems of awareness and seizure potential, limit their use as sole agents in many situations. In general, the opiates are a useful adjunct to a local anesthetic technique or other hypnotic agents and relaxants in securing the airway emergently.

REFERENCES

1. Janssen PAJ. The development of new synthetic narcotics. In: Estafanous FG, ed. *Opioids in Anesthesia*. Boston: Butterworth; 1984:37–44.
2. Scott JC, Ponganis KV, Stanski DR. EEG quantitation of narcotic effect: the comparative pharmacodynamics of fentanyl and alfentanil. *Anesthesiology* 1985;62:235.
3. Scott JC, Cooke JE, Stanski DR. Electroencephalographic quantitation of opioid effect: comparative pharmacodynamics of fentanyl and sufentanil. *Anesthesiology* 1991;74:34.
4. Shafer SL, Varvel JR. Pharmacokinetics, pharmacodynamics, and rational opioid selection. *Anesthesiology* 1991;74:53.
5. Hug CC, Murphy MR. Tissue redistribution of fentanyl and termination of its effects in rats. *Anesthesiology* 1981;55:369.
6. Pert CB, Snyder SH. Opiate receptor: demonstration in nervous tissue. *Science* 1973;179:1011.
7. Akil H, Watson SJ, Young E, Lewis ME, Khachaturian H, Walker LM. Endogenous opioids: biology and function. *Annu Rev Neurosci* 1984:7:223.
8. Stein C. Peripheral mechanisms of opioid analgesia. *Anesth Analg* 1973;76:182.
9. Stefano GB, Scharrer B. Endogenous morphine and related opiates, a new class of chemical messengers. *Adv Neuroimmunol* 1994;4:57.
10. Molina PE, Abumrad NN. Metabolic effects of opiates and opioid peptides. *Adv Neuroimmunol* 1994;4:105.
11. Murkin JM. Central analgesic mechanisms: a review of opioid receptor physiopharmacology and related antinociceptive systems. *J Cardiothorac Vasc Anesth* 1991;5:268.
12. Ling GSF, Spiegel K, Lockhart SH, Pasternak GW. Separation of opioid analgesia from respiratory depression: evidence for different receptor mechanisms. *J Pharmacol Exp Ther* 1995;232:149.
13. Pleuvry BJ. Opioid receptors and their ligands: natural and unnatural. *Br J Anaesth* 1991;66:370.
14. Pleuvry BJ. Opioid receptors and their relevance to anaesthesia. *Br J Anaesth* 1993;71:119.
15. Pasternak GW. Pharmacological mechanisms of opioid analgesics. *Clin Neuropharmacol* 1993;16:1.
16. Dickenson AH. Mechanisms of the analgesic actions of opiates and opioids. *Br Med Bull* 1991;47:690.
17. Tiseo PJ, Inturrisi CE. Attenuation and reversal of morphine tolerance by the competitive N-methyl-D-aspartate receptor antagonist, LY274614. *J Pharmacol Exp Ther* 1992;264:1090.

18. Portoghese PS. The role of concepts in structure-activity relationship studies of opioid ligands. *J Med Chem* 1992;35:1927.
19. Chen Y, Mestek A, Liu J, Yu L. Molecular cloning and functional expression of a mu-opioid receptor from rat brain. *Mol Pharmacol* 1993;44:8.
20. Yasuda K, Raynor K, Knong H, et al. Cloning and functional comparison of κ and δ opioid receptors from mouse brain. *Proc Natl Acad Sci U S A* 1993;90:6736.
21. Kieffer BL, Befort K, Gaveriaux-Ruff C, Hirth CG. The δ-opioid receptor: isolation of a cDNA by expression cloning and pharmacological characterization. *Proc Natl Acad Sci U S A* 1994;91:1193.
22. Reisine T, Brownstein MJ. Opioid and cannabinoid receptors. *Curr Opin Neurobiol* 1994;4:406.
23. Russell WJ, Morris RG, Frewin DB, Drew SE. Changes in plasma catecholamine concentrations during endotracheal intubation. *Br J Anaesth* 1981;53:837.
24. Derbyshire DR, Chmielewski A, Fell D, Vater M, Achola K, Smith G. Plasma catecholamine responses to tracheal intubation. *Br J Anaesth* 1983;55:855.
25. Fox EJ, Sklar GS, Hill CH, Villanueva R, King BD. Complications related to the pressor response to endotracheal intubation. *Anesthesiology* 1977;47:524.
26. Reitan JA, Stengert KB, Wymore ML, Martucci RW. Central vagal control of fentanyl-induced bradycardia during halothane anesthesia. *Anesth Analg* 1978;57:31.
27. Atweh SF, Kuhar MJ. Autoradiographic localization of opiate receptors in rat brain I. Spinal cord and lower medulla. *Brain Res* 1977; 124:53.
28. Sebel PS, Bovil JG. Cardiovascular effects of sufentanil anesthesia. *Anesth Analg* 1982;61:115.
29. Chraemmer-Jorgensen B, Hertel S, Strom J, Hoilund-Carlsen PF, Bjerre-Jepsen K. Catecholamine response to laryngoscopy and intubation. *Anaesthesia* 1992;47:750.
30. Black TE, Kay B, Healy TEJ. Reducing the haemodynamic responses to laryngoscopy and intubation. *Anaesthesia* 1984;39:883.
31. Cork RC, Weiss JL, Hameroff SR, Bentley J. Fentanyl preloading for rapid-sequence induction of anesthesia. *Anesth Analg* 1984;63:60.
32. Kautto U-M. Attenuation of the circulatory response to laryngoscopy and intubation by fentanyl. *Acta Anaesthesiol Scand* 1982;26:217.
33. Iyer V, Russell WJ. Induction using fentanyl to suppress the intubation response in the cardiac patient: what is the optimal dose? *Anaesth Intensive Care* 1988;16:411.
34. Crosby ET, Miller DR, Hamilton PP, Martineau RJ, Bouchard A, Wellington J. A randomized double-blind comparison of fentanyl and sufentanil-oxygen anesthesia for abdominal aortic surgery. *J Cardiothorac Anesth* 1990;4:168.
35. Miller DR, Wellwood M, Teasdale SJ, et al. Effects of anaesthetic induction on myocardial function and metabolism: a comparison of fentanyl, sufentanil and alfentanil. *Can J Anaesth* 1988;35:219.
36. Philbin DM, Rosow CE, Schneider RC, Koski G, D'Ambra MN. Fentanyl and sufentanil anesthesia revisited: how much is enough? *Anesthesiology* 1990;73:5.
37. Bailey PL, Streisand JB, East KA, et al. Differences in magnitude and duration of opioid-induced respiratory depression and analgesia with fentanyl and sufentanil. *Anesth Analg* 1990;70:8.
38. Davidson JAH, Gillespie JA. Tracheal intubation after induction of anaesthesia with propofol, alfentanil and I.V. lignocaine. *Br J Anaesth* 1993;70:163.
39. Hug CC. Does opioid "anesthesia" exist? *Anesthesiology* 1990;73:1.
40. Sjogren P, Eriksen J. Opioid toxicity. *Curr Opin Anaesthesiol* 1994; 7:465.
41. Smith NT, Benthuysen JL, Bickford RG, et al. Seizures during opioid anesthetic induction—are they opioid-induced rigidity? *Anesthesiology* 1989;71:852.
42. de Lange S, Boscoe MJ, Stanley TH, Pace N. Comparison of sufentanil-O_2 and fentanyl-O_2 for coronary artery surgery. *Anesthesiology* 1982;56:112.
43. Safwat AM, Daniel D. Grand mal seizure after fentanyl administration [Letter]. *Anesthesiology* 1983;59:78.
44. Rao TL, Mummaneni N, El-Etr AA. An unusual response to intravenous fentanyl administration [Letter]. *Anesth Analg* 1982;61:1020.
45. Strong WE, Matson M. Probable seizure after alfentanil. *Anesth Analg* 1989;68:692.
46. Brian JE Jr, Seifen AB. Tonic-clonic activity after sufentanil [Letter]. *Anesth Analg* 1987;66:481.
47. Molbegott LP, Flashburg MH, Karasic HL, Karlin BL. Probable seizures after sufentanil. *Anesth Analg* 1987;66:91.
48. Tempelhoff R, Modica PA, Bernardo KL, Edwards I. Fentanyl-induced electrocorticographic seizures in patients with complex partial epilepsy. *J Neurosurg* 1992;77:201.
49. Kofke WA, Garman RH, Tom WC, Rose ME, Hawkins RA. Alfentanil-induced hypermetabolism, seizure and histopathology in rat brain. *Anesth Analg* 1992;75:953.
50. Askitopoulou H, Whitwam JG, Al-Khudhairi D, Chakrabarti M, Bower S, Hull CJ. Acute tolerance to fentanyl during anesthesia in dogs. *Anesthesiology* 1985;63:255.
51. Bovill JG, Sebel PS, Wauquier A, Rog P, Schuyt HC. Influence of high-dose alfentanil anaesthesia on the electroencephalogram: correlation with plasma concentrations. *Br J Anaesth* 1983;55:199s.
52. Schwartz JA, Koenigsberg MD. Naloxone-induced pulmonary edema. *Ann Emerg Med* 1987;16:1294.
53. Olsen KS. Naloxone administration and laryngospasm followed by pulmonary edema. *Intensive Care Med* 1990;16:340.
54. Michaelis LL, Hickey PR, Clark TA, Dixon WM. Ventricular irritability associated with the use of naloxone hydrochloride. *Ann Thorac Surg* 1974;18:608.
55. Ngai SH, Berkowitz BA, Yang JC, Hempstead J, Spector S. Pharmacokinetics of naloxone in rats and in man: basis for its potency and short duration of action. *Anesthesiology* 1976;44:398.
56. Yealy DM, Paris PM, Kaplan RM, Heller MB, Marini SE. The safety of prehospital naloxone administration by paramedics. *Ann Emerg Med* 1990;19:902.
57. Kaplan JL, Marx JA. Effectiveness and safety of intravenous nalmefene for emergency department patients with suspected narcotic overdose: a pilot study. *Ann Emerg Med* 1993;22:187.
58. Foley KM. Opioids. *Neurol Clin* 1993;11:503.
59. Rout CC, Rocke DA. Effects of alfentanil and fentanyl on induction of anaesthesia in patients with severe pregnancy-induced hypertension. *Br J Anaesth* 1990;65:468.
60. Ashton WB, James MFM, Janicki P, Uys PC. Attenuation of the pressor response to tracheal intubation by magnesium sulphate with and without alfentanil in hypertensive proteinuric patients undergoing caesarean section. *Br J Anaesth* 1991;67:741.
61. Dann WL, Hutchinson A, Cartwright DP. Maternal and neonatal responses to alfentanil administered before induction of general anaesthesia for caesarean section. *Br J Anaesth* 1987;59:1392.
62. Hanowell LH, Thurston JD, Behrman KH, Disbrow EA. Alfentanil administered prior to endotracheal suctioning reduces cerebral perfusion pressure. *J Neurosurg Anesthesiol* 1993;5:1.
63. Bailey PL, Pace NL, Ashburn MA, Moll JWB, East KA, Stanley TH. Frequent hypoxemia and apnea after sedation with midazolam and fentanyl. *Anesthesiology* 1990;73:826.

PART IV

Advanced Airway Techniques

Airway Management, edited by
L.H. Hanowell, M.D. and R.J. Waldron, M.D.,
Lippincott-Raven Publishers, Philadelphia © 1996.

CHAPTER 13

The Laryngeal Mask Airway

Joseph R. Brimacombe, Alison M. Berry, and Suanne M. Daves

INTRODUCTION

The laryngeal mask airway (LMA) was designed by Brain in 1981, following anatomic studies of the upper airway in human cadavers (1). It evolved from the search for an airway that was more practical than the face mask (FM), less invasive than the tracheal tube (TT), and could be used as an airway intubator. The LMA became commercially available in the UK in 1988, following an extensive research and development program that included 60 different prototypes (Fig. 1). Compared with the FM, LMAs generally provide a clearer airway, with improved oxygenation/end-tidal CO_2, remote airway access [e.g., magnetic resonance imaging (MRI), computed tomography (CT) scans], and a lower incidence of airway obstruction events. Its advantages over the TT include no need to directly visualize the larynx or to produce 100% muscle relaxation, minimization of physiologic responses to intubation, less invasion of the lower respiratory tract, avoidance of the risks of endobronchial or esophageal intubation, and less trauma to local tissues. Disadvantages are that the LMA does not protect the lungs from regurgitated gastric contents and is not suitable for high airway pressure ventilation or prolonged ventilation (e.g., ICU patients).

The LMA had been used in an estimated 20 million anesthetics in over 60 countries by mid-1994 (Fig. 2). It has been in use in the US since December 1992, and is currently available in six sizes. These range from masks for premature neonates (2) to those for large adults (Table 1). The principle use of the LMA is in elective surgery, where common usage rates outside the US are in the range of 30% to 60% of all general anesthetics given, being highest in ambulatory/day surgery centers. Numerous case reports indicate its ability to rescue patients from difficult airway situations, even where extreme hypoxia has intervened. It has been included by the American Society of Anesthesiologists in the algorithm for management of the difficult airway (3). Use of the LMA as an emergency airway device for relatively unskilled "first responders" and in the emergency room setting is still being investigated.

J. R. Brimacombe: Department of Anaesthesia and Intensive Care, Queensland University, Cairns Base Hospital, Cairns, Queensland, Australia 4870.
A. M. Berry: Nambour Hospital, Nambour, Australia.
S. M. Daves: Department of Anesthesiology, University of California, Irvine Medical Center, Orange, California 92668.

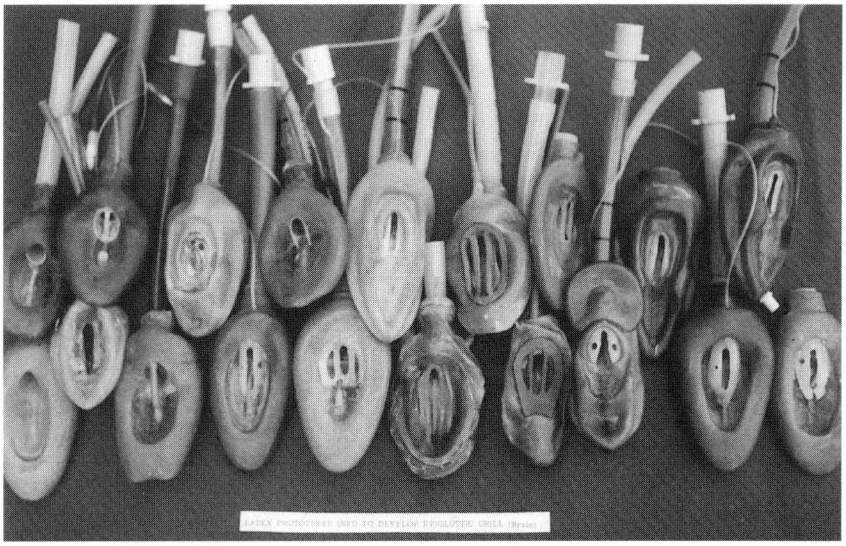

FIG. 1. Early LMA prototype. There were over 60 prototypes tested during the development phase 1981–1988.

The purpose of this chapter is to provide an overview of the LMA and a practical guide to its use in the management of difficult airway.

FEATURES OF THE LMA

Design

The LMA is composed of medical-grade silicone rubber and is reusable, being sterilized by steam autoclaving. It consists of a tube opening at the distal end into the lumen of a small elliptical mask that has an inflatable outer rim. Two vertical elastic bars are present across the distal opening to prevent obstruction of the tube by the epiglottis. When placed, the cuff portion sits in the hypopharynx at the interface between the gastrointestinal and respiratory tracts, where it forms a circumferential low pressure seal around the glottis (Fig. 3). This has the advantage of providing conditions suitable for controlling ventilation while avoiding invasion of the larynx and esophagus (4). However, the presence of the cuff tip blocking the upper esophageal sphincter (UES) does not form a barrier against regurgitated gastric contents. The large-bore tube and the ability to bypass upper airway structures (5,6) allow a lower resistance pathway to respiration than do the FM and Guedel airway (7) or the corresponding-sized TT (8,9).

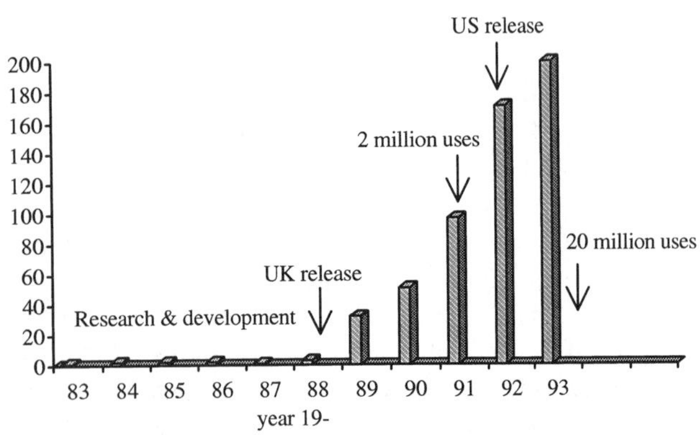

FIG. 2. The growth of LMA publications 1983–1993.

Physiology

The LMA is a relatively "noninvasive airway," compared with the TT, and causes minimal disturbance of the cardiovascular and respiratory systems. Insertion is relatively unstimulating due to avoidance of instrumentation and manipulation of structures associated with noxious reflex responses(10). The hemodynamic stress response to LMA insertion is less pronounced than during tracheal intubation (11), and less anesthetic is required to tolerate the LMA once *in situ* (10). Resistance to airflow of the standard LMA is less than that of the corresponding TT tube (8) although work of breathing during intermittent positive pressure ventilation (IPPV) is not reduced (12). Overall, there is a reduced incidence of laryngeal spasm (13) when compared with incidences pre- and posttracheal intubation. Insertion of the LMA does not cause a significant bacteremia when compared to nasal intubation (14). It has been suggested that the presence of the LMA in the hypopharynx may cause a reflex reduction in lower esophageal sphincter pressure (15–17), but this has not been confirmed by other workers (18–20) and is of unlikely clinical significance(21).

Anatomic Features

The LMA distorts pharyngeal architecture, increasing the AP diameter at the level of the tongue and epiglottis

TABLE 1. *Description of different sizes of laryngeal mask airway devices*

Mask size	Patient weight (kg)	ID/OD (mm)	Length (cm)	Cuff volume (ml)	Largest TT (ID, mm)	FOB size (mm)
1	<6.5	5.25/8.0	10	2–5	3.5	2.7
2	6.5–20	7.0/11.0	11.5	7–10	4.5	3.5
2.5	20–30	8.4/13.0	12.5	12–15	5.0	4.0
3	30–70	10/15.0	19	15–20	6.0 cuffed	5.0
4	70–90	10/15.0	19	25–30	6.0 cuffed	5.0
5	>90	11.5/16.5	20	35–40	7.5 cuffed	6.5

ID/OD, internal diameter/external diameter; FOB, fiberoptic bronchoscope.

(22). In its final position, the distal rim of the cuff lies above the upper esophageal sphincter at the approximate level of the cricoid cartilage and is too large to pass into the esophagus. Superiorly, the proximal part of the cuff lies under the base of the tongue, and the lateral margins of the LMA lie in the piriform fossae. Radiologic (23), fiberoptic (24), CT (25), and nuclear magnetic resonance (NMR) (22) studies have revealed that that the actual position of the LMA *in situ* often varies from the ideal, even when function is excellent. The epiglottis rests within the bowl of the mask or under the proximal cuff, but in 13% to 60% of adults (26,27) may become downfolded over the vocal cords as the mask is inserted into place. This is more likely if insertion techniques rather than the currently recommended one are employed (27). The esophagus is visible in the bowl of the mask in 0% to 10% (24,27,28). This may be related to poor insertion technique or to overpressure (>25 cm H_2O) applied by ventilation, which may displace the LMA and thus expose the esophagus (29). Dye studies have demonstrated that the LMA cuff acts as an airtight throat pack and forms an effective seal across the pharynx, preventing aspiration from the oropharynx (30) downward into the trachea.

INSERTION COMMENTS

Technique of Insertion

Laryngeal mask airway insertion is best carried out with the head in the "sniffing" position, with slight additional head extension (Fig. 4). However, it can also be inserted with the head maintained in the neutral position by halo (31) or manual-in-line traction (32), and in patients with abnormal cervical spines (33,34). Laryngeal mask airway placement may be possible in patients with limited mouth opening if the interdental distance is >1.5 cm. The LMA is inserted along the path taken by a food

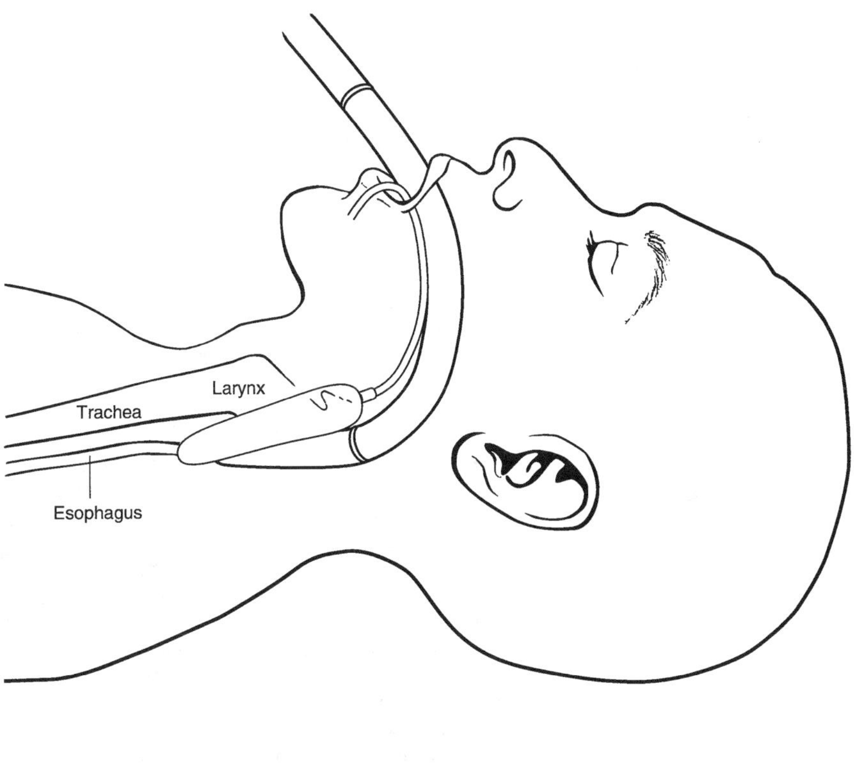

FIG. 3. Schematic representation of position of LMA in hypopharynx. The LMA sits at the junction of the respiratory tract and gastrointestinal tract.

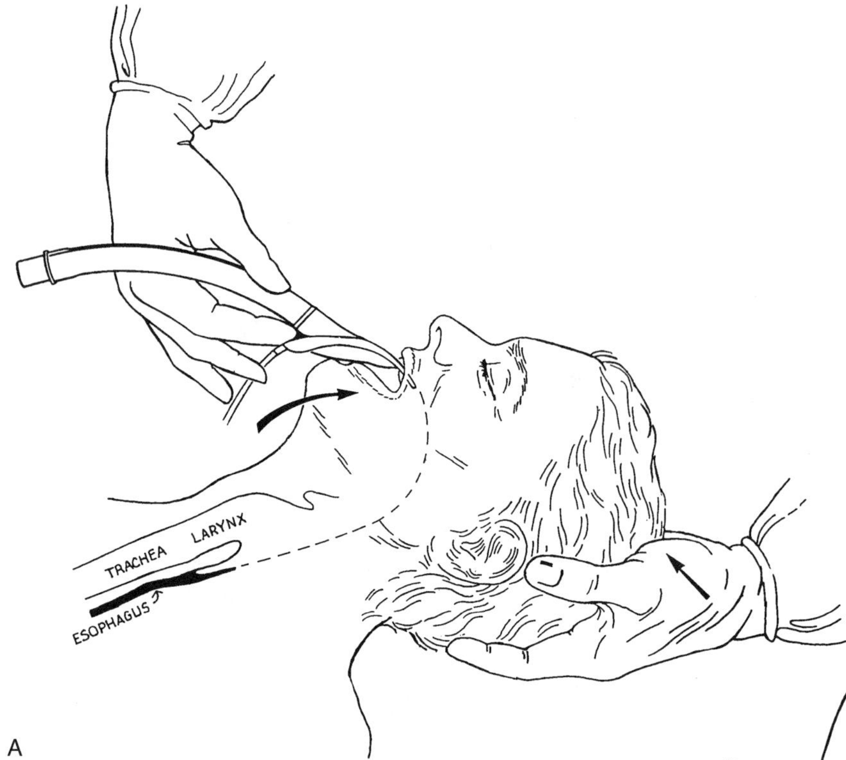

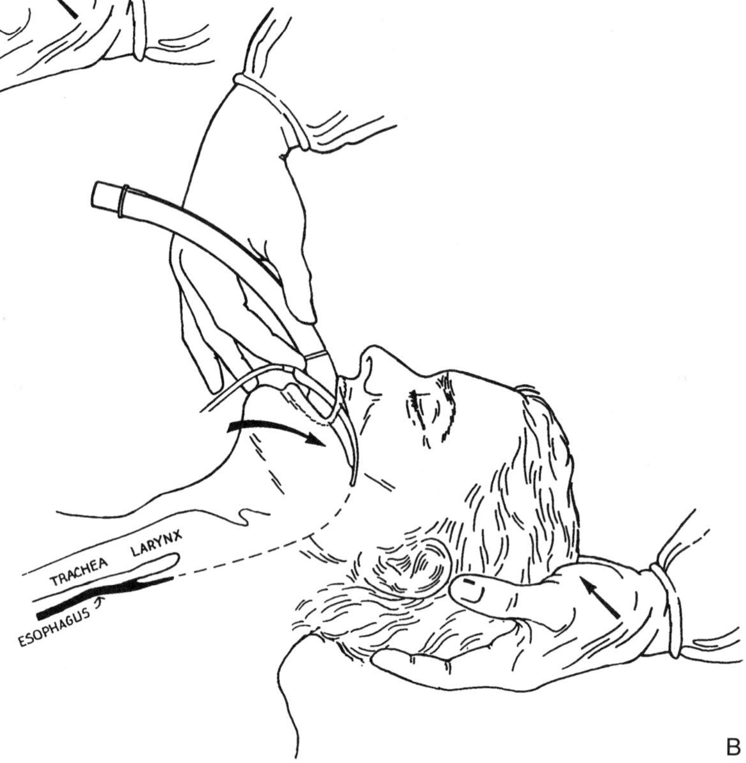

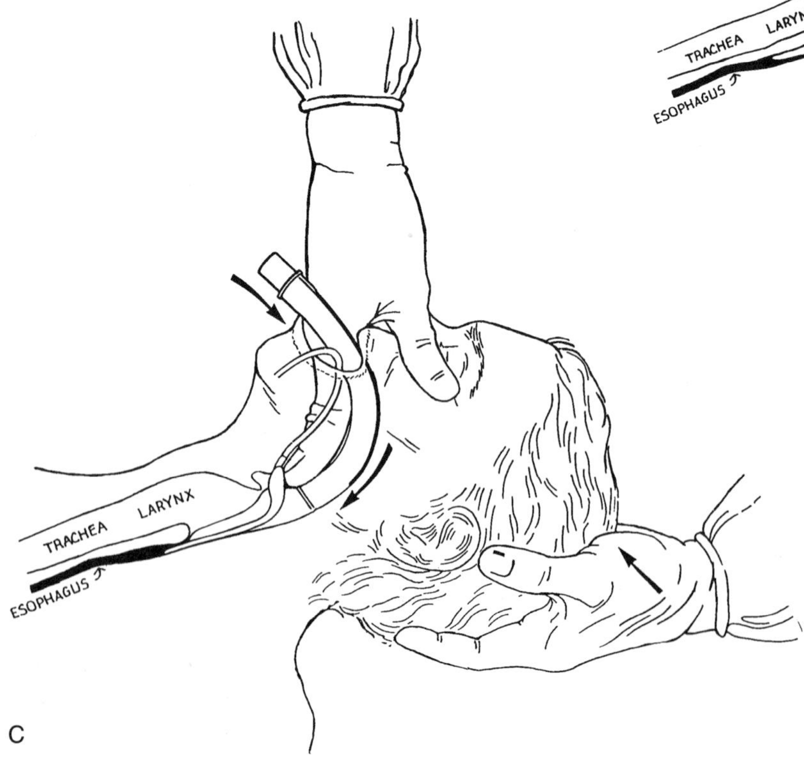

FIG. 4. Illustration sequence for LMA insertion*. **A:** To obtain optimal placement in the hypopharynx with its surrounding musculature, the appropriate sized LMA should be inserted with reflexes obtunded by either general or topical anesthesia with the head and neck in the standard intubating position. The cuff should be fully deflated and lubricated on its posterior surface. The intention is to follow the line of the palato-pharyngeal curve as indicated. **B:** Under direct vision and holding the LMA at the mask-tube junction between the index finger and thumb, press the mask tip upwards against the hard palate to flatten it out. **C:** Keeping the neck flexed and head extended, press the mask into the palato-pharyngeal curve and advance the mask into the oro-pharynx and along the posterior pharyngeal wall using the index finger. It is important that as you advance the mask into the pharynx to ensure the tip remains flattened and avoids the tongue. **D:** Continue pushing with the index finger until the mask is guided into position. If required, the LMA can be pushed into final

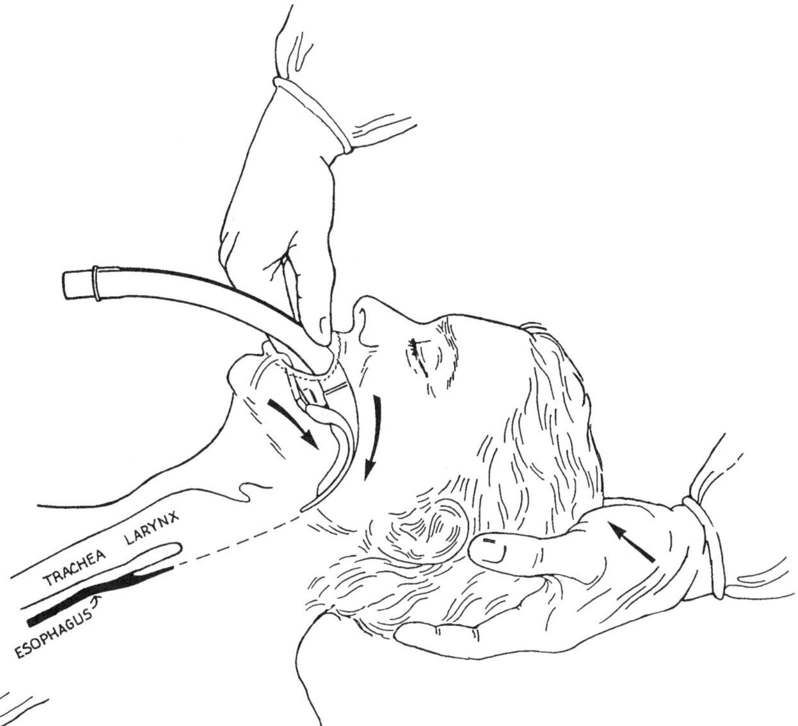

D

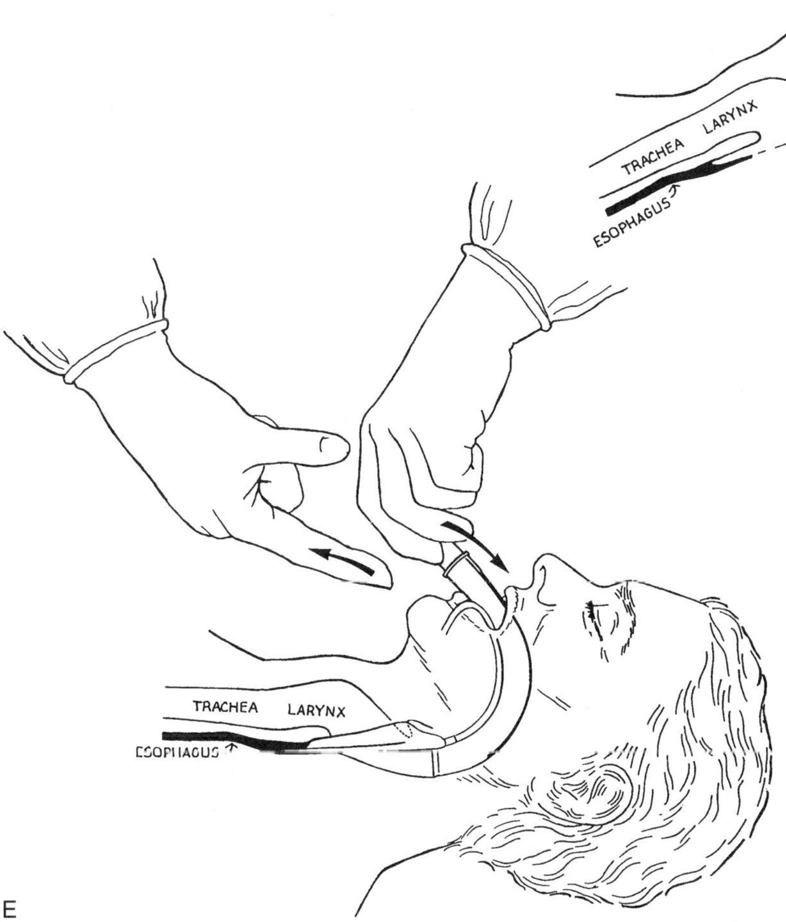

E

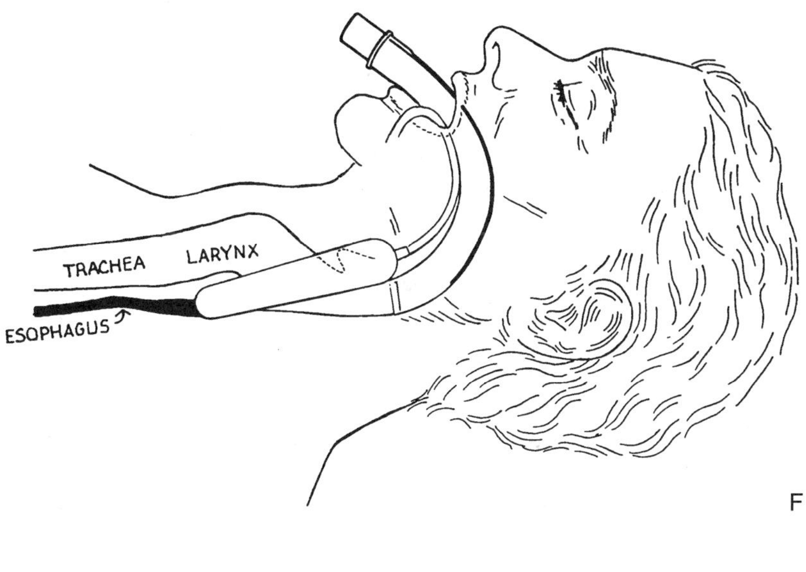

F

position by pressing along the shaft with the other hand once the mask has circumvented the oropharyngeal inlet. **E:** Now grasp the tube firmly with the other hand and then withdraw the index finger from the pharynx. Press gently downward with this other hand to ensure the mask is fully inserted. **F:** Inflate the mask with the recommended volume of air. Do not touch the LMA while inflating unless the position is obviously unstable. Normally the mask should be allowed to rise up slightly out of the hypopharynx as it is inflated, to find its correct position.

*Note: The most common problem encountered during insertion is difficulty in passing the LMA downwards behind the tongue and this usually reflects poor insertion technique. The most common error is failure to maintain a constant centrifugal force with the index finger against the curve of the hard palate and posterior oropharynx until the LMA passes down into the hypopharynx. From: Brain AIJ. *The Use of the LMA in cardiopulmonary resuscitation handbook,* with permission.

TABLE 2. *Anatomic and functional signs of correct placement*

Anatomic	Functional
Swelling in thyroid region at inflation	Observation of reservoir bag
Outward movement of LMA tube at inflation	Gentle hand ventilation
Cuff not visible in mouth	Auscultation of lungs and side of neck
Tube protruding <8 cm above teeth	Auscultation of left hypochondrium[a]
Black marking in midline and cranial	Capnography
Fiberoptic laryngoscopy via LMA	Esophageal detector device

[a]During intermittent positive pressure ventilation to detect gastric insufflation.
LMA, laryngeal mask airway.

TABLE 3. *Some alternative insertion techniques*

Slight lateral approach
Initially inverted like a Guedel airway
Jaw thrust
Laryngoscope
Thumb insertion technique (if access restricted)
Semi-inflated cuff (awake insertion)

bolus during the normal swallowing reflex, with the posterior surface pressed into the hard palate by the index finger mimicking the action of the tongue to achieve smooth advancement into the pharynx. Maintained posterior pressure applied centrifugally allows the flattened LMA to slide over the back of the tongue, avoiding anterior structures such as the epiglottis, arytenoids, and glottis. First-time successful insertion rates vary with experience and technique but should reach over 96% as the early learning curve is achieved. In experienced hands, the LMA is inserted and functions well at the first attempt in 98% of patients within 20 sec and with Mallampati scores of 1–4. If failure occurs on initial insertion, the LMA may be quickly prepared again for reinsertion. Anatomic and functional signs of correct placement are listed in Table 2.

A wide number of alternative insertion techniques and aids have been described (n=23) (27). The standard technique appears to offer superior results in terms of function and final anatomic position in adults (27). This is an important consideration when using the LMA as an aid to intubation because optimal views of the vocal cords are achieved where there is less epiglottic downfolding. Recent cadaver studies have shown that adoption of the correct head position for insertion, smooth deflation of the LMA with a posterior tip, and adherence to the swallowing principle of insertion will cause the LMA to follow the ideal posterior pathway to its final position over the semiinflated, anterior tip and "midshaft push" techniques (Brain, *personal communication,* 1994). It is likely that the standard technique is also superior in pediatric patients (35), although some authors have recommended the semiinflated (36) or Guedel airway (37) techniques for inexperienced LMA users in children. Alternative techniques may be useful where the standard technique fails or is inappropriate (Table 3).

Cricoid Pressure

As the tip of the LMA cuff lies at a variable depth behind the cricoid cartilage (CC), the application of cricoid pressure (CP) may potentially reduce the ease of insertion of the LMA and also hinder subsequent passage of a TT through the LMA. Once *in situ*, the presence of the LMA does not compromise cricoid pressure (38), but CP reduces the successful first-time insertion rates from 94% to 79% (39). There is some evidence to show that the mode of application of CP may be a factor in impeding placement, with three large studies using single-handed manual CP showing that CP has little effect (24, 40,41), and two smaller studies using bimanual CP suggesting that LMA insertion is markedly impeded (42,43). In one of the latter studies, there was gross deterioration of the view of the vocal cords, which significantly obstructed subsequent passage of a fiberoptic bronchoscope and subsequent intubation (43). In two of the single-handed CP studies, there was only a slight but insignificant deterioration in fiberoptic view. The presence of CP also considerably affects successful blind intubation through the LMA, and single-handed CP drops the first-time success rate of blind passage of a TT by 50% (41). Anterior tipping of the laryngeal inlet by the CP may be an associated factor (24) (Fig. 5). The application of CP has been noted to cause mechanical cord closure on one occasion (44).

Training

Most complications of tracheal intubation by paramedics are related to prolonged intubation attempts and esophageal placement, with first-attempt success rates of 50% to 60% (45,46). Studies conducted under controlled conditions in the operating room have demonstrated that unskilled personnel insert the LMA more rapidly and reliably than they insert the TT (47,48) and that it is superior to a bag and mask (49) in anesthetized patients. Reinhart (50) found that health care providers who already had TT experience placed an LMA and achieved effective ventilation faster and more reliably than with a TT in the same anesthetized and paralyzed patients. The only studies to date conducted in the field are those involving ward nurses acting as first responders to a cardiac arrest

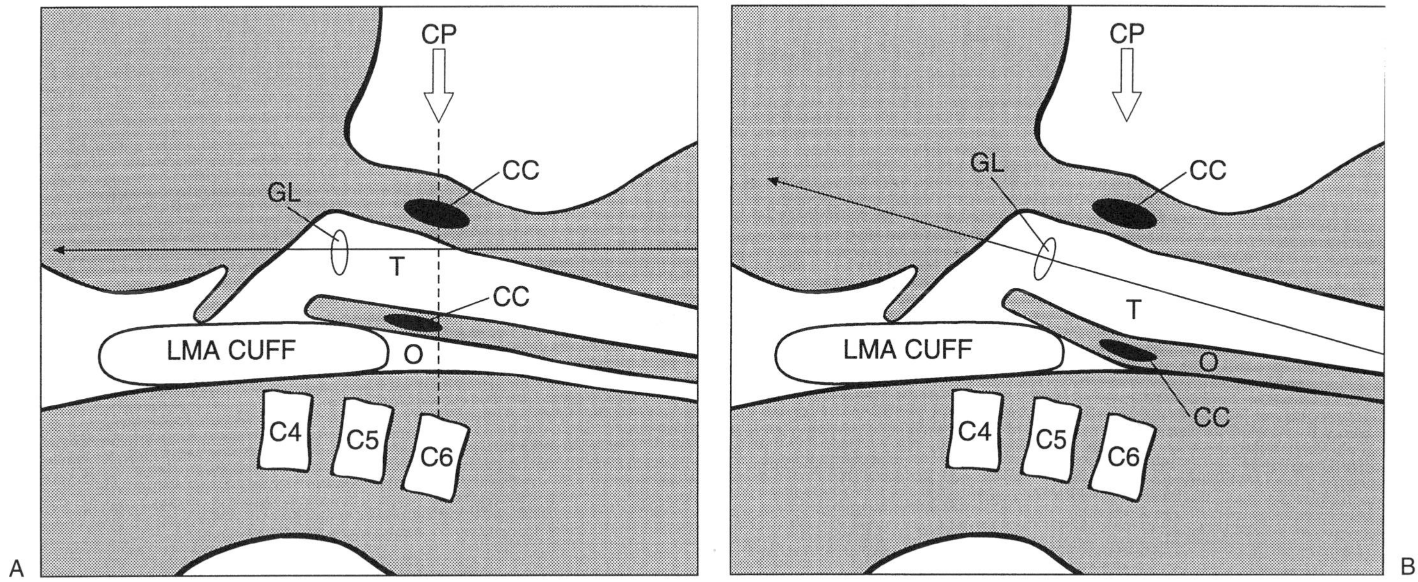

FIG. 5. The effect of cricoid pressure on glottic position. **A:** Before cricoid pressure applied. **B:** After cricoid pressure applied.

situation when bag and mask would normally be employed (51,52). First-attempt successful LMA insertion rates were 76% in the latter study, with overall success rates of 84% to 94%. Unfortunately, tests of aspiration were not specifically used in these studies, but regurgitation generally occurred prior to LMA insertion. Evidence that physicians who are nonanesthesiologists find the LMA a useful adjunct for management of airway problems comes from a study of neonatal resuscitation, where residents received training from an anesthesiologist and successfully inserted all LMAs at the first attempt in 21 neonates (53).

Training programs should be standardized to ensure complete coverage of LMA usage and should include formal lectures, adherence to guidelines in the instruction manual and video, and experience in LMA insertion in an intubating mannequin prior to practical experience in the operating room (54). Some form of certification and continued training would also be desirable (54). The best insertion technique to teach will be the one that most reliably ensures correct placement and good function on the first attempt, with a minimum of complications. At the present time, evidence continues to support the teaching of the standard technique for adult patients. Alternative techniques should be reserved for when the standard technique fails (e.g., in tonsillar hypertrophy, limited mouth opening) or if, having gained experience with the standard technique, the individual has greater success with an alternative. The Resuscitation Council (UK) has recently implemented formal training of paramedics to use the LMA in the field, and the results of auditing from this study will have implications for the future use of the LMA by nonanesthesiologists.

USE IN ROUTINE/ELECTIVE ANESTHESIA

The LMA is compatible with most ventilatory modes, including spontaneous breathing to which continuous positive airways pressure (CPAP) or inspired pressure support may be added, or positive pressure ventilation (PPV). Maximum achievable airway pressures for PPV are variable but, generally, most patients with normal lung compliance may be ventilated to airway pressures of 20–25 cm H_2O (55,56). Tidal volumes of 8–10 ml/kg and low inspiratory flow rates will generally achieve adequate ventilation (12). Factors influencing maximum leak pressure and seal around the larynx include choosing the largest LMA appropriate for the patient, placing the LMA optimally, avoiding overinflation of the LMA cuff, and maintaining low lung compliance by monitoring neuromuscular blockade and depth of anesthesia (57). If leak around the cuff occurs, light pressure applied temporarily over the front of the neck may resolve the loss of seal. If the leak persists, auscultation of the anterolateral part of the neck or fiberoptic laryngoscopy may be useful in differentiating between malposition or degrees of glottic closure (58). While there is no firm evidence that the use of PPV with the correctly inserted LMA increases the risk of gastric insufflation, the presence of an audible leak may indicate some passage of air into the stomach (Table 4).

Indications

The LMA is routinely used in circumstances where the patient is not at risk of aspiration and where faultless ventilation is not mandatory. Studies comparing the LMA to

TABLE 4. *Troubleshooting guide*

Problem	Likely causes	Solutions
Failure to insert LMA	Inadequate anesthesia	Ensure deep anesthesia
	Suboptimal head/neck position • Incorrect mask deflation • Failure to press LMA into palato-pharyngeal curve during insertion	Ensure correct insertion technique, try alternative technique
	Cricoid pressure (CP)	Temporarily release CP
	Pathology, e.g., large tonsils	Try alternative insertion technique
Laryngeal spasm and coughing	Inadequate anesthesia	Deepen anesthesia
	Tip impaction against glottis	Check LMA position • Reposition if necessary
	Aspiration	See Brimacombe and Berry, ref. 21.
Mask leaks, or unable to manually ventilate the lungs	Inadequate anesthesia • Glottic closure • Low lung compliance	Check anesthetic depth
	Malpositioned mask: • Rotation • Wrong cuff inflation volume • Folded back on itself	Check LMA position (Table 2) • Reinsert if necessary
	High airway pressures	Reduce airway pressure: • Lower tidal volume • Lower inspiratory flow rate • Muscle relaxation
High $PeCO_2$	Respiratory depression:	
	Drug induced	Reduce MAC, avoid further opiates
	Low minute volumes	Assist ventilation
Displaced after insertion	Inadequate anesthetic depth	Deepen anesthesia
	Pulled or twisted tube	Avoid circuit dragging, appropriate fixation
Problems during recovery	Removal of LMA at inappropriate anesthetic depth	Remove LMA deep or when patient opens mouth to command
	Oral secretions entering larynx on cuff deflation	Deflate LMA as it is removed, or remove still inflated
	Patient moved or stimulated	Avoid patient stimulation
	LMA occluded by biting	Use bite block pre emergence
	Regurgitation	

LMA, laryngeal mask airway; MAC, minimum alveolar concentration.

the FM and Guedel airway have proven the superiority of the LMA in terms of preserving oxygen saturation levels and avoiding adverse airway events (59–61). Adverse airway events such as difficult placement and laryngeal spasm occur less frequently with the LMA than with the TT (13) (Table 5). Studies on general use of the LMA from the UK indicate a pattern of use whereby 60% of patients with an LMA are spontaneously breathing and 40% are ventilated, with a range of uses through peripheral orthopedic, plastic, ophthalmologic, general, and gynecologic surgeries (62). More specialized uses of the LMA include remote anesthesia (63), adenotonsillectomy (64), molar extractions (65), laser pharyngoplasty (66), bronchoscopy (28,67), and surgery to the large airways such as tracheostomy (68) and percutaneous tracheostomy (69). Successful use of the LMA for up to 8 hours has been reported (70), and no LMA-related patient morbidity occurred in a study specifically examining cuff pressures in cases of 1–2 hours in duration (71).

Contraindications

The LMA does not isolate the respiratory tract from the gastrointestinal tract; therefore, the lungs are not protected from regurgitated gastric contents. A metanalysis of 547 LMA publications to September 1993 suggested an incidence of 2/10,000 during elective anesthesia (21). These are comparable figures to those found for elective anesthesia with either the FM or the TT (72). Those aspirations occurring with an LMA *in situ* can generally be linked to inappropriate use and failure to follow the recommendations for use. The LMA is contraindicated in patients at risk of aspiration due to the presence of a full stomach, hiatal hernia, morbid obesity, intestinal obstruction, delayed gastric emptying (recent trauma with concurrent opioid medication), and in patients unable to give accurate histories. It is relatively contraindicated in patients with low airway compliance, upper airway obstruction, and uncontrolled bleeding diatheses. Use of the

TABLE 5. *The ratio of adverse events for tracheal intubation and the LMA*

Adverse event	TT (%)	LMA (%)	Ratio TT:LMA
Clinically significant problems (13)	3.4	0.9	3.8
Laryngeal spasm	0.38	0.12	3.2
Aspiration	0.017	0.02	0.85
Sore throat	50	10	5
Laryngeal trauma (127)	6.2	—	—
BP/HR increase on insertion	25	5	5
IOP increase on insertion	25	10	2.5
Coughing during recovery	60	2	30

LMA, larygeal mask airway; TT, tracheal tube; BP/HR, blood pressure/heart rate; IOP, intraocular pressure.

LMA for intraabdominal procedures (73) and laparoscopic surgery (74) is controversial.

Difficult Airway

Most circumstances of failed intubation are associated with an inability to view the vocal cords. Some authorities consider that laryngoscopy is often suboptimal, unnecessarily increasing the incidence of failed intubation (75). The chief advantages of the LMA in the difficult airway situation are:

1. Reliance on direct vision of the vocal cords for successful airway control is removed.
2. Only obtunded airway reflexes (not full muscle relaxation) are required for placement and function.
3. The LMA can usually be easily inserted in the presence of abnormalities of supraglottic anatomy.

The LMA is useful because it can generally be inserted within a few seconds, and the first-attempt success rate is high. If it were to fail in a patient with a difficult airway, little time would be lost in proceeding along the algorithm to cricothyroid puncture. Tracheal intubation, even in skilled hands, may require three or more attempts in 2% of patients in urban teaching hospitals (76). Unlike the edema and bleeding associated with repeated attempts at intubation, LMA insertion is associated with a low incidence of laryngeal and other tissue trauma. Laryngeal mask airway insertion is readily achieved in awake patients who are adequately prepared with topical anesthesia, with or without administration of sedation and a drying agent (67,77).

There are numerous case reports and two studies (78,79) indicating that LMA insertion is readily achieved in patients with abnormal airways. Insertion is independent of anatomic features used to predict (80,81) or score (80) difficult intubation and is usually unaffected by manual-in-line traction (32) or the presence of a hard collar (31). The LMA has been inserted in the presence of halo traction (34), in the prone position (82), and where access was otherwise impossible in major trauma (83). Conversely, infraglottic problems (and double-handed cricoid pressure) may impede LMA placement (42,43); the LMA is not recommended in cases of acute epiglottitis. As a result, the LMA has been incorporated into difficult airway algorithms by the American Society of Anesthesiologists (3) and the Australian Incident Monitoring Study group (84).

Anticipated Difficult Airway

Although there have been no large multicenter trials on the usefulness of the LMA in the many varieties of pathology related to the anticipated difficult airway, there are many case reports of its successful use in both adults and children in a wide variety of airway problems (Table 6). In patients in whom difficult or impossible intubation is anticipated, the LMA may be used either alone as the definitive airway or as an aid to oral intubation. The options are to insert the LMA either under general anesthesia or with the patient awake and the airway topicalized. Asai and Morris (85) and others suggest that LMA insertion and intubation under topical anesthesia and sedation are safer in the predicted difficult airway. Some authors argue that the LMA should not be used as a definitive airway, in case the need for urgent intubation arises intraoperatively, and that it may not function adequately in a substantial minority of patients (86,87). There are certain clinical situations in which an adequately placed LMA might be exchanged for a TT: if high airway pressure ventilation, prolonged ventilation, prevention of pulmonary contamination, or oropharyngeal surgery are required. Data taken from 2359 patients undergoing rou-

TABLE 6. *Some airway problems managed with the laryngeal mask airway*

Failed obstetric intubation
Rheumatoid arthritis, cervical spondylitis, ankylosing spondylitis
Oral tumor, spinal tumor
Facial burns
Neck contracture and instability
Calcinosis universalis
Acromegaly
Ossification of the posterior longitudinal ligament
Fractured jaw
Treacher-Collins, Pierre Robin, Cri-du-chat, Goldenhar, Edwards, and Hurler's syndromes
Kugelberg-Welander disease
Impossible patient access for laryngoscopy—trauma, halo traction
Laryngeal polyposis
Lingual tonsillar hyperplasia

tine surgery indicated that the LMA had to be abandoned in only 0.4% in favor of a TT (62). It is important that, if the LMA is used without intubation, the operator be prepared for urgent fiberoptic intubation or cricothyroid puncture, should the need arise. When a case of known impossible intubation is encountered, the use of the LMA on its own should probably be considered to have the same indications as do other non-TT anesthetics.

Unanticipated Difficult Airway

The LMA is included in the ASA algorithm as a nonsurgical alternative airway in the failed intubation or failed FM ventilation situation. The success of the LMA in rescuing patients from an unanticipated difficult airway situation depends in part on the following factors: familiarity of the operator with the device in routine clinical practice, adherence to basic principles of failed intubation drills, appreciation of the interaction between cricoid pressure and the LMA, prior experience with intubation through the LMA.

If used following a failed intubation in a patient with a potentially full stomach, the risk of aspiration should be reduced once hypoxia is relieved (88). However, once the immediate crisis situation is relieved, further management should be directed at ensuring that the airway remains secure. An algorithm has been proposed for the use of the LMA in a patient with a potentially full stomach in whom intubation has proved impossible (89) (Fig. 6). Once oxygenation has been restored, several options may be considered. In many cases, the safest option will be to wake the patient with CP maintained and revert to an awake intubation or regional technique. If this is not feasible and surgery must continue, then CP can be maintained after LMA insertion for the duration of the operation. Cricoid pressure has been maintained for 2 hours in an obstetric patient breathing spontaneously with no aspi-

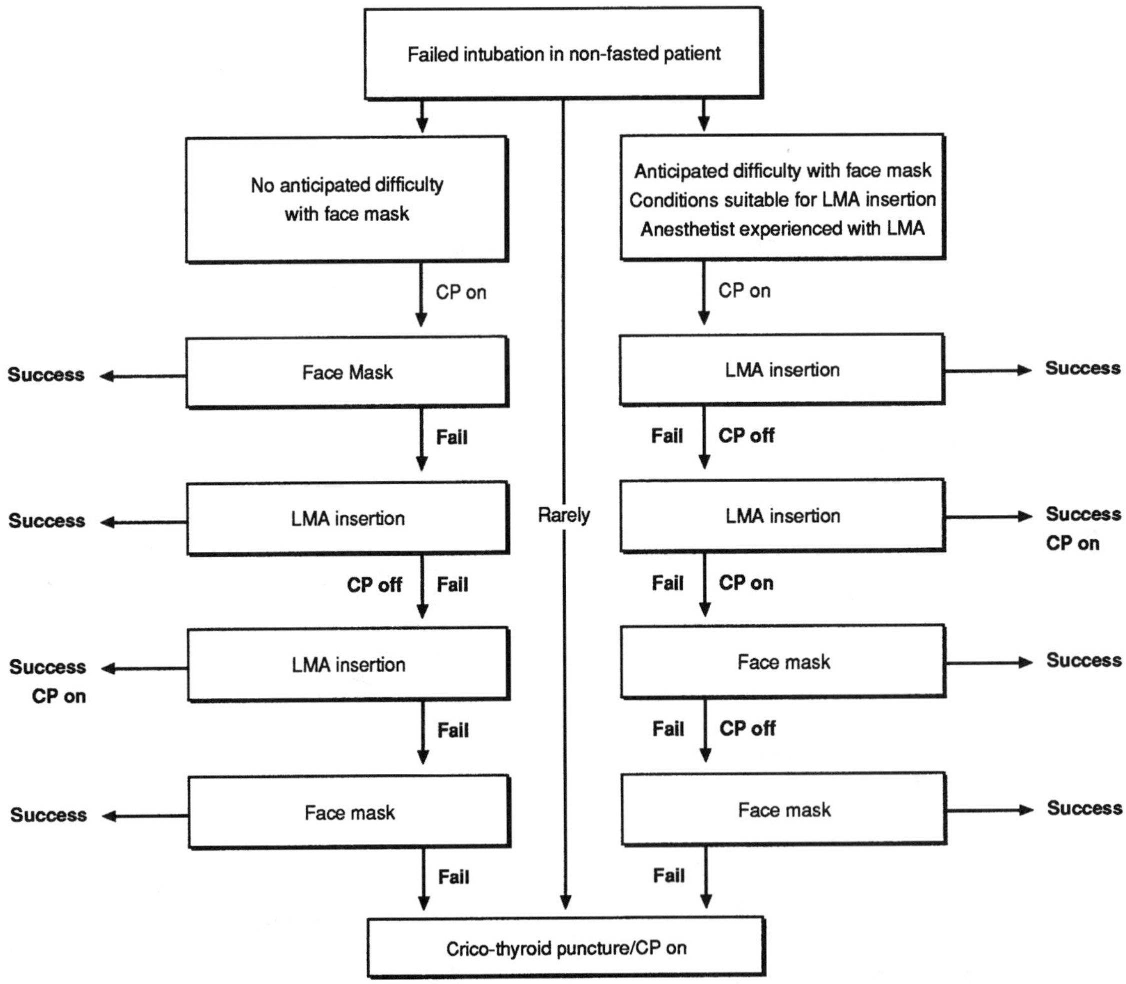

FIG. 6. Algorithm for use of the LMA during failed intubation in a non-fasted patient. Reproduced and modified with permission from the International Anesthesia Research Society.

ration (90). It is not known whether SV or PPV is the safer option in terms of risk of regurgitation. The concern is that PPV may lead to gastric dilatation, but certainly FM ventilation with maintained CP has been proven to be effective, and this should also be true for the LMA. If SV is used, lightening of anesthesia should be avoided as glottic narrowing may result in negative intrathoracic pressure and siphoning of gastric fluid. There have been no incidences of aspiration among the eight published cases of use of the LMA in obstetrics where the operation has continued using SV, and CP has been maintained throughout. Swayne and Greenslade demonstrated the effectiveness of CP with an LMA *in situ* following a failed obstetric intubation. Once intubation through the LMA had been achieved, release of CP led to regurgitation (91).

The trachea may be intubated either blindly or fiberoptically; however, the results of blind intubation through the LMA are not dependable enough for the technique to be considered a satisfactory option. The reported success rates for blind passage of a TT in patients with normal airways are 30% to 93% within 2 min, and up to three attempts may be required, which implies that the risks of esophageal intubation and repeated desaturation are too high (92). Fiberoptic intubation in patients with normal airways has a high first-attempt success rate, but the presence of a downfolded epiglottis or the presence of CP may hinder the fiberoptic view.

TABLE 7. *Comparisons of emergency airway equipment*

Description	LMA	TT	FM	ETC	EOA
Ease of use	+++	+	++	+	+
Protection against aspiration[a]	+	+++	0	++	++
Safe drainage of gastric contents	0	+++	0	++	++
Functions when blindly passed into trachea	NA	Yes	NA	Yes	No
Functions when blindly passed into esophagus	NA	No	NA	Yes	Yes
Requires effective FM fit	No	No	Yes	No	Yes
Pediatric sizes available	Yes	Yes	Yes	No	No
Cardiorespiratory stability	+++	+	+++	+	+
Aid to intubation	Yes	NA	No	No	No
Ventilation availability	++	+++	+	++	+

[a] Both gastric contents and oropharyngeal contamination.
LMA, laryngeal mask airway; TT, tracheal tube; FM, face mask; ETC, esophageal tracheal combitube; EOA, esophageal obturator airway.

The place of the LMA, when taken in the context of other techniques, is unknown. Percutaneous transtracheal jet ventilation (TTJV) is extremely effective and well tested (93) but has been associated with a 29% complication rate in the emergency situation (94). Experience with the esophageal tracheal combitube (ETC) and TTJV during failed intubation is limited, and neither device is used in routine anesthetic practice (95,96). A limited study of use of the combitube in routine anesthetic practice where the patients had normal airways demonstrated a failure to ventilate in two patients; there have been no studies of the use of the combitube in the abnormal airway (97) (Table 7).

AIRWAY INTUBATION

The curved LMA tube is shaped to direct the passage of a TT into the trachea (Fig. 7), and in up to 96% of cases the vocal cords will be visible directly below the aperture bars of the LMA (27). In some patients, the vocal cord view may be obscured by a downfolded epiglottis. The ease of access to the vocal cords and trachea, and the ability to monitor adequacy of respiration and to perform patient ventilation while intubating make the LMA useful as an aid to intubation. For successful intubation, the pharyngolaryngeal reflexes must be sufficiently obtunded to allow passage of a TT. It is possible to use topical anesthesia for both LMA insertion and intubation via the LMA (98) or to insert the LMA under local anesthesia and use it to aid intubation following induction of general anesthesia (78).

There are two limiting features of the LMA as an aid to intubation. The internal diameter of the LMA tube will accommodate only a relatively small cuffed TT, due in part to the extra bulk of the TT pilot balloon. This is sufficient to ventilate most patients, but if a larger bore TT is needed for ICU ventilation, for example, the problem can be resolved by the use of a tube changer, the split LMA, or the intubating LMA (ILMA) (Fig. 8). Secondly, in taller patients, the cuff of the TT may not be long enough to pass down the length of the LMA and then through the vocal cords (99). When the TT is inserted to its full length through the LMA, the distance at the teeth will generally be about 21 cm. It is useful to keep readily available the longer, size 6 mm, microlaryngeal tube (Mallindkrodt Medical, Athlone, Ireland) if more TT length is required. Removal of the LMA over the TT may be difficult following successful intubation and is generally thought unnecessary. If LMA removal is desired, it can be accomplished using a second TT as an extender (100,101) or Magills forceps (102) to hold the TT in place. Maltby suggests that if the patient is extubated deep, it is an advantage to leave the LMA in place, since this will reduce the risk of laryngeal spasm requiring airway intervention during emergence from anesthesia (103).

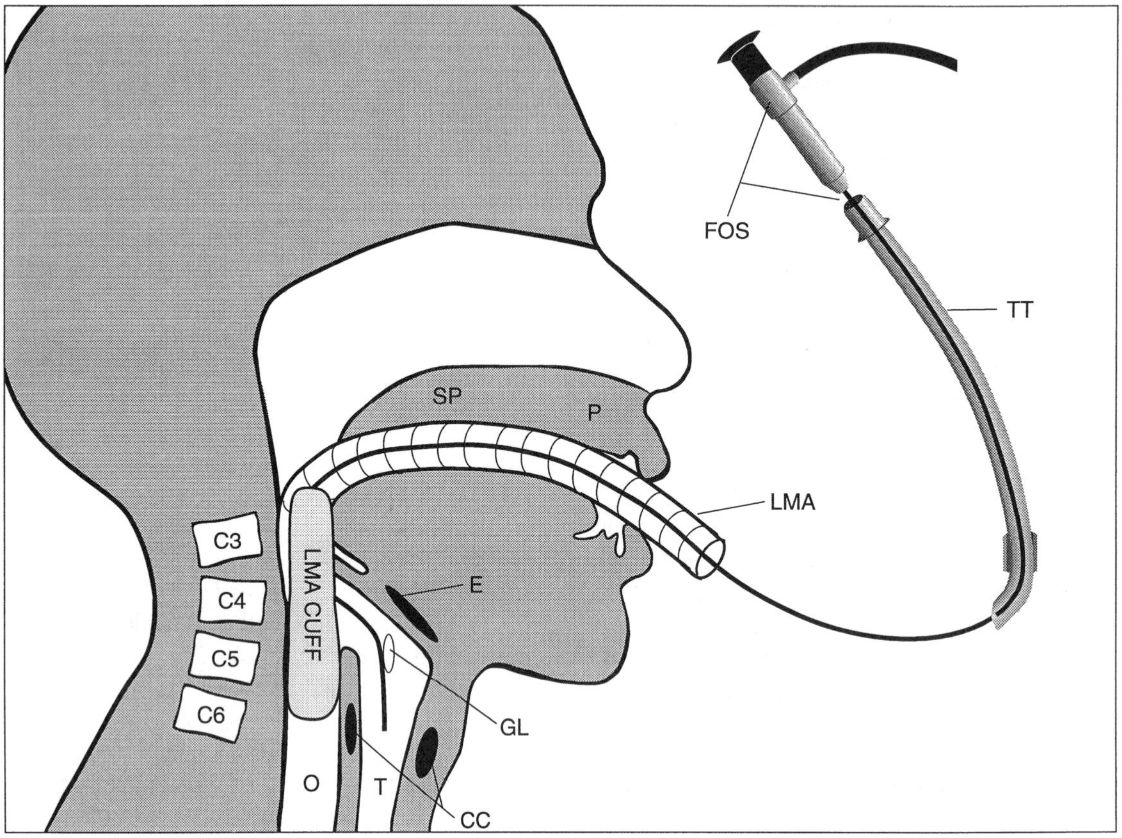

FIG. 7. LMA primed with tracheal tube and fiberoptic bronchoscope. FOS, fiberoptic scope; E, epiglottis; GL, glottis; CC, cricoid cartilae; T, trachea; O, esophagus; P, palate; SP, soft palate.

Techniques of Intubation Through the LMA

Blind Techniques

Reported success rates for blind intubation via the LMA (Fig. 8) vary between 0% (104) and 93% (92), depending on technique, experience, the number of attempts taken, and the equipment chosen. Heath and Allagain (41) found that blind passage of a size-6 cuffed tube was successful in 90% of anesthetized, paralyzed patients. Cricoid pressure reduced the success rate to 56%. The type of TT, the orientation of the TT bevel, and manipulation of the patient's head and neck may affect success rates. The success rate on the first attempt using the Portex TT has been reported as 60% with no head manipulation (92). The advantage of blind intubation is that it does not require availability of or familiarity with the fiberoptic scope or other intubating aids. The disadvantages are those of any blind technique in that it may be time-consuming, misplacement may result in trauma, and there is a risk of esophageal intubation. The presence of a downfolded epiglottis obstructing the cords would tend to make blind intubation more difficult and hazardous.

Introduction of a stylet or a bougie blindly into the trachea is possible, followed by removal of the LMA and passage of a full-size TT over the intratracheal device. Successful blind passage of a gum elastic bougie (GEB) has been reported in both awake (105) and anesthetized patients (106) in adults (84%) (107) and children (88%) (108). Success may be increased by pointing the tip anteriorly and then rotating it by 180° when it enters the trachea (107). Although successful use of tube changers has been reported in awake (109) and anesthetized patients (110), two limited studies have demonstrated variable success rates of 0% (104) and 30% (111). Tube changers are thicker and stiffer than the normal bougie, making them more likely to follow a posterior path and enter the esophagus.

Fiberoptic Techniques

Visually guided techniques for intubation using the LMA have predictably higher success rates of 90% to 100% with a single attempt. Intubation is usually rapidly achieved with minimal risk of trauma and esophageal intubation. There are numerous case reports of the successful use of a fiberoptic scope (FOS) to aid intubation via the LMA in patients with abnormal airways (112, 113). The most common method is to prime the FOS with a small, well-lubricated TT, which is advanced into place once the scope is in the trachea (Figs. 7,9). Two small

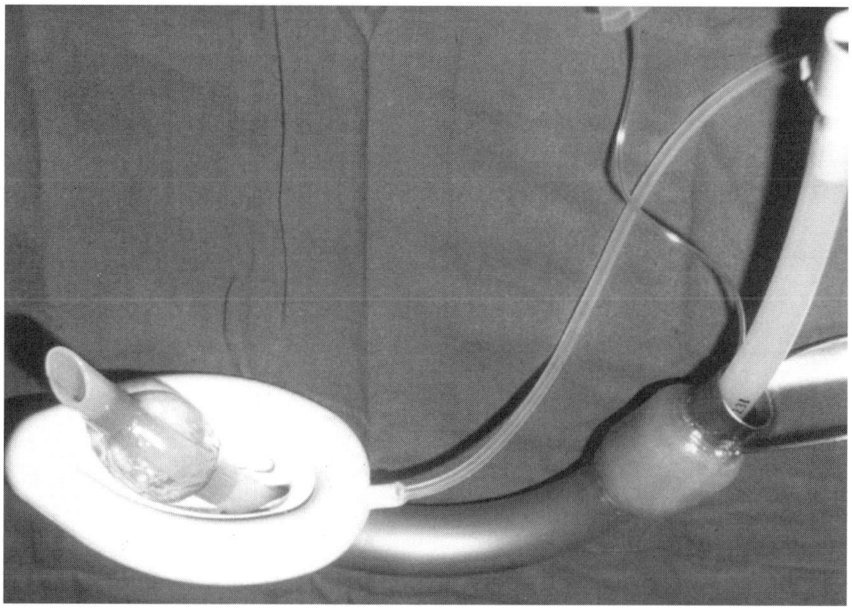

FIG. 8. The new prototype intubating LMA.

studies have investigated the use of the fiberscope/tracheal tube (FO/TT) combination in patients with abnormal airways. Kadota et al. (79), using a long PVC tube primed with the FOS, successfully intubated five of five adult patients (three had severe rheumatoid arthritis, one a tongue malignancy, and one ossification of the posterior longitudinal ligament) (79). In a more extensive study, Silk et al. (78) used the FO/TT in 48 patients with anticipated intubation difficulty. The technique was successful in 96% (46/48); failures resulted from one problem with LMA insertion and one failure to pass the TT.

It is useful to practice the technique of fiberoptic laryngoscopy through the LMA to gain experience in orientation and manipulation of the scope. Initial valuable experience can be gained using an intubating mannequin.

EMERGENCY MEDICINE APPLICATIONS OF THE LMA

There is interest in the possible use of the LMA in emergency situations by nonanesthetists involved in airway management; this includes emergency room physicians, paramedics, and "first responder" nurses. The advantages of the LMA for first responders are that it is relatively easy to insert and the risks of esophageal and right main bronchus intubation are avoided. However, the relative risks of aspiration and inability to achieve high pressure ventilation have not as yet been defined in this patient population. These limitations imply that it should be regarded as a device providing temporary airway support, but not as a replacement for a TT except in life-threatening situations. It is possible that the LMA will find a role in emergency room management of suspected cervical spine injury as it may be inserted with the head maintained in the neutral position (31,33,34,113, 114) and without general anesthesia. A recent multicenter study found that, after a training program, ward nurses obtained satisfactory chest expansion after LMA insertion in 86% of cases during CPR. In 7% of these, subsequent intubation by an anesthetist proved impossible in the ward setting, and ventilation was continued through the LMA (51). Two cases have been reported of its successful use in providing emergency airway control in trapped victims of traffic accidents where access to the patients was limited, making laryngoscopy impossible (83). The Resuscitation Council (UK) has approved the training of "paramedical staff" in the use of the LMA, and a UK comprehensive trial will shortly commence on its use in the field. Until the results of such trials are available on large numbers of patients, the precise role of the LMA in the emergency situation is uncertain. It would seem essential, however, that LMAs are available in the emergency room for management of difficult airway situations.

Patient Transport

Loss of airway control during transportation may present enormous management difficulties, even in the presence of experienced personnel. Even an intubated patient may occasionally suffer a TT-related incident and urgently require another form of airway control (115, 116). Restricted access, constant movement, and noise may make reintubation and FM ventilation not just difficult, but impossible. The appropriately sized LMA should be immediately available on the difficult airway tray during transport of critically ill patients, both within and between hospitals.

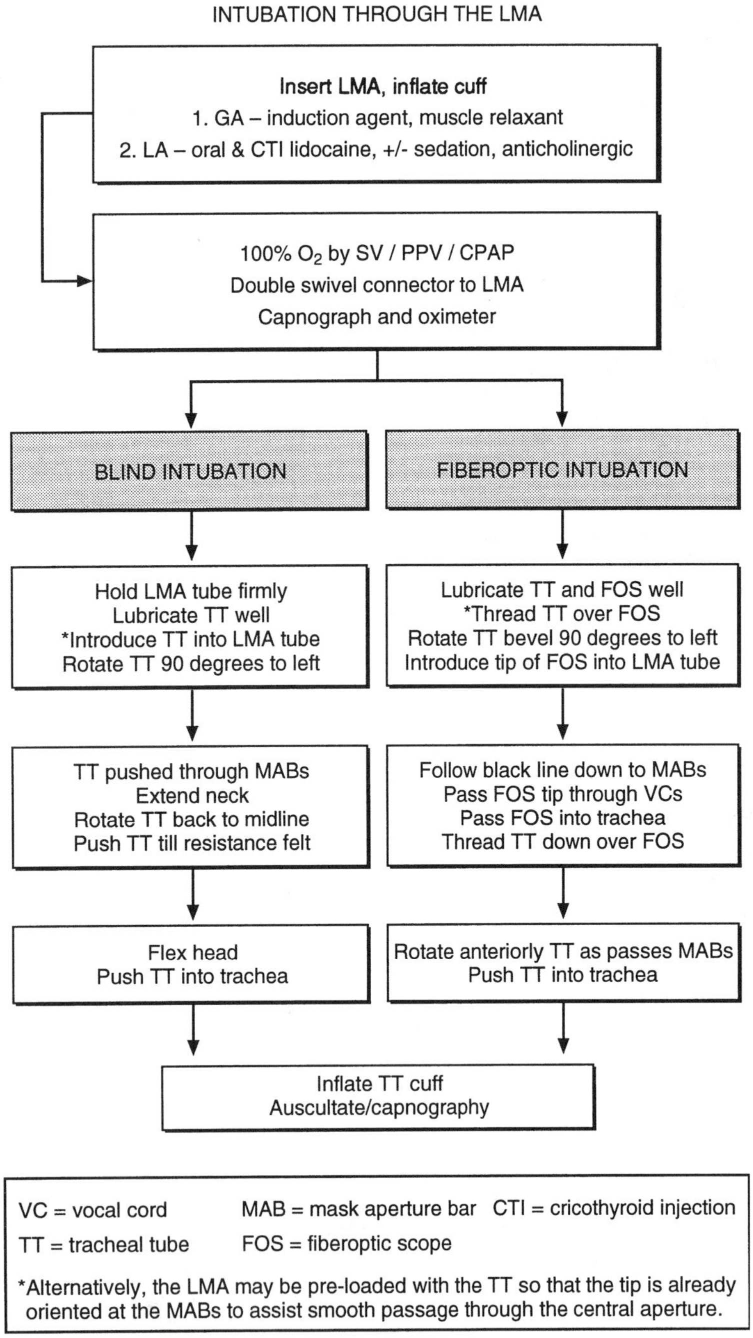

FIG. 9. Flow chart—use as airway intubator—blind and guided.

Pediatric/Neonatal Resuscitation

Although the use of the LMA in neonatal anesthetic practice has not been established, it is developing a role in neonatal resuscitation. In small obstetric units with less than 500 deliveries per annum, 43% of resuscitations after vaginal delivery and 24% after Cesarean section are performed by nonphysician personnel (117). The majority of personnel resuscitating neonates in small obstetric units are so infrequently exposed to advanced resuscitation techniques that they have difficulty maintaining proficiency (118). Resuscitation is necessary in up to 80% for those whose birth weight is less than 1.5 kg (119). The size-1 LMA is available for infants/neonates (<6.5 kg), and early studies during anesthesia suggest that insertion is successful in 68% at the first attempt and 32% at the second (120). Tests on neonatal intubation training models have shown that midwives and junior doctors can obtain a clear airway more rapidly with the LMA than with the TT and with fewer failures (121). In a prospective study, LMA-trained neonatologists were able to initially resuscitate 21/21 neonates with the LMA, and in all cases insertion was successful at the first attempt (53). Oxygenation and restoration of heart rate occurred in each neonate within 30 sec. Potential limitations are that the LMA may not be suitable for removal of meconium aspiration and may be inadequate for neonates who require high airway pressures. No studies have yet been performed on pediatric resuscitation with the LMA.

Intensive Care

There is only anecdotal evidence concerning the specific use of the LMA in the ICU, but there are potential applications in this setting. The LMA can be inserted under topical anesthesia; little sedation is required to tolerate the procedure. The wide-bore tube offers a low resistance pathway to spontaneous respiration, and CPAP has been applied comfortably in a patient (122). The LMA may be useful in certain patients where reintubation is undesirable and the airway requires only simple support (123). Its use, however, would depend on the patient having an empty stomach. In theory, chest physiotherapy may be difficult, since turning and suctioning might precipitate laryngospasm and regurgitation. Other potential ICU applications of the LMA would be its use as an aid to difficult intubation, as an emergency airway, and as an aid to bronchoscopy for removal of sputum plugs (124). Tracheostomy can be performed with the LMA (68), which avoids the risk of TT cuff rupture and the need to withdraw the airway during surgery. Endoscopically guided percutaneous tracheostomy, performed in the ICU, is now a common technique in the UK and in Australia. A guidewire is inserted in the trachea over which dilators are passed to place a tracheostomy tube (125). Tracheostomy can also be performed with fiberoptic guidance via the LMA in selected patients. The advantage of the LMA over the TT is a better view of the trachea, avoiding interference with the surgical field (69) and misplacement of the guidewire.

SUMMARY/CONCLUSIONS

In the few years since its release, the LMA has been widely accepted as a general purpose airway in routine anesthesia, as well as in the difficult airway situation. There are many case reports of its life-saving use in the patient who can be neither intubated nor mask-ventilated. Its impact on resuscitation techniques in adults and in neonates is under investigation. Further research is clearly required to define the role of the LMA in emergency medicine, to decide the safety issues in this context, and to determine the level of initial and continued training needed. Training in its use should be considered by anyone involved in airway management and particularly by emergency room and ICU personnel. Finally, new designs of the LMA are being studied. The gastro-LMA (GLMA) is intended to offer improved protection of the lungs against regurgitated gastric contents while offering a higher pressure seal for controlling ventilation (126). The intubating LMA will allow intubation with a larger diameter TT and removal of the device after intubation.

SUGGESTED READING LIST

Brimacombe J, Shorney N. The laryngeal mask airway—a review and update. In: Kaufman L, ed. *Anaesthesia Review*, vol 10. London: Churchill Livingstone, 1993:183–202.

White DC. The laryngeal mask—a non-invasive airway. *Eur J Anaesthesiol* 1991;4:1–4.

Benumof JL. Laryngeal mask airway—indications and contraindications. *Anesthesiology* 1992;77:843–846.

Wilson IG. The laryngeal mask airway in paediatric practice. *Br J Anaesth* 1993;70:124–125.

McEwan AI, Mason DG. The laryngeal mask airway. *J Clin Anesth* 1992; 4:252–257.

Leach AB, Alexander CA. The laryngeal mask—an overview. *Eur J Anaesthesiol* 1991;4:19–31.

Brimacombe J. AANA Journal course: update for nurse anesthetist. IV. The laryngeal mask airway: a review for the nurse anesthetist. *Am Assoc Nurse Anesthet J* 1992;60:490–499.

Pennant JH, White PF. The laryngeal mask airway. Its uses in anesthesiology. *Anesthesiology* 1993;79:144–163.

Brimacombe J, Berry A, Brain A. The laryngeal mask airway. *Anesth Clin North Am*, in press.

REFERENCES

1. Brain AIJ. The development of the laryngeal mask—a brief history of the invention, early clinical studies and experimental work from which the laryngeal mask evolved. *Eur J Anaesthesiol* 1991;4:5–17.
2. Brimacombe J. The use of the laryngeal mask airway in very small neonates. *Anesthesiology* 1994;81:1302.
3. Practice guidelines for management of the difficult airway—a report by the American Society of Anesthesiologists Task Force on Management of the Difficult Airway. *Anesthesiology* 1993;78:597–602.
4. White DC. The laryngeal mask—a non-invasive airway. *Eur J Anaesthesiol* 1991;4:1–4.
5. Drummond GB. Influence of thiopentone on upper airway muscles. *Br J Anaesth* 1989;63:12–21.
6. Fouke JM, Strohl KP. Effect of position and lung volume on upper airway geometry. *J Appl Physiol* 1987;63:375–380.
7. Marsh AM, Nunn JF, Taylor SJ, Charlesworth CH. Airway obstruction associated with the use of the Guedel airway. *Br J Anaesth* 1991; 67:517–523.
8. Ooi R, Soni N. The work of ventilation imposed by the laryngeal mask airway. *Anesthesiology* 1993;79:A499.
9. Al-Hasani A. Resistance to constant air flow imposed by the standard laryngeal mask, the reinforced laryngeal mask airway and RAE tubes. *Br J Anaesth* 1993;71:594–596.
10. Wilkins CJ, Cramp PG, Staples J, Stevens WC. Comparison of the anesthetic requirement for tolerance of laryngeal mask airway and endotracheal tube. *Anesth Analg* 1992;75:794–797.
11. Wilson IG, Fell D, Robinson SL, Smith G. Cardiovascular responses to insertion of the laryngeal mask. *Anaesthesia* 1992;47:300–302.
12. Berry A, Verghese C. Changes in pulmonary mechanics during IPPV with the laryngeal mask airway compared to the tracheal tube. *Anesth Analg* 1994;78:S38
13. Haden RM, Pinnock CA, Campbell RL. The laryngeal mask for intraocular surgery. *Br J Anaesth* 1993;71:772
14. Brimacombe J, Shorney N, Swainston R, Bapty G. The incidence of bacteriemia following laryngeal mask insertion. *Anaesth Intensive Care* 1992;20:484–485.
15. Barker P, Langton JA, Murphy PJ, Rowbotham DJ. Regurgitation of gastric contents during general anesthesia using the laryngeal mask airway. *Br J Anaesth* 1992;69:314–315.
16. Rabey PG, Murphy PJ, Langton JA, Barker P, Rowbotham DJ. Effect

of the laryngeal mask airway on lower oesophageal sphincter pressure in patients during general anesthesia. *Br J Anaesth* 1992;69:346–348.
17. Owens T, Robertson P, Twomey K, Doyle M, McShane AJ. Incidence of gastroesophageal reflux with the laryngeal mask. *Anesthesiology* 1993;79:A1053
18. Brimacombe J, Berry A. Regurgitation and the laryngeal mask airway. *Br J Anaesth* 1993;70:381
19. Vanner RG. Regurgitation and the laryngeal mask airway. *Br J Anaesth* 1993;70:380
20. El Mikatti N, Luthra AD, Healy TEJ, Mortimer AJ. Gastric regurgitation during general anesthesia in the supine position with the laryngeal and face mask airways. *Br J Anaesth* 1992;68:529P–530P.
21. Brimacombe J, Berry A. The incidence of aspiration associated with the laryngeal mask airway—a meta-analysis of published literature. *J Clin Anesth* 1995;7:295–305.
22. Shorten GD, Opie NJ, Graziotti P, Morris I, Khangure M. Assessment of upper airway anatomy in awake, sedated and anesthetised patients using magnetic resonance imaging. *Anaesth Intensive Care* 1994;22: 165–169.
23. Nandi PR, Nunn JF, Charlesworth CH, Taylor SJ. Radiological study of the laryngeal mask. *Eur J Anaesthesiol* 1991;4:33–39.
24. Brimacombe J. Cricoid pressure and the laryngeal mask airway. *Anaesthesia* 1991;46:986–987.
25. Goudsouzian NG, Denman W, Cleveland R, Shorten G. Radiologic localization of the laryngeal mask airway in children. *Anesthesiology* 1992;77:1085–1089.
26. Payne J. The use of the fiberoptic laryngoscope to confirm the position of the laryngeal mask. *Anaesthesia* 1989;44:465
27. Brimacombe J, Berry A. Insertion of the laryngeal mask airway—a prospective study of four techniques. *Anaesth Intensive Care* 1993; 21:89–92.
28. Du Plessis MC, Marshall Barr A, Verghese C, Lyall JRW. Fiberoptic bronchoscopy under general anesthesia using the laryngeal mask airway. *Eur J Anaesthesiol* 1993;103:363–365.
29. Pothmann W, Fullekrug B, Schulte am Esch J. Fiberoptic determination of the position of the laryngeal mask. *Anaesthesist* 1992;41: 779–784.
30. John RE, Hill S, Hughes TJ. Airway protection by the laryngeal mask—a barrier to dye placed in the pharynx. *Anaesthesia* 1991;46: 366–367.
31. Pennant JH, Pace NA, Gajraj NM. Role of the laryngeal mask airway in the immobile cervical spine. *J Clin Anesth* 1993;5:226–230.
32. Brimacombe J, Berry A. Laryngeal mask airway insertion. A comparison of the standard verses neutral position in normal patients with a view to its use in cervical spine instability. *Anaesthesia* 1993;48: 670–671.
33. Logan A. Use of the laryngeal mask in a patient with an unstable fracture of the cervical spine. *Anaesthesia* 1991;46:987
34. Lee JJ, Yau K, Barcroft J. LMA and respiratory arrest after anterior cervical fusion. *Can J Anaesth* 1993;40:395–396.
35. Wilson IG. The laryngeal mask airway in paediatric practice. *Br J Anaesth* 1993;70:124–125.
36. O'Neill B, Caramico L, Templeton JJ, Schreiner MS. Inflated vs. deflated insertion of the laryngeal mask airway in infants and children. *Anesthesiology* 1993;79:A1188
37. McNicol LR. Insertion of the laryngeal mask airway in children. *Anaesthesia* 1991;46:330
38. Strang TI. Does the laryngeal mask airway compromise cricoid pressure? *Anaesthesia* 1992;47:829–831.
39. Brimacombe J, Berry A, White A. Single versus double handed cricoid pressure for LMA insertion. *Br J Anaesth* 1994;72:732–733.
40. Brimacombe J, White A, Berry A. Effect of cricoid pressure on ease of insertion of the laryngeal mask airway. *Br J Anaesth* 1993;71:800–802.
41. Heath ML, Allagain J. Intubation through the laryngeal mask—a technique for unexpected difficult intubation. *Anaesthesia* 1991;46: 545–548.
42. Ansermino JM, Blogg CE. Cricoid pressure may prevent insertion of the laryngeal mask airway. *Br J Anaesth* 1992;69:465–467.
43. Asai T, Barkley K, Power I, Vaughan RS. Cricoid pressure impedes placement of the laryngeal mask airway and subsequent tracheal intubation. *Br J Anaesth* 1994;72:47–51.
44. Brimacombe J, Berry A. Mechanical airway obstruction following cricoid pressure with the laryngeal mask airway. *Anesth Analg* 1994; 78:604–605.
45. Stewart RD, Paris PM, Pelton GH, Cannon GM. Field endotracheal intubation by paramedical personnel. *Chest* 1984;85:341
46. Vertesi L. The paramedic ambulance: a Canadian experience. *Can Med Assoc J* 1978;119:25
47. Pennant JH, Walker MB. Comparison of the endotracheal tube and laryngeal mask in airway management by paramedical personnel. *Anesth Analg* 1992;74:531–534.
48. Davies PRF, Tighe SQ, Greenslade GL, Evans GH. Laryngeal mask airway and tracheal tube insertion by unskilled personnel. *Lancet* 1990;336:977–979.
49. Martin PD, Cyna AM, Hunter WAH, Henry J, Pamayya GP. Training nursing staff in airway management for resuscitation—a clinical comparison of the face mask and laryngeal mask. *Anaesthesia* 1993;48: 33–37.
50. Reinhart DJ, Simmons G. Comparison of placement of the laryngeal mask airway with endotracheal tube by paramedics and respiratory therapists. *Ann Emerg Med* 1994;24:260–263.
51. Stone BJ, Leach AB, Alexander CA, Ruffer DR, McBeth C, Warwick JP, Baskett PJF, Nicholls E, Prior-Willeard PFS, Verghese C, Jago RH. The use of the laryngeal mask airway by nurses during cardiopulmonary resuscitation—results of a multicentre trial. *Anaesthesia* 1994;49:3–7.
52. Leach A, Alexander CA, Stone B. The laryngeal mask in cardiopulmonary resuscitation in a district general hospital: a preliminary communication. *Resuscitation* 1993;25:245–248.
53. Paterson SJ, Byrne PJ, Molesky MG, Seal RF, Finucane BT. Neonatal resuscitation using the laryngeal mask airway. *Anesthesiology* 1994;80:1248–1253.
54. Brimacombe J, Berry A, Fletcher D. A training program for laryngeal mask airway removal in the PACU. *J Post Anaes Nurs* 1993;8:236–237.
55. Devitt JH, Wenstone R, Noel AG, O'Donnell RRT. The laryngeal mask airway and positive-pressure ventilation. *Anesthesiology* 1994; 80:550–555.
56. Graziotti PJ. Intermittent positive pressure ventilation through a laryngeal mask airway—is a nasogastric tube useful? *Anaesthesia* 1992;47:1088–1089.
57. Brimacombe J, Berry A. Size selection and the sixth LMA. *J Clin Anesth* 1995;7:265–266.
58. Brimacombe J. Laryngoscopy through the LMA—a useful skill to acquire. *Anaesth Intensive Care* 1992;20:535
59. Johnston DF, Wrigley SR, Robb PJ, Jones HE. The laryngeal mask airway in paediatric anesthesia. *Anaesthesia* 1990;45:924–927.
60. Smith I, White PF. Use of the laryngeal mask airway as an alternative to a face mask during outpatient arthroscopy. *Anesthesiology* 1992; 77:850–855.
61. Watcha MF, Garner FT, White PF. Perioperative conditions with face mask—oral airway or laryngeal mask airway during bilateral myringotomy in children. *Anesth Analg* 1993;76:S456
62. Verghese C, Smith TGC, Young E. Prospective survey of the use of the laryngeal mask airway in 2359 patients. *Anaesthesia* 1993;48: 58–60.
63. Grebenik CR, Ferguson C, White A. The laryngeal mask airway in pediatric radiotherapy. *Anesthesiology* 1990;72:474–477.
64. Webster AC, Morley-Forster PK, Dain S, Ganapathy S, Ruby R, Au A, Cook MJ. Anesthesia for adenotonsillectomy: a comparison between tracheal intubation and the armoured laryngeal mask airway. *Can J Anaesth* 1993;40:1171–1177.
65. Goodwin A, Ogg TW, Lamb W, Adlam D. The reinforced laryngeal mask airway in dental day surgery. *Ambulatory Surg* 1993;1:31–35.
66. Brimacombe J, Sher M, Berry A. The reinforced laryngeal mask airway for laser pharyngoplasty. *Anaesthesia* 1993;48:1105
67. Brimacombe J, Newell S, Swainston R, Thompson J. A potential new technique for awake fiberoptic bronchoscopy—use of the laryngeal mask airway. *Med J Aust* 1992;156:876–877.
68. Thomson KD. Laryngeal mask airway for elective tracheostomy. *Anaesthesia* 1992;47:76
69. Dexter TJ. The laryngeal mask airway: a method to improve visualisation of the trachea and larynx during fiberoptic assisted percutaneous tracheostomy. *Anaesth Intensive Care* 1994;22:35–39.
70. Brimacombe J, Shorney N. The laryngeal mask airway and prolonged balanced anesthesia. *Can J Anaesth* 1993;40:360–364.
71. Brimacombe J, Berry A. Laryngeal mask airway cuff pressure and position during anesthesia lasting 1–2 hours. *Can J Anaesth* 1994;41: 589–593.

72. Kallar SK. Aspiration pneumonitis: fact or fiction? *Probl Anesth* 1988;2:29–36.
73. Brimacombe J. The laryngeal mask airway for intra abdominal surgery. *J Clin Exp Med* 1994;171:949–951.
74. Brimacombe J. Laparoscopy and the laryngeal mask airway. *Br J Anaesth*, in press.
75. Benumof JL. Difficult laryngoscopy: obtaining the best view. *Can J Anaesth* 1994;41:361–365.
76. Rose DK, Cohen MM. The airway: problems and predictions in 18,500 patients. *Can J Anaesth* 1994;41:372–383.
77. Brimacombe J, Tucker P, Simons S. The laryngeal mask airway for awake diagnostic bronchoscopy—a study of 200 consecutive patients. *Eur J Anaesthesiol* 1995;12:357–361.
78. Silk JM, Hill HM, Calder I. Difficult intubation and the laryngeal mask. *Eur J Anaesthesiol* 1991;4:47–51.
79. Kadota Y, Oda T, Yoshimura N. Application of a laryngeal mask to a fiberoptic bronchoscope-aided tracheal intubation. *J Clin Anesth* 1992;4:503–504.
80. Mahiou P, Narchi P, Veyrac P, Germond M, Gory G, Bazin G. Is laryngeal mask easy to use in case of difficult intubation? *Anesthesiology* 1992;77:A1228.
81. Brimacombe J, Berry A. Mallampati classification and laryngeal mask insertion. *Anaesthesia* 1993;48:347.
82. McCaughey W, Bhanumurthy S. Laryngeal mask placement in the prone position. *Anaesthesia* 1993;48:1104–1105.
83. Greene MK, Roden R, Hinchley G. The laryngeal mask airway. Two cases of prehospital trauma care. *Anaesthesia* 1992;47:688–689.
84. Williamson JA, Webb RK, Szekely S, Gillies ERN. Difficult intubation: an analysis of 2000 incident reports. *Anaesth Intensive Care* 1993;21:602–607.
85. Asai T, Morris S. Elective use of the laryngeal mask in patients with difficult airways. *Can J Anaesth* 1993;40:1221–1222.
86. Todesco J, Dodd C, Tudor Williams R, Williams PJ, Bailey PM. Laryngeal mask airway: defining the limits. *Can J Anaesth* 1993;40: 816–818.
87. Benumof JL. Laryngeal mask airway and difficult intubation. *Anesthesiology* 1993;78:995.
88. Johnston IG, Restall J. The laryngeal mask airway. *J Br Assoc Immediate Care* 1989;12:3–4.
89. Brimacombe J, Berry A, White A. An algorithm for use of the laryngeal mask airway during failed intubation in the patient with a full stomach. *Anesth Analg* 1993;77:398–399.
90. Brimacombe J, Berry A. The laryngeal mask airway for obstetric anesthesia and neonatal resuscitation. *Int J Obstet Anesth* 1994;3: 211–218.
91. Kokkinis K. The use of the laryngeal mask airway in CPR. *Resuscitation* 1994;27:9–12.
92. Lim SL, Tay DHB, Thomas E. A comparison of three types of tracheal tube for use in laryngeal mask assisted blind orotracheal intubation. *Anaesthesia* 1994;49:255–257.
93. Benumof JL, Scheller MS. The importance of transtracheal jet ventilation in the management of the difficult airway. *Anesthesiology* 1989;71:769–778.
94. Smith RB, Babinski M, Klain M, Pfaaffle H. Percutaneous transtracheal ventilation. *J Am Coll Emerg Phys* 1976;5:765–770.
95. Lawlor M, Johnson C, Weiner M. Airway management in obstetric anesthesia. *Int J Obstet Anesth* 1993;3:225–232.
96. Benumof JL. Management of the difficult adult airway—with special emphasis on awake tracheal intubation. *Anesthesiology* 1991;75: 1087–1110.
97. Green KS, Beger TH. Proper use of the combitube. *Anesthesiology* 1994;81:513–514.
98. Dasey N, Mansour N. Coughing and laryngospasm with the laryngeal mask. *Anaesthesia* 1989;44:865.
99. Asai T, Latto IP, Vaughan RS. The distance between the grill of the laryngeal mask airway and the cords. Is conventional intubation through the laryngeal mask safe? *Anaesthesia* 1993;48:667–669.
100. Chadd GD, Walford AJ, Crane DL. The 3.5/4.5 modification for fiberscope-guided tracheal intubation using the laryngeal mask airway. *Anesth Analg* 1992;75:307–308.
101. Zagnoev M, McCloskey J, Martin T. Fiberoptic intubation via the laryngeal mask airway. *Anesth Analg* 1994;78:813–814.
102. Goldie AS, Hudson I. Fiberoptic tracheal intubation through a modified laryngeal mask. *Paediatr Anaesth* 1992;2:344
103. Maltby JR, Neil SG. Laryngeal mask airway and difficult intubation. *Anesthesiology* 1993;78:994–995.
104. Watai Y, Salem MR, Tartaglione A, Joseph NJ. Facilitation of blind intubation through the laryngeal mask airway by the the self-inflating bulb. *Anesth Analg* 1994;79:A628.
105. McCrirrick A, Pracilio JA. Awake intubation: a new technique. *Anaesthesia* 1991;46:661–663.
106. Chadd GD, Ackers JW, Bailey PM. Difficult intubation aided by the laryngeal mask airway. *Anaesthesia* 1989;44:1015.
107. Allison A, McCrory J. Tracheal placement of a gum elastic bougie using the laryngeal mask airway. *Anaesthesia* 1990;45:419–420.
108. White AP, Billingham IM. Laryngeal mask guided tracheal intubation in paediatric anesthesia. *Paediatr Anaesth* 1992;2:265.
109. Carey MF, Smith J, Cooney CM. Laryngeal mask to aid tracheal intubation. *Anaesthesia* 1991;46:1083.
110. Hasham FM, Andrews PJD, Juneja MM, Ackermann III WE. The laryngeal mask airway facilitates intubation at Cesarean section. A case report of difficult intubation. *Int J Obstet Anesth* 1993;2:181–182.
111. Brimacombe J, Berry A. Placement of the Cook airway exchange catheter via the laryngeal mask airway. *Anaesthesia* 1993;48:351–352.
112. Smith JE, Sherwood NA. Combined use of laryngeal mask airway and fiberoptic laryngoscope in difficult intubation. *Anaesth Intensive Care* 1991;19:471–472.
113. Asai T. Fiberoptic tracheal intubation through the laryngeal mask airway in an awake patient with cervical spine instability. *Anesth Analg* 1993;77:404.
114. Calder I, Ordman AJ, Jackowski A, Crockard HA. The Brain laryngeal mask airway. An alternative to emergency tracheal intubation. *Anaesthesia* 1990;45:137–139.
115. Anonymous Guidelines for the transfer of critically ill patients. Guidelines Committee of the American College of Critical Care Medicine; Society of Critical Care Medicine and American Association of Critical-Care Nurses Transfer Guidelines Task Force. *Crit Care Med* 1993;21:931–937.
116. Kanter RK, Tompkins JM. Adverse events during interhospital transport: physiologic deterioration associated with pretransport severity of illness. *Pediatrics* 1989;84:43–48.
117. Standards and guidelines for cardiopulmonary resuscitation (CPR) and emergency cardiac care (ECC). VI. Neonatal advanced life support. *JAMA* 1986;255:2969–2973.
118. Gibbs CP, Krischer J, Peckham BM, Sharp H, Kirschbaum TH. Obstetric anesthesia: a national survey. *Anesthesiology* 1986;65:298–306.
119. Emergency Cardiac Care Committee and Subcomittees AH. Guidelines for cardiopulmonary resuscitation and emergency cardiac care. VII. Neonatal resuscitation. *JAMA* 1994;268:2276–2281.
120. Dubreuil M, Laffon M, Plaud B, Penon C, Ecoffey C. Incidence of complications with size 1 laryngeal mask. *Anesthesiology* 1992;77: A1174.
121. Lavies NG. Use of the laryngeal mask airway in neonatal resuscitation. *Anaesthesia* 1993;48:352.
122. Fullekrug B, Pothmann W, Druge G. Unkonventioneller Einsatz der Kehlikopfmaske zur Therapie einer postoperativen, atelektasenbedingten ateminsuffizienz. *Anasth Intensivther Notfallmed* 1993;28: 187–189.
123. Salib YM. The use of the laryngeal mask airway in intensive care. *Today's Anaesthetist* 1989;4:268.
124. Mabuchi N. Laryngeal mask airway in the ICU. *J Clin Exp Med* 1992; 162,12,9:876–878.
125. Miyasaka K. Laryngeal mask airway in pediatric anesthesia. *J Clin Exp Med* 1992;162,12,9:872–875.
126. Brain AIJ, Verghese C, Strube P, Brimacombe J. A new laryngeal mask prototype—preliminary evaluation of seal pressures and glottic isolation. *Anaesthesia* 1995;50:42–48.
127. Harmer M. Complications of tracheal intubation. In: Latto IP, Rosen M, eds. *Difficulties in tracheal intubation*. London: Bailliere Tindall, 1987:36–48.

Airway Management, edited by
L.H. Hanowell, M.D. and R.J. Waldron, M.D.,
Lippincott-Raven Publishers, Philadelphia © 1996.

CHAPTER 14

The Esophageal-Tracheal Combitube

Douglas R. Mest

HISTORY AND INTRODUCTION

In order to appreciate the utility of the esophageal-tracheal Combitube (Combitube™, Sheridan-Kendall Catheter Corporation, Argyle, New York), one must first understand its history. This device is a significant improvement over the old esophageal obturator airway (EOA), a blindly placed airway device that was popular with paramedics in the 1970s and early 1980s for airway management of out-of-hospital patients (1,2,3).

Although easy to learn and simple to use, the EOA had two distinct problems that eventually led to significantly decreased usage. First of all, a proper mask fit was difficult to obtain after the device was inserted. This often resulted in inadequate ventilation of the patient owing to leak of air around the face mask. The second and more lethal problem involved unrecognized tracheal placement of the EOA. In this situation, the patient could not be ventilated (4,5,6). This scenario resulted in several deaths, and the EOA was largely replaced by endotracheal intubation by paramedical personnel.

The esophageal-tracheal Combitube overcomes these two difficulties by combining the functions of an EOA and that of a traditional endotracheal tube.

D.R. Mest: Long Beach Community Medical Center, and Department of Anesthesiology, University of California, Irvine Medical Center, Orange, California 92668.

DESIGN FEATURES

Packaging

The Combitube comprises two separate, clear polyvinyl chloride (PVC) tubes, longitudinally fused, with a standard 15-mm airway connector on the proximal end of each tube (Fig. 1). It is prepackaged with a 140-cc syringe, predrawn to 100 cc, and a 20-cc syringe, predrawn to 15 cc (Fig. 2). The 140-cc syringe has a color-coded blue dot to emphasize its use with the blue pilot balloon, which attaches to the oropharyngeal balloon. A 12F suction catheter is also provided.

Combitube Design

The Combitube is designed to be able to be used in most patients taller than 5 feet (153 cm). The distal curvature approximates the adult human hypopharynx. Correct placement depth in the majority of patients is indicated when two black marks on the proximal portion of the Combitube are located between the patient's teeth. At this depth, the oropharyngeal balloon tends to be in the proper position, although there are some patients in whom this does not occur (see Placement Confirmation). The outer diameter of the distal end of the Combitube is 41F (13 mm), which is approximately the size of a No.

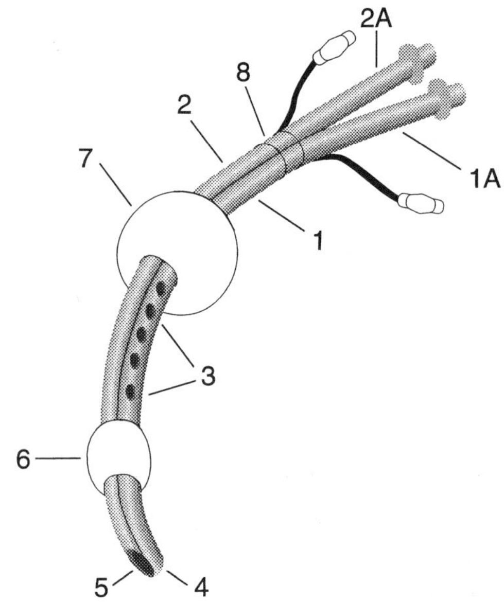

FIG. 1. Components of the esophageal-tracheal Combitube. *(1)* Occluded "esophageal obturator" lumen. *(1A)* Longer, blue tube for No. 1 lumen. *(2)* "Tracheal" lumen. *(2A)* Shorter, clear tube for No. 2 lumen. *(3)* Perforations of No. 1 lumen. *(4)* Distal blind end of No. 1 lumen. *(5)* Open end of No. 2 lumen. *(6)* Distal cuff. *(7)* Oropharyngeal balloon. *(8)* Black printed rings indicating correct depth of insertion. (From Frass M, et al. Ventilation via the esophageal-tracheal combitube in a case of difficult intubation. *J Cardiothorac Anesth* 1987;1: 566, with permission.)

10.0 endotracheal tube. There are two inflatable balloons on the Combitube:

1. A proximal, 100-cc latex oropharyngeal balloon that is resistant to damage from broken teeth
2. A 15-cc PVC balloon near the distal tip (Fig. 1)

Inflation of the specially designed oropharyngeal balloon produces an airtight seal so that ventilation is not hampered by escape of gases through the mouth or nose. The problems of a difficult mask fit, which complicated the use of the old EOA, are thus resolved. Another benefit of this oropharyngeal balloon is that by pressing against the hard palate, it anchors the Combitube in place and makes it difficult to dislodge.

Lumen No. 1 (Fig. 1) has a longer proximal end that is colored blue and has an occluded distal tip. Eight small (7 × 3-mm), oval-shaped holes in lumen No. 1 are located between the two balloons. Lumen No. 2 (Fig. 1) is clear, with a shorter proximal end and a patent distal tip. It is possible to ventilate the trachea through this lumen if the the Combitube is placed tracheally. Otherwise, this lumen serves as a suction port for gastric contents.

The esophageal portion of the Combitube is also much shorter than the old EOA, theoretically decreasing the chance of esophageal rupture. This is especially important in patients with left atrial dilatation who have lateral deviation of the lower half of the esophagus (7,8,9). The likelihood of esophageal rupture is also decreased by the presence of the second, open lumen of the Combitube. This lumen acts to allow the pressure caused by contraction of the stomach against a closed distal esophagus to be relieved. With these factors in mind, the esophageal-tracheal Combitube was submitted and received final FDA approval as an airway device in January of 1988.

INSERTION AND PLACEMENT

Published reports have documented the effectiveness of this device in routine surgery (10,11), during cardiopulmonary resuscitation (8,12), and during mechanical ventilation in the intensive care unit (13). However, the main use of the esophageal-tracheal Combitube is for emergent airway control (8,12,14). Direct laryngoscopy and endotracheal intubation are technical skills that need constant renewal and practice. Although relatively simple to learn to use (15), the Combitube still requires some continuing education, especially in situations of infrequent usage (16). Ongoing studies are being performed to assess the Combitube as an alternative to endotracheal intubation by paramedical personnel during prehospital care (17).

Insertion Technique

It is recommended that the integrity of both balloons be checked prior to insertion. Although not mandatory, many practitioners feel that it is easier to insert the Combitube after the tip has been lubricated. It is important to avoid excess lubrication near the ventilating eyes, as this could lead to obstruction of airflow. In patients with large amounts of blood or vomitus, it is almost never necessary to lubricate the Combitube.

Placement of the esophageal-tracheal Combitube is most readily performed with the head in a neutral, semi-flexed position. The back of the patient's tongue and lower jaw are held between the thumb and forefinger of the person inserting the tube, and a mandible thrust is performed. Following this, the Combitube is inserted blindly with gentle dorsocaudal pressure until the two black marks on the proximal shaft are adjacent to the teeth (or alveolar ridge in edentulous patients). Care should be taken to insure that neither balloon is damaged by broken teeth or debris that might be present. Alternatively, a laryngoscope can be used to place the Combitube under direct vision. It is important to note that one should not attempt to place the Combitube preferentially in the trachea. This is not necessary and defeats the purpose of the device. The laryngoscope should be used solely as an aid to move the back of the tongue out of the way of the Combitube.

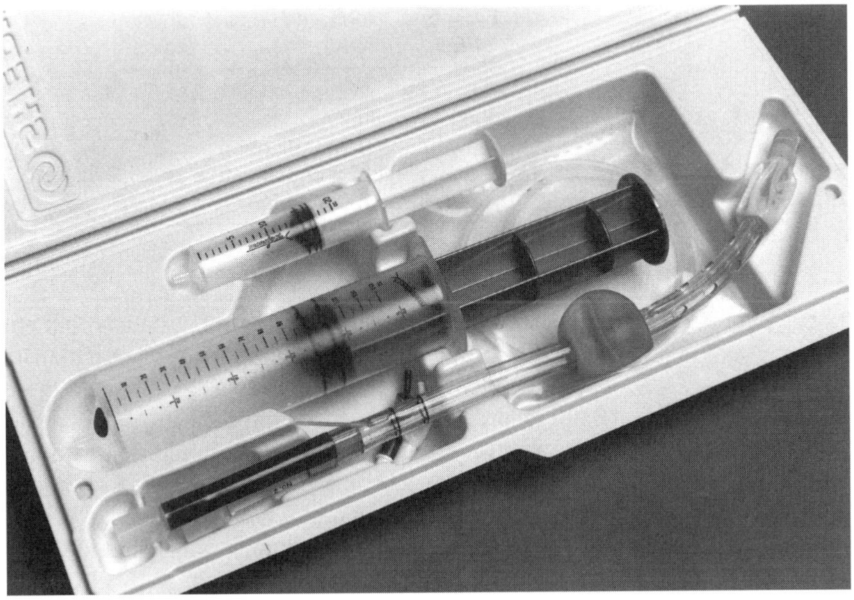

FIG. 2. Packaged esophageal-tracheal Combitube showing predrawn syringes.

Placement Confirmation

Once the esophageal-tracheal Combitube is inserted, the distal and oropharyngeal balloons are inflated. The proximal oropharyngeal balloon is inflated first by instilling 100 cc of air using the large 140-cc syringe provided. The blue pilot balloon of the oropharyngeal balloon is labeled "No. 1." At this stage, the esophageal-tracheal Combitube may "pop out" or move cephalad approximately 1 cm as it adjusts to the correct position. In this position, the proximal margin of the balloon is pressing against the posterior hard palate and fills the space between the soft palate and the base of the tongue. This position anchors the Combitube strongly and inhibits forward or backward movement. It should be emphasized that significant resistance is encountered during inflation of this latex balloon. Furthermore, the sensation experienced when its pilot balloon is inflated is very different from that experienced with PVC balloons of other airway devices because of its different compliance. The entire 100 cc should be instilled to ensure an adequate seal of the oropharynx. The special design of the oropharyngeal balloon allows the same amount of air to be instilled independently of the patient's size. Hyperinflation experiments have documented that further expansion of the proximal balloon occurs into the oral cavity rather than towards the epiglottis (18). Once the oropharyngeal balloon has been inflated, the more distal cuff is inflated to form a distal seal using the smaller syringe provided. This cuff is inflated with 10 to 15 cc of air.

Because there is a high probability (94% to 98%) of esophageal placement (10), the blue lumen, labeled "No. 1," is ventilated first (Fig. 3). This blue or esophageal lumen is blocked distally. Thus, by ventilating through this lumen, air is forced out through the eight perforations back up toward the oropharyngeal balloon. Since the oropharyngeal balloon forms a seal preventing escape of air through the nose and mouth and the distal cuff seals the esophagus, the air passes around the epiglottis and into the trachea. Auscultation should reveal presence of breath sounds over the lung fields and absence of breath sounds over the epigastrium. In the operating room setting, capnography is also useful to confirm adequate ventilation. If ventilation via the blue (No. 1) lumen fails to produce adequate chest movement and breath sounds

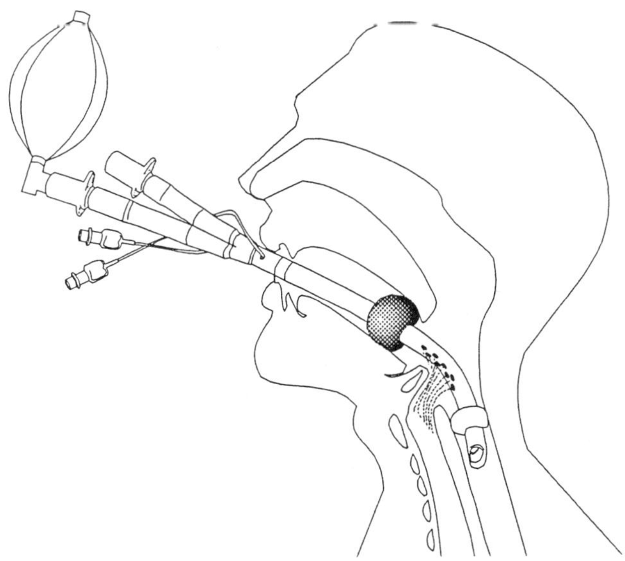

FIG. 3. Esophageal-tracheal Combitube in the esophageal position. (From Eichinger S, et al. Airway management in a case of neck impalement: use of the oesophageal-tracheal Combitube airway. *Br J Anaesth* 1992;68:534, with permission.)

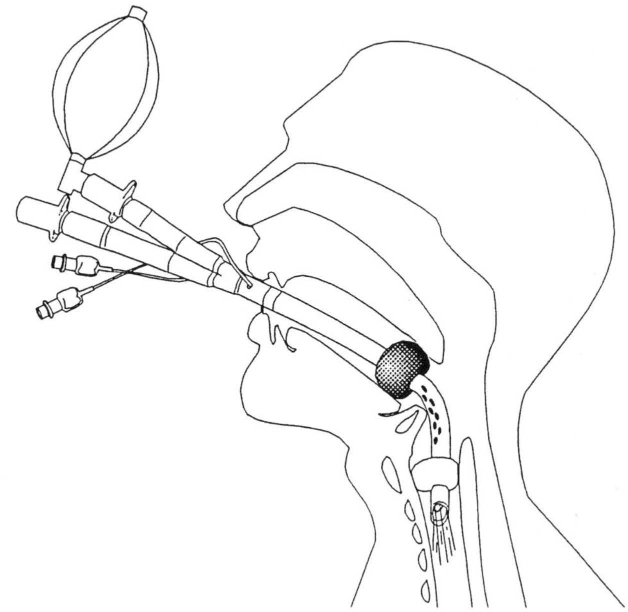

FIG. 4. Esophageal-tracheal Combitube in the tracheal position. (From Eichinger S, et al. Airway management in a case of neck impalement: use of the oesophageal-tracheal Combitube airway. *Br J Anaesth* 1992;68:535, with permission)

over the lung fields, then it is assumed that the Combitube is in the trachea. Ventilation should be changed to the open, clear No. 2 lumen (Fig. 4). In this position, the esophageal-tracheal Combitube functions as a standard endotracheal tube. It is important to note that when changing from the No. 1 (blue) lumen to the No. 2 (clear) lumen, the position of the esophageal-tracheal Combitube is not moved or altered (Table 1).

If there are no breath sounds by either of the two maneuvers listed above, then a quick attempt can be made to manipulate the Combitube further. First, more air can be added to the oropharyngeal balloon (up to a total of 160 cc may be instilled) to form a more complete seal of the oropharynx. After doing this, ventilation is again attempted through the blue (No. 1) lumen. If there are still no breath sounds, then both cuffs are deflated and the esophageal-tracheal Combitube should be removed. The entire process is then reattempted (Fig. 5).

Malpositions of the Combitube have been reported (19). In two patients, the Combitube was inserted to the black marks, following the manufacturer's specifications. Upon inflation of both cuffs, no ventilation was possible via either lumen. It was proposed that the esophageal-tracheal Combitube had been inserted too deeply for these patients; the oropharyngeal balloon actually became a laryngeal balloon, which, when inflated, pushed the epiglottis into or over the tracheal lumen. After deflating both cuffs, pulling the tube back 3 cm, and reinflating both cuffs, ventilation was successful via the blue lumen. It should be noted that both patients reported were over 5 feet tall (Table 2), which is the minimum height requirement for usage of the Combitube. This report serves to emphasize the fact that while the Combitube is easy to insert and use, it is not foolproof. Clinical judgment should always be exercised during insertion.

TABLE 1. *Clinical guidelines for use of Esophageal-tracheal Combitube*

Insertion
Place head in neutral position.
Lift chin.
Use laryngoscope to lift tongue AWAY (NOT to attempt to visualize vocal cords).
Apply gentle pressure.
Patient must be flaccid (paralysis in elective surgery).
Cuff inflation
Use entire 100 cc for No. 1 balloon.
ETC will "pop out" 1 cm.
Ventilation
Ventilate No. 1 lumen first.
Chance of esophageal placement is 94% to 98%.
DO NOT manipulate ETC/head when changing ventilation from lumen No. 1 to lumen No. 2.
Blue lumen is blocked.

TABLE 2. *Contraindications for use of Esophageal-tracheal Combitube*

Patient height of less than 5 feet
Intact gag reflex
Known esophageal disease
Prior ingestion of caustic substances
Upper airway obstruction

Ventilation and Oxygenation

Ventilation/oxygenation via the esophageal-tracheal Combitube has been compared directly with that obtained with endotracheal intubation in several crossover

TABLE 3. *PaO_2 in cardiac arrest patients*

	Initial airway	Second airway[a]
	Esophageal-tracheal Combitube	Endotracheal airway
Group 1 PaO_2	141.6 ± 43.1*	119.2 ± 39.9
	Endotracheal airway	Esophageal-tracheal Combitube
Group 2 PaO_2	117.4 ± 16.0	145.8 ± 13.3*

From Frass M et al. The esophageal-tracheal Combitube: preliminary results with a new airway for CPR. *Ann Emerg Med* 1987;16:769.

PaO_2, mean arterial oxygen tension in mm Hg ± standard deviation.

[a] Second airway inserted 20 minutes after initial airway.

*$p < 0.001$.

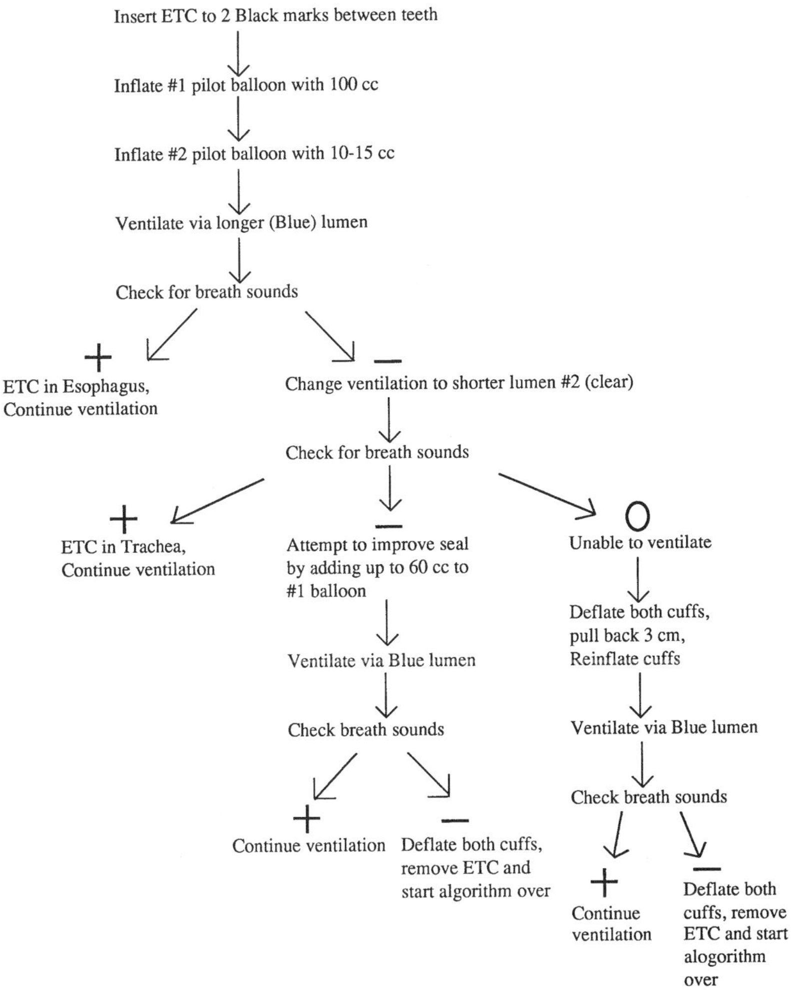

FIG. 5. Esophageal-tracheal Combitube (ETC) placement algorithm.

studies (8,10,12,15), and at least one study has compared it with mask ventilation (11). The studies have involved either elective surgical patients (10,11) or cardiopulmonary arrest patients (8,12,15). Using the same ventilatory parameters, oxygenation has consistently and significantly improved with the Combitube as compared with standard endotracheal intubation (Table 3). There has been no difference in oxygen tension of patients ventilated by bag valve mask vs. the esophageal-tracheal Combitube. A further study measuring ventilatory pressures has revealed a small positive end expiratory pressure (PEEP) effect of approximately 2 cm H_2O (11) accompanying use of the Combitube, attributed to a slightly prolonged expiratory flow via the perforations in the esophageal lumen. There is no difference in intrinsic PEEP levels generated during mask ventilation and ventilation via the Combitube, and similar PaO_2 levels are observed with these two methods of ventilation. There is no chance for right main bronchial intubation with the esophageal-tracheal Combitube, another potential reason for improved oxygenation with the Combitube as compared with endotracheal intubation. Although there is a statistically significant difference in oxygenation via the Combitube vs. endotracheal intubation, the clinical significance of this has been questioned (20).

Findings regarding $PaCO_2$ levels and pH related to use of the Combitube are inconsistent. $PaCO_2$ levels are higher with mask ventilation when compared with both the Combitube and endotracheal intubation. The corollary of this is that the pH levels are also lower with mask ventilation. This difference is caused by the greater anatomic dead space that occurs with mask ventilation. Air leakage is also highest with mask ventilation, providing less effective ventilation and therefore higher levels of $PaCO_2$. In terms of ventilatory capabilities of the Combitube versus endotracheal intubation, all published studies except one show statistically similar levels of $PaCO_2$ (Table 4). However, the majority of these same studies show a significant decrease in pH (Table 4). A confounding variable may be the design of the initial studies. In all but one study, patients with pulmonary disease (chronic obstructive pulmonary disease, pneumonia) were excluded. This exclusion may have masked a greater degree of difference in ventilation, although in the one study that did not exclude patients with chronic obstructive pulmonary disease, similar levels of $PaCO_2$ and pH were found.

TABLE 4. *pH and PCO_2 in cardiac arrest patients*

		Initial airway	Second airway[a]
		Esophageal-tracheal Combitube	Endotracheal airway
Group 1	pH	7.24 ± 0.1*	7.30 ± 0.1
	PCO_2	36.8 ± 3.5	36.3 ± 2.9
		Endotracheal airway	Esophageal-tracheal Combitube
Group 2	pH	7.28 ± 0.1*	7.21 ± 0.1
	PCO_2	36.4 ± 3.4	35.5 ± 3.7

From Frass M, Frenzer R, Rauscha F, et al. Ventilation with the esophageal-tracheal Combitube in cardiopulmonary resuscitation: promptness and effectiveness. *Chest* 1988;93: 782.

PCO_2, mean arterial carbon dioxide tension in mm Hg ± standard deviation.

[a]Second airway inserted 20 to 30 minutes after initial airway.

*$p < 0.001$.

TABLE 5. *Time to successful intubation in cardiac arrest patients*

		Initial airway	Second airway[a]
		Esophageal-tracheal Combitube	Endotracheal airway
Group 1	time[b]	27.3 ± 8.4*	39.0 ± 14.9
		Endotracheal airway	Esophageal-tracheal Combitube
Group 2	time[b]	39.7 ± 10.0	28.0 ± 4.8*

From Frass M, Frenzer R, Rauscha F, et al. Ventilation with the esophageal-tracheal Combitube in cardiopulmonary resuscitation: promptness and effectiveness. *Chest* 1988;93: 782.

[a]Second airway inserted 20 to 30 minutes after initial airway.

[b]Seconds ± standard deviation.

*$p < 0.001$.

The best conclusion from the available literature is that the Combitube provides excellent oxygenation and similar ventilation as compared with standard endotracheal intubation. Endotracheal intubation remains the preferred method for airway management. Unfortunately, endotracheal intubation is not always possible. The esophageal-tracheal Combitube is an acceptable alternative for effective ventilation and oxygenation in such situations. More subtle questions related to the efficiency of ventilation with the Combitube become irrelevant in the setting of the difficult airway where no ventilation is possible.

Training

A benefit of the Combitube is the reportedly short time to adequate placement (approximately 20 to 35 seconds). This is significantly shorter than the time required for endotracheal tube placement according to a crossover study of patients undergoing in-hospital cardiopulmonary resuscitation (12) (Table 5). In this study, the practitioners had experience with both airway devices. The Combitube was successfully placed 10 to 15 seconds more quickly than the endotracheal tube. Compared with endotracheal intubation, the skills required for Combitube placement do not need to be reinforced as often. Therefore, the difference in time to insertion between the Combitube and an endotracheal tube may be even greater in personnel who infrequently perform laryngoscopy.

The skills required for insertion of the Combitube are also more easily learned than those necessary for direct laryngoscopy. In a study involving intensive care unit nurses receiving only 2 hours of theory and mannequin demonstration, the Combitube was successfully placed in 16 of 17 cardiopulmonary arrest patients within 30 seconds (15). This suggests that paramedical personnel, with the proper training, can successfully use the Combitube to ventilate such patients as an alternative to intubation. By contrast, in a different study involving paramedics in a nonurban emergency medical system, there was only a 70% success rate of insertion of the esophageal-tracheal Combitube (21). However, the authors indicated that the training was flawed and the angle of insertion improper. There was also a relatively high rate of inadequate skills retention, further suggesting initially inadequate knowledge and training. Other experience with the Combitube by paramedical personnel has been more promising. In a series of 258 patients, the emergency medical system of Québec, Canada, reported a 98% insertion success rate (Dr. Daniel Lefrançois, written communication, 1994).

USES AND INDICATIONS

Cardiopulmonary Resuscitation

The prompt establishment of a patent airway and adequate ventilation during cardiopulmonary resuscitation is essential (22).

Cervical Spine Abnormalities

Another possible advantage of the Combitube over endotracheal intubation is that there is no need for neck movement with placement of the Combitube. This theoretically decreases the risk of cervical spine injuries in trauma victims (23) as well as in other surgical patients at risk, such as those with rheumatoid arthritis, in which subluxation of the atlantoaxial joint can occur (18).

Difficult Airways

While endotracheal intubation remains the preferred method of securing a patent airway, the Combitube has proved to be a valuable alternative in a number of clinical situations in which direct laryngoscopy has proved impossible. Since insertion of the Combitube does not require visualization of the larynx, the presence of blood and/or vomitus does not prevent its successful insertion. Case reports include the use of the Combitube in a patient whose neck was impaled by a piece of fence (24). Other case reports have described the use of the Combitube in cases of excessive bleeding associated with thrombolytic therapy (25) and cervical hematoma from inadvertent carotid puncture complicating central line placement (26).

In addition to its applications in trauma cases, the Combitube is one of three nonsurgical techniques for emergency airway ventilation in the American Society of Anesthesiologists (ASA) difficult airway algorithm (27) (Fig. 6). It has been estimated that direct visualization of the vocal cords and subsequent endotracheal intubation are impossible in between 15 and 35 patients per 10,000 (14). The two other techniques available in the "cannot intubate-cannot mask ventilate" setting are transtracheal jet ventilation (TTJV) and the laryngeal mask airway (LMA). Transtracheal jet ventilation requires special equipment and some degree of skill in locating the cricothyroid membrane, especially in obese patients with short necks (16). For these reasons, it has been suggested that the Combitube or LMA be tried prior to TTJV (20,28). The laryngeal mask airway, although often easy to place, does not protect against aspiration nor allow ventilation with peak pressures greater than approximately 20 cm H_2O (29). Therefore, in those at risk for aspiration, such as obese, obstetric, or emergency patients, the Combitube offers advantages over the LMA in terms of emergent airway control.

Once the esophageal-tracheal Combitube is in position and adequate ventilation and oxygenation have been achieved, a more definitive airway can be attempted. This can be accomplished by deflating the oropharyngeal balloon with a syringe (air is aspirated with a syringe attached to the pilot balloon of the oropharyngeal balloon) and performing direct laryngoscopy for endotracheal intubation around the Combitube. With the urgency of providing a patent airway and adequate oxygenation resolved by Combitube placement, a previously difficult (or failed) intubation may become more manageable (successful). The presence of the Combitube can also act as a guide to prevent esophageal intubation. If direct laryngoscopy is not successful, then other maneuvers (oral fiberoptic intubation using a mouth guide, nasal

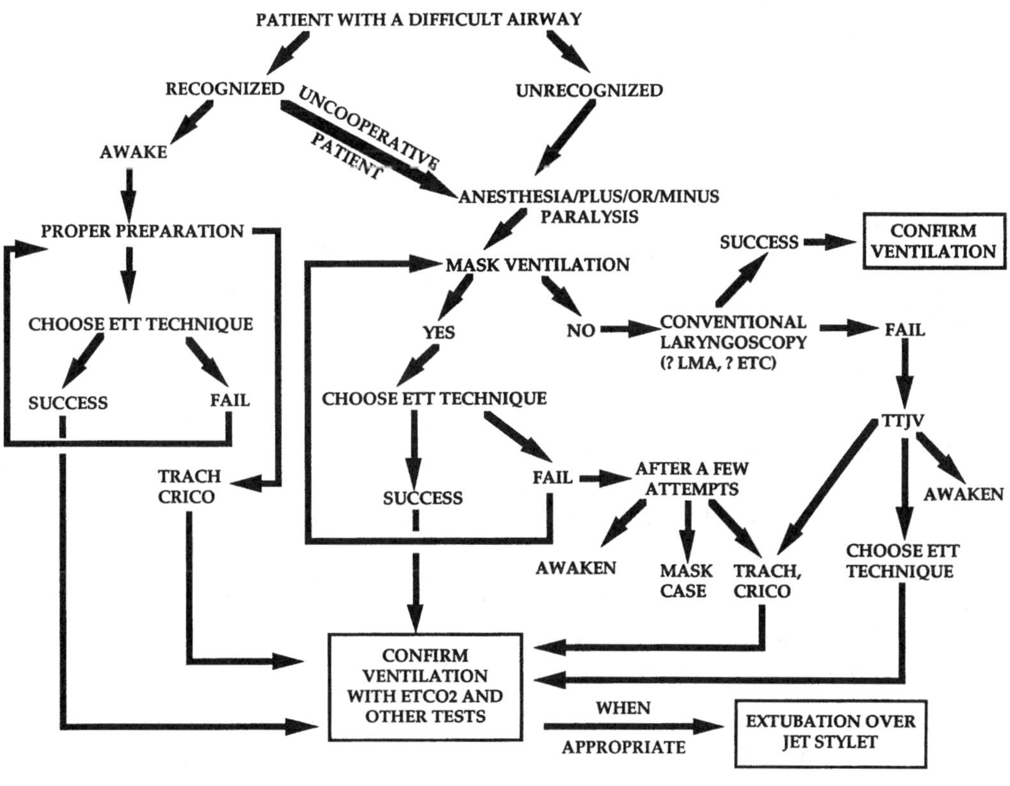

FIG. 6. American Society of Anesthesiologists (ASA) difficult airway algorithm. (From ASA Task Force. Practice guidelines for management of the difficult airway. *Anesthesiology* 1993;78:600, with permission.)

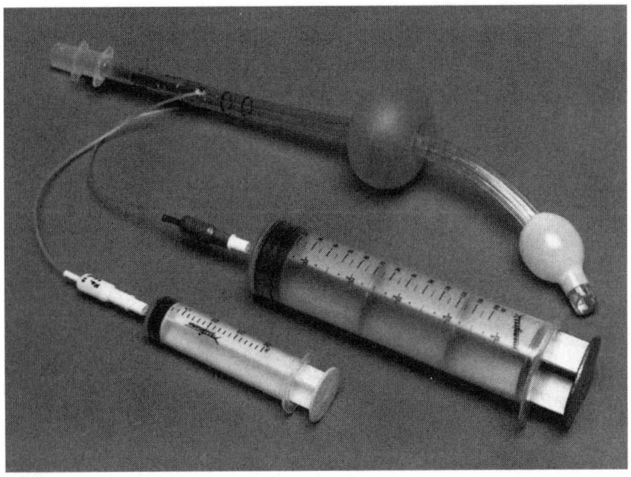

FIG. 7. Assembled esophageal-tracheal Combitube with both proximal and distal cuffs inflated.

fiberoptic intubation, or transillumination using a lighted stylet) can be attempted. Once an endotracheal tube is properly placed, the distal cuff of the Combitube is deflated. The Combitube can then be safely removed while the oropharynx is continuously suctioned. If there is difficulty in performing successful endotracheal intubation, then the oropharyngeal balloon can simply be reinflated for continued use of the Combitube. It is very important that the distal cuff of the Combitube remain inflated during any airway manipulation prior to endotracheal intubation (Fig. 7). This is necessary to prevent aspiration in the event of regurgitation.

If there is tracheal placement of the esophageal-tracheal Combitube, there is no immediate need to replace it with a standard endotracheal tube. The oropharyngeal balloon is simply deflated and the patient ventilated via the open (clear) lumen. If one is concerned about the size of the Combitube in the trachea (outer diameter distally is that of the largest-size double-lumen endotracheal tube) or the relatively small size of the open lumen (approximately that of a No. 5.5 endotracheal tube), a tube changer may be inserted through the No. 2 clear lumen and the Combitube exchanged for a standard endotracheal tube. The obvious hazard is the real potential for losing a relatively secured airway. Thus, if it is absolutely necessary to obtain a larger, more permanent airway for long-term ventilation, the literature suggests that the patient receive a formal tracheostomy performed under ideal conditions in an operating room setting (30). Careful clinical judgment must be used to select the appropriate method to establish a new airway after prior insertion of a Combitube.

Avoidance of Laryngeal Apparatus

It has also been suggested (18) that the Combitube can be used for elective airway management in individuals such as speakers, announcers, and singers, who rely on their voices and are afraid of possible damage to their vocal cords during endotracheal intubation. This may be possible with the Combitube, however, the laryngeal mask airway provides the same benefits for these patients and appears to be much better tolerated. The exception to the use of the LMA in these cases would be those patients considered to be at risk for aspiration.

CONTRAINDICATIONS AND PRECAUTIONS

Contraindications

Currently there are two sizes of esophageal-tracheal Combitubes, which account for the main absolute contraindication to use of the Combitube: a patient height of less than 4 feet (123 cm). The smaller model of the esophageal-tracheal Combitube (Combitube S.A., "small adult") has only recently been introduced. It should be useful in patients between 4 and 5 feet tall who are more than 11 to 12 years of age. Other contraindications include an intact gag reflex, since such patients will not tolerate the oropharyngeal cuff. If patients become responsive or agitated while the Combitube is in place, then they will require neuromuscular relaxation if prior ventilation has been effective. Alternatively, the Combitube can be removed if their clinical condition permits safe removal. If spontaneous ventilation returns, the oropharyngeal balloon can be deflated and the patient allowed to breath around the Combitube. Also, the presence of esophageal disease or prior ingestion of caustic substances contraindicate placement of an esophageal-tracheal Combitube. This contraindication is based on the concern for potential rupture of, or bleeding from, the esophagus; however, this complication has not yet been reported (10). A final contraindication is upper airway obstruction, such as the presence of a foreign body, severe glottic edema, or epiglottitis (Table 2).

Precautions and Concerns

Overall, there is a relatively small published clinical experience with use of the Combitube. The Combitube has been inserted in over 300 patients in various published studies with no reported complications (15). The EOA, on the other hand, has been used in over 1.5 million patients. There are several concerns regarding routine use of the esophageal-tracheal Combitube. Perhaps the greatest impediment to routine use of the Combitube is the past problems encountered with the EOA. Although the esophageal-tracheal Combitube has some features in common with the EOA, it has been specifically designed to avoid its potential complications.

There is also some concern regarding nasopharyngeal, oropharyngeal, or tracheal mucosal damage or edema with the use of this airway device. However, in case studies involving patients who were mechanically ventilated via the Combitube for 2 to 8 hours, there has been no gross evidence on autopsy of any mucosal injury (13,31). Other limited autopsy data have failed to reveal any microscopic or macroscopic evidence of aspiration, nor any injury to the mouth, pharynx, or esophagus (13). Nevertheless, as usage of this device increases, the potential for reports of damage to the airway may also increase.

As stated before, when the esophageal-tracheal Combitube is in the esophageal position, the trachea cannot be suctioned. Except in the rare patient with excessive secretions or need for bronchoscopy, this does not appear to be problematic. In addition, the added small PEEP effect actually tends to improve oxygenation. Finally, the esophageal-tracheal Combitube is a single-use airway device that currently sells for approximately $48.00 in the United States. This could preclude its routine daily use.

TROUBLESHOOTING

There are several important points to be emphasized regarding the placement of the Combitube. First of all, the clear lumen can be used for suctioning gastric contents with the enclosed 12F catheter when the Combitube is placed in the esophagus (up to 98% occurrence). Obviously, if the esophageal-tracheal Combitube is in the esophagus, it is impossible to suction the trachea. This has not, however, been shown to cause a clinically significant problem during its use. Other important reminders are that when the Combitube is placed, it does not matter whether it has been placed in the trachea or the esophagus. It is merely important to verify position (esophageal vs. tracheal) so that the appropriate lumen can be utilized to ventilate and oxygenate the patient. Although a laryngoscope blade can be used to move the base of the tongue out of the way during placement, it should not be used to attempt to locate the larynx. It is very important to keep the Combitubes in the midline during its insertion. This helps to avoid any blind pockets, such as the vallecula. One way of helping to ensure a midline course is to have an assistant put gentle pressure on both sides of the anterior neck during insertion. Finally, the head should be placed in a neutral position, not the routine sniffing position that is best for endotracheal tube placement.

Probably the most important factor in terms of successful placement of the esophageal-tracheal Combitube is adequate education and training. The Combitube, although relatively easy to use and insert, does require some degree of familiarity. Insertion of the Combitube into mannequins should be practiced until there is relative ease of insertion. Once this is accomplished, it is suggested that trainees place the Combitube in a few elective, fasted patients who appear to have relatively normal airway anatomy. (Appropriate consent, supervision, and credentials of personnel are, of course, necessary.) This is the only certain way to become familiar enough with the device in the clinical setting to be comfortable with its use for emergency airway management. It should be emphasized that when using the Combitube in an elective case, it is important to ensure that the patient is paralyzed to prevent any response to the oropharyngeal balloon. The rate of successful insertion of any airway device depends on prior experience with that device. The esophageal-tracheal Combitube is no exception.

SUMMARY AND CONCLUSIONS

In conclusion, the esophageal-tracheal Combitube is a quick, easy-to-use, emergency airway device. It has advantages for patients in whom manipulation of the cervical spine is hazardous or impossible (e.g., trauma, rheumatoid arthritis), and for patients at risk for aspiration (e.g., cesarean section, morbid obesity) (19). Once in place, it provides sufficient ventilation and oxygenation as compared with routine endotracheal intubation. In addition, endotracheal intubation can be performed around the Combitube without fear of losing the airway. The main disadvantage is that there are currently only two sizes available and, therefore, it should not be used in patients less than 4 feet tall.

One should practice inserting the esophageal-tracheal Combitube under controlled conditions before attempting its use with a difficult airway. With experience, the practitioner then will have another nonsurgical option for air way management when faced with the patient who can neither be intubated or mask ventilated.

REFERENCES

1. DonMichael TA. Comparison of the esophageal obturator airway and endotracheal intubation in prehospital ventilation during CPR. *Chest* 1985;87:814.
2. Meislin HW. The esophageal obturator airway: a study of respiratory effectiveness. *Ann Emerg Med* 1980;9:54.
3. Smith JP, Bodui BI, Seifkin A, et al. The esophageal obturator airway: a review. *JAMA* 1983;250:1081.
4. Bass RR, Allison EJ, Hunt RC. The esophageal obturator airway: a reassessment of use by paramedics. *Ann Emerg Med* 1982;11:358.
5. Gertler JP, Cameron DE, Shea K, Baker CC. The esophageal obturator airway: obturator or obtundator? *J Trauma* 1985;25:424.
6. Yancey W, Wears R, Kamajian G, et al. Unrecognized tracheal intubation: a complication of the esophageal obturator airway. *Ann Emerg Med* 1980;9:18.
7. Crippen D, Olvey S, Graffis R. Gastric rupture: an esophageal obturator airway complication. *Ann Emerg Med* 1981;10:370.
8. Frass M, Frenzer R, Rauscha F, Weber H, Pacher R, Leithner C. Evaluation of esophageal tracheal combitube in cardiopulmonary resuscitation. *Crit Care Med* 1986;15:609.
9. Harrison EE, Nord HJ, Beeman RW. Esophageal perforation follow-

ing use of the esophageal obturator airway. *Ann Emerg Med* 1980; 9:21.
10. Frass M, Frenzer R, Zdrahal F, Hoflehner G, Porges P, Lackner F. The esophageal tracheal combitube: preliminary results with a new airway for CPR. *Ann Emerg Med* 1987;16:768.
11. Frass M, Rödler S, Frenzer R, Ilias W, Leithner C, Lackner F. Esophageal tracheal combitube, endotracheal airway, and mask: comparison of ventilatory pressure curves. *J Trauma* 1989;29: 1476.
12. Frass M, Frenzer R, Rauscha F, Schuster E, Glogar D. Ventilation with the esophageal tracheal combitube in cardiopulmonary resuscitation—promptness and effectiveness. *Chest* 1988;93:781.
13. Frass M, Frenzer R, Mayer G, Popovic R, Leithner C. Mechanical ventilation with the esophageal tracheal combitube (ETC) in the intensive care unit. *Arch Emerg Med* 1987;4:219.
14. Benumof JL. Management of the difficult adult airway. *Anesthesiology* 1991;75:1087.
15. Staudinger T, Brugger S, Watschinger B, Roggla M, Dielacher C, Lobl T, Fink D, Klauser R, Frass M. Emergency intubation with the combitube: comparison with the endotracheal airway. *Ann Emerg Med* 1993;72:1573.
16. Banyai M, Falyer S, Röggla M, Brugger S, Staudinger T, Frass M, et al. Emergency intubation with the combitube in a grossly obese patient with bull neck. *Resuscitation* 1993;26:271.
17. Johnson JC, Atherton GL. The esophageal tracheal combitube. *JEMS* 1991;May:29.
18. Frass M, Johnson JC, Atherton GL, Fruhwald FX, Traindl O, Schwaighofer B, Leithner C. Esophageal tracheal combitube (ETC) for emergency intubation: anatomical evaluation of ETC placement by radiography. *Resuscitation* 1989;18:95.
19. Green KS, Beger TH. Proper use of the combitube. *Anesthesiology* 1994;81:513.
20. Wissler R. The esophageal-tracheal combitube. *Anesthesiol Rev* 1993;20:147.
21. Atherton GL, Johnson JC. Ability of paramedics to use the combitube in prehospital cardiac arrest. *Ann Emerg Med* 1993;22:1263.
22. Hammargren Y, Clinton JE, Ruiz E. A standard comparison of esophageal obturator airway and endotracheal tube ventilation in cardiac arrest. *Ann Emerg Med* 1985;14:953.
23. Majernick TG, Bieniek R, Houston JB, et al. Cervical spine movement during orotracheal intubation. *Ann Emerg Med* 1986;15:417.
24. Eichinger S, Schreiber W, Heinz T, Kier P, Dufek V, Goldin M, Leithner C, Frass M. Airway management in a case of neck impalement: use of the oesophageal tracheal combitube airway. *Br J Anaesth* 1992;68:534.
25. Klauser R, Röggla G, Pidlich J, Leithner C, Frass M. Massive upper airway bleeding after thrombolytic therapy: successful airway management with the combitube. *Ann Emerg Med* 1992;21:431-433.
26. Bigenzahn W, Pesau B, Frass M. Emergency ventilation using the combitube in cases of difficult intubation. *Eur Arch Otorhinolaryngol* 1991;248:129.
27. American Society of Anesthesiologists Task Force on Management of the Difficult Airway. Practice guidelines for management of the difficult airway. *Anesthesiology* 1993;78:597.
28. Jantzen JAH, Gouldson R, Giesecke AH. Airway management for the trauma patient. *Semin Anesth* 1993;12:192.
29. Griffen RM, Hatcher IS. Aspiration pneumonia and the laryngeal mask airway. *Anaesthesia* 1990;45:1039.
30. Wiltschke C, Kment G, Swoboda H, Knöbl P, Frass M, et al. Ventilation with the combitube during tracheostomy. *Laryngoscope* 1994; 104:763.
31. Frass M, Frenzer R, Zahler J, Ilias W, Leithner C. Ventilation via the esophageal tracheal combitube in a case of difficult intubation. *J Cardiothorac Anesth* 1987;1:565.

Airway Management, edited by
L.H. Hanowell, M.D. and R.J. Waldron, M.D.,
Lippincott-Raven Publishers, Philadelphia © 1996.

CHAPTER 15

Laryngoscope Blades and Lighted Stylets

Sheila D. Cooper

INTRODUCTION

Components of a Laryngoscope

The basic components of a laryngoscope are the handle, blade, and light source. The two main categories of handles consist of the *L* type and the *U* type. The *U* type introduced by Jackson (see later section) has been abandoned in favor of the *L* type, which is lighter and less bulky. Most handles lie at a right angle to the blade but there have been several modifications of the angle of the handle to the blade to facilitate entry of the blade into the oropharynx in specific clinical situations (i.e., Polio blade to intubate patients in an iron lung machine) that diminish the tendency to utilize the upper incisors as a fulcrum during direct laryngoscopy. The handle can be further classified based on the method of attachment to the blade. There are permanently attached blades (rarely found today) and "hook-on" folding blades. This hook-on or hinged folding mechanism not only facilitates attachment of the blade to the handle but contains an automated switch to provide illumination from the light source when the blade is lifted into the working position.

S. D. Cooper: Department of Anesthesia, University of California, San Diego Medical Center, San Diego, California 92103.

The earliest laryngoscope utilized proximal lighting, i.e., the light sources came from a point between the laryngoscopist and the laryngoscope. Examples of commonly used proximal light sources included head-mirrors, head-lamps, and electric lights directed into the oropharynx by a prism or mirror. The invention of the electric light bulb carrier by Einhorn in 1902 led to the introduction of distal lighting in 1907 by Jackson, which provided illumination to the blade tip. In 1913, Janeway incorporated the battery into the handle to power the light source, which has become a standard for laryngoscopes used by anesthesiologists (1). Morch's laryngoscope (2) incorporated the light source in the handle so that blades of any design can be attached to the handle.

The blade itself is composed of the spatula, flange, and tip. The spatula is designed to compress and manipulate the soft tissues of the lower jaw to facilitate a direct line of vision past the upper incisors and around the bulk of the tongue to get a view of the larynx during direct laryngoscopy. The long axis of the spatula is either straight or curved in all or part of its length. The flange projects off the side of the spatula to deflect tissues out of the line of vision during laryngoscopy. The flange is a component of the cross-sectional shape of the blade, and this shape varies from blade to blade; from no flange so that the blade resembles a straight or curved tongue depressor

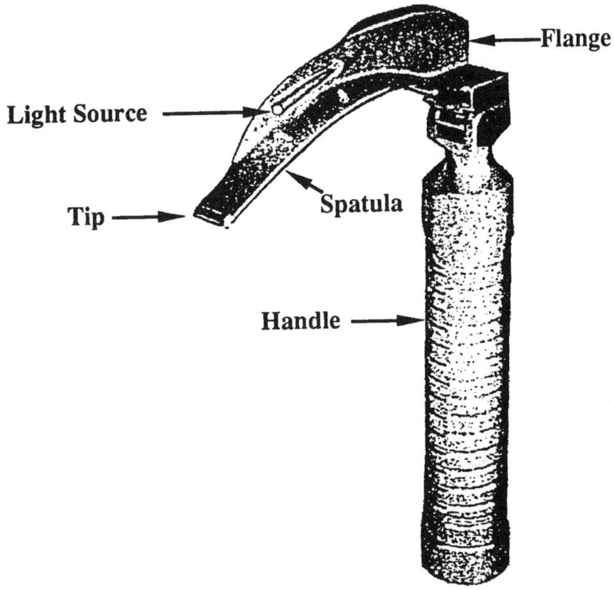

FIG. 1. The components of a laryngoscope.

(e.g., the double-angle blade) to a completely closed tube or *O*-shaped blade. Intermediate cross-sectional curves include a *C*, a flattened *C*, a *U* turned on its side, or a *Z* in reverse (i.e., **Σ**). The vertical height of the cross-sectional shape of a blade is occasionally referred to as the *step*.

The blade tip is designed to either directly or indirectly elevate the epiglottis to facilitate a view of the larynx. The tip of straight blades is one of multiple designs; it has been ridged, curved, slotted, and hooked in an effort to directly lift the epiglottis more effectively. Solutions to aid in indirect elevation of the epiglottis have included various curved and angled blades to blades that have bifid tips that straddle the hyoepiglottic ligament in the vallecula. The blade tip or "beak" is blunt and thickened to prevent trauma to the oropharyngeal tissues and is either flat, curved, or slightly uplifted. Figure 1 illustrates the basic components of a laryngoscope.

The Original Direct Vision Laryngoscopes

Over 50 descriptions of laryngoscope blade designs have been published since William MacEwan, a distinguished surgeon of the Glasgow Royal Infirmary, first passed a tube through the mouth into the trachea using his fingers as the guide in 1878. This method of intubation by palpation continued for several decades, and even in experienced hands it was an uncertain and often traumatic event. Although indirect laryngoscopy using a mirror antedated MacEwan's experience [a method originally used by Manuel Garcia in 1854 and then Turck and Czermak (3)], many clinicians had the misconception that it would be impossible to visualize the vocal cords directly while passing an endotracheal tube (ETT), due the geometric relationship between the mouth and the vocal cords. This notion was dispelled by the introduc-

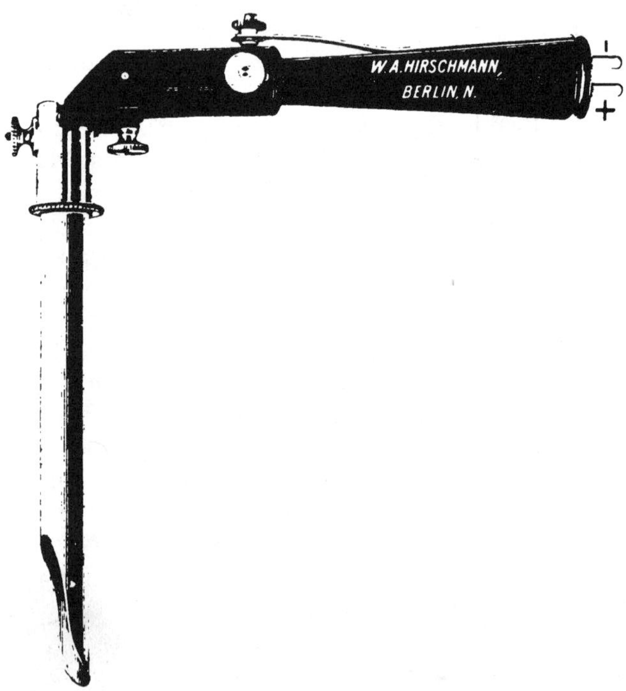

FIG. 2. Kirstein's original autoscope.

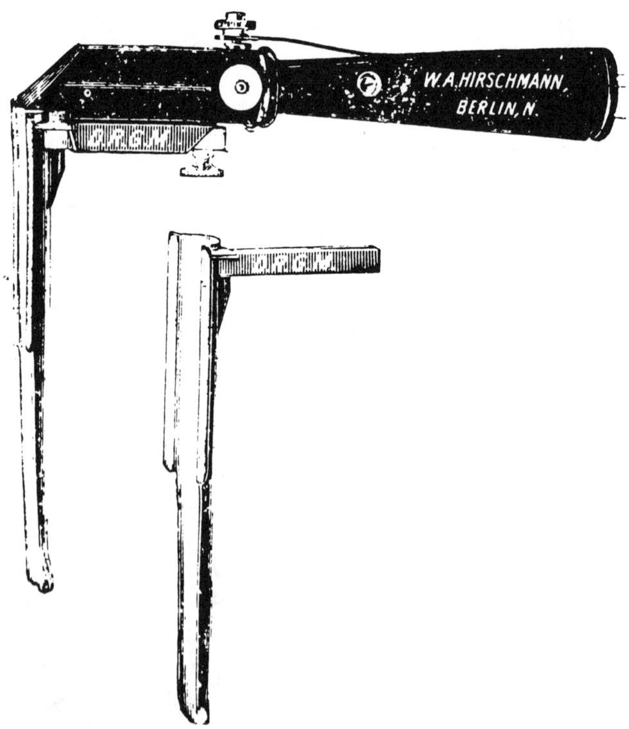

FIG. 3. Kirstein's modified autoscope. The standard blade is attached to the handle and the intralaryngeal blade is shown separately.

tion of the first direct vision laryngoscope by Alfred Kirstein in Berlin in 1895.

Kirstein's "autoscope" was the forerunner of the modern laryngoscope. It was developed after Kirstein's colleague Rosenheim had informed him that an esophageal scope had accidentally slipped into the trachea, giving rise to a perfect view of the bronchial bifurcation. From this information, Kirstein devised a reproducible method of viewing the larynx directly. His initial device consisted of a 25-cm esophagoscope attached to an electroscope (an electric hand lamp) that was used as the handle (Fig. 2) (4). He termed this combination electroscope/esophagoscope the *autoscope*. Due to the concern about the pressure the autoscope placed on the upper incisors and the marked neck extension necessary for direct laryngoscopy, he modified the original autoscope by replacing the cylindrical esophagoscope with one of two different designs of semicircular blades (Fig. 3), which are strikingly similar to those described in the 1940s by Macintosh (5) and Miller (6). Kirstein's other claim to fame was his appreciation of proper positioning of the patient's head, and he was most certainly the first to describe what is now referred to as the *sniff* or McGill position.

Gustav Killian, a pupil of Kirstein, enthusiastically supported his concepts and used this auto- or laryngoscope. He was not only the first to introduce a tube into the trachea but also used the Kirstein laryngoscope to aid in the first successful extraction of a foreign body from the right mainstem bronchus via the translaryngeal route on March 30, 1897. He subsequently performed other successful foreign body translaryngeal extractions using a suspension laryngoscope, and he is commonly referred to as the father of bronchoscopy (7). The Kirstein direct vision laryngoscope initially had no light attached to it and was used in conjunction with an electric light that was reflected down the lumen by a prism. Electrical wires trailed from the laryngoscope to a separate battery box, and eventually the cord was passed through the hollow handle of the instrument. This arrangement continued until 1913 when the battery itself was housed in the handle, making the entire apparatus self-contained and much easier to handle (8).

The development of the ordinary hand laryngoscope can be attributed to multiple individuals, most notably, Chevalier Jackson in 1907. His straight-bladed laryngoscope with the *O*-shaped flange had a *U* type handle that looked like three sides of a square with the lifting handgrip parallel to the blade. This facilitated exposure of the larynx without applying direct pressure to the upper teeth (Fig. 4) (9). The Jackson laryngoscope became a standard instrument for laryngeal examinations and was utilized to directly inspect the vocal cords prior to intubation, a technique advocated by Charles Elsberg, a New York surgeon, in 1912. Jackson pointed out that the use of a gag (e.g., a suspension laryngoscope), commonly employed by other laryngoscopists of that day, should be abandoned because a sufficiently anesthetized patient should not need one and wide gagging defeats exposure of the larynx by jamming the mandible. He also commented that "the most important thing of all is the position of the patient, and next to that comes recognition of the epiglottis, and then

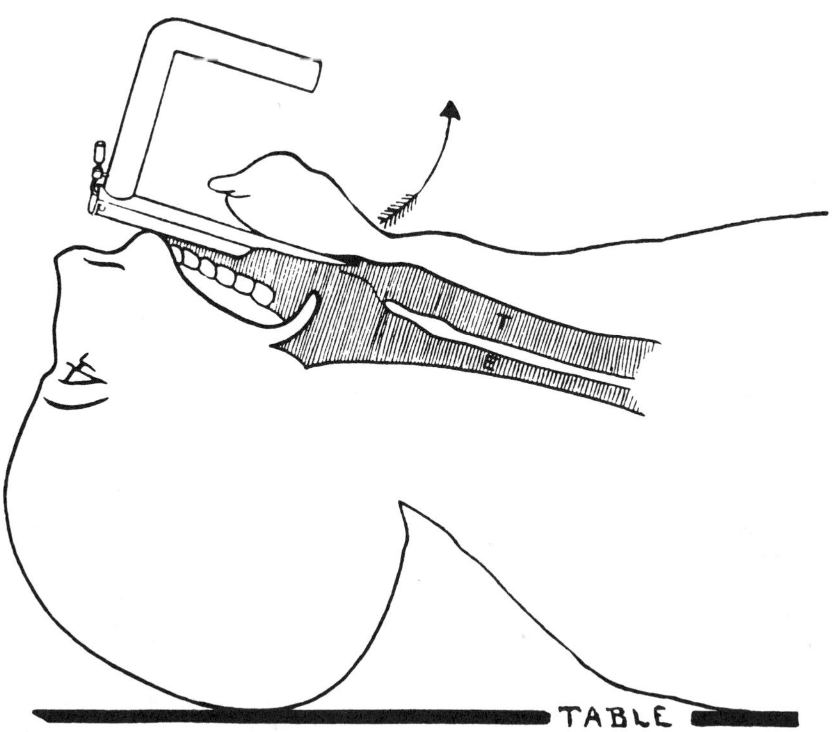

FIG. 4. The Jackson laryngoscope positioned in the oropharynx. The arrow illustrates the direction of motion that should be imparted on the laryngoscope blade to assist in exposure of the larynx and insertion of an endotracheal tube.

the application of a proper lifting motion of the hyoid bone which all aid in exposing the larynx." (9)

The use of the straight *O*-shaped Jackson blade continued for many years despite the introduction of a slightly curved *O*-shaped blade attached to an *L*-type handle by Henry Janeway, another American surgeon, in 1913 (10, 11). His instrument was notable for the first laryngoscope to have an internal light source powered by batteries contained in the handle. The use of *O*-shaped tube-like blades was a carryover from the esophagoscope used in the late nineteenth century. This closed tube was either slotted or segmented to facilitate its removal after the introduction of a bronchoscope. As the laryngoscope became more commonly used for orotracheal intubation, the lateral segment was removed completely (usually on the right side) so that the blade became *C*-shaped.

The best known examples of the original *C*-shaped straight blades are the Magill (1920) and Flagg (1928) laryngoscopes. In an effort to decrease the amount of volume the blade occupied in the oropharynx, the *C* shape was flattened in the upper portion (i.e., the flat *C* shape) [Elam (1935), Murphy (ca. 1940), Miller (1941), Wis-Foregger (ca. 1940)] and in the upper and lower curves (i.e., to produce a lateral *U* shape) [Bruening (1909), Guedel (1927), Waters-Hipple (ca. 1940)]. Other changes in the shape of the flange cross-sectional area included a reverse *Z*-shape (Ƹ) [Seldon (1938), Macintosh (1943)] and a shallow upside-down and reversed *L* (˥) [Bennett (1943)]. Despite the many modifications of laryngoscopes, particularly the blade shape, only the Macintosh and Miller laryngoscope blades introduced in the 1940s have achieved lasting popularity.

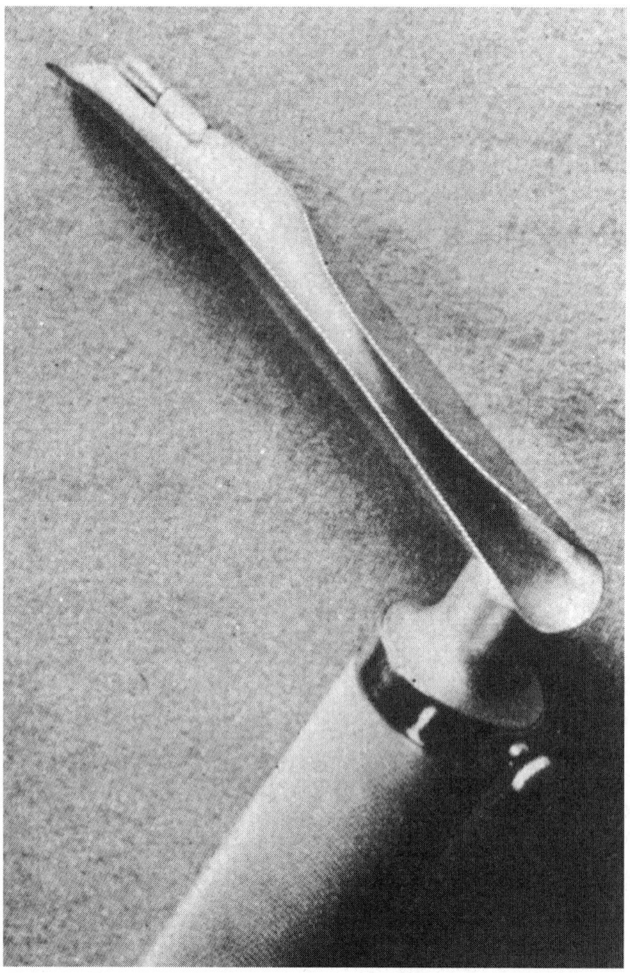

FIG. 5. The original Miller laryngoscope blade. Note the long, narrow shape.

The Miller Laryngoscope Blade

By 1941 Miller recognized that existing laryngoscopes were too thick at the base, thereby increasing the risk of trauma to the teeth. He additionally noted that the blade tips did not have the proper shape to lift the epiglottis, the blades were often too short, the curve of the blades were too distal, and the flat bottom tended to push the tongue against the floor of the mouth, thereby inhibiting adequate exposure in "difficult" patients (i.e., those with a deep throat, thick tongue, or prominent upper incisors) (6). To overcome these deficiencies, Miller designed a laryngoscope that is longer, rounded on the bottom, smaller at the tip, has a shallower base, and has an extra curve beginning 2 inches from the distal tip (Fig. 5). These changes resulted in less required mouth opening and allowed for freer anterior movement of the mandible so that when the small round end of the blade presses up against the tongue and the distal tip entraps the epiglottis,

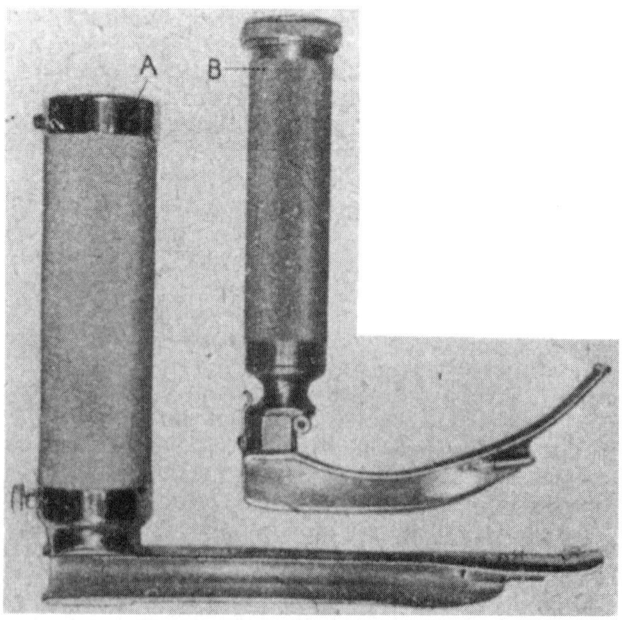

FIG. 6. A: The standard Miller long straight laryngoscope blade. **B:** The Macintosh short curved blade.

a channel is created through which the larynx is exposed. Miller noted that although the epiglottic entrapment technique of intubation is utilized, the decrease in required mouth opening limited the area for tube manipulation, so that it is often necessary to use a stylet in order to pass a larger ETT. Since its introduction, the Miller blade has become the standard to which other subsequently developed laryngoscope blades are compared.

The Macintosh Laryngoscope Blade

Although his original laryngoscope blade was fashioned after a Boyle-Davis gag, Macintosh recognized the limitations of a suspension laryngoscope and in 1943 introduced his sharply curved blade specifically designed not to entrap the epiglottis (Fig. 6). He quotes Human (12) as advising that in some cases the blade of the laryngoscope should be passed only until the epiglottis comes into view and then the ETT should be guided behind the epiglottis into the trachea. The Macintosh laryngoscope blade is introduced into the right side of the mouth, pushing the tongue to the left and is advanced until the distal tip of the short curved blade rests in the glossoepiglottic fold (vallecula) (Fig. 7). Upward traction is exerted on the base of the tongue by lifting the laryngoscope to elevate the epiglottis upward, facilitating exposure of the larynx (Fig. 8). If the tongue

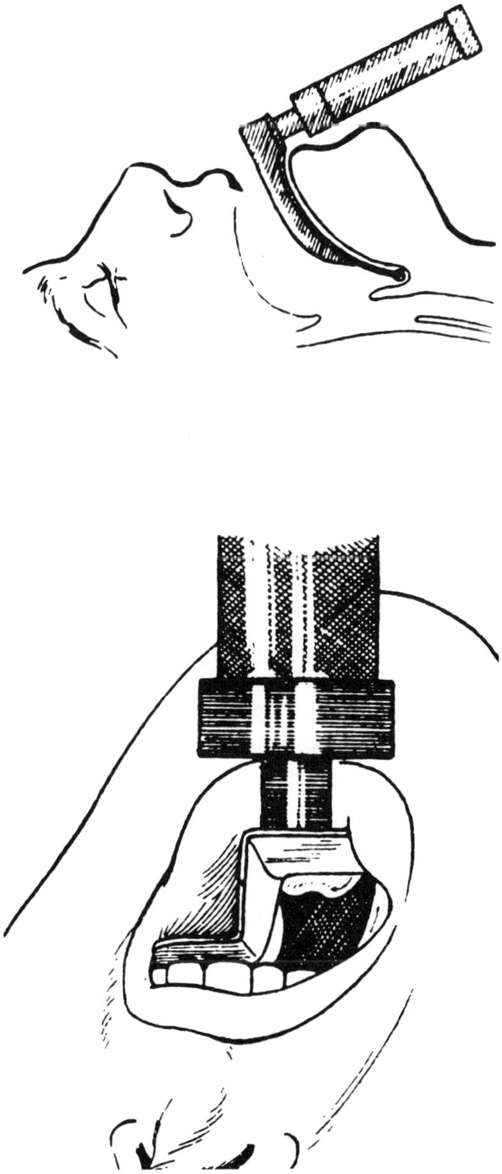

FIG. 7. Correct positioning and view obtained prior to lifting the Macintosh laryngoscope blade.

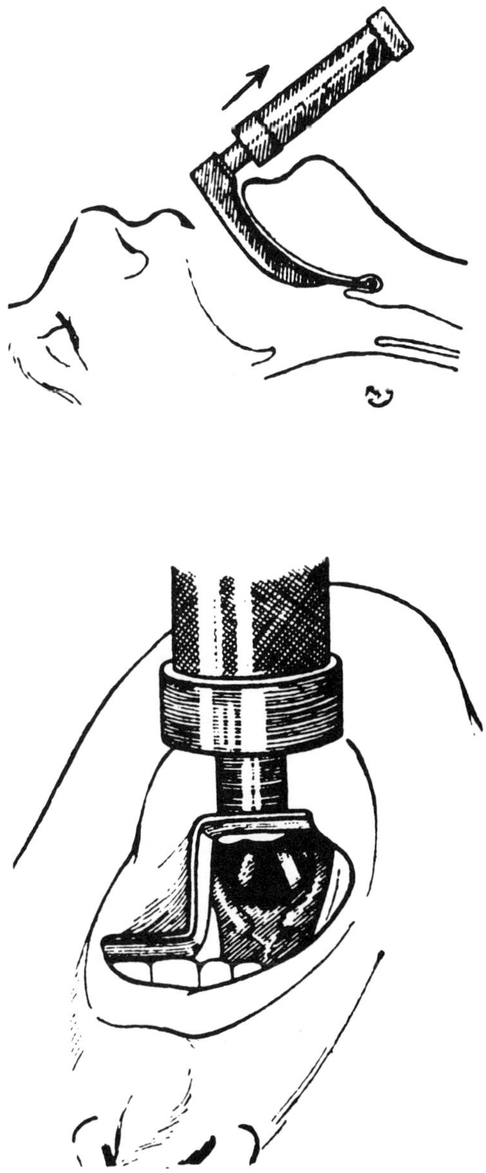

FIG. 8. The direction of motion applied to the Macintosh laryngoscope blade and the view obtained of the larynx.

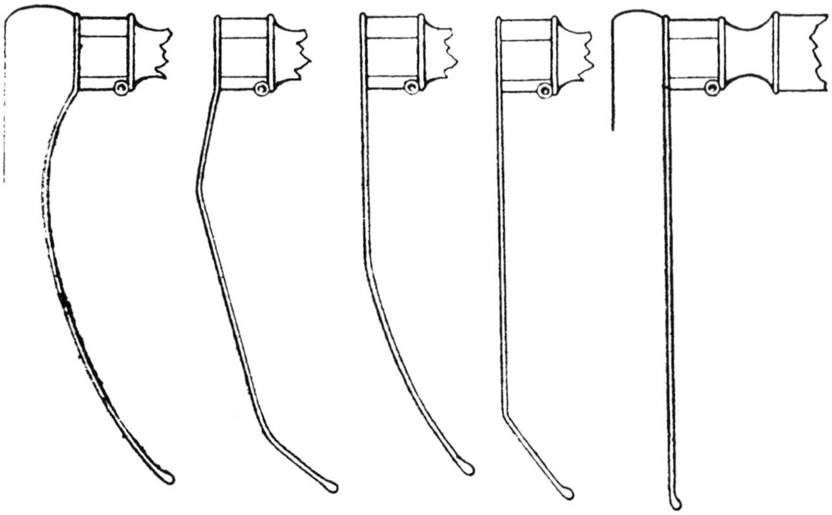

FIG. 9. The range of blade curvatures Sir Robert Macintosh experimented with in developing the final version of the Macintosh blade *(far left).*

is not adequately retracted to the left and bulges over the blade, the view of the larynx is obscured. Due to the diminished blade contact with the extensively innervated epiglottis, Macintosh claimed it could be utilized under a lighter plane of anesthesia. He also claimed that his blade design resulted in less risk of damage to the teeth, owing to its completely open top section. He further explained that the shape of the blade did not matter greatly, provided it did not go beyond or make contact with the epiglottis and that the degree of curvature accommodated the natural curve of a Magill-type ETT. In fact, he used blades ranging from those with a well-marked curve to those that were perfectly straight (Fig. 9) (13). Many refinements followed from different inventors. A hinge was incorporated between the blade and handle by the Welch-Allyn Company so that the blade could be folded against the handle, allowing for easy transportation (14). An automated switch was later incorporated into the hinge mechanism to provide illumination from the light source when the blade is lifted into the working position. The Foregger Company was given the right to copy the Macintosh laryngoscope blade for the North American market in 1943. The inventors (Macintosh and Mr. Salt, the senior chief technician of the Nuffield Department of Anaesthetics) sent a prototype to Foregger, expecting their engineers to refine it, only to discover later that the blade had been marketed in its original form.

From the principle three laryngoscope blade types—straight blade (Jackson), curved tip (Miller), and curved (Macintosh)—many modifications have been proposed because even in the most experienced hands, there were still occasional patients in whom intubation was found to be difficult or impossible with existing technics. Most of these modifications were attempts to overcome specific anatomic variations of the mouth or pharynx that contribute to intubation difficulties. A broad categorization of these variations includes: an anterior larynx, limited mouth opening, decreased size of the infra-oral cavity, immobile or unstable cervical spine, and a large or protruding sternal region (15). In order to emphasize clinical function, the more effective and more commonly used adult laryngoscope blades developed since the introduction of the Miller and Macintosh blades are organized into these categories. Although they are placed in a specific category based on the primary anatomic variation that they were designed to overcome, there is considerable overlap such that many of the blades might fit under multiple categories. Where appropriate, this is elaborated on in the following sections.

MODIFICATIONS OF LARYNGOSCOPE BLADES BASED ON SPECIFIC ANATOMIC VARIATIONS

The Anterior Larynx

Siker Laryngoscope Blade

Description

In addition to assisting with exposure of an anterior larynx, the Siker blade (1959) was developed to overcome other anatomic variations, such as a recessed mandible, prominent and/or overriding upper incisors (buck teeth), and an increased tongue size, all of which contributed to intubation difficulty (16). Siker incorporated a mirror onto the blade that is positioned 3 inches from the distal tip (Fig. 10). The blade distal to the mirror makes an angle of 135° to the 2.5-inch proximal portion. The mirror is attached to the blade via a copper jacket that facilitates conduction of the patient's heat to minimize fogging of the mirror during exhalation.

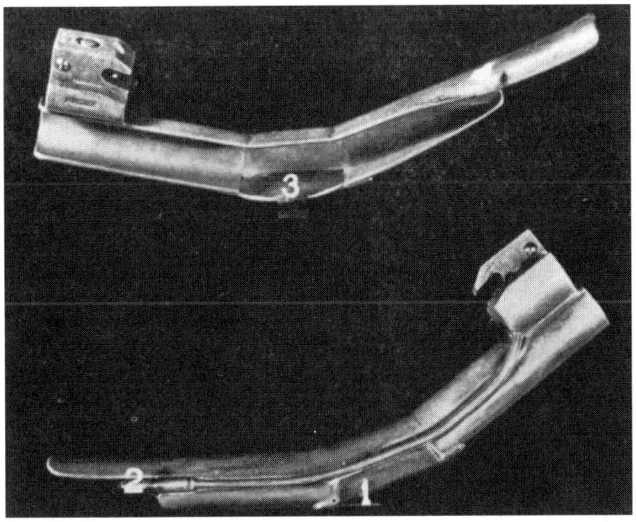

FIG. 10. The Siker mirror laryngoscope. 1, Copper jacket; 2, Light source; 3, Stainless steel mirror.

Technique

The original description of the technique for using this laryngoscope cautioned that the operator become conditioned to viewing and working with inverted structures, since the mirror reflects an inverted image. Keeping this in mind, the blade is inserted in the usual manner, pushing the tongue to the left side, with the operator looking through the proximal mirror to view the structures at the distal end of the blade. Once the oropharyngeal curve is negotiated, the epiglottis appears in the lower portion of the mirror and is then elevated with the tip of the blade. When a view of the vocal cords is obtained, an ETT is inserted with the aid of the stylet to help direct it around the curvature of the laryngoscope blade. As the ETT is passed through the laryngeal inlet, the reflected image in the mirror will appear as though the tube is moving in a posterocaudad direction. When the tip of the ETT passes through the cords, the laryngoscope is removed and intubation is completed by threading the ETT off the stylet and into the trachea.

Clinical Experience

Initial experience by Siker with his blade was extremely favorable. Out of one hundred randomly selected patients who required endotracheal intubation, laryngoscopy was successfully performed in all but one patient. This one failure was attributed to the large size of the blade; the distal tip was in the larynx prior to the mirror entering the oral cavity. Furthermore, Siker cited three cases in which laryngoscopy and intubation were easily accomplished with his blade where the "classical" (Miller) and Macintosh laryngoscope blades had failed (16). The primary disadvantage of this instrument is that extensive practice is required to become adept at its use, thereby necessitating a committed period of learning, even in the hands of very experienced laryngoscopists. The Siker laryngoscope blade is rarely used today.

Belscope

Description

The Belscope is an angulated, straight-bladed laryngoscope bent forward 45° at the midpoint and is available in three lengths (6.7, 8, and 9 cm from tip to angle) (Fig. 11) (17). It was designed to combine the attractive features of both straight and curved laryngoscope blades and is similar conceptually to the Siker blade; a prism mechanism provides an indirect view of the larynx to assist with difficult intubations. When the angle of the blade blocks a view of the larynx, the prism is utilized to "see" around this corner and to provide an indirect view of the glottic opening. This may be easier to conceptualize than the inverted image obtained by looking in the mirror with the Siker blade. In contrast to the Siker blade, it is less bulky and has an inverted, *L*-shaped cross-section (as opposed to the *C*-shaped cross section of the Siker blade), so that in the majority of laryngoscopies a direct view of the larynx is obtained, making it useful for routine intubations as well. Compared to the Macintosh blade, the Belscope

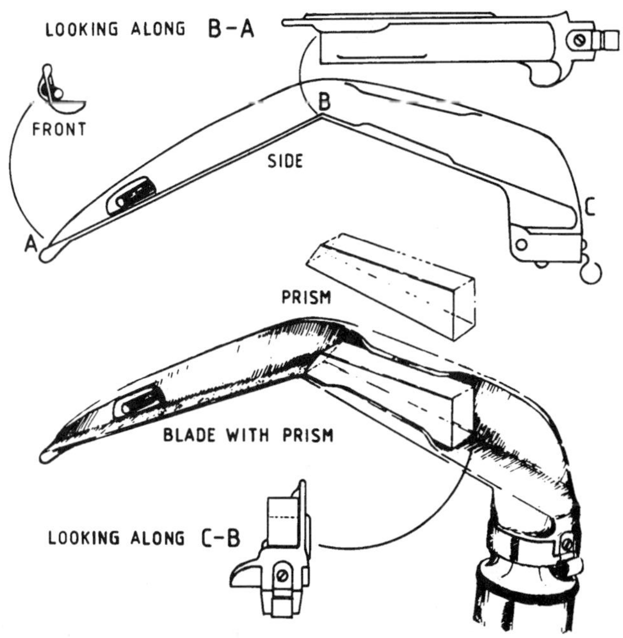

FIG. 11. Scale drawings of the "Belscope" angulated laryngoscope. **Upper:** Looking forward from the angle along the distal part of the blade in direction B-A. **Lower:** Prism in position on the blade. When the prism is utilized, a view of the larynx is obtained by looking down line C-B through the prism.

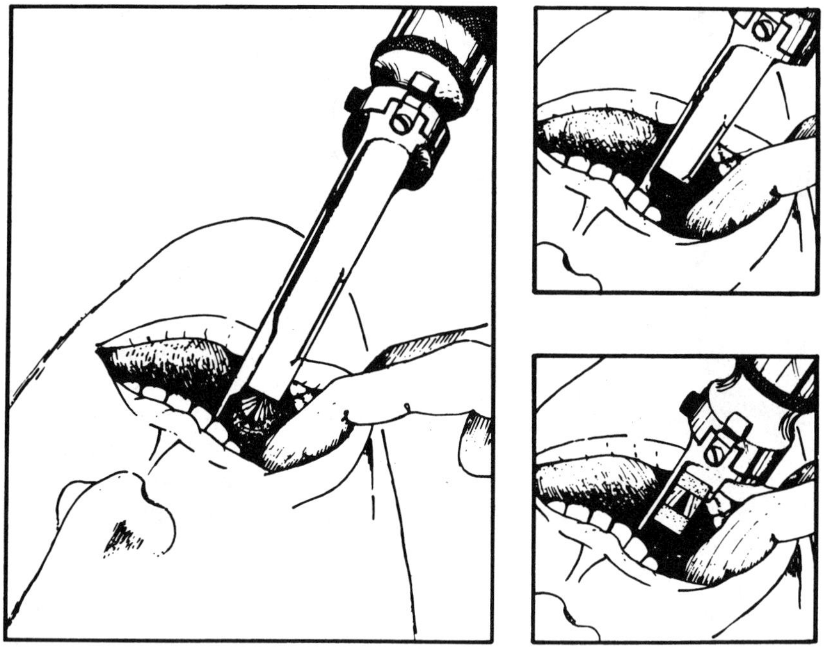

FIG. 12. The angulated laryngoscope in the oropharynx facilitating a direct view of the larynx *(left)*. An illustration of the uncommon situation where oropharyngeal tissues push the laryngoscope angle back into the pharynx, obscuring a view of the larynx *(upper right)*. Attachment of the prism affords an indirect view of the larynx in this situation *(lower right)*.

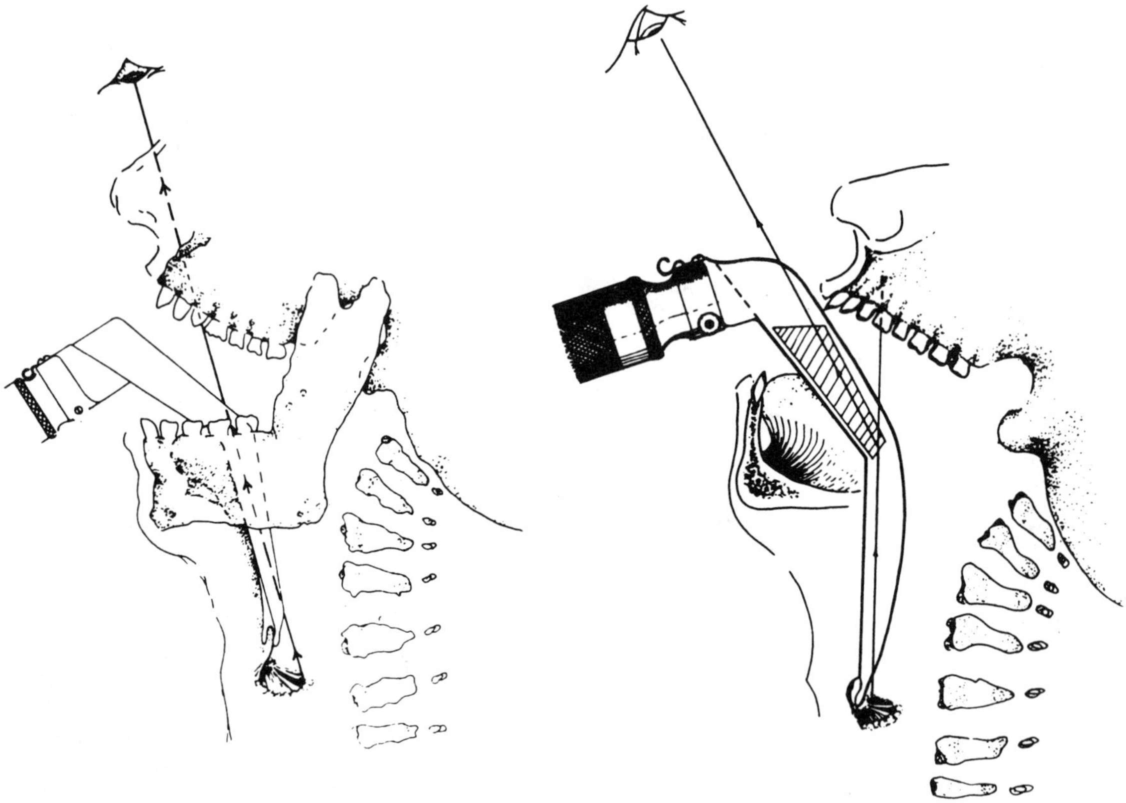

FIG. 13. In the majority of laryngoscopies with the Belscope, a view of the posterior commissure (and usually much more) is seen when the lip is pulled upward and outward by looking down the right side of the maxilla *(left)*. In difficult laryngoscopies, when the laryngoscope angle cannot be pulled forward sufficiently for direct viewing of the larynx, attachment of the prism will provide an indirect view around the corner *(right)*.

has a significantly smaller step with a shorter vertical component, and this, in combination with the inverted *L*-shaped cross section, leaves more room to manipulate an ETT in the oropharynx.

Technique

Without Prism. For the majority of laryngoscopies, the Belscope is used much like a conventional, straight laryngoscope blade. The tip of the blade traps the epiglottis so that the view is obtained by looking down the straight part of the distal end of the flange (Fig. 12).

With Prism. If the laryngoscope blade has been optimally placed and the view is still impaired (as in the patient with limited atlanto-occipital extension, a short mandible, or a large tongue), the prism is utilized, which, when looking through the proximal end (Fig. 13), will provide an indirect view of the larynx. The prism rotates the image of the larynx by 34°, which often necessitates the use of a curved stylet to direct the tip of the ETT anteriorly. When the prism is used, it is important to prevent fogging, either by using a commercial antifog preparation or by warming the prism in a towel prior to attaching it to the blade.

Clinical Experience

Bellhouse's clinical experience in over 4000 intubations has been favorable; he has been successful with both routine as well as known difficult intubations in patients with major anatomic abnormalities such as poor neck extension, short mandible, and large tongues. The longest blade was used in 80% of cases, the medium blade in 20% of cases, and the shortest blade in 5 cases per 1000 (0.5%). This angulated laryngoscope was designed for the prism but is advantageous for routine intubations without the prism, as well. In fact, the prism has been found to be necessary only 3 times per 1000. Experience from other evaluators has also been favorable, but comparison studies with other similar laryngoscope blades are lacking (18). An important caveat men-

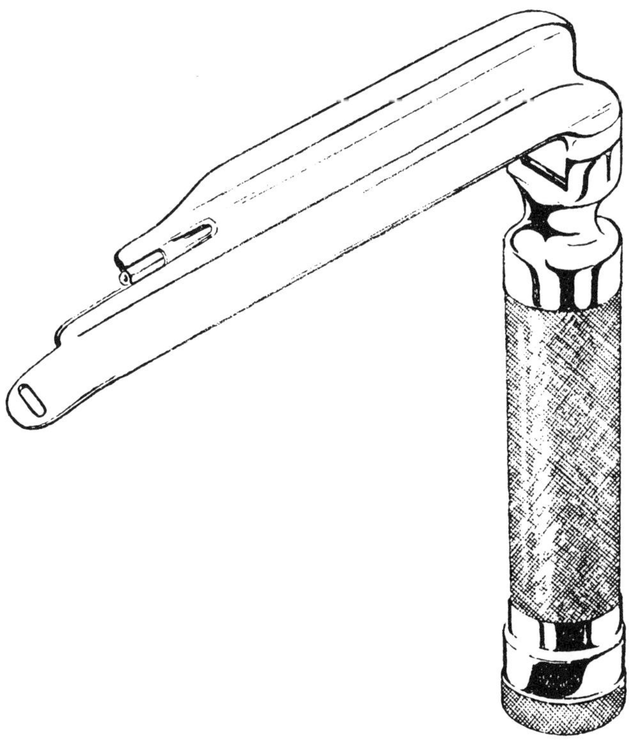

FIG. 14. The Soper laryngoscope.

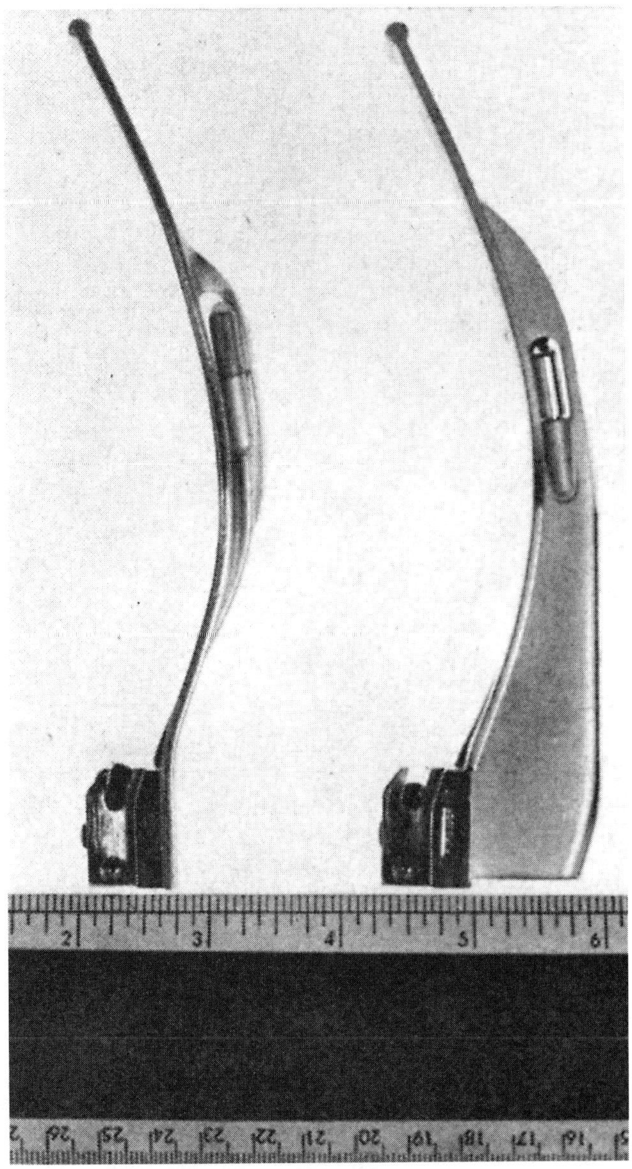

FIG. 15. The Bizzarri-Giuffrida laryngoscope blade *(left)* compared to the Macintosh laryngoscope blade *(right)*. The Bizzarri-Giuffrida blade is substantially thinner with essentially no vertical component. This aspect dramatically reduces potential damage to the teeth.

tioned by all users is that the angulated blade feels different than other blades and, therefore, that practice is essential. In fact, Bellhouse himself recommends that 50 intubations should be performed without the prism, followed by another 20 or 30 with the prism before the user can be expected to be comfortable with the blade.

Limited Mouth Opening

Soper Laryngoscope Blade

The Soper blade was introduced in 1947 and although quoted as the first true derivative of the Macintosh laryngoscope, its shape is similar to the Miller blade. This blade was developed as a result of the perceived disadvantages of the Macintosh laryngoscope; elevating the epiglottis indirectly did not always result in exposure of the cords, especially when there was a large, "flabby" epiglottis. It was also found that, although the laryngeal opening was visualized, it was often necessary to use a "stiffener" inside the ETT to manipulate it around the curvature of the blade (19).

The Soper laryngoscope (Fig. 14), like the Macintosh, has a *Z*-shaped section on the flange instead of the older, *C*-shaped section. However, the blade portion is straight and similar in length to the Miller. It is designed to elevate the epiglottis in the usual way and has a slot built into the tip, which is intended to prevent the epiglottis from slipping off the blade. Two sizes, adult and child, were available from the Longworth Scientific Instrument Company in Oxford, England. This laryngoscope was never very popular and now serves only as a point of historical interest.

Bizzarri-Giuffrida Laryngoscope Blade

The first radical change in the shape of the Macintosh laryngoscope was proposed by Bizzarri and Giuffrida in 1958 (20). They modified the shape, based on the frequent contact that the vertical flange on the original Macintosh made with the upper incisors during laryngoscopy, especially in patients with limited mobility of the mandible. In an effort to overcome this problem, they eliminated the vertical component entirely (Fig. 15). Their experience in over 200 patients found this blade particularly useful in patients with protruding incisors, receding jaws, large bull necks, and in patients with an anteriorly positioned larynx. Other than their initial report, little data is available on this blade with regard to clinical evaluation.

Improved Vision Macintosh Laryngoscope Blade

When Sir Robert Macintosh first presented his laryngoscope blade in 1943, it was curved and had a markedly flattened midportion. Since its inception, the flattened

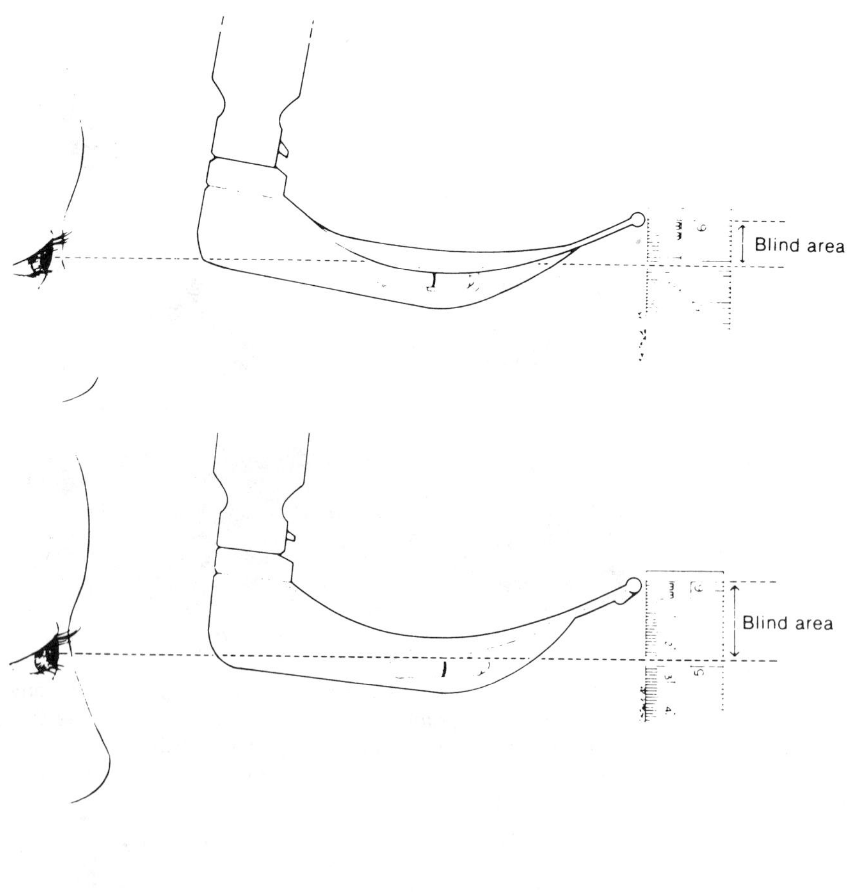

FIG. 16. A schematic illustrating from a side view the improved line of vision with the "improved vision" Macintosh as indicated on the ruler *(top)* compared to the standard Macintosh laryngoscope *(bottom)*.

midportion disappeared, and the blade has assumed a curved shape that was retained largely due to manufacturing considerations (14). Unfortunately, the curve in the midportion often inhibits visualization of the larynx, especially in patients with prominent teeth, receding jaws, or poor cervical spine mobility. The improved vision (IV) Macintosh laryngoscope sought to correct this perceived disadvantage by replacing the convex curvature with a concave midportion curvature, while maintaining the curved appearance of the outer edge (Fig. 16) (21). Limited clinical experience has demonstrated improved visibility, although no formal clinical trials have been performed. This laryngoscope blade is manufactured by, and is available from, Anesthesia Medical Specialties™ (Santa Fe Springs, California).

Kawahara Laryngoscope Blade

In response to the difficulty experienced in performing endotracheal intubation in the patient with a fractured mandible, ankylosis of the jaw, tumor of the neck, or malformation of the orofacial region, Kawahara et al. evaluated a laryngoscope equipped with fiberoptics as an alternative to their usual intubating techniques in these clinical situations (e.g., awake blind nasal intubation, retrograde intubation, or intubation utilizing a flexible fiberoptic bronchoscope) (22). The flexible, fiberoptic bronchoscope was considered their method of choice, which, as the authors correctly point out, requires extensive training and practice to become skilled in its use. This new laryngoscope is composed of a curved blade—slightly more curved than a standard Macintosh blade—with an attached fiberoptic eyepiece at the proximal end (Fig. 17).

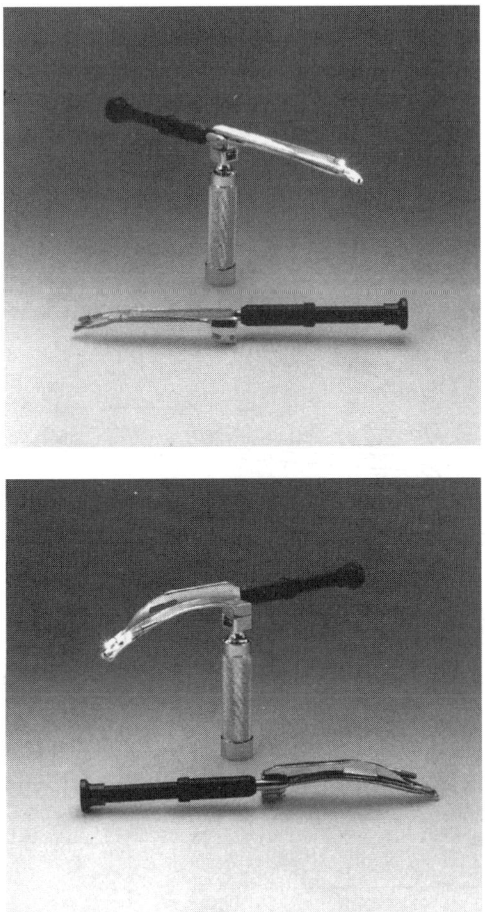

FIG. 17. The Kawahara laryngoscope with fiberoptics; Miller *(top)* and Macintosh *(bottom)*.

To use this fiberoptic laryngoscope, the lens is first defogged and focused; the blade is then inserted into the oropharynx in the standard fashion. It is advanced until the epiglottis comes into view through the eyepiece. The glottis is then visualized by elevating the epiglottis slightly with the distal blade tip. Once the glottic opening comes into focus, the ETT is advanced through the vocal cords. Because the glottis is viewed indirectly, it is initially cumbersome and spatially difficult to advance the ETT through the vocal cords but, with practice, it is reported to become easier. The reported advantage of this blade is that neither extensive mouth opening nor extreme hyperextension of the neck are necessary for successful intubation. No clinical comparison studies have been performed.

Double-Angle Laryngoscope Blade

The Double-angle blade (prototype made by Anesthesia Medical Specialties™, Cerritos, California, US patent pending) was designed by Choi (23) in an effort to combine the advantageous features of the Miller and Macintosh laryngoscope blades, while eliminating their disad-

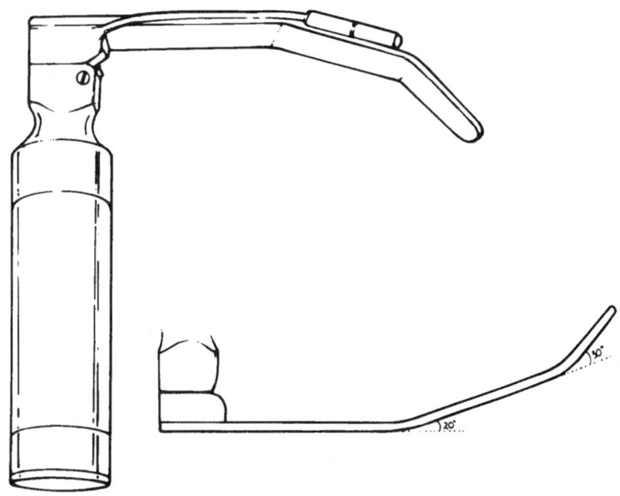

FIG. 18. The Double-angle blade with 30° and 20° incremental curvatures.

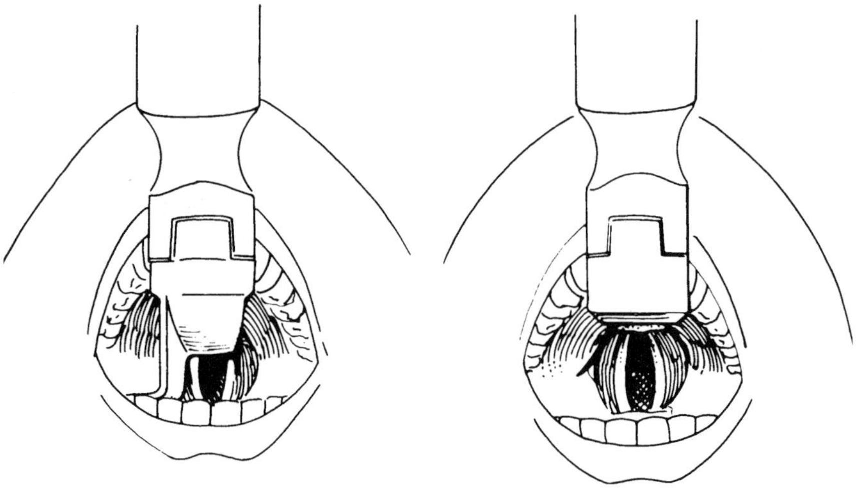

FIG. 19. Schematic comparison of the Macintosh *(left)* and double-angle *(right)* blades. The nonflanged, double-angle blade improves vision and provides more room for passage of an ETT, and should reduce the risk of tooth damage.

vantages. This blade incorporates two incremental curves, 20° and 30°, which allow for visualization of an anteriorally situated larynx without having to tilt the laryngoscope posteriorly. The vertical flange was eliminated entirely to reduce the risk of tooth damage and to create more room for intubation. The blade tip is also wider and flatter, allowing easier manipulation of a large tongue or floppy epiglottis (Fig. 18).

The blade is introduced into the oropharynx in the standard fashion, and visualization of the glottis is achieved, either directly by lifting the epiglottis or indirectly by placing the blade tip in the vallecula. Elimination of the flange is thought to decrease damage to the upper incisors, while maintaining the ability to displace the tongue out of the line of vision (Fig. 19). The simplicity of this blade is its most attractive feature, but it must be tested clinically prior to widespread recommended use.

Small Infra-Oral Cavity

Bainton Pharyngolaryngoscope

Description

In 1987, Bainton (24) introduced to the anesthesia community a new laryngoscope blade that he had designed specifically for use in patients with pharyngeal obstructions. The etiology of acute upper airway obstruction includes laryngopharyngeal neoplasm, infection, complication following neck trauma and surgery, and various other conditions that can lead to life-threatening swelling and edema. In these situations, a standard, nontubular laryngoscope blade cannot provide sufficient viewing space, since the mucosa and/or scar tissue envelopes the blade, obliterating both the viewing space and the light source on direct laryngoscopy. Several ENT tubular laryngoscopes (Jackson®, Holinger®, Jako®, Dedo-Pilling Co., Washington, Pennsylvania) exist that create space within the pharynx and have an intraluminal light source that prevents the edematous tissue from obstructing the illumination. The problem with these laryngoscope blades is that they are too long to facilitate

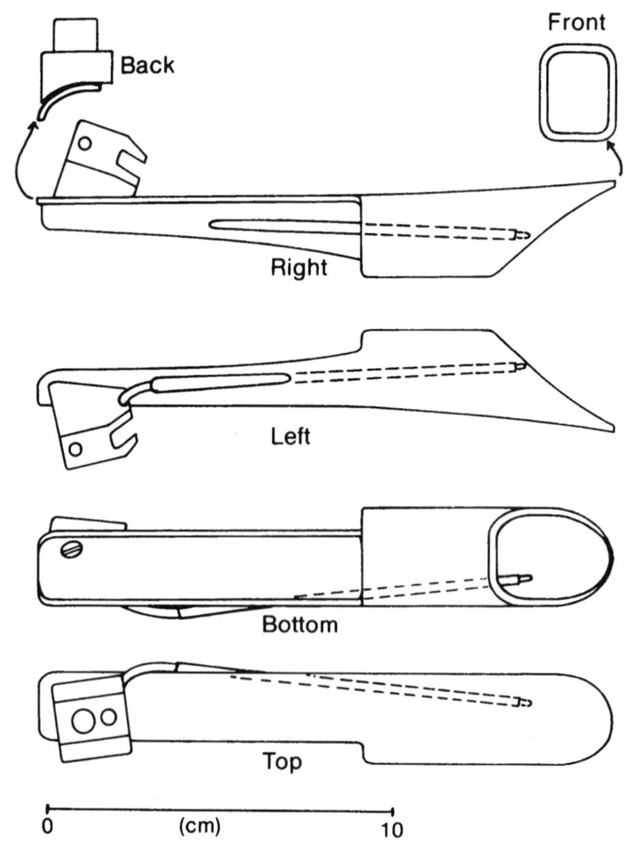

FIG. 20. Scale drawings of the Bainton tubular pharyngolaryngoscope.

easy passage of an ETT; as the ETT is inserted, the view is obstructed. Also, it is difficult to stabilize the position of the ETT during removal of these laryngoscopes. Therefore, Bainton developed a pharyngolaryngoscope that achieved the following objectives:

1. Creates pharyngeal space using a tubular design.
2. The tubular structure optimizes the passing of endotracheal tubes through or around the blade into the larynx.
3. It fits onto existing standardized light handles.

The Bainton pharyngolaryngoscope (model 52-2220, Pilling Instruments, Fort Washington, Pennsylvania) resembles a standard straight blade with a 7-cm tube incorporated onto the distal portion. A dual fiberoptic light source is recessed within the lumen to protect it from secretions and obstruction by the surrounding oropharyngeal tissue (Fig. 20). The distal tip of the blade is beveled at a 60° angle, creating an oval opening. An inside diameter (ID) of 8.0 or smaller ETT is easily accommodated through the tubular lumen without significantly obstructing the view.

Technique

The intubation technique is similar to that for any straight blade. It is inserted in the right side of the mouth by pushing the tongue to the left and advancing until the distal tip entraps the epiglottis. Once the glottic opening is visualized, an ETT without an adaptor is placed through the tubular lumen and passed through the vocal cords. The ETT cuff is then inflated and the stylet is removed from the ETT. The blade is carefully removed from the mouth as the operator's right hand stabilizes the ETT (Fig. 21).

Clinical Experience

This laryngoscope blade was first tested in a dog that was injected with a saline solution in the pharyngeal submucosa and at the base of the tongue to simulate an edematous pharynx. Visualization of the larynx was easily accomplished with the new blade, whereas both the Guedel and Macintosh laryngoscope blades failed to produce an adequate view. Other clinical experience by Bainton included twelve patients with edematous pharynges and one with a bleeding pharyngeal tumor in whom this blade successfully produced a view of the larynx while other blades failed. Bainton's experience has not been repeated in any formal clinical trials, but his patient trials have emphasized several important features of the pharyngolaryngoscope. First, the tubular portion of the blade must extend to the tip so that the tip remains in the visual field during insertion; otherwise, it will get lost in the edematous tissue. Second, the internal diameter of the tubular portion should be approximately 20 mm to create sufficient viewing space as well as to prevent obstruction of the laryngeal view when the ETT is inserted. Finally, the length of the tubular portion should be limited to the pharynx; longer tubes extending into the mouth are more difficult to manage.

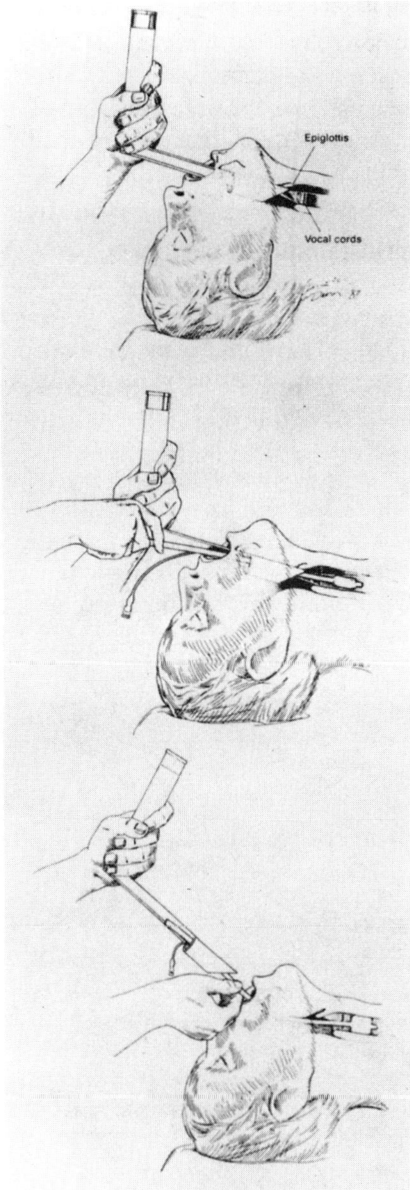

FIG. 21. Schematic of the intubation technique with the Bainton tubular pharyngolaryngoscope. **Upper:** The tubular portion, pictured in the cutaway, fits within the pharyngeal space. The tip of the blade elevates the epiglottis to permit a view of the larynx. **Middle:** An ETT without an adapter (stylet optional) is inserted into the tubular portion of the blade and advanced into the larynx. The ETT cuff is inflated. **Lower:** The syringe and stylet are removed from the ETT and the pharyngolaryngoscope is withdrawn from the mouth. The right hand of the operator stabilizes the ETT as the blade is elevated over the proximal end of the ETT and the cuff pilot tube.

Although there is very little clinical research in support of this blade, some anesthesiologists have found the Bainton pharyngolaryngoscope useful in the obstetrical suite, particularly for the occasional pre-eclamptic parturient requiring an urgent general anesthetic with rapid sequence intubation.

Immobile/Unstable Cervical Spines

Direct laryngoscopy is the easiest, quickest, and surest method of endotracheal intubation, but it requires flexion of the cervical spine and altanto-occipital extension for alignment of the oral, pharyngeal, and laryngeal axes to create a direct line of vision from the mouth to the vocal cords. There are situations when such patient positioning is impossible or contraindicated: in patients with a fused cervical spine or with cervical spine instability following injury. In elective situations, fiberoptic bronchoscopy is probably the preferred method of intubation. In an emergency setting, a rapid sequence induction with in-line manual axial traction has been recommended as a stabilization maneuver (25). As emphasized by Hastings and Mark (26) in a subsequent study, the potential for neck movement does exist with this approach; however, neurologic sequelae are infrequent. Several new laryngoscopes address this concern.

Bullard Laryngoscope

Description

The Bullard laryngoscope (BL) (Circon, ACMI, Stamford, Connecticut) is one of these new intubating devices. This rigid instrument functions as an indirect fiberoptic laryngoscope, and the blade portion is designed to match the anatomical airway. This feature negates the need for manipulation of the patient's head and neck to visualize the larynx, an obvious advantage in patients with cervical

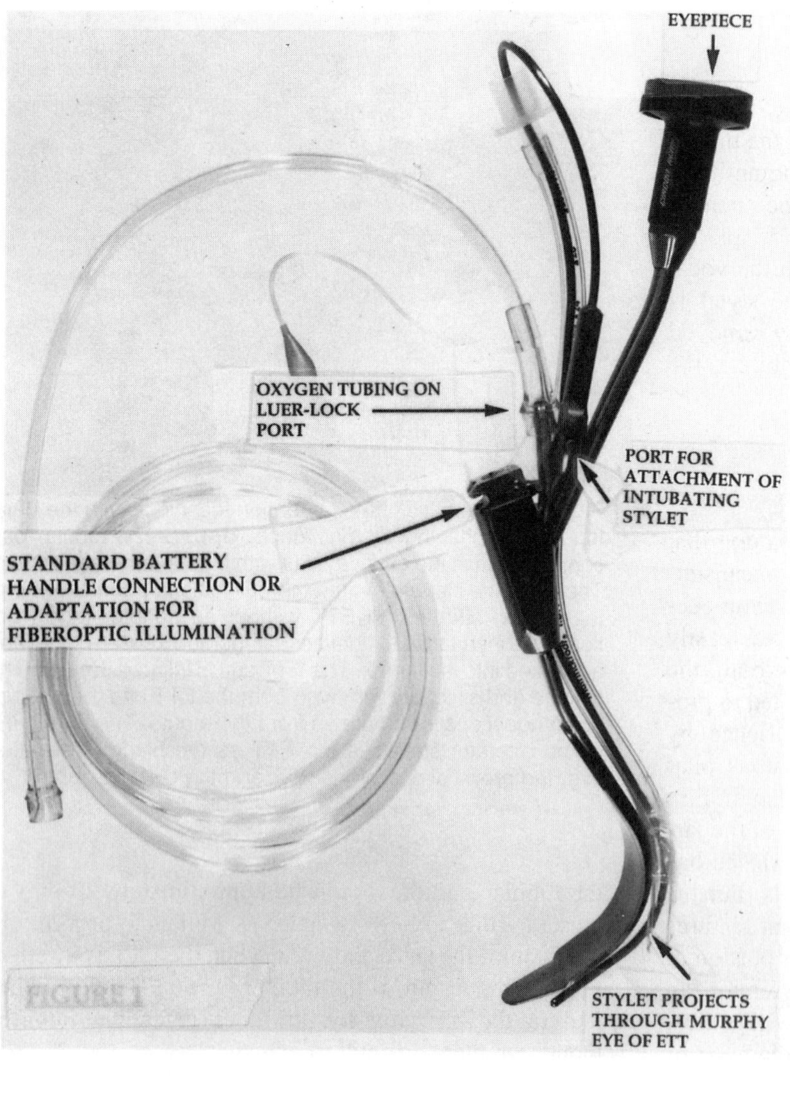

FIG. 22. The Bullard laryngoscope is shown with the new intubating stylet. A 3.7-mm channel is incorporated into the laryngoscope which is bifurcated at its proximal end. One port is equipped with a Luer-lock fitting for attachment of a three-way stopcock to provide suction, insufflation of oxygen or the application of local anesthetics. The other port of the bifurcation accepts the proximal end of the dedicated, nonmalleable intubating stylet. An endotracheal tube (ETT) is positioned on the well lubricated stylet so that the distal end of the stylet projects through the Murphy eye of the ETT. Removal of the ETT adapter will enable proximal positioning of the ETT on the stylet, thereby reducing the amount of mouth opening required for blade insertion. The stylet then clips onto its designated port so that when it is correctly attached, the stylet/ETT apparatus hugs the right side of the posterior surface of the blade.

spine pathology. Specific features of this blade include: length, 13.2 cm; width, 1.3 cm; radius of curvature, 3.4 cm; and blade thickness, 0.64 cm. The fiberoptic bundle is positioned along the posterior aspect of the blade, and the distal end of the fiber comes to within 26 mm of the distal tip of the blade, placing the endoscopist's eye in the posterior pharynx. This facilitates excellent visualization of the larynx. Other features include a bifurcated 3.7-mm channel incorporated into the laryngoscope at its proximal end. One port of the bifurcation is equipped with a Luer-lock fitting for attachment of a three-way stopcock to provide suction or insufflation of oxygen or installation of local anesthetics. The other port of the bifurcation accepts the proximal end of a newer, dedicated, nonmalleable intubating stylet, the newest device to aid in intubation (Fig. 22). The original intubating mechanisms included: (a) a styletted ETT shaped to mimic the curve of the Bullard blade; (b) an ETT with a directional tip (e.g., Endotrol®; Mallinckrodt Critical Care, Glensfalls, New York); and (c) use of the Bullard intubating forceps, a thumb-lever-activated device that allows the operator to advance the intubating forceps into the larynx and release the ETT once it is through the vocal cords. The intubating forceps have recently been abandoned in favor of the nonmalleable intubating stylet.

Technique

To use the intubating stylet, the ETT must be preloaded prior to attaching the stylet onto the laryngoscope. The stylet is well-lubricated and, after removal of the ETT adapter, the ETT is positioned on the stylet so that the distal end of the stylet projects through the Murphy eye of the ETT. The ETT can then either be advanced proximally over the length of the stylet if there is limited mouth opening or left in position near the distal tip of the blade. The stylet clips onto a designated port on the BL, so that when it is correctly attached, the stylet/ETT apparatus lies along the right side of the posterior spine of the blade. Since the new intubating stylet hugs the posterior surface of the blade, the BL must be used like a modified Miller blade; the epiglottis is retracted against the posterior tongue. If the epiglottis is not retracted, the ETT will impact the vallecula as it is advanced off the stylet.

The technique of intubation with the BL is in the following manner (Fig. 23). The BL, held in the left hand, is inserted into the mouth in the horizontal plane; once it clears the tongue, the blade is rotated to a vertical plane by allowing it to slide around the midline of the tongue. The laryngoscope is then momentarily dropped into the posterior pharynx, and with a scooping motion, gentle

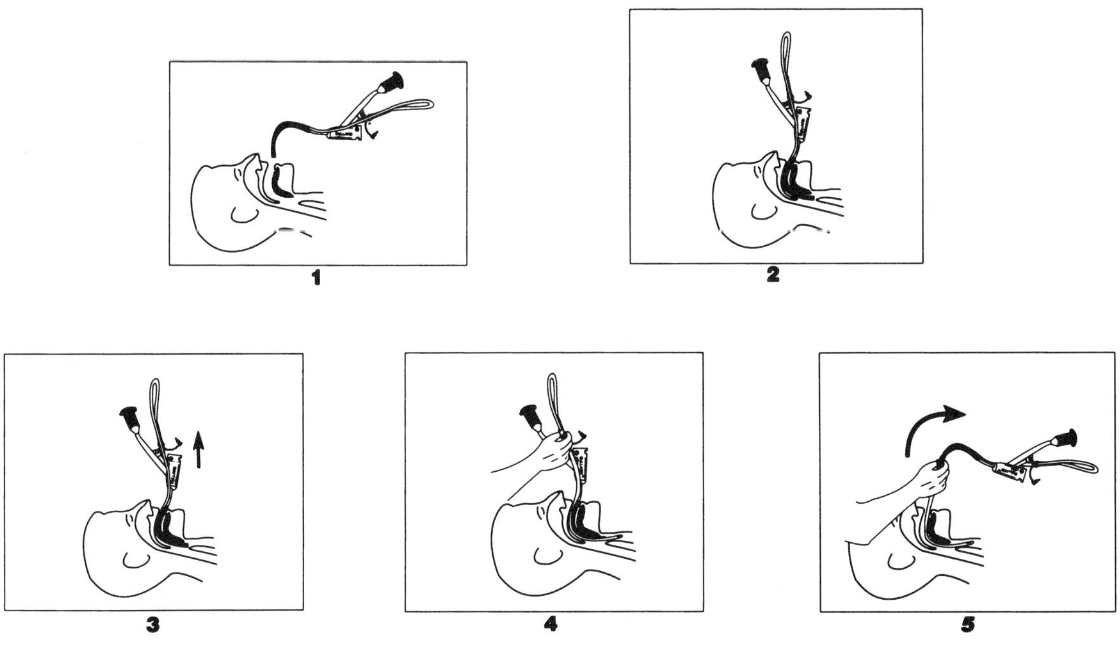

FIG. 23. The panels illustrate the intubation technique with the new intubating stylet. **1:** The Bullard laryngoscope (BL) with a preloaded, attached intubating stylet is inserted into the oral cavity in the horizontal plane; less than 7 mm of opening between the teeth is required when the endotracheal tube (ETT) is positioned on the proximal end of the stylet. **2:** The handle is rotated to the vertical plane, allowing the blade to slide around the tongue. The blade is then allowed to momentarily drop into the posterior pharynx. **3:** The blade is elevated against the tongue's dorsal surface with upward pressure on the handle so that the epiglottis is trapped by the blade, exposing the glottic opening. **4:** The ETT is advanced off the stylet through the glottic opening and into the trachea. Placement is initially visually confirmed. **5:** Securing the ETT at the proximal end, the BL and the intubating stylet are removed by rotating the unit forward, back to the horizontal plane and gently lifting it out of the oral cavity.

traction is applied in the vertical plane to lift the blade up against the posterior surface of the tongue. Either the epiglottis or the vocal cords will come into view. If the epiglottis is the only structure visualized with initial blade insertion, the blade is dropped back into the posterior pharynx; the application of a more pronounced scooping motion on the blade is made in an attempt to position the laryngoscope under the epiglottis and obtain a clear, unobstructed view of the glottic opening and vocal cords. With the stylet pointed directly at the glottic opening, the ETT is advanced off the stylet with the right hand and through the laryngeal aperture until the cuff passes just beyond the vocal cords under direct vision. The BL is then removed; the right hand stabilizes the ETT and the left hand rotates the blade from a vertical to a horizontal plane, taking care that the stylet remains in close contact with the blade to avoid injury to the teeth or face upon removal of the device.

Clinical Experience

Several authors have described their experiences with the BL. Bjoraker (27) detailed the characteristics of the BL and described the three original intubating techniques recommended by the manufacturer, mentioned previously. He concluded that, although the BL affords excellent visualization of the glottis, serious commitment and training are necessary to become skillful at intubation with any one of these intubating techniques. Dyson et al. (28) compared the learning curves of first-year anesthesia residents using both the fiberoptic bronchoscope and the BL in a mannequin modified to make intubation difficult. They found that the time course for proficiency using either device was similar, but passage of the ETT through the laryngeal aperture took longer with the BL (using one of the three originally described intubation techniques). Borland and Casselbrant (29) used the pediatric BL in 93 patients (ages 1 day to 10.7 years), 64 with normal airway anatomy and 29 with known abnormal upper airway anatomy. Intubation was successful in 97% of the cases (intubation technique not mentioned); difficulty occurred in two patients with excessive secretions and, in a third patient, intubation failed as a result of a small mouth that did not allow adequate space to direct and insert the endotracheal tube. Saunders and Giesecke (30) reported the use of the BL in a variety of circumstances, including patients with uncomplicated airways (n=40), cervical spine instability (n=5), rapid sequence intubations (n=10), and awake patients (n=3). In the first three patient groups there was an 88% intubation success rate in under 24 sec by passing a styletted ETT freehand. For unexplained reasons, three intubations failed in the group with uncomplicated airways, and they were intubated by other, unspecified means. All three awake intubation attempts (5% of all study patients) failed secondary to poor visualization; in these patients, intubation was accomplished by, again, other unspecified means. Gorback (31) presented five case reports of successful intubation with the BL in which a styletted ETT was passed freehand in adults with unusual airway anatomy (grade III and IV airways, limited temporomandibular joint mobility, and limited cervical spine mobility). He concluded that, although there might be a steep learning curve, the BL is a worthwhile addition to any anesthesiologist's armamentarium in approaching a potentially difficult airway.

Most recently, Cooper et al. (32) determined that the optimal intubating mechanism with the BL was the new

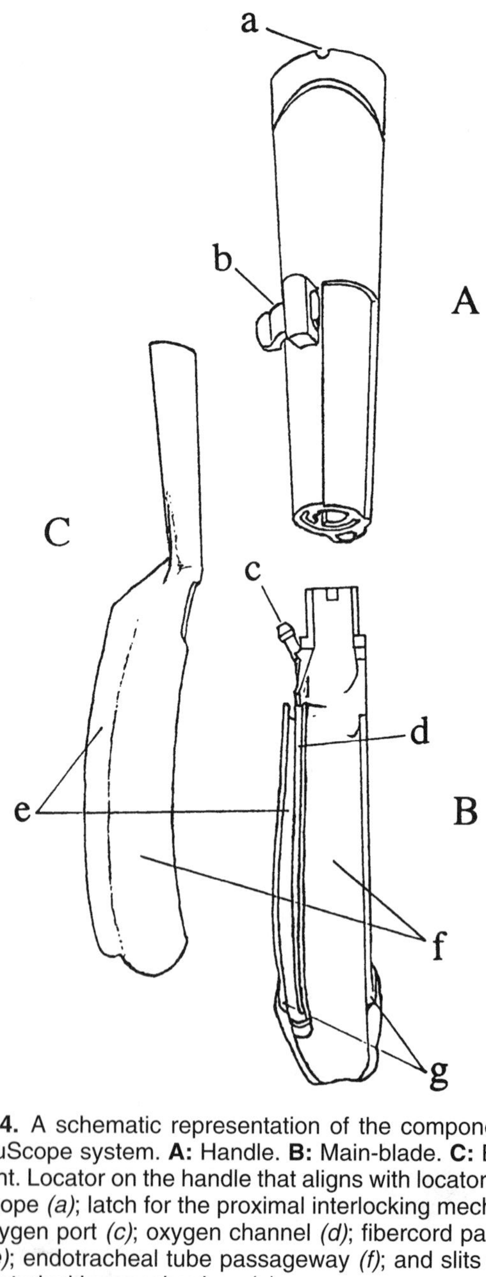

FIG. 24. A schematic representation of the components of the WuScope system. **A:** Handle. **B:** Main-blade. **C:** Bivalve element. Locator on the handle that aligns with locator on the fiberscope *(a)*; latch for the proximal interlocking mechanism *(b)*; oxygen port *(c)*; oxygen channel *(d)*; fibercord passageway *(e)*; endotracheal tube passageway *(f)*; and slits for the distal interlocking mechanism *(g)*.

dedicated intubating stylet; fewer attempts were required and it took less time to successful tracheal intubation compared to the original three intubating mechanisms. Their results also suggested that time to successful intubation with the BL using the intubating stylet was not affected by the conventional laryngoscopic grade; it was just as easy (and difficult) to intubate a conventional, grade I laryngoscopic view patient (full glottic view) as it was to intubate a conventional, grade III laryngoscopic view patient (visualization of just the epiglottis) with the BL. There were two failed intubations with the BL (3%) due to an inability to trap the epiglottis. Based on their results and the results of other investigators, the BL may be uniquely useful in trauma patients with uncleared cervical spines and in other patients when the head and neck cannot be manipulated (32). Of interest, Hastings et al. (33) recently found that some, albeit minimal, neck movement does occur when using the BL for intubation. Whether or not this results in any neurologic sequelae is not yet known, but preliminary results show this blade to be quite favorable in patients with cervical spine pathology.

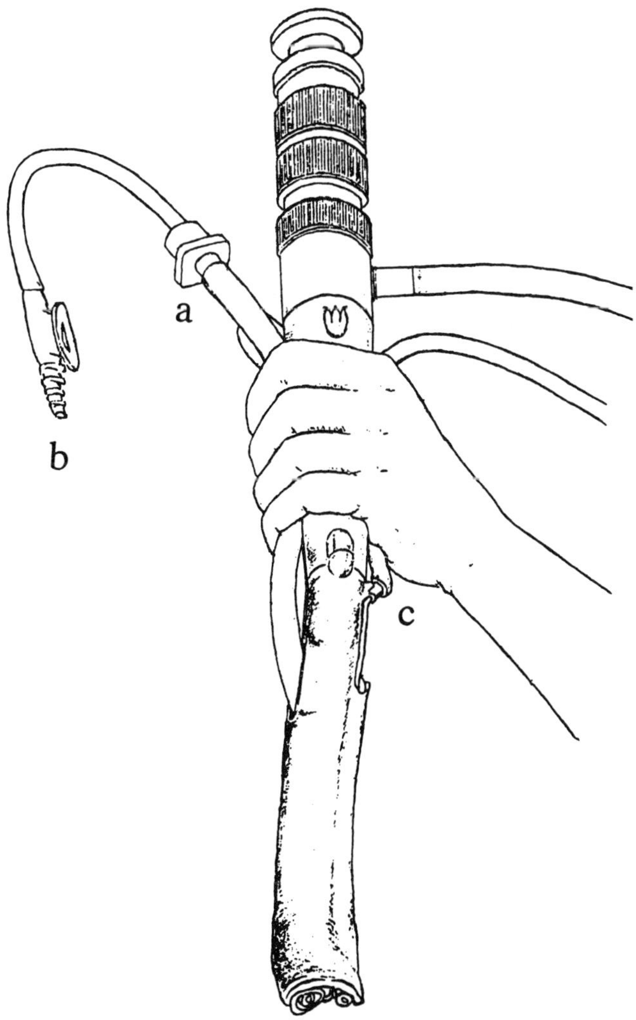

FIG. 25. The WuScope System with the rigid and flexible portion fitted together and properly assembled with *(a)* an endotracheal tube (ETT) in the ETT passageway, *(b)* a suction catheter in the ETT lumen, and *(c)* oxygen tubing connected to the oxygen port.

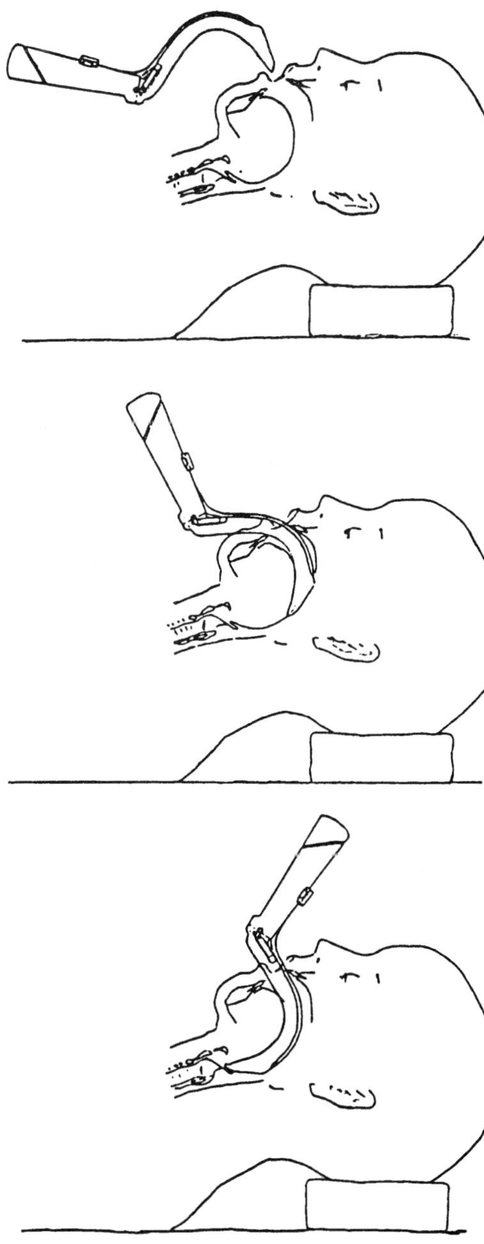

FIG. 26. A schematic of the technique for orotracheal intubation with the WuScope system. **Upper:** With the patient's head in the neutral position, the device is introduced into the patient's mouth in the horizontal axis at the midline, often using a tongue depressor to aid with insertion. **Middle:** Maintaining a midline position, the blade is rotated around the tongue until the handle reaches a vertical position. **Lower:** Once the glottis is in view, the ETT and distal blade are aligned with the glottic opening and the ETT is advanced through the tubular blade until the cuff is observed to pass beyond the vocal cords.

The WuScope System

Description

The WuScope System (Achi Corp., Dublin, California) is similar to both the tubular pharyngolaryngoscope and the BL. This system consists of a rigid blade portion and a separate, flexible fiberoptic portion (Olympus fiberscope LF-1, LF-2 or rhinolaryngoscope ENF-P3 are recommended) (Figs. 24,25). When assembled, the laryngoscope is essentially a tubular, curved, bivalved rigid blade with an incorporated flexible fiberscope as its optical guide. The assembly is somewhat complex for the beginner, but after a few trial-and-error sessions, this task is readily accomplished. A detailed description of the assembly is nicely outlined in the instruction manual available from the manufacturer. Currently, there are two adult sizes available.

Technique

The WuScope System is suitable for tracheal intubations in awake or anesthetized patients, through the oral or nasal route. The technique for orotracheal intubation is strikingly similar to that for the BL. Maintaining the patient's head in the neutral position, the device is introduced into the patient's mouth at the midline with the help of a tongue depressor, much like inserting an oral airway. Holding the handle with the left hand, it is gradually rotated around the contour of the tongue until the handle reaches a vertical position (Fig. 26). It is recommended that the user look through the eyepiece as soon as the tip of the blade enters the oropharynx in order to follow the progress as the blade is rotated. Experience has revealed that maintaining a midline position, with proper orientation of the airway structures as the blade is advanced, greatly facilitates laryngeal inlet exposure. Once the vocal cords come into view, the ETT and distal blade are aligned with the glottis, and the ETT is advanced through the tubular main blade until the cuff is visually observed to pass through the vocal cords. The inventors report that first passing a suction catheter through the vocal cords may serve as a reliable conduit to aid in alignment of the ETT with the glottis. The WuScope blade is then disassembled and carefully removed from the patient's mouth while holding the ETT firmly in place. Once the usual steps have been taken to confirm the intratracheal location of the ETT, it is secured.

The shape of the blade and its fiberoptic viewing ability preclude the need for alignment of the upper oral airway in order to visualize the larynx. This feature is advantageous when head and neck manipulation are contraindicated (i.e., suspected or known unstable cervical spine injuries). The tubular aspect of the main blade helps create viewing space when tumors, trauma, edema, or inflammation obscure the posterior pharynx. This tubular portion also contains the fiberoptic bronchoscope and protects the optics from being obscured by blood, secretions, or soft oropharyngeal tissues.

Clinical Experience

Wu and Chou (34), the inventors, have extensive experience with this intubating system, having achieved great success in their clinical trials. They have found it useful in awake or anesthetized patients in routine as well as dif-

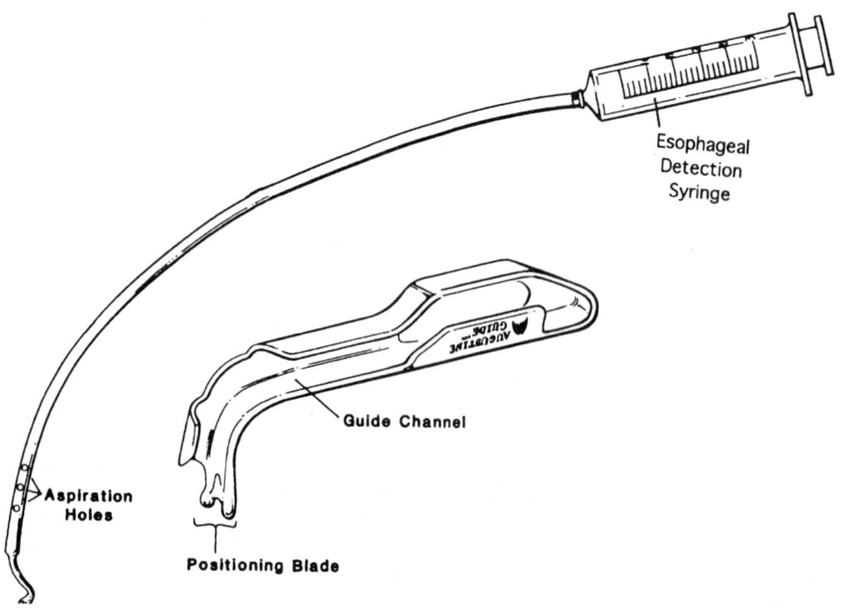

FIG. 27. The components of the Augustine Guide; the Augustine stylet *(top)* and the intubation guide *(bottom)*.

ficult intubations. Theoretically, "unexpected difficult intubation" will not exist if the WuScope System is used routinely. Limitations for its use include: limited mouth opening (TMJ disease, rheumatoid arthritis) and extreme fixed flexion neck deformity. Reported complications are similar to those with the use of other rigid laryngoscopes: sore throat, chipped teeth, and mucosal injury. Other than the inventors' clinical experience, there are no published data on the use of the WuScope System. Obviously, more experience is necessary before it can be recommended for widespread clinical use.

The Augustine Guide

Description

Another intubation device that is rapidly gaining in popularity is the Augustine Guide (AG; Augustine Medical Inc., Eden Prairie, Minnesota), originally designed for blind orotracheal intubation. The AG is a two-piece device that is constructed of medical-grade plastic and consists of an intubation guide and stylet (Fig. 27). The intubation guide is curved in shape and is designed to follow around the back of the tongue and fit into the vallecula. The distal edge has a midline indentation and two lateral bulbous protrusions. When the leading or distal edge is properly seated in the vallecula, the midline indentation straddles the hyoepiglottic ligament, and the lateral bulbous protrusions lock into the recesses of the vallecula, setting beneath the hyoid bone. Proper positioning is verified by palpating lateral movements of the hyoid bone when the intubation guide is moved from side to side. A hollow guide channel runs alongside the interior and underside of the intubation guide. When properly oriented, the guide channel is positioned directly opposite the glottic opening. The stylet has an *S*-shaped, molded tip with six aspiration holes (three on each side) and is connected to a 35-ml syringe. It is utilized as an esophageal detector device and as a guide to facilitate easy passage of the ETT.

Technique

Prior to blade insertion into the oropharynx, the well-lubricated intubating stylet is placed through a 7.0-, 7.5-, or 8.0-mm ID ETT. The *S*-shaped, molded portion of the stylet is then advanced to the edge of the open tip of the ETT, and the ETT and stylet are inserted into the guide channel of the AG (Fig. 28). A special bite block is included with the AG to facilitate introduction of the device into the mouth.

The intubation technique involves opening the mouth and inserting the bite block between the molars on the right to ensure that the mouth remains open. Once the bite block is properly positioned, a 4×4 gauze is used to pull the tongue up out of the patient's mouth. The preloaded AG is then inserted into the oropharynx. The leading edge is advanced toward the vallecula by rotating the guide handle from a horizontal to a vertical position until it is at 90° to the plane of the face (similar to positioning the BL and WuScope System). To ensure proper placement of the AG in the vallecula, the hyoid bone is palpated and the guide handle is gently moved from side to side. The hyoid bone will move if the guide is correctly seated in the glossoepiglottic fold (Fig. 29). The stylet is then gently advanced into the larynx until the syringe contacts the ETT connector. If an obstruction is met, gentle probing may be necessary until the stylet advances easily. The plunger of the syringe is then aspirated to its full volume. Free and easy return of air confirms suc-

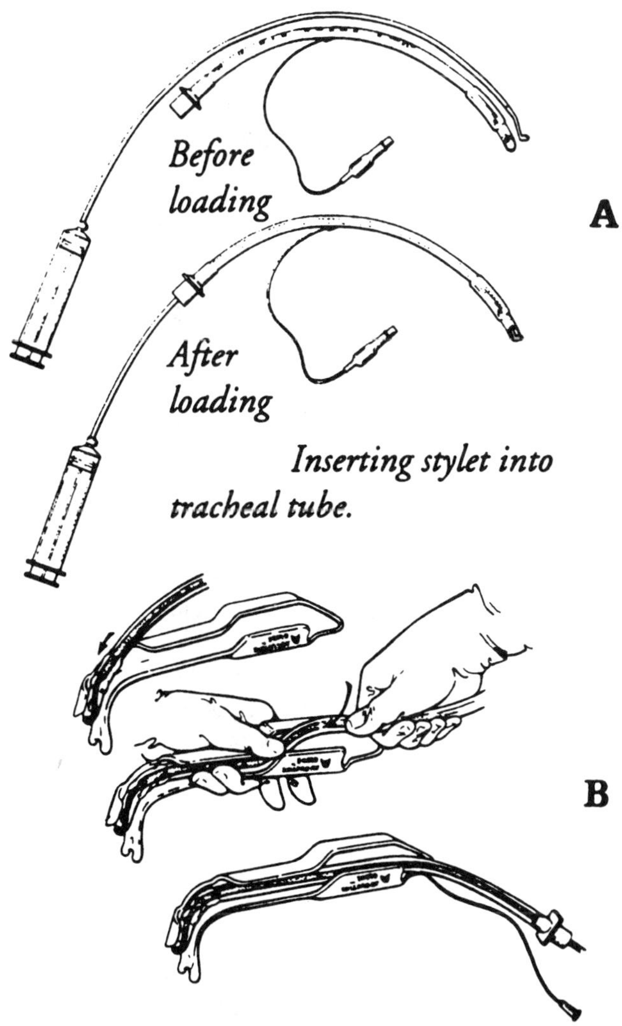

FIG. 28. Schematic of guide preparation. **A:** The stylet is lubricated well and placed through a 7.0-, 7.5-, or 8.0-mm ID ETT. **B:** The *S*-shaped molded portion of the stylet is then advanced to the edge of the open tip of the ETT and the ETT and stylet are inserted into the guide channel of the Augustine Guide.

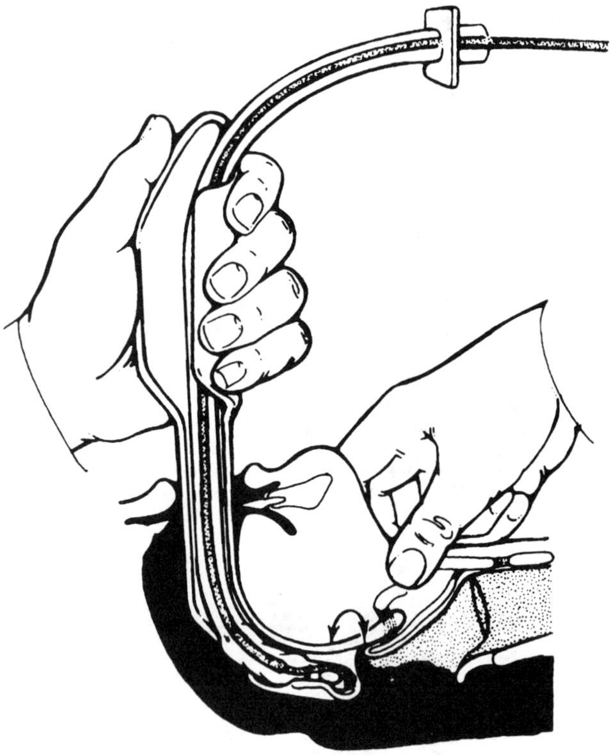

FIG. 29. The guide inserted into the vallecula. Palpable movement of the hyoid bone with gentle side-to-side motion of the guide indicates the guide is properly engaged in the vallecula around the hyoepiglottic ligament.

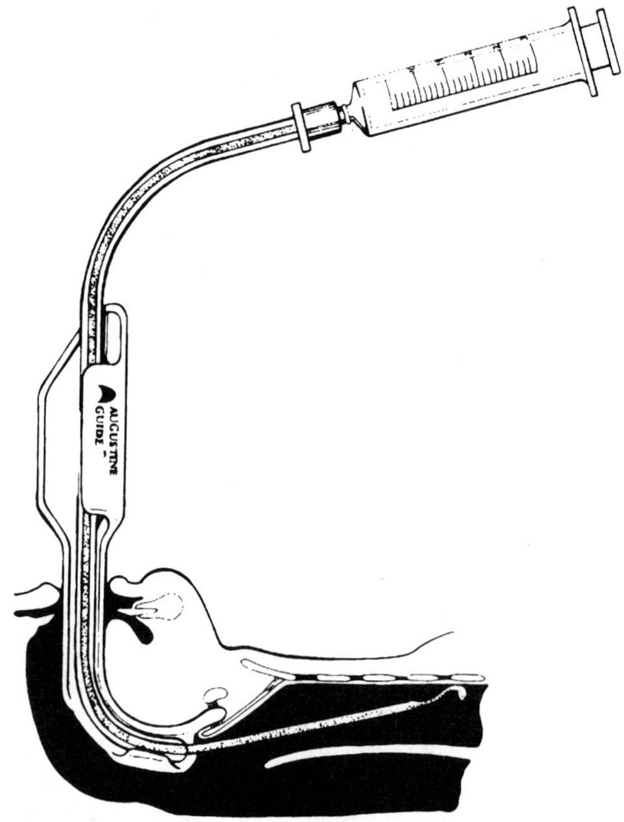

FIG. 30. The stylet is used to locate the trachea. Free return of air with syringe aspiration with no vacuum-like resistance indicates an intratracheal location.

cessful placement of the stylet in the trachea (Fig. 30). Any resistance to aspiration or recoil with release of the plunger implies that the soft muscular walls of the esophagus are being sucked over the perforations in the stylet, creating a vacuum.

Once the intratracheal position of the stylet is verified, the right hand grasps the AG handle, while the left hand disengages the ETT from the guide channel and advances it over the stylet into the trachea (Fig. 31). Rotation of the AG may be necessary if resistance is encountered. The intubation guide and stylet are carefully removed, and verification of proper ETT placement is accomplished using conventional criteria.

Clinical Experience

The AG has been shown to facilitate rapid, blind, orotracheal intubation in adults (no pediatric version is available) (35,36). A recent report described the successful use of the AG in patients with normal airways who presented for operations under general anesthesia (37). They found that the AG was a safe and effective device in achieving rapid, blind, orotracheal intubation in 94% of patients studied. Since this is a blind intubating device, blood, vomitus, and secretions in the oropharynx that would obscure direct vision with conventional laryngoscopy or fiberoptic bronchoscopy do not pose a problem. In addition, head and neck manipulation are not required to achieve successful intubation with this device. This makes the device uniquely useful in patients with known or suspected cervical spine injury (38). It has also been found to be useful in intubating the trachea of an adult with Treacher-Collins syndrome (39).

The primary disadvantage is that it is a blind technique. However, the reliability of correct placement with the esophageal detector device (the stylet) has been established (35). In addition, Augustine has recently developed a prototype that incorporates fiberoptic viewing capability onto the standard AG. It is currently undergoing clinical trials (Fig. 32). In addition, many anesthesiologists have evolved a technique wherein a flexible fiberoptic bronchoscope (FOB) is independently passed down the ETT in a correctly positioned AG, converting the blind technique to a fiberoptic one; the ETT is advanced over the FOB into the trachea under direct vision (40). The AG appears to be a promising new tool to add to the anesthesiologist's armamentarium for managing difficult airway problems.

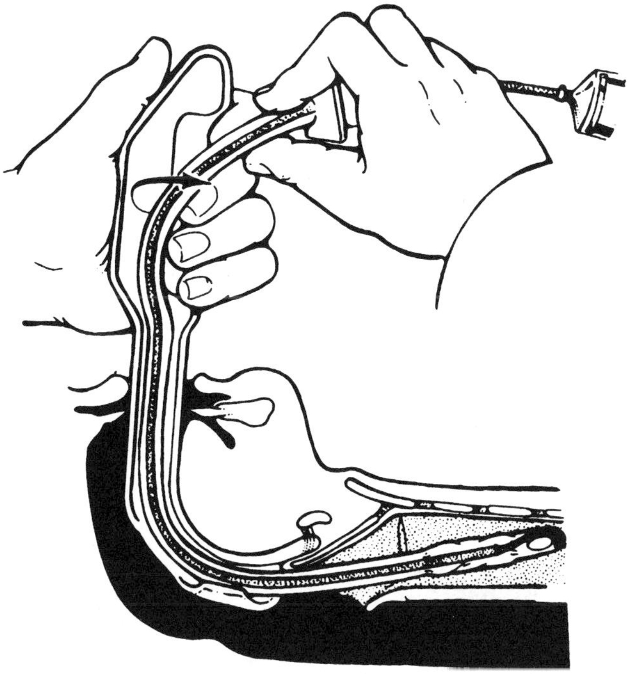

FIG. 31. The ETT is firmly grasped to stabilize it while it is detached from the guide.

Enlarged Sternal Region

The curved Macintosh laryngoscope (5) is at a right angle to the blade. It is the most widely used instrument for direct viewing of the larynx in a variety of patients, including obstetrical patients. However, parturients requiring general anesthesia present problems that affect the ease of intubation, including the risk of aspiration, airway edema, and engorged and enlarged breasts. To prevent aspiration, a rapid sequence induction with the application of cricoid pressure (the Sellick maneuver) is employed. The combination of an assistant's hand on the cricoid cartilage and the patient's enlarged breasts may make insertion of the laryngoscope blade difficult. Many solutions to overcome this problem have been proposed, including:

1. Removing the blade from the handle and reconnecting it after it is inserted into the oropharynx (41).
2. Using a short laryngoscope handle (42).
3. Inserting the blade into the corner of the patient's mouth with the handle parallel to the patient's shoulder and then rotating it to the correct position (43–45).
4. Altering the angle the blade makes with the handle.

These techniques have been utilized not only in the obstetrical population but also for obese patients, patients with kyphosis and severe barrel-chest deformity, and patients with short necks.

The Polio Laryngoscope Blade

The use of a Polio blade, originally designed for intubating the tracheas of patients in iron lung machines, has been one suggestion to overcome these problems (Fig. 33) (46–48). However, the very obtuse angle it forms with the handle makes it difficult to apply pressure to the tongue in the correct direction to facilitate a view of the glottic opening; therefore, it is not easy to use.

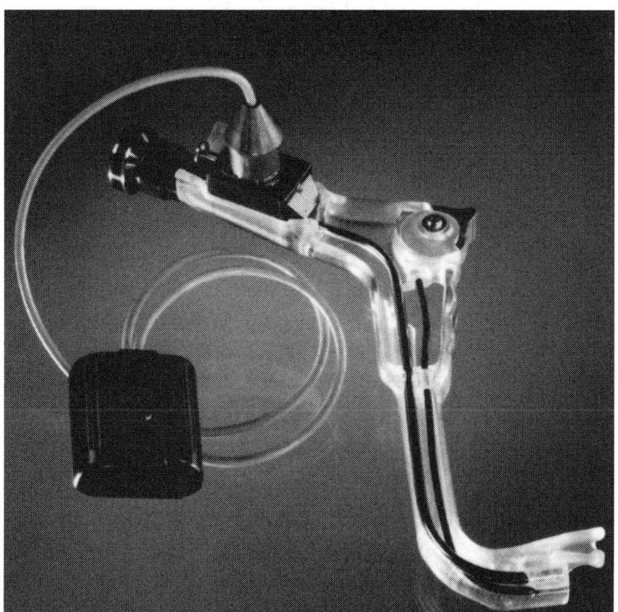

FIG. 32. The Augustine Guide fiberoptic device.

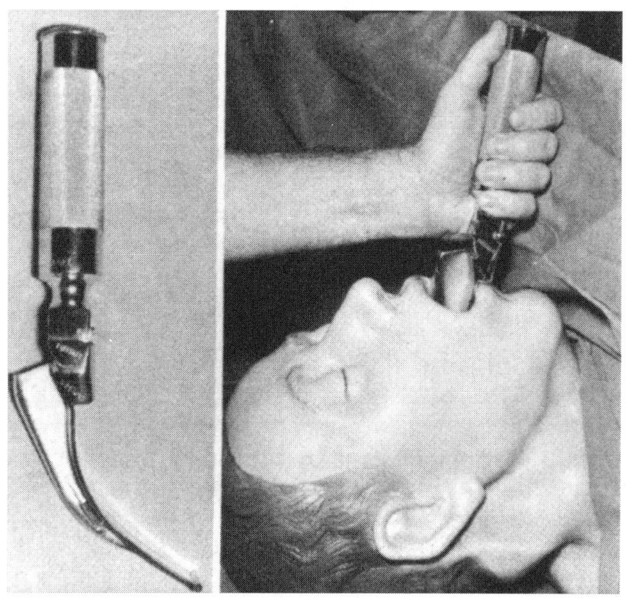

FIG. 33. The Polio blade *(left)* inserted into the patient's mouth *(right)*.

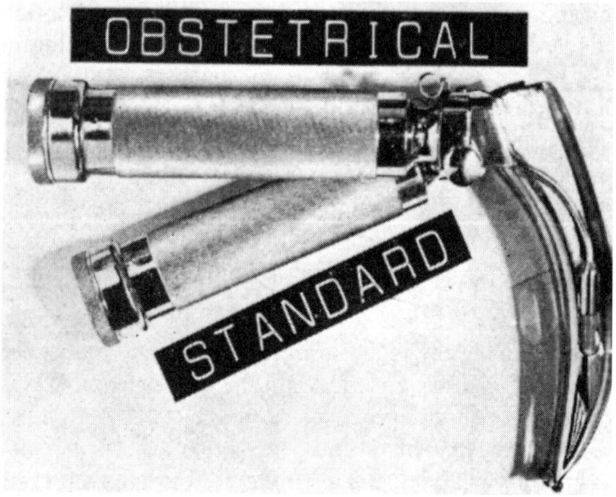

FIG. 34. Comparison of angles of obstetrical and standard laryngoscope handles with superimposed blades.

Kessel Laryngoscope Blade

Kessel (49) took a standard Macintosh laryngoscope blade and varied the fitting so that it came off the handle at approximately 110° (Fig. 34). In his experience, it did not feel different than the standard Macintosh. It did not impinge on either the chest wall or the hand of the assistant applying cricoid pressure during airway intubation. It is manufactured by Pen Medic Ltd. in New Zealand and apparently is distributed by HI Clements Pty, Ltd. in Australia.

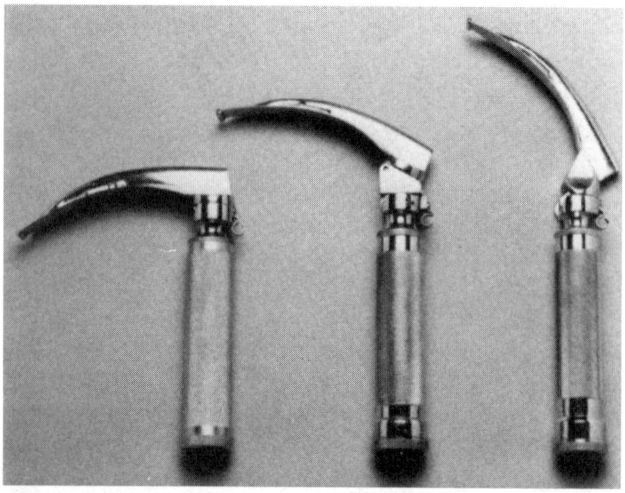

FIG. 35. Comparison of the standard Macintosh arrangement *(left)*, the standard laryngoscope with the adapter in place *(middle)* and the Polio blade *(right)*.

Jellicoe and Harris Adapter

Jellicoe and Harris (50) further modified the standard Macintosh arrangement by interposing an adapter between the laryngoscope handle and the blade. This adapter tilts the angle between the blade tip and handle to 90°, a marked increase over the 58° angle between the blade tip and handle of the standard Macintosh laryngoscope (Fig. 35). This enables introduction of the blade tip in the vertical plane while maintaining the handle in the horizontal plane, easily clearing the patient's chest and the assistant's hand on the cricoid cartilage. This adapter will fit onto any standard laryngoscope handle and is widely used in the obstetrical population in England.

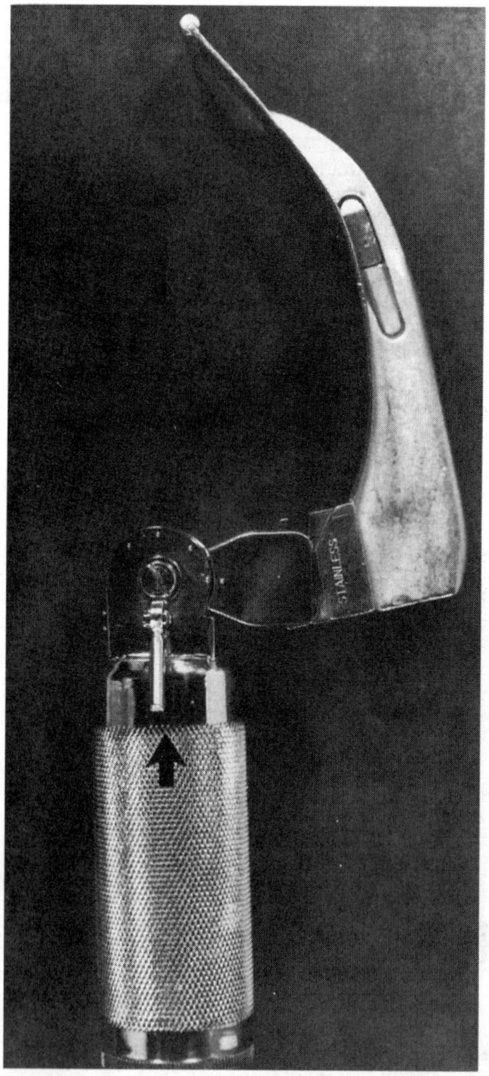

FIG. 36. The adjustable laryngoscope handle. A blade lock *(arrow)* allows positioning of the blade at 180°, 135°, 90°, or 45° to the handle.

Patil and Stehling Laryngoscope Handle

An extension of this idea is the adjustable laryngoscope handle that allows positioning of the Macintosh blade at four different angles to the handle, 180°, 135°, 90°, and 45° (Fig. 36) (51). If the handle contacts the patient's chest upon initial insertion of the blade into the mouth, the lock on the handle (Fig. 36, *arrow*) is released until the blade position lies parallel to the handle (180° angle); after it is inserted into the patient's mouth, the blade–handle angle is readjusted to 90° and standard laryngoscopic technique follows.

Yentis Laryngoscope Blade

The solution proposed by Yentis was the development of a laryngoscope adapter that maintains the normal angle between the handle and blade but allows lateral rotation of the laryngoscope handle (Fig. 37)(52). The adapter is a 2.5×2.5×2.5-cm block that fits between a standard screw-fit Penlon laryngoscope handle and the Macintosh blade. When the blade is inserted into the patient's mouth, the handle is pointing 90° to the right, avoiding contact with the patient's chest and/or an assistant's hand (Fig. 38). The handle is then swiveled back to its normal position and laryngoscopy is performed in the standard fashion. This device might also be uniquely advantageous for intubating patients in the left lateral decubitus position.

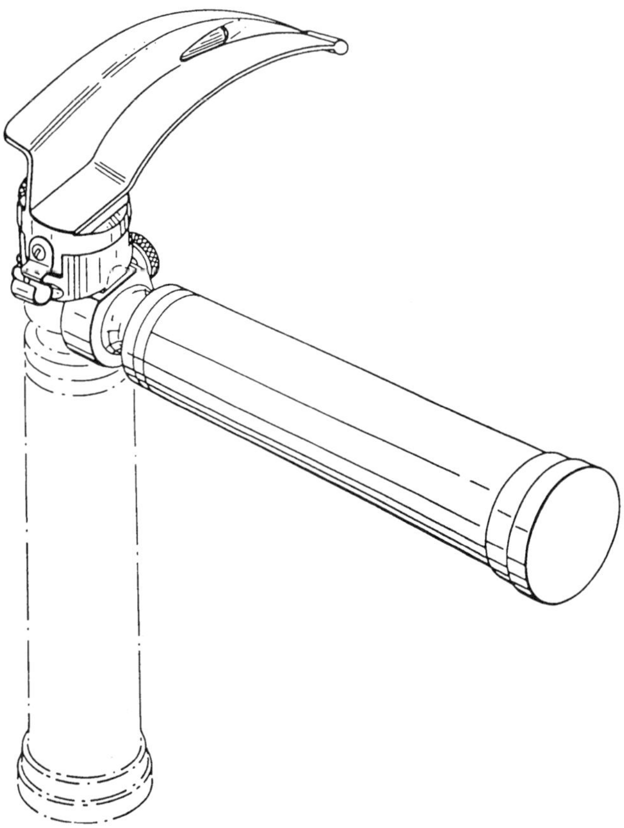

FIG. 37. The laryngoscope and adapter assembled illustrating the lateral pivoting ability.

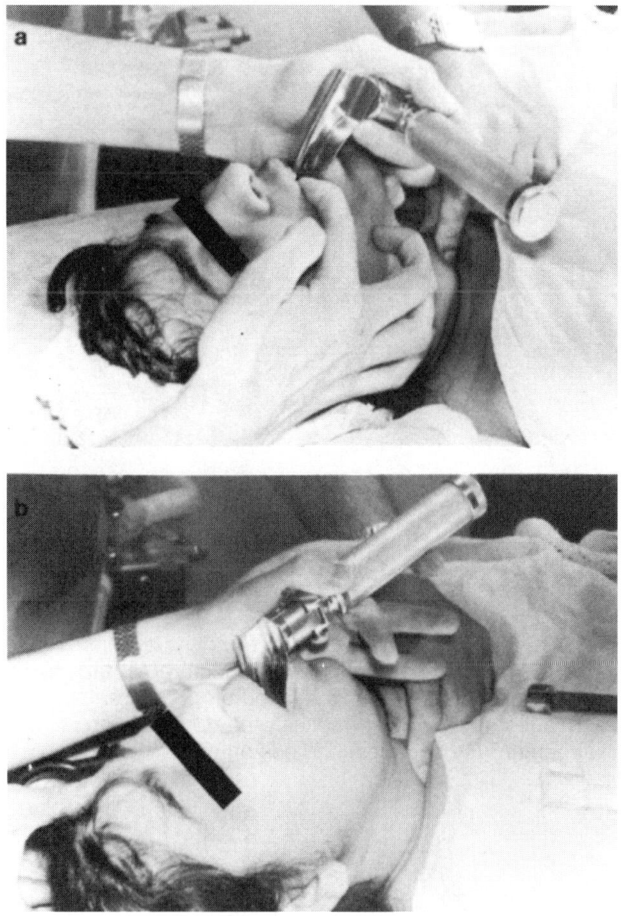

FIG. 38. The pivoting adapter in use. **a:** Insertion of the blade into the patient's mouth. **b:** The handle in the normal position.

Dhara and Cheong Adapter

Another adjustable multiple angle laryngoscope adapter was developed by Dhara and Cheong (53). Their adapter also fits onto a standard laryngoscope handle and, unlike the Patil adapter, it allows the operator to choose from a wider variety of clinically useful angles (180°, 150°, 130°, 110°, 90°, and 65°) single-handedly (Fig. 39). The adapter hooks onto a standard laryngoscope handle on one end, and another, similar arrangement is on the opposite end for attachment of a Macintosh laryngo-

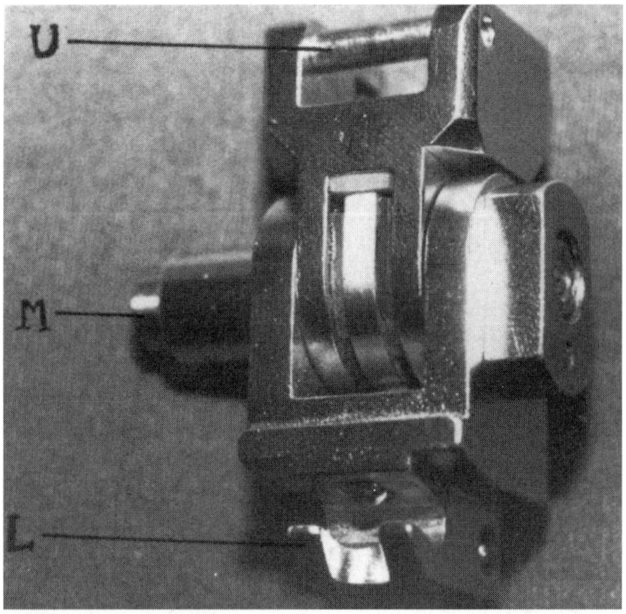

FIG. 39. The adapter. A hook-on arrangement fits onto a standard laryngoscope handle *(L)*. A push-rod in the middle section *(M)* operates a spring-loaded pin, which engages or disengages the rotating mechanism. On the top, a bar arrangement *(U)* engages the hook-on type of laryngoscope blade.

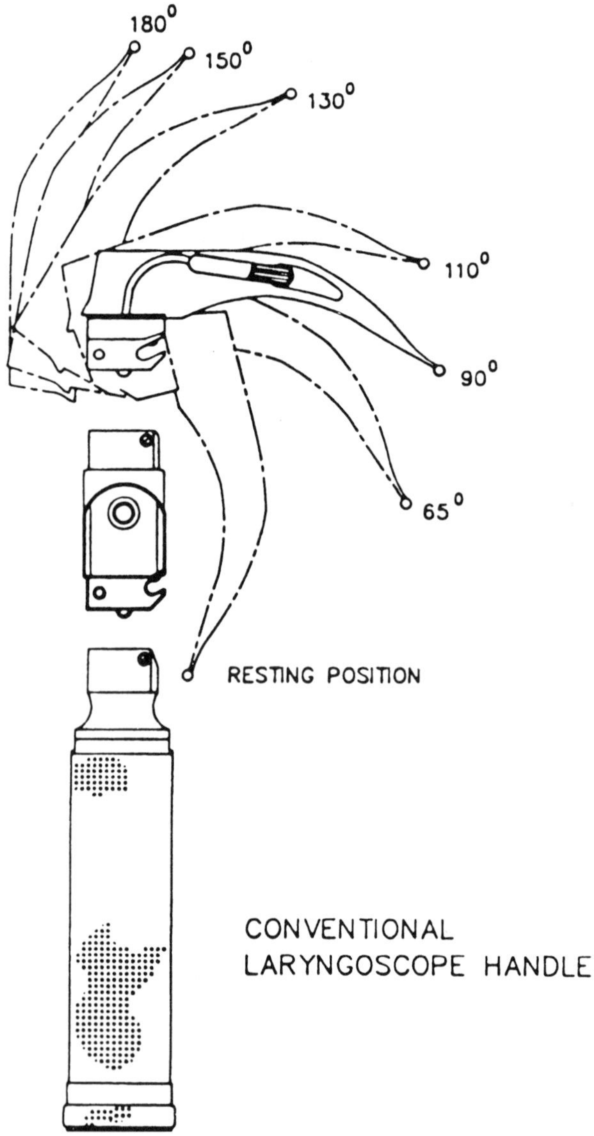

FIG. 40. The adapter illustrating the available angles.

scope blade. The rotating mechanism is operated by a push-rod connected to a spring-loaded pin in the middle of the adapter (Fig. 40). The laryngoscope is held and used in the standard fashion with the operator's left hypothenar eminence positioned very near the push-rod. If the clinical situation dictates, pressure from the hypothenar area toward the handle will release the rotating mechanism; when the blade reaches the desired angle, the blade is locked in position by releasing the push-rod. The inventors have found this device to be "convenient and easy to use in difficult clinical situations" (53) but no other formal clinical experience has appeared in literature.

LIGHTED STYLETS

History

The placement of ETTs under direct vision using a rigid laryngoscope blade has been the standard method for intubation for more than 50 years. Even with the introduction of multiple new rigid laryngoscope blades that were designed to specifically address anatomic variations that have been found to contribute to intubation difficulty, the inability to manage a difficult airway successfully is responsible for as many as 30% of anesthesia-related deaths in the United States (54,55). Preoperative airway assessment using the Mallampati classification (56), assessing the amount of atlanto-occipital joint extension (57,58), and measuring the mandibular space anterior to the larynx (59) are good, but not perfect, predictors of difficult intubation. This has led to the search for alternative techniques for intubation. One such technique is transillumination through the tissues of the neck, using a strong light from a special light source (illuminating stylet = lightwand = lighted stylet).

Sir Robert Macintosh was the first to report tracheal transillumination as an aid to intubation in 1957 (60). His device was an 18-in-long malleable introducer that was made to project beyond the end of the ETT. It was composed of an outer portex tubing that carried electrical wires within the lumen to illuminate the tip. The flexible casing also contained a copper wire that added to its mal-

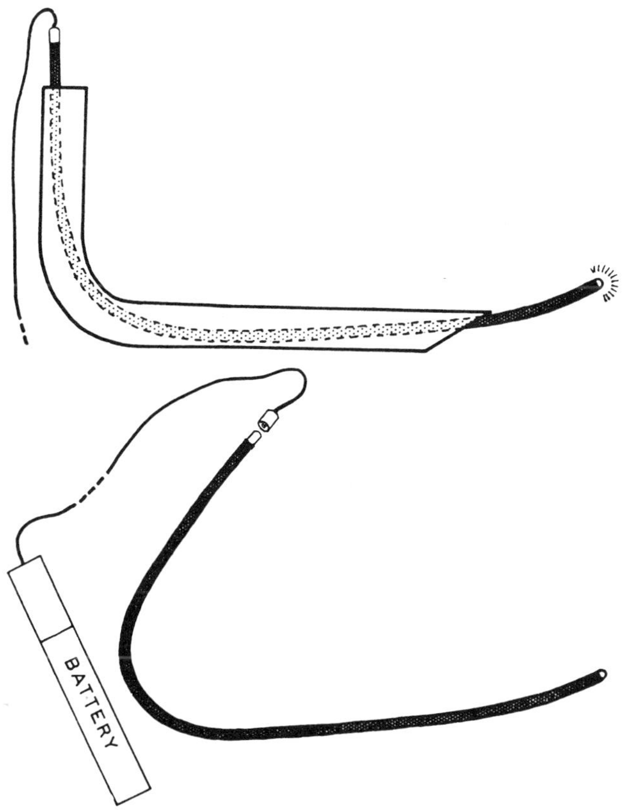

FIG. 41. Sir Robert Macintosh's malleable introducer *(bottom)* inserted into an endotracheal tube with the tip illuminated *(top)*.

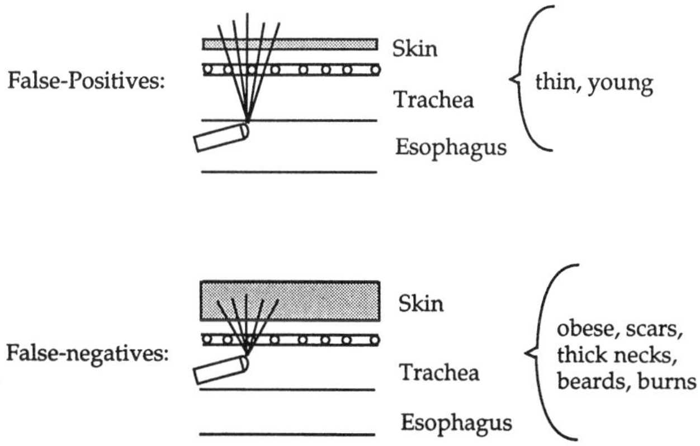

FIG. 42. Transillumination of the soft tissues of the neck in the anterior/posterior plane to differentiate esophageal from tracheal placement may be problematic for the extremes of physical habitus, such as the very thin or young (false-positive) and the morbidly obese or patients with very thick necks (false-negative).

leability in adapting to a particular clinical situation. The proximal end connected to a standard pocket battery (Fig. 41). This device was used in conjunction with direct laryngoscopy; the ETT was passed under direct vision with the light on the distal end of the stylet, providing additional illumination or serving as a backup source, should the light source of the laryngoscope fail.

In 1959, Berman (61) introduced another malleable stylet attached to an ordinary pen flashlight with a light at the end. He used his stylet as Macintosh did, primarily as an illumination aid during direct laryngoscopy. That same year, a flexible, lighted stylet was used to facilitate blind nasotracheal intubation (62). The first blind orotracheal intubation utilizing the tracheal transillumination technique was not reported until 1978 by Ducrow (63). He utilized red rubber endotracheal tubes that obscured the transillumination effect, necessitating dimming or turning off the room lighting. He also stated that the lighted stylet should not be placed within an ETT; he preferred to put the stylet in a catheter over which an ETT was passed. Rayburn (64) introduced the term *lightwand* in 1979 and recommended that it be used within an ETT. With the introduction of clear plastic endotracheal tubes, enthusiasm for this technique rose abruptly.

Theory

The theory behind tracheal transillumination for blind intubation is that as the endoscopist inserts the ETT containing the lighted stylet, transillumination will appear abruptly as the bulb passes the bulk of the tongue and epiglottis, just superior to the thyroid cartilage. Once the larynx is entered, a pronounced jack-o'-lantern effect is produced, which is occasionally more prominent if the ambient light is decreased (64). If the lighted stylet enters the esophagus, the light will appear dimmed; if deviation occurs laterally, the light is clearly off the midline. Since the light source is contained within the ETT lumen, it is presumed that the tube has passed through the glottic opening when transillumination of the larynx occurs; the trachea is then intubated by simply advancing the ETT off the stylet. A 96% accuracy in determining tube position (trachea, esophagus, upper airway) by physicians and paramedics in an average of 5 sec has been demonstrated using preplaced tubes in adult cadavers (65). Tube location was identified in two planes almost without exception, whereas the third plane, that of anterior-posterior depth (to differentiate esophageal from tracheal placement), may be problematic for the extremes of physical habitus, such as the very thin or young (false-positive) and the morbidly obese or patients with very thick necks (false-negative). In general, any condition that enhances or obscures the transillumination effect will lead to failure with this technique (Fig. 42).

Anesthesia

Some type of anesthesia is required to intubate the trachea electively. General anesthesia is not mandatory for this type of intubation technique. An awake intubation is the alternative; the minimum area that must be anesthetized includes the posterior third of the tongue to the mid-trachea. This can be achieved through the application of topical lidocaine (2% to 4%) or tetracaine (0.3% to 0.5%) and/or supplemental nerve blocks of the glossopharyngeal and superior laryngeal nerves. The glossopharyngeal nerve supplies the sensory innervation to the pharynx, tonsils, and posterior third of the tongue (66). The internal branch of the superior laryngeal nerve supplies the sensory innervation to the epiglottis, aryepiglottic folds, and mucous membrane of the larynx down to the false cords. In addition, a transtracheal block might be considered to provide anesthesia to the lower larynx. Another consideration for an awake intubation is administration of a vagolytic agent, atropine or glycopyrrolate, that not only helps to prevent a vagally mediated bradycardia in response to airway manipulation but will also promote bronchodilation and augment the application of local anesthetic by drying the oropharyngeal mucous membranes. Sedation is often not necessary if the upper airway has been well topicalized, but it is acceptable as long as it is titrated to maintain meaningful patient contact, i.e., the patient must be cooperative and able to follow directions. Finally, supplemental oxygen and adequate monitoring (at a minimum, ECG and pulse oximetry) are always advised.

Commercially Available Lighted Stylets

The technique for tracheal transillumination intubation has evolved with the introduction of new lighted stylets with subtle design changes. Commercially available lighted stylets include disposable [Flexi-lum™ surgical light (Linvatec Corporation, Largo, Florida) and Tube-Stat™ lighted stylet (Concept Corporation, Clearwater, Florida)], partially disposable [Trachlight™ stylet and tracheal lightwand (Laerdal Medical Corporation, Armonk, New York) and Imagica™ Fiberoptic Lighted Stylet (Fiberoptic Medical Products, Inc., Allentown, Pennsylvania)], and nondisposable versions [Fiberoptic Lighted Intubation Stilette and "The Shuttle"—Fiberlightview™ Lighted Stilette (patent pending) (Anesthesia Medical Specialties™, Santa Fe Springs, California)]. The design differences and the technique for intubation by tracheal transillumination for each of these devices will be discussed in the following sections.

The Disposable Lighted Stylets

Description

The Flexi-lum™ surgical light and Tube-Stat™ lighted stylet are similar in design. Both stylets have a solid state battery handle that carries a copper stylet ensheathed in

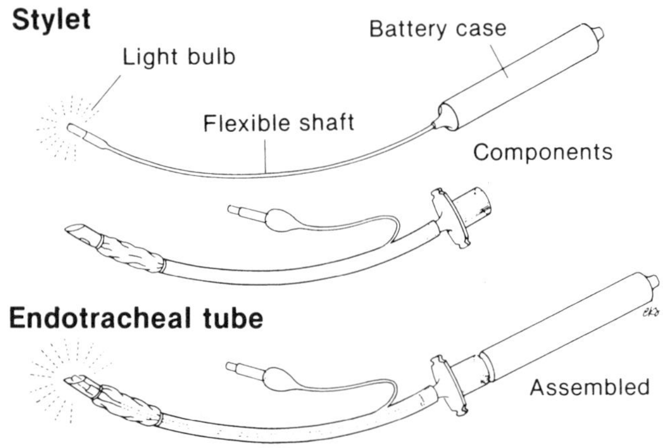

FIG. 43. A schematic of the Flexi-lum™ surgical light and Tube-Stat™ lighted stylet with labeled components *(top)* and inserted into an endotracheal tube (ETT) *(middle)* with the light bulb positioned within the lumen of the ETT, close to the distal tip *(bottom)*.

tough plastic (Fig. 43). The bulb is located on the distal end, and the light is operated by turning a switch on the proximal end of the handle. The Flexi-lum™ device was specifically designed as a surgical light and was never intended to be used as a stylet. In fact, its use has been abandoned, due to several known and one reported serious complication; the bulb became disconnected from the end of the surgical light and lodged in the right mainstem bronchus of a patient, requiring bronchoscopic removal (67–69). The device has since been redesigned to function specifically as an intubating stylet. The changes in design consisted of enclosing the wire and bulb together in a uniform polymer armor from bulb to battery case and incorporating a much brighter light to aid in transillumination. This new stylet is the Tube-Stat™ lighted stylet, and no further problems with detaching parts have been reported. The Tube-Stat™ costs about $30 and, with the nonreplaceable batteries, can be used approximately 30 times, a cost of $1 per use. It is available in two lengths, 25 and 33 cm. The longer model is more flexible and is intended for nasotracheal intubation. The increased malleability allows the tube to negotiate the small radius curvature at the posterior border of the palate.

Technique

Preparation of the Tube-Stat™ Lighted Stylet. A well-lubricated stylet is inserted into an appropriately sized ETT (5.0 mm or larger, the bulb diameter = 3.7 mm) so that it is positioned just within the lumen of the tube and the bulb does not project beyond the distal tip. Next, the arc that the stylet must make around the tongue and over the epiglottis into the larynx is estimated from the patient's submental mandibular-hyoid distance. This is accomplished by having the patient extend the neck as far

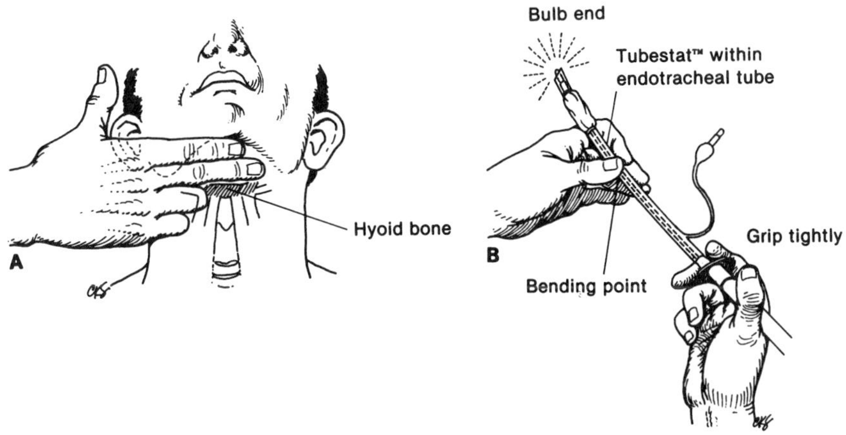

FIG. 44. Preparation of the Tube-Stat™ lighted stylet. **A:** With the patient's head fully extended, the submental mandibular-hyoid distance is measured. **B:** The shaft of the stylet is bent equal to this distance from the distal stylet tip.

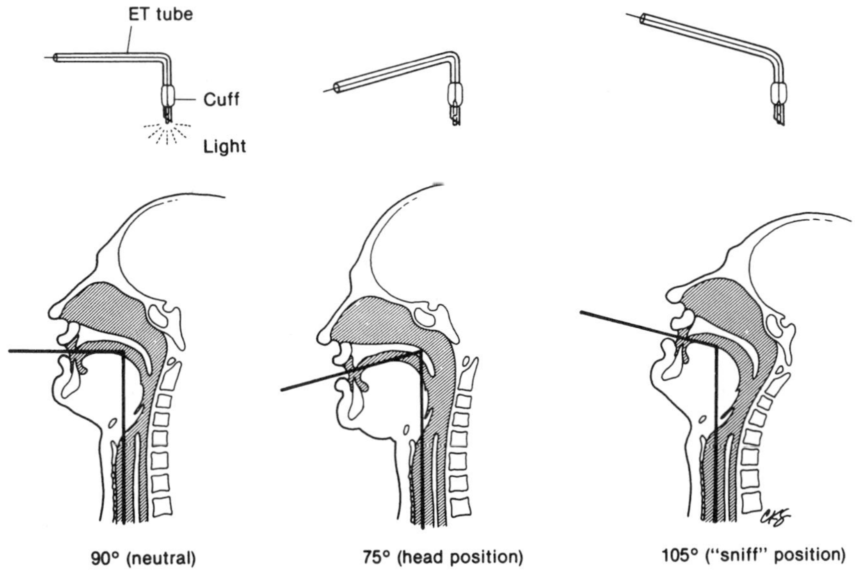

FIG. 45. The angle of the bend in the stylet is dependent on the patient's head position. With the patient's head neutral *(left)*, the angle should approximate a tight 90° arc; with the patient's head flexed, less than a 90° bend is necessary and with the patient's head extended, greater than 90° is required.

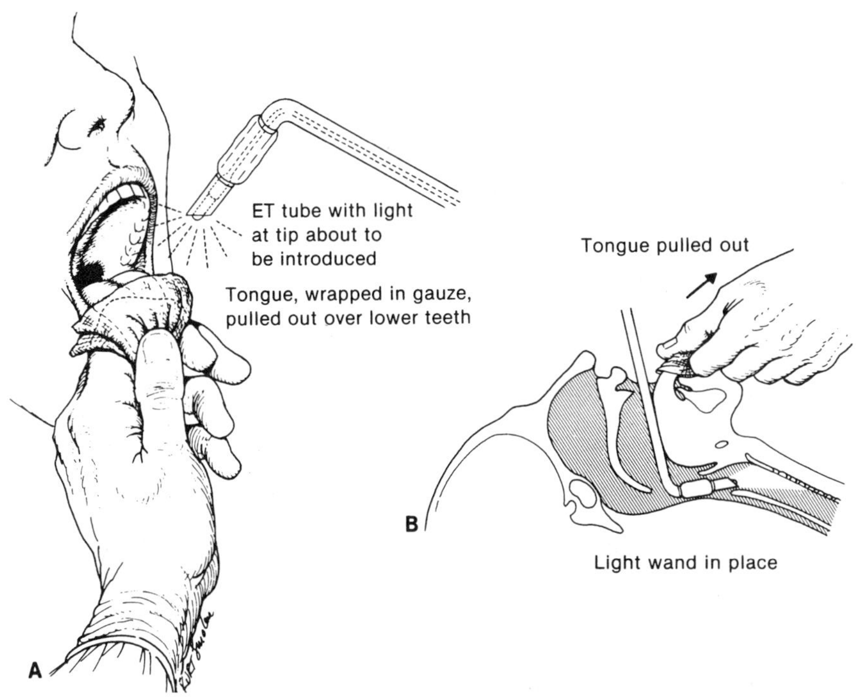

FIG. 46. Prior to inserting the lighted stylet, the tongue must be brought out of the patient's mouth and pulled out over the lower teeth. **A:** The awake cooperative patient can assist with this maneuver. **B:** When the patient is under general anesthesia, use of a gauze pad greatly facilitates this task.

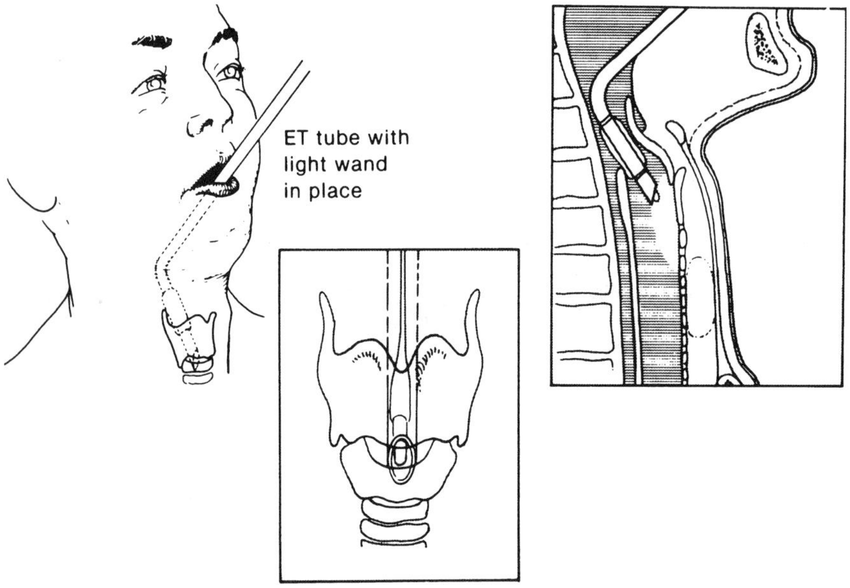

FIG. 47. With the lighted stylet correctly positioned, abrupt transillumination will appear superior to the thyroid cartilage. If the ambient light is decreased, the transillumination has been likened to a jack-o'-lantern effect.

as possible and measuring the distance from the tip of the mentum to the hyoid bone. The shaft of the stylet is then flexed equal to this distance from the distal tip of the stylet (Fig. 44). The angle of the bend in the stylet is crucial and is entirely dependent on head position. If the patient's head and neck are in the neutral position, the angle should approximate 90°; with the patient's head flexed, an angle of less than 90° is necessary. If the patient's head is extended, an angle of greater than 90° is required (Fig. 45).

Intubation with the Tube-Stat™ Lighted Stylet. Once the lighted stylet has been prepared, it is ready to be inserted into the oropharynx. If the patient is awake and cooperative, he/she should be asked to stick out his/her tongue; if the patient is uncooperative or under general anesthesia, the tongue is grasped with a piece of gauze and pulled out over the lower teeth (Fig. 46). Copious secretions can greatly increase the difficulty of this task; if this technique is anticipated and there is no contraindication, prior administration of an antisialagogue is helpful.

The tube and stylet are held in the horizontal plane with the long axis parallel to the patient. They are then inserted into the oropharynx in the midline or from the side of the mouth. The device is rotated around the curvature of the tongue, observing for abrupt transillumination as the light appears superior to the thyroid cartilage. If the ambient light is decreased, transillumination is usually much more obvious and has been likened to a jack-o'-lantern effect (Fig. 47). If the light is midline but appears dimmed, the lighted stylet probably entered the esophagus, and a combination of gentle withdrawal and lifting will create a popping sensation as the tip of the stylet enters the glottic orifice, producing tracheal transillumination. It is occasionally helpful to purposely orient the lighted stylet in the right piriform fossa because the brightness and definition of light transmitted in this location is very consistent with that observed when the lighted stylet is intratracheal. Williams has recommended his Airway Intubator™ to be a useful splint and guide to keep the lighted stylet midline by preventing lateral movement. In the correct position, it also keeps the ETT from going posteriorly into the esophagus, which facilitates quick and easy insertion into the larynx, decreasing the amount of time to successful intubation (69,70,71).

Once tracheal transillumination is identified, the ETT is advanced off the stylet. With the stylet in the proper position, it is pointing at the anterior wall of the thyroid cartilage. If the tube and stylet are advanced as a unit, the distal end will impact the anterior larynx, inducing trauma to the mucosa. Therefore, it is important to hold the lighted stylet in a static position with one hand while the other hand advances the ETT off the stylet (Fig. 48). As the tube enters the trachea, the light in the neck may appear to separate and form an expanding dumbbell as the ETT enters the thorax. The stylet is then removed and the usual steps should follow to confirm tracheal intubation.

Clinical Experience

Both the Flexi-lum™ and Tube-Stat™ lighted stylets have been reported to be successful alternative intubation devices. Shortly after Ducrow's (63) initial report of blind orotracheal intubation with the lighted stylet, Rayburn (64) wrote that he had been using a very similar technique for "years" under general anesthesia with a relaxant and, more commonly, using regional anesthesia. He found this technique extremely successful, and intu-

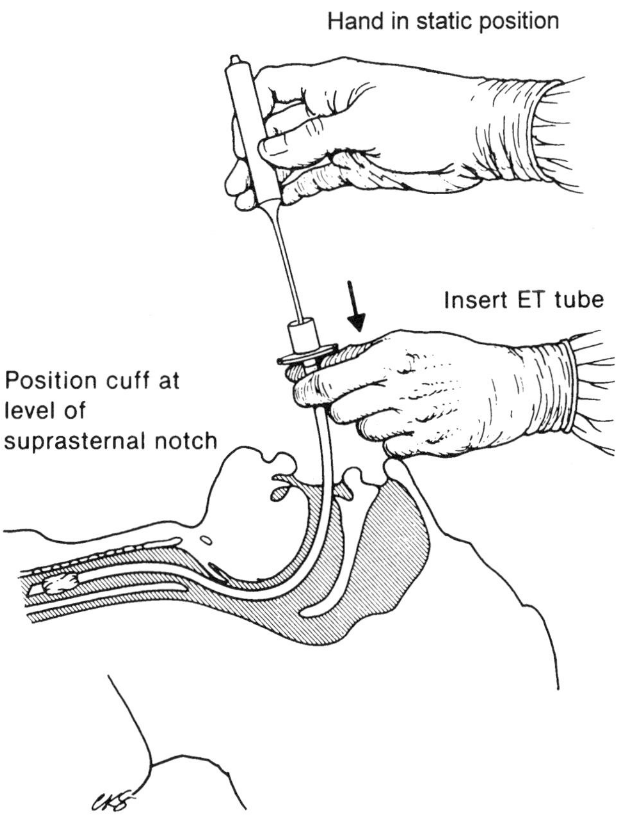

FIG. 48. The endotracheal tube is advanced off the lighted stylet with one hand, while the lighted stylet is held in the static position with the other hand.

bation was accomplished in "seconds" with a minimum of practice. Problems he encountered with this technique were usually due either to inadequate regional anesthesia or to an improper curve at the distal end of the ETT and stylet, preventing easy entry into the trachea. He reported no complications and was successful in intubating patients when the neck could not be extended (burn strictures, unstable cervical spines), in cases of large oropharyngeal tumors where there was not enough room in the mouth for a laryngoscope, and in patients with congenital syndromes where visualization of the larynx was difficult by conventional methods (Treacher-Collins, Pierre-Robin).

Other reports of success with the Flexi-lum™ and Tube-Stat™ followed, including its use for guided orotracheal intubation in the prehospital setting (68,69,72,73). Failure of this technique was attributed to marked obesity (73), excessive ambient light (73), and copious vomitus in the oropharynx, which obscured the light (73). Ellis et al. (74) were the first to compare blind orotracheal intubation using transillumination of the neck tissues with the Tube-Stat™ lighted stylet to conventional, direct-vision laryngoscopy in a randomized, prospective study in the operating room. They reported a 100% success rate in the 40 patients intubated with the lighted stylet; 11 patients (22%) required 2 attempts, and 3 patients (6%) required 3 attempts, with an average intubation time of 11–72 sec. No major complications and no soft tissue or dental trauma occurred.

Fox et al. (75) subsequently compared intubation with the Flexi-lum™ surgical light to a blind nasal approach in awake patients with regard to efficacy, speed, and incidence of complications. Their study demonstrated that the patients in the lightwand group required significantly fewer attempts and less time to successful intubation compared to the blind nasal approach. In addition, less trauma occurred in the patients intubated with the lightwand, attributed primarily to avoidance of the nares. These investigators and others believe that use of a lightwand for nasal intubation is too traumatic, although other investigators have found a useful role for the lighted stylet to nasally intubate apneic patients (76). Stone et al. (67) reported a complication of nasotracheal intubation with the Flexi-lum™ lighted stylet; the lightwand bulb disconnected from the distal stylet upon its removal from the ETT, lodging in the patient's right lung and necessitating bronchoscopic removal. Other reported complications with the use of the Tube-Stat™ and Flexi-lum™ lighted stylets include cricoarytenoid dislocation (77), nonspecific tissue trauma (73), and arytenoid dislocation (78).

Several studies have also shown lighted stylets to be useful devices for positioning endotracheal tubes. The gold standard to assess tube position is a chest roentgenogram, particularly after emergency intubations (79). However, this is expensive and time-consuming. A useful and inexpensive alternative is transtracheal illumination, which has been found to be useful and accurate in optimal tracheal tube placement (80,81). With proper cuff positioning, the maximum point of transillumination was found to be visible just distal to the cricoid cartilage; this equated to a distance from the tip of the endotracheal tube to the carina of 3.7–5 cm.

The Partially Disposable Lighted Stylets

Trachlight™ Stylet and Tracheal Lightwand

Description. The Trachlight™ stylet and tracheal lightwand consists of a disposable stylet that attaches to a nondisposable handle. The stylet differs from other lighted stylets in several ways; it is longer, has a brighter bulb at the tip with the light beam pointed both anteriorly and downward into the airway, a retractable inner rigid wire that can be removed to convert the lightwand to a flexible instrument suitable for nasal intubation, and a longer stylet portion that enables its use with tubes of standard length (82). The stylet attaches to the handle via a ratchetlike mechanism, and its position is adjusted on the handle by a release arm situated on the proximal end.

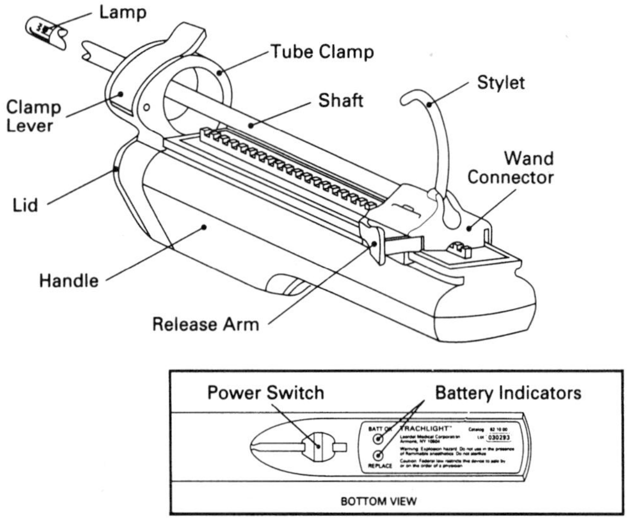

FIG. 49. Components of the Trachlight™ stylet and tracheal lightwand.

A tube clamp is located on the distal end of the handle and is designed to fit a standard 15-mm ETT adapter. A clamp lever on the tube clamp secures the ETT in position. The handle contains three AAA batteries to power the light source. The power switch for the light control is located on the underside of the handle, along with a light indicator that illuminates when the batteries require replacement (Fig. 49).

Technique.

Stylet preparation. Prior to attaching the stylet to the handle, the metal rod within the stylet is snapped into the wand connector (Figs. 49, 50A). Once secured, the release arm is squeezed (Fig. 50A, *arrow 1*) and the wand connector is slid onto the back of the handle (Fig. 50A, *arrow 2*) so that the stylet projects through the tube clamp and the grooves engage on both sides. Next, a well-lubricated ETT is slid over the distal end of the stylet until the 15-mm adapter on the ETT enters the tube clamp (Fig. 50B, *arrow 1*). The clamp lever is then closed to secure the ETT (Fig. 50B, *arrow 2*) in position. The lamp on the distal end of the stylet is positioned on the wand connector by squeezing the release arm until it is just proximal to the bevel within the lumen of the ETT. Aligning the cm markings on the ETT with the corresponding markings on the stylet ensures that the stylet does not project beyond the tip of the ETT.

Orotracheal intubation. For orotracheal intubation, a bend in the wand is made prior to inserting the device into the patient's mouth. A "bend here" marking is located on the stylet, but as previously discussed, it is important to measure each patient's hyomental distance in order to accurately estimate the arc the stylet must make around the tongue to enter the trachea. In addition, the angle of the bend is dependent on the head position of the patient. If the patient's head is neutral, the angle of the bend should approximate a tight 90°. Once the tube/Trachlight™ is prepared, the light is switched on to ensure that it is working properly; it is important to check that the green "BATT OK" indicator light is on and functioning.

To insert the tube/Trachlight™ into the oropharynx, the tongue must be lifted up and out of the patient's mouth, pulling it over the lower teeth. The device is inserted from the right corner of the patient's mouth and rotated around the back of the tongue. The device is brought to the midline and gently advanced while observing for abrupt transillumination at the laryngeal prominence (Fig. 51A). Once a bright glow is seen in the midline, it is advanced another 1–2 cm until resistance is met. At this point, the glow should have moved just below the laryn-

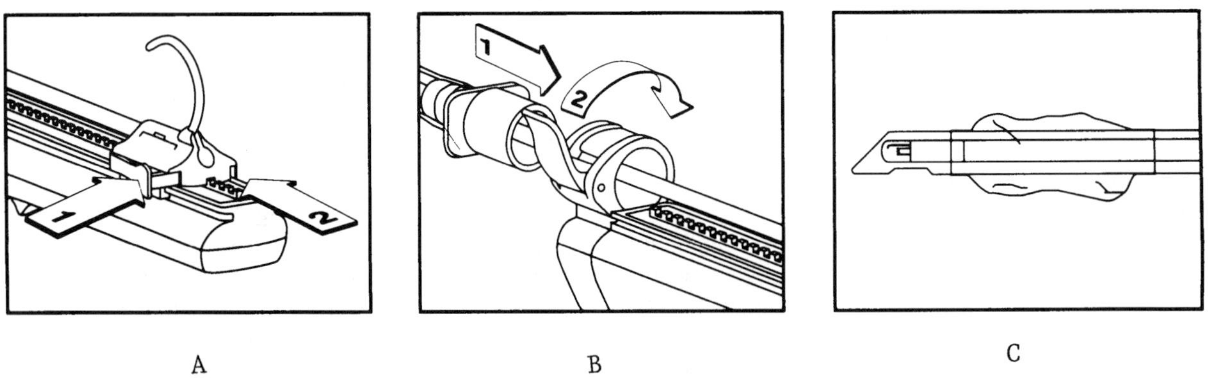

FIG. 50. A: To attach the stylet to the handle, the metal rod is snapped into the wand connector and once secured, the release arm is squeezed *(arrow 1)* and the wand connector is slid onto the back of the handle until the grooves engage on either side *(arrow 2)*. **B:** A well-lubricated endotracheal tube (ETT) is advanced over the stylet *(arrow 1)* and pushed into the tube clamp. It is secured in place by the clamp lever *(arrow 2)*. **C:** The release arm on the wand connector (see Fig. 49) is squeezed to adjust the position of the stylet within the ETT so that the lamp sits just proximal to the bevel within the tube lumen.

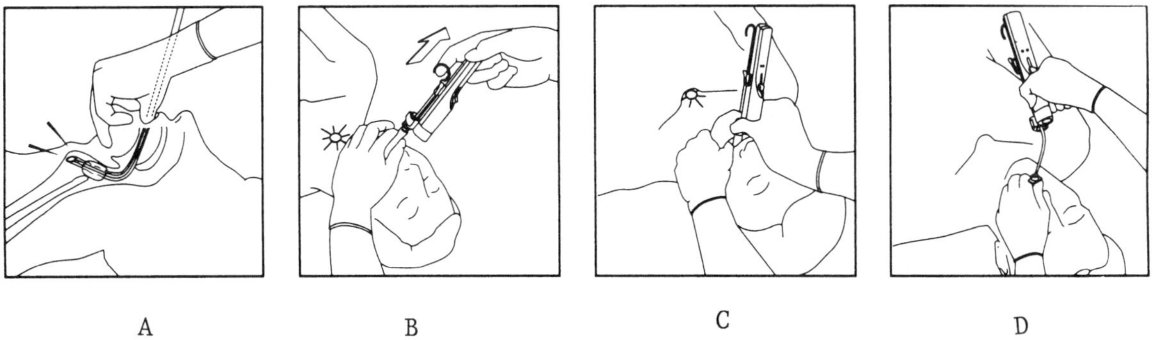

FIG. 51. A: Trachlight™ orotracheal intubation. The tongue is lifted up and out of the patients mouth over the lower teeth and a correctly bent (see Figs. 44,45) tube/Trachlight™ is inserted in the midline around the tongue, observing for transillumination at the laryngeal prominence. **B:** When a glow is observed in the correct location, the metal rod is retracted out of the stylet approximately 10 cm. **C:** The tube/Trachlight™ is advanced until the glow just begins to disappear under the sternum. **D:** The tube is held against the patient's lips, the clamp lever is unlocked and the Trachlight™ is removed.

geal prominence and should have become brighter and smaller. This indicates that the tip has passed through the vocal cords and is pressed up against the anterior trachea. If the light appears dimmer or if no glow is observed with advancement of the stylet, the tip probably entered the esophagus. If the glow appears laterally, the tube/Trachlight™ is gently withdrawn until transillumination is observed in the midline. Once 30 sec has elapsed, the lamp will begin blinking "as a reminder to ventilate the patient and minimize heat." (83) Turning the power switch off and then on will quickly restore the light source, but the distal lamp tip will warm with repeated similar maneuvers. This emphasizes the importance of keeping the stylet within the ETT lumen so that the lamp does not make contact with the oropharyngeal mucosa.

Once transillumination is observed below the laryngeal prominence, the tube is held tightly against the patient's teeth or lips, and the metal rod is retracted out of the stylet approximately 10 cm (Fig. 51B). This increases the flexibility of the distal tip, which minimizes the trauma to the tracheal mucosa when the tube/Trachlight™ is advanced into the trachea. Positioning is completed by advancing the entire apparatus until the glow just begins to disappear behind the sternum. In this position, the tube tip is halfway through the vocal cords to the carina (Fig. 51C). Intubation is completed by holding the tube against the patient's teeth, releasing the clamp lever to unlock the ETT, and then removing the Trachlight™ (Fig. 51D). The usual confirmatory steps should follow to assure tracheal intubation.

Nasotracheal intubation. The Trachlight™ can also be utilized for nasotracheal intubation. The technique is similar to orotracheal intubation, with a few minor alterations. Prior to attaching the stylet to the handle, the retractable inner metal rod is completely removed. After attaching the stylet to the handle, a well-lubricated stylet is positioned within the ETT, as previously described. If a directional tip (e.g., Endotrol®, Mallinckrodt, Inc., Glens Falls, New York) ETT is used, the lamp is recessed approximately 0.5 cm from the proximal edge of the bevel to prevent the lamp from protruding beyond the tip of the tube when traction is exerted on the loop which directs the tip of the ETT anteriorly.

The tube tip and cuff are lubricated well to facilitate entry into the nares. The tube bevel should be against the septum or the floor of the nasal cavity as it is advanced into the nasal passage. The entire device is advanced until a well-defined bright glow is observed just below the laryngeal prominence. If a directional tip ETT is utilized, it may help guide the tube tip anteriorly into the trachea. Intubation is completed as described for orotracheal intubation.

Clinical Experience. Clinical studies on the use of the Trachlight™ are limited to preliminary investigations presented in abstract form by one primary investigator, Dr. Orlando Hung from Dalhousie University in Halifax, Canada. He and his collaborators have found the Trachlight™ lighted stylet to be useful for intubation in patients with known difficult airways (84) (e.g., previous failed intubation, cervical spine instability, ankylosing temporomandibular joints, morbidly obese patients), for nasotracheal intubation (85), and for determining optimal ETT positioning following intubation (86). In addition, they found no significant difference in time to intubation or any significant change in mean arterial pressure or heart rate following intubation (87) with the Trachlight™ compared to direct laryngoscopy. Lastly, they found this device to be simple to use, as demonstrated by novice intubators who took half the time to intubation, had fewer failures, and reported less trauma with fewer sore throats in patients whose tracheas were intubated with the Trachlight™, compared to direct laryngoscopy (88).

The Imagica™ Fiberoptic Lighted Stylet

Description. The Imagica™ Fiberoptic Lighted Stylet (Fiberoptic Medical Products, Inc., Allentown, Pennsylvania) consists of a 10-foot-long, flexible fiberoptic light guide that has the last 40 cm covered in malleable annealed surgical stainless steel. The light guide connects to any standard light source (including Wolf, Stortz, ACMI, Olympus, etc.). A disposable sheath covers the malleable portion of the light guide. This sheath is made of frosted PVC with the distal end completely sealed and the other end fitted with a Luer-lock attachment for connection to the light guide. The sealed end of the sheath diffuses the light in a 360° pattern. Plastic fibers within the light guide transmit xenon light to emit an extremely bright light. In fact, the Imagica™ Fiberoptic Lighted Stylet emits the brightest light of any of the commercially available lighted stylets. The sheath also has cm markings to help position the stylet within the ETT lumen.

The stylet comes in two sizes, small for 2.5- to 4.0-mm ID ETT and large to accommodate 4.5- to 10.0-mm ETT. The fiberoptic light guide costs $89 and can be used innumerable times, although it may fatigue and break if bent repeatedly in the same location. The PVC disposable sheath sells for $2.95 and is discarded after each use. The light guide can be totally submerged for cold (Cidex) sterilization or can be gas (ETO) sterilized.

Technique.

Preparation of the stylet. The proximal end of the light guide is attached to a standard light source (see above) and a clean disposable sheath is locked in place (Luer-lock) over the distal malleable stylet. A well-lubricated, appropriately sized ETT is positioned over the sheath, and the cm markings on the sheath are aligned with the same cm markings on the ETT. With proper alignment, the distal end of the stylet will not project beyond the tip of the tube. The ETT is secured in place by a pluglike adapter that fits into the proximal 15-mm ETT adapter and locks onto the stylet.

Intubation. The technique for orotracheal intubation is identical to that described for the Tube-Stat™ lighted stylet. The brighter xenon light emitted from the distal tip of the Imagica™ Fiberoptic Lighted Stylet projects a much more prominent transillumination effect which precludes the need to reduce ambient lighting, an obvious advantage when this is not possible. Nasotracheal intubation is not recommended, due to the rigidity of the stainless steel stylet.

Clinical Experience. The Imagica™ Fiberoptic Lighted Stylet is a relatively new device on the market and, although no formal clinical studies have been performed, personal experience has found this device to be easy to use, with the special advantage of an extremely bright light source that greatly enhances the transillumination effect.

The Nondisposable Lighted Stylets

Fiberoptic Lighted Intubation Stilette

Description. The Fiberoptic Lighted Intubation Stilette supplied by Anesthesia Medical Specialties™ is a nondisposable lighted stylet (Fig. 53). It is made of aircraft-quality metal that surrounds the fiberoptic light bundles and is encased from bulb to battery case. Two standard AA batteries power the incandescent light source. This lighted stylet is available in adult and pediatric versions (pediatric fits down to a 4.0-mm ID ETT). The cost is approximately 2–3 times that of a disposable lighted stylet (e.g., the Tube-Stat™), but this stylet should, theoretically, last forever. The risk of infection from reuse of this lighted stylet is minimized by the ability to satisfactorily sterilize it by submerging the malleable stylet portion in cold Cidex solution. Gas (ETO) sterilization has not been recommended.

Technique. The technique of this stylet is identical to those described for the Tube-Stat™ and Imagica™ Fiber-

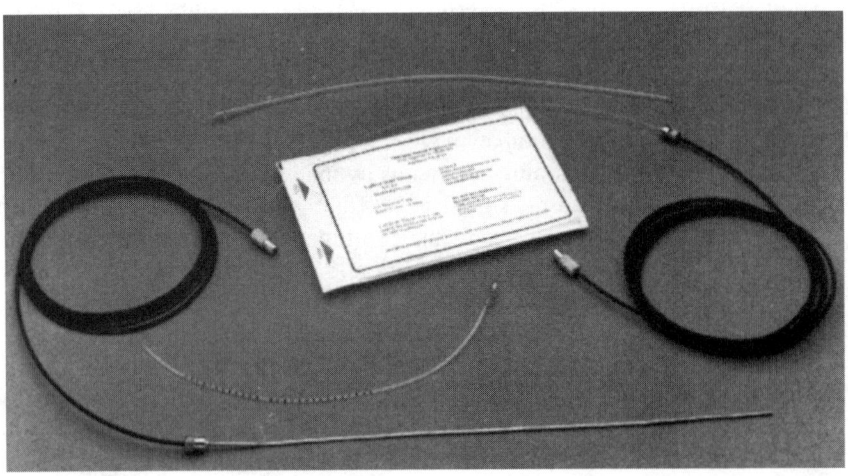

FIG. 52. The Imagica™ Fiberoptic Lighted Stylet in adult *(left, bottom)* and pediatric *(right, top)* sizes. A disposable PVC sheath *(middle)* fits over the distal malleable stainless steel portion.

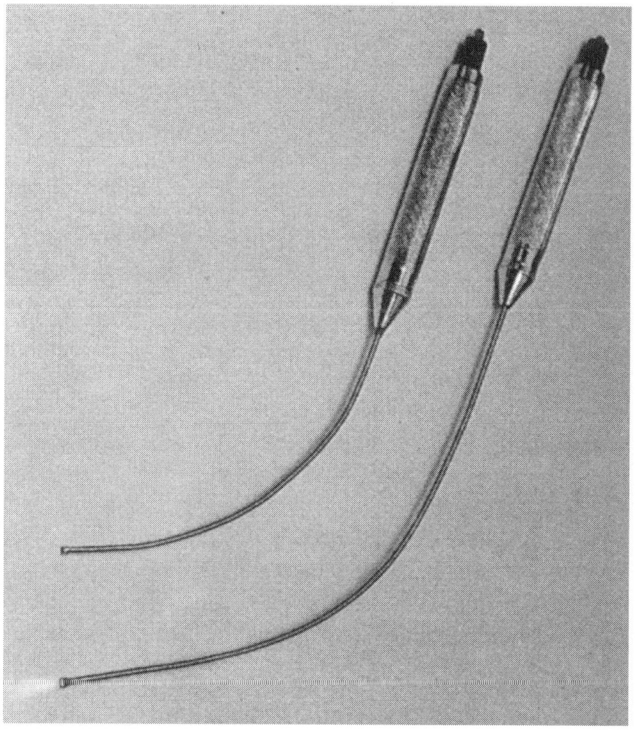

FIG. 53. The nondisposable adult *(right)* and pediatric *(left)* Fiberoptic Lighted Intubation Stilettes.

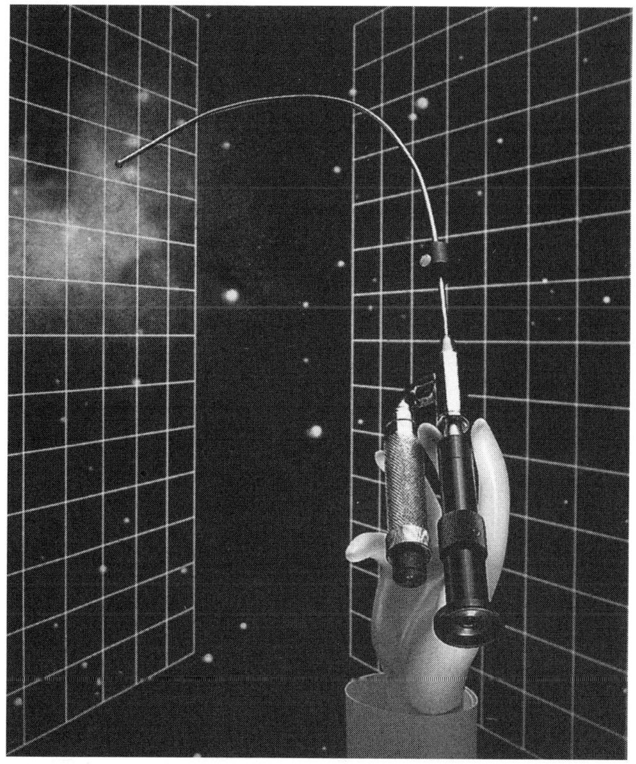

FIG. 54. "The Shuttle"—Fiberlightview™ Lighted Stilette with the viewing lens on the proximal end of the malleable stylet.

optic Lighted Stylet. The brightness of illumination provided by the light source is approximately equivalent to the Tube-Stat™ lighted stylet; both are inferior light sources compared to the halogen light emitted from the Trachlight™ lighted stylet and the xenon light emitted from the Imagica™ Fiberoptic Lighted Stylet.

Clinical Experience. No formal clinical studies have appeared in the literature with this device.

"The Shuttle"—Fiberlightview™ Lighted Stilette

Description. The most recently introduced lighted stylet to the anesthesia community is "The Shuttle"—Fiberlightview™ Lighted Stilette (patent pending). It is identical to the Fiberoptic Lighted Intubation Stilette, also supplied by Anesthesia Medical Specialties™, except that it has a viewing lens on top of the stylet and is designed for use in conjunction with direct laryngoscopy, not only to increase illumination but to also provide a clear view of the larynx by means of the viewing lens (Fig. 54). This indirect viewing capability is an obvious advantage when a direct view is obstructed on direct laryngoscopy. The malleable stylet is made of stainless steel and is operated with standard batteries or can be attached to an external light source (AS-150, Anesthesia Medical Specialties™, Santa Fe Springs, California). For teaching purposes, a coupler charged device (CCD) camera can additionally be attached to the viewing lens to display images of the airway on a monitor (AS-2000, Anesthesia Medical Specialties™, Santa Fe Springs, California). Both adult and pediatric versions are available (adult is 33 cm in length and fits 4.5-mm ID ETT minimum; the pediatric lighted stylet is 21 cm in length and fits 3.5-mm ID ETT minimum). The malleable stylet can be submerged in cold Cidex solution for sterilization; gas sterilization is not recommended. "The Shuttle"—Fiberlightview™ Lighted Stilette sells for approximately $925.

Technique. This lighted stylet was designed for use as an illumination and optical guide during direct laryngoscopy and not as a device for performing blind orotracheal intubation based on transillumination of the soft tissues of the neck. If it were inserted blindly into the oropharynx, the viewing capability would be lost because the surrounding oropharyngeal tissues would collapse over the distal lens.

After focusing the lens and lubricating the stylet well, it is inserted into an appropriately sized ETT, much like a standard malleable stylet. The light source is illuminated, and standard direct laryngoscopy is performed. The increased illumination provided by the Fiberlightview™ Lighted Stilette is designed to aid with direct visualization of the larynx to facilitate intubation. If direct sight of the laryngeal inlet is obstructed on direct laryngoscopy, the intubationist looks through the viewing lens on the lighted stylet and manipulates the ETT, in an effort to increase the field of visualization. Once an indirect view of the larynx is obtained, the ETT is advanced through the vocal cords, off the lighted stylet.

Clinical Experience. The indirect viewing capability of this device may assist with difficult intubations as well as reduce trauma during intubation. However, no clinical studies have been performed on the utility and efficacy of this device.

CONCLUSION

Most patients can be intubated with one of the three principle laryngoscope blade types; the straight blade (Jackson), the curved tip (Miller), or the curved blade (Macintosh). However, despite careful preinduction assessment of the airway, there are still occasional patients in whom intubation is difficult or impossible with these conventional laryngoscope blades. When this situation occurs, many options exist, including using one or more of the blades or lighted stylets discussed. The best choice is the one that the intubationist is most familiar with. The basis of design of new intubating devices ranges from individual clinical experience to x-ray (89,90) and anatomic studies, as well as the use of an animal model (24); overall, it has been a relatively arbitrary process. In fact, Sikes aptly stated that "accessories for endotracheal anaesthesia are without end. There is no living anaesthetist who holds the distinction of not having designed one or more devices." (91) It is essential that every anesthesiologist gain experience with several different devices or techniques designed to address specific anatomic variations that contribute to intubation difficulties, so that when an airway management problem occurs, it can be approached in a knowledgeable, confident manner.

REFERENCES

1. Collins VJ. *Endotracheal Anesthesia: Basic Considerations in Principles of Anesthesiology*, 2nd edition. Philadelphia: Lea and Febegson, 1976.
2. Gillespie NA. *Equipment and Apparatus in Endotracheal Anesthesia*. Madison, WI: University of Wisconsin Press, 1963.
3. Fink BR. *The Human Larynx—a Functional Study*. New York: Raven Press, 1975;9–12.
4. Hirsch NP, Smith GB, Hirsch PO. Alfred Kirstein, pioneer of direct laryngoscopy. *Anaesthesia* 1986;41:42–45.
5. Macintosh RR. A new laryngoscope. *Lancet* 1943;1:205.
6. Miller RA. A new laryngoscope. *Anesthesiology* 1941;2:317–320.
7. Zollner F. Gustav Killian, father of bronchoscopy. *Arch Otolaryngol* 1965;82:656–659.
8. Chapter 7. The Cheerful Centenarian, or the Founder of Laryngoscopy. In: Sykes WS: *Essays on the first hundred years of anaesthesia, Volume 2.* Huntington, New York: Robert E. Kreiger Publishing Co., 1972;95–111.
9. Jackson C. The technique of insertion of intratracheal insufflation tubes. *Surg Gynecol Obstet* 1913;17:507–509.
10. Janeway HH. Intratracheal anesthesia from the standpoint of the nose, throat and oral surgeon with a description of a new instrument for catheterizing the trachea. *Laryngoscope* Nov 1913;23:1082–1090.
11. Calverly RK. Intubation in anaesthesia. In: Atkinson RS, Boulton TB, eds. *The History of Anesthesia*. Parthenon Publishing Group, Royal Society of Medical International Congress and Symposium Series No. 134, 1989;333–341.
12. Human JU. *Blind Intubation and the Signs of Anaesthesia*. London, 1941;57.
13. Macintosh RR. Laryngoscope blades. *Lancet* 1944;1:485.
14. Jephcott A. The Macintosh laryngoscope. A historical note on its clinical and commercial development. *Anaesthesia* 1984;39:474–479.
15. McIntyre JNR. Laryngoscope design and the difficult adult tracheal intubation. *Can J Anaesth* 1989;36:94–98.
16. Siker ES. A mirror laryngoscope. *Anesthesiology* 1956;17:38–42.
17. Bellhouse CP. An angulated laryngoscope for routine and difficult tracheal intubation. *Anesthesiology* 1988;69:126–129.
18. Mayall RM. The Belscope for management of the difficult airway. *Anesthesiology* 1992;76:1059–1060.
19. Soper RL. A new laryngoscope for anaesthetists. *BMJ* 1947;1:265.
20. Bizzarri DV, Giuffrida JG. Improved laryngoscope blade designed for ease of manipulation and reduction of trauma. *Anesth Analg* 1958; 37:231–232.
21. Racz GB. Improved vision modification of the Macintosh laryngoscope. [Letter to the editor] *Anaesthesia* 1984;39:1249–1250.
22. Kawahara M, Takeshita T, Akitu S. A new model of laryngoscope equipped with fiberoptics. *Anesth Prog* 1989;36:70–71.
23. Choi JJ. A new double-angle blade for direct laryngoscopy. *Anesthesiology* 72:576, 1990.
24. Bainton CR. A new laryngoscope blade to overcome pharyngeal obstruction. *Anesthesiology* 1987;67:767–770.
25. Grande CM, Barton CR, Stene JK. Appropriate techniques for airway management of emergency patients with suspected spinal cord injury. *Anesth Analg* 1988;67:714–715.
26. Hastings RH, Marks JD. Airway management for trauma patients with potential cervical spine injuries. *Anesth Analg* 1991;l73:471–482.
27. Bjoraker DG. The Bullard intubating laryngoscopes. *Anesthesiol Rev* 1990;XVII(5):64–70.
28. Dyson A, Harris J, Bhatta K. Rapidity and accuracy of tracheal intubation in a mannequin: comparison of the fiberoptic with the Bullard laryngoscope. *Br J Anaesth* 1990;65:268–270.
29. Borland LM, Casselbrant M. The Bullard laryngoscope: a new indirect oral laryngoscope (pediatric version). *Anesth Analg* 1990;70: 105–108.
30. Saunders PR, Giesecke AH. Clinical assessment of the adult Bullard laryngoscope [abstract]. *Can J Anaesth* 1989;36:518–519.
31. Gorback MS. Management of the challenging airway with the Bullard laryngoscope. *J Clin Anesth* 1991;3:473–377.
32. Cooper SD, Benumof JL, Ozaki GT. Evaluation of the Bullard laryngoscope using the new intubating stylet: comparison with conventional laryngoscopy. *Anesth Analg* 1994;79:965–970.
33. Hastings RH, Vigil CC, Hanna R, Yang BY, Sartoris DJ. Cervical spine movement during laryngoscopy with the Bullard, Macintosh and Miller laryngoscopes. *Anesthesiology*. in press.
34. Wu T, Chou H. A new laryngoscope: the combination intubating device. *Anesthesiology* 1994;81(4):1085–1086.
35. Kovac AL. The Augustine guide: a new device for blind orotracheal intubation. *Anesthesiol Rev* 1993;1:25–29.
36. Krafft P, Fitzgerald R, Pernarstorfer T, Kapral S, Weinstabl C. A new device for blind oral intubation in routine and difficult airway management. *Eur J Anaesthesiol* 1994;11:207–212.
37. Carr RJ, Belani KGB. Clinical assessment of the Augustine guide for endotracheal intubation. *Anesth Analg* 1994;78:983–987.
38. Cicala RS, Grande CM, Stene JK, Behringer EC. Emergency and elective airway management for trauma patients. *Textbook of Trauma Anesthesia and Critical Care*. Baltimore: Mosby, 1993;368–369.
39. Kovac AL. Use of the Augustine stylet anticipating difficult tracheal intubation in Treacher-Collins syndrome. *J Clin Anesth* 1992;4:409–412.
40. LaTourette P, Patil VU. The Augustine guide as a fiberoptic bronchoscopic guide. *Anesth Analg* 1993;76:1164–1165.
41. Bourke DL, Lawrence J. Another way to insert a Macintosh blade. *Anesthesiology* 1983;39:80.
42. Datta S, Briwa J. Modified laryngoscope for endotracheal intubation of obese patients. *Anesth Analg* 1981;60:120–121.
43. Kubota Y. Mammomegaly and intubation. *Anaesthesia* 1982;37:779–780.

44. Kay NH. Mammomegaly and intubation. *Anaesthesia* 1982;37:221.
45. Jephcott A. Mammomegaly and intubation—the Polio blade. *Anaesthesia* 1982;37:780.
46. Wilson J, Kerr M. *Operative Obstetrics*, 10th ed. London: Balliere-Tindall, 1982;243.
47. Lagade MRG, Poppers PJ. Revival of the Polio laryngoscope blade. *Anesthesiology* 1982;57:545.
48. Weeks DB. A new use for an old blade. *Anesthesiology* 1974;40:200–201.
49. Kessel J. A laryngoscope for obstetrical use: an obstetrical laryngoscope. *Anaesth Intensive Care* 1977;5:265–266.
50. Jellicoe JA, Harris NR. A modification of a standard laryngoscope for difficult tracheal intubation in obstetric cases. *Anaesthesia* 1984;39: 800–802.
51. Patil VU, Stehling LC, Zauder HL. An adjustable laryngoscope handle for difficult intubations. [Letter to the Editor] *Anesthesiology* 1984;60:609.
52. Yentis SM. A laryngoscope adaptor for difficult intubation. *Anaesthesia* 1987;42:764–766.
53. Dhara SF, Cheong TW. An adjustable multiple angle laryngoscope adaptor. *Anaesth Intensive Care* 1991;19:243–245.
54. Bellhouse CP, Dore C. Criteria for estimating likelihood of difficulty of endotracheal intubation with MacIntosh laryngoscope. *Anaesth Intensive Care* 1988;16:329–337.
55. Benumof JL, Scheller MS. The importance of transtracheal jet ventilation in the management of the difficult airway. *Anesthesiology* 1989;71:769–778.
56. Mallampati SR, Gatt SP, Gugino LD, Desai SP, et al. A clinical sign to predict difficult tracheal intubation: a prospective study. *Can J Anaesth* 1985;32:429–434.
57. White A, Kander PL. Anatomical factors in difficult direct laryngoscopy. *Br J Anaesth* 1975;47:488.
58. Nichol HL, Zack B. Difficult laryngoscopy: the "anterior" larynx and the atlanto-occipital gap. *Br J Anaesth* 1983;55:141–144.
59. Rocke DA, Murray WB, Rout CC, Gouws E. Relative risk analysis of factors associated with difficult intubation in obstetric anesthesia. *Anesthesiology* 1992;77:67–73.
60. Macintosh R, Richards H. Illuminated introducer for endotracheal tubes. *Anaesthesia* 1957;12:223–225.
61. Berman RA. Lighted stylet. *Anesthesiology* 1959;20:382–383.
62. Yamamura H, Yamamoto T, Kamiyama M. Device for blind nasal intubation. *Anesthesiology* 1959;20:221.
63. Ducrow M. Throwing light on blind intubation. *Anaesthesia* 1978;33: 827–829.
64. Rayburn RL. Light wand intubation. *Anaesthesia* 1979;34:677–678.
65. Stewart RD, et al. Use of a lighted stylet to confirm correct endotracheal tube placement. *Chest* 1987;92:900–903.
66. Burton S, Williams JD. Glossopharyngeal nerve block. *Arch Otolaryngol* 1971;93:186–188.
67. Stone DJ, et al. A complication of lightwand-guided nasotracheal intubation. *Anesthesiology* 1984;61:780–781.
68. Stewart RD, Ellis DG. Lighted stylet and endotracheal intubation. *Anesthesiology* 1987;66:851.
69. Williams RT, Stewart RD. Transillumination of the trachea with a lighted stylet. *Anesth Analg* 1986;65:543.
70. Williams RT. Lighted stylet and endotracheal intubation. II. *Anesthesiology* 1987;66:851–852.
71. Hammer M, Garry B. Transillumination of the trachea with Flexi-lum™. *Anesth Analg* 1985;64:91.
72. Weis FR, Hatton MN. Intubation by use of the light wand: experience in 253 patients. *J Oral Maxillofac Surg* 1989;47:577–580.
73. Vollmer TP, Stewart RD, Paris PM, Ellis D, Berkebile PE. Use of a lighted stylet for guided orotracheal intubation in the prehospital setting. *Ann Emerg Med* 1985;14:324–328.
74. Ellis DG, Jakymec A, Kaplan RM, Stewart RD, Freeman JA, et al. Guided orotracheal intubation in the operating room using a lighted stylet: a comparison with direct laryngoscopic technique. *Anesthesiology* 1986;64:823–826.
75. Fox DJ, Castro T, Rastrelli AJ. Comparison of intubation techniques in the awake patient: the Flexi-lum™ surgical light (lightwand). *Anesthesiology* 1987;66:69–71.
76. Verdile VD, Chiang JL, Bedger R, Stewart RD, Kaplan R, Paris PM. Nasotracheal intubation using a flexible lighted stylet. *Ann Emerg Med* 1990;19:506–510.
77. Debo RF, Colonna D, Dewerd G, Gonzalez C. Cricoarytenoid subluxation: complication of blind intubation with a lighted stylet. *Ear Nose Throat J* 1989;68:517–519.
78. Szigeti CL, Baeuerle JJ, Mongan PD. Arytenoid dislocation with lighted stylet intubation: case report and retrospective review. *Anesth Analg* 1994;78:185–186.
79. Brunel W, Coleman DL, Schwartz DE, Peper E, Cohen NH. Assessment of routine chest roentgenograms and physical examination to confirm endotracheal tube position. *Chest* 1989;96:1043–1045.
80. Mehta S. Transtracheal illumination for optimal tracheal tube placement. A clinical study. *Anaesthesia* 1989;44:970–972.
81. Stewart RD, LaRosee A, Kaplan RM, Ilkhanipour K. Correct positioning of an endotracheal tube using a flexible lighted stylet. *Crit Care Med* 1990;18:97–99.
82. Stevens S, Hung OR. A new instrument for airway transillumination-design features and technique for use. *Can J Anaesth* 1992; 39:A86.
83. *Trachlight™ Stylet and Tracheal Lightwand Instruction Manual.* Armonk, NY: Laerdal Medical Corporation, revised 1/94.
84. Hung OR, Stevens SC, Pytka S, Morris I, et al. Clinical trial of a new lightwand device for intubation in patients with difficult airway. *Can J Anaesth* 1992;39:A147.
85. Hung OR, Shields K, Stewart RD. Optimal position of the tip of the endotracheal tube following intubation. *Anesthesiology* 1993;79: A1084.
86. Hung OR, Stevens SC, Hawboldt G. Light-guided vs. laryngoscopic intubation in surgical patients: clinical trial of a new lightwand device. Presented at Canadian Anaestetists Society meeting *(abstract)* 1993.
87. Hung OR, Pytka S, Murphy MF, Launcelott GO, et al. Comparative hemodynamic changes following laryngoscopic or lightwand intubation. *Anesthesiology* 1993;79:A497.
88. Hung OR, Pytka S, Murphy MF, Stewart RD. *An Improved Intubation Technique for Novice Intubators: Clinical Trial of a New Lightwand.* [Abstract] Society of Academic Emergency Medicine, 1993.
89. Fink BR. Roentgenographic studies of the oropharyngeal airway. *Anesthesiology* 1957;18:711–718.
90. Gabuya R, Orkin LR. Design and utility of a new curved laryngoscope blade. *Anesth Analg* 1959;38:364–369.
91. Sykes NS. *Essay on the First Hundred Years of Anesthesia*, vol 2. Edinburgh: E & S Livingstone, 1961;Ch7.

Airway Management, edited by
L.H. Hanowell, M.D. and R.J. Waldron, M.D.,
Lippincott-Raven Publishers, Philadelphia © 1996.

CHAPTER 16

Perioperative Bronchoscopy

Judith C. F. Hwang, Leland H. Hanowell, John M. Mott,
David A. White, and Peter G. Moore

GUIDELINES FOR BRONCHOSCOPY

In 1987, the American Thoracic Society (ATS) published guidelines for fiberoptic bronchoscopy (FOB) (1). This position statement addressed the following aspects related to perioperative bronchoscopy: 1) diagnostic purposes, 2) therapeutic uses, 3) research applications, 4) conditions involving increased risk, 5) contraindications, and 6) specific comments. Specific guidelines are given for various aspects of bronchoscopy. Extracting from these guidelines the aspects of diagnosis and therapy most important to the use of bronchoscopy for airway management, the practitioner is left with the clinical indications for bronchoscopy listed in Tables 1 and 2.

A number of conditions, cited in the ATS position paper on bronchoscopy, are considered to impose greater risk for performance of bronchoscopy (Table 3). These include an uncooperative patient, hypoxemia, uremia, immunosuppression, debilitation, malnourishment, and/or bleeding. Additionally, patients with angina, arrhythmias, superior vena cava syndrome, lung abscess, pulmonary hypertension, asthma, partial tracheal obstruction, and/or coagulopathy are designated as being at increased risk for complications during bronchoscopic procedures. Contraindications to bronchoscopy are listed in Table 4.

These guidelines from the ATS advise that bronchoscopy is but one aspect of overall management. Bronchoscopy should not be performed for pulmonary hygiene if less invasive means for removal of secretions suffice (e.g., standard suctioning, postural drainage). Rigid bronchoscopy is the method of choice for the patient with massive hemoptysis who requires bronchoscopic evaluation (2).

J. C. F. Hwang, L. H. Hanowell, J. M. Mott, D. A. White, and P. G. Moore: Department of Anesthesiology, University of California, Davis School of Medicine and Medical Center, Sacramento, California 95817.

TABLE 1. *Indications for diagnostic fiberoptic bronchoscopy*

Assessing airway patency
Detecting airway injury
Bronchial tear
Inhalational injury
Determining etiology of hemoptysis
Assessing endotracheal tube placement
Obtaining sputum for culture

TABLE 3. *Risk factors for complications during fiberoptic bronchoscopy*

Uncooperative patient	Pulmonary hypertension
Recent myocardial infarction	Lung abscess
Unstable angina	Immunosuppression
Arrhythmias	Superior vena cava syndrome
Asthma	Debility
Hypoxemia	Advanced age
Hypercarbia	Bleeding diathesis
Need for mechanical ventilation	Uremia
Bronchial obstruction	

THE FIBEROPTIC BRONCHOSCOPE: EQUIPMENT DESIGN

The bronchoscope is constructed of fiberoptic bundles and cables encased in a slender, waterproof sheath from the handle to the tip. The distal, working portion of the bronchoscope, the tip, consists of a specialized bending section with a flexible covering. This region, 3 to 6 cm in length, has hinges and anchor points for the two cables from the handle. The cable system permits manipulation of the tip of the bronchoscope by adjustments at the handle, the operating end of the bronchoscope. Movement of the tip is limited to one plane. Bending generally can occur up to 180° in one direction, and often to 120° in the opposite direction.

As depicted in Fig. 1, within the sheath, there are usually two fiberoptic bundles, which carry the illumination for viewing and a single optical-fiber bundle. Depending on the type of bronchoscope, there are generally two light-fiber bundles and one to three channels. The channels are of sufficient caliber to permit suctioning of secretions, small clots of blood, and particulate matter from the airway. The channels are also large enough to permit passage of instruments. The operating end of the bronchoscope has a port to which suction is attached or through which medications or saline lavage can be injected. Sometimes an additional port is available for injection of lavage or medications. The suction channel can also be used to administer oxygen if the bronchoscope is used in patients to whom oxygen cannot be conveniently administered by another route.

Fiberoptic Fibers

Flexible fiberoptic bundles consist of numerous glass fibers that are 10 to 12 μm in diameter. There is a lower limit on fiber size because of physical and optical limitations. In general, the fiber core cannot be less than 5.0 μm in diameter for two reasons. As the diameter of the fiber core approaches the wavelength of visible light (0.2 to 0.8 μm), the efficiency of light transmission diminishes. Additionally, from a practical point of view, allowing for the thickness of the cladding and the packing of the fibers, the minimum total fiber diameter is approximately 5 μm because of the manufacturing process. The endoscopes used for bronchoscopy have optical bundles (total of all fibers) approximately 1.5 mm in diameter composed of approximately 10,000 to 15,000 fibers.

Each individual fiber is "clad" or coated with a 1- to 2-μm layer of glass having a refractive index different from that of the core, allowing complete trapping of the transmitted light within a fiber by internal reflection. Without this cladding, the light rays from one fiber could leave the fiber and/or cross to other fibers, causing decreased light transmission and a degradation of the image.

The properties of fiberoptics that have made them useful in medicine are their ability to allow for numerous reflections of light within the fiber with little loss in light transmission and their flexibility. The high efficiency of light transmission by a properly constructed fiber occurs because of 1) the high purity of the glass and 2) the cladding of the fiber core with a glass of lower refractive index. At the interface of the two glasses, the light within the fiber reflects back within the core and continues to travel within the fiber. The flexibility is achieved by producing a bundle of very thin fibers that are secured only at the ends, allowing the fibers to slide during flexing of the bundle.

TABLE 2. *Indications for therapeutic fiberoptic bronchoscopy*

Management of difficult intubation
Removal of secretions and mucous plugs
Removal of foreign bodies and clots

TABLE 4. *Contraindications to fiberoptic bronchoscopy*

Lack of consent
Inability to oxygenate
Inadequate facility to deal with complications
Inexperienced operator without direct supervision

Construction of the Bronchoscope

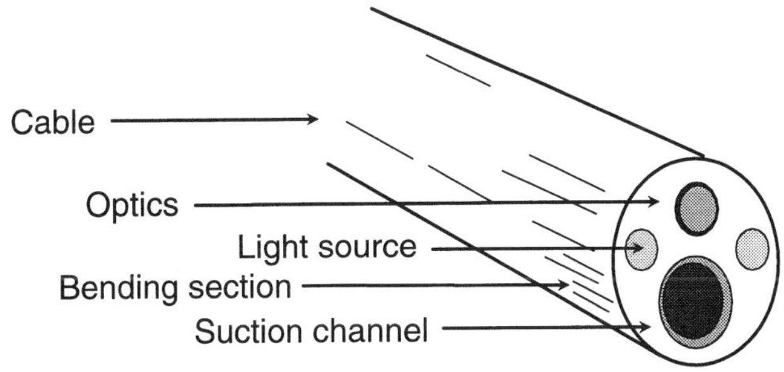

FIG. 1. Tip of a conventional bronchoscope with channels for optics, light source, and suction (medication or lavage.) (Courtesy of Dr. David A. White.) From: Waldron RJ, Hanowell LH, Grande CM. Blunt airway trauma. In: *Seminars in Anesthesia.* Philadelphia: W.B. Saunders; 1994:13:136, with permission.

Image Transmission

The light entering the fiber is trapped, and after many reflections off the wall (up to 10,000 reflections per meter), it emerges uniformly distributed over the exit face of the fiber. As a result of the repeated internal reflections, the transmitted information of any given fiber is a blurred "average" of that which entered the fiber.

A key requirement of fiberoptic transmission of images is that the fibers at each end of the bundle be identically aligned to ensure coherency of light transmission; otherwise, the image is scrambled. Small mismatching of fiber position degrades the image substantially. Destruction of one or more light-transmitting fibers results in black spots in the image of the airway.

The resolution of the optical bundle depends on the diameter of the fiber core, the thickness of the cladding (and therefore fiber diameter), and the alignment of fibers within the bundle. Thinner fibers, and therefore greater numbers of fibers within a bundle, produce improved image resolution.

Distal End

A focused image at the distal end of the fiberoptic bundle is transmitted to the proximal end in "pixels" or small "quanta" formed by each fiber. The size and number of these pixels naturally depend on the size and number of fibers within the fiberoptic bundle. Since each fiber does not produce an exact replica of the original image but rather a blurred "average" of the image, the resolution of the image depends on the size and number of the fibers.

The field of view depends on the optics of the objective lens located on the distal end of the bronchoscope, which can produce a wide-or narrow-angle view. The size of the transmitted image depends in part on the number of fibers, with a greater number of fibers necessary for a wider field of view.

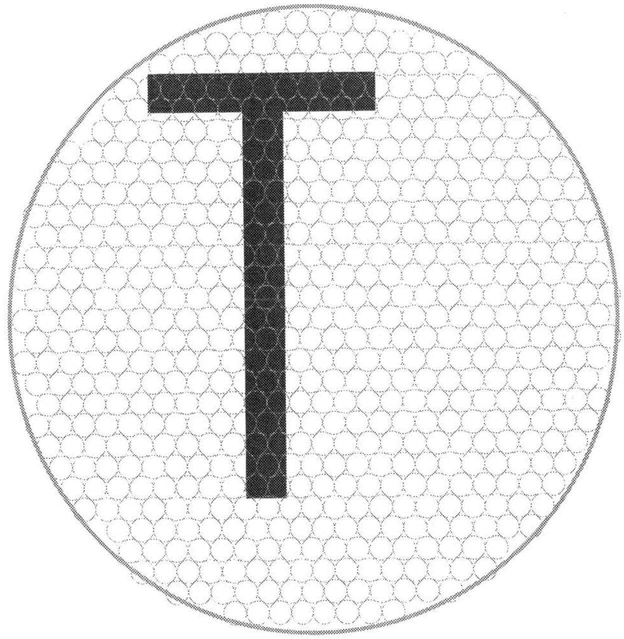

FIG. 2. Image of *T* as seen by the distal portion of a bronchoscope.

Proximal End

Since the viewed image is a result of "averaging" of the initial image within each fiber, whether the viewed image is a faithful representative of the initial image depends on the size and number of fibers and the magnification of the viewed image. For example, the viewed image in a bronchoscope with relatively few, large fibers becomes a distorted "granular" depiction of the original subject (Figs. 2 and 3).

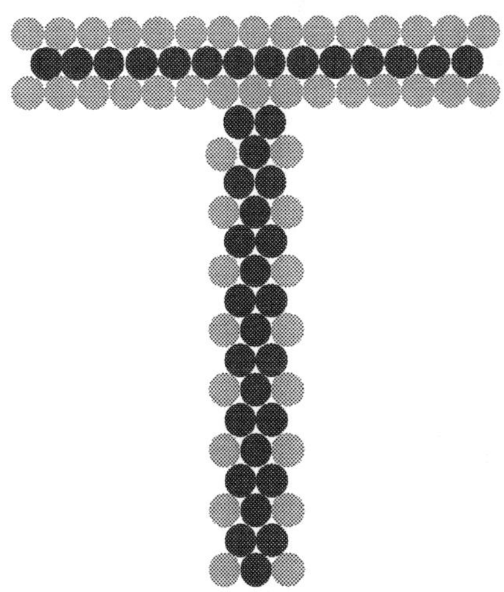

FIG. 3. Image of *T*, as seen at the proximal end of a bronchoscope, has a distorted, "granular" appearance resulting from "averaging" of the initial image (Fig. 2).

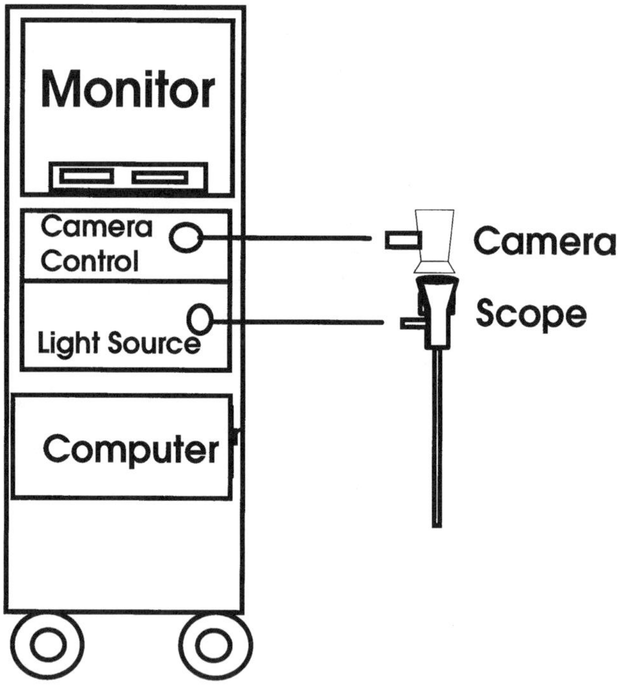

FIG. 4. Bronchoscopic techniques incorporate video equipment to display images on a monitor. Images can be recorded on videotape and retrieved for storage as computer files. From: Waldron RJ, Hanowell LH, Grande CM. Blunt airway trauma. In: *Seminars in Anesthesia.* Philadelphia: W.B. Saunders; 1994:13;136, with permission.

An eyepiece magnifies the image. The size of the image without magnification is that of the optical-bundle diameter (1.5 mm). Image magnification, while necessary for viewing, is limited by the resolution of the fiberoptic system, since a low-resolution system is further degraded by magnification.

Video camera equipment permits display of bronchoscopic images on a television monitor. These images are often recorded or can be stored as computer graphic files for archiving and labeling of anatomic findings. Such video systems (Fig. 4) are portable, enhance the teaching of bronchoscopy, and are commonplace in operating rooms and intensive care units.

Light Source

A light source is necessary to illuminate the field; halogen and xenon light sources are commonly used. Although halogen is more economical, a xenon source provides much brighter light for a given temperature. In addition, for photography the xenon light source is preferred. A flash capability is helpful for still-frame photography, while a continuous bright source is necessary for video imaging.

The light-transmission bundles do not need to be coherent since no image is reproduced. The bundles and fibers generally are larger and therefore less expensive to produce.

Heat from the light source can be transmitted down a fiberoptic bundle. Although not generally a problem with bronchoscopy, it is important to realize this potential hazard. There have been numerous cases of fires being ignited by placing the light bundle of rigid endoscopes on surgical drapes, a clear indication of the potential hazard.

Use and Abuse

Damage and wear of bronchoscopes are a serious issue because repairs are costly. Repair costs for a fiberoptic bronchoscope can surpass the bronchoscope's initial cost within a short time if care is not taken to become familiar with its construction and the most common mechanisms of damage; these are listed in Table 5.

Kirkpatrick and colleagues (3) described the findings of a survey of bronchoscopists with respect to damage to equipment. Sixty-two percent of all damage could be attributed to improper handling, especially in association with biopsy forceps, brushes, or needles. Sixty-four percent of the damage to bronchoscopes was deemed to have been preventable. The average period during which bronchoscopes were unavailable for clinical service during repair was approximately 4 weeks, and average cost of repair amounted to nearly U.S.$3000 per occurrence.

The fiberoptic bundle is most commonly damaged. The damage occurs from twisting, crushing, or excessive bending. Fractured fibers appear as black dots on the bronchoscopic field of view. As the relative number of these fractured fibers increases, the image becomes degraded to the point where the optical bundle needs to be replaced. Similar damage to the light-transmitting bundles obviously decreases the intensity of light reaching the objects within view. Even with normal use, a few fiberoptic fibers can be expected to break over time.

Damage to the sheath of the bronchoscope can be avoided by careful instrumentation. A suitable lubricant should be used during placement of the fiberoptic bronchoscope through the airtight diaphragm of a swiveling adapter (Fig. 5). Such adapters permit the continued administration of oxygen to patients during bronchoscopic intubation as well as continued mechanical ventilation during anesthesia and critical care. To prevent

TABLE 5. *Common causes of damage to fiberoptic bronchoscope*

Excessive bending
Twisting against resistance
Closing drawer of cart on sheath of bronchoscope
Patient biting bronchoscope
Use of brush or biopsy forceps

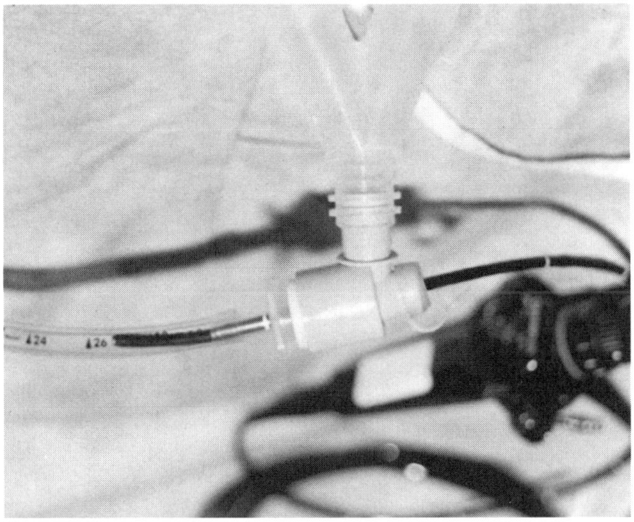

FIG. 5. Passage of a bronchoscope through a self-sealing adapter and then into the endotracheal tube. The adapter is attached to the circuit of an anesthesia machine or mechanical ventilator so that oxygenation and ventilation are not interrupted during bronchoscopy. From: Hanowell LH, Junod FL (eds). *Pulmonary care of the surgical patient.* Armonk, New York: Futura Publishing Co.; 1994:64, with permission.

shearing between the diaphragm and the bronchoscope, lubricant is generally applied to the site where the bronchoscope enters the diaphragm.

Damage to the bending mechanism is probably one of the more common forms of damage to fiberoptic bronchoscopes. Generally, repairs cost in excess of U.S.$1000. The damage occurs most commonly within the endotracheal tube. Care must be taken to advance the tip of the bronchoscope beyond the point of last visualization of the endotracheal tube to assure emergence of the bronchoscope prior to bending of the tip. Conversely, the tip must be in neutral position (i.e., not flexed) before the bronchoscope is withdrawn through the endotracheal tube. Additionally, excessive pressure on the bending mechanism must be avoided during manipulation. With experience, the operator develops a sense of the proper resistance to movement of the tip, and the use of excess force can usually be avoided.

Leakage of fluid within the bronchoscope often causes severe damage, requiring complete rebuilding of the bronchoscope at a cost greater than U.S.$3000. The flexible, waterproof cover of the bending section is a potential "weak" point in the construction of endoscopes, in that this is where a leak may occur from continual "wear and tear." The tip sheath is also vulnerable to damage during rotation of the bronchoscope while the tip is in a tight position or from pulling the flexed tip into the endotracheal tube. Other reasons for fluid ingress include immersing inappropriate portions of the bronchoscope during cleaning or not following proper procedure prior to immersing. Leak testing of the bronchoscope before cleaning is critical to extending its life; this detects such a hazard before damage occurs.

Thorough familiarity with equipment, anatomy of the upper airway and bronchial tree, airway management, and technical procedures is essential for appropriate and safe use of bronchoscopes. Substantial training and experience in these areas are required to minimize the downtime and expense of bronchoscope repair and, still more importantly, to ensure patient safety. Adherence to the manufacturer's guidelines and a commonsense approach to use of the bronchoscope can also help to minimize expensive repairs.

CLINICAL ASPECTS OF BRONCHOSCOPY

Bronchoscopy is employed perioperatively in a variety of circumstances, including airway placement (fiberoptic intubation), assessment of airway position (placement of airway dividers for thoracic surgical procedures), diagnosis of perioperative and trauma-related compromise, bacteriologic/histopathologic diagnosis, and alleviation of airway obstruction by clotted blood (trauma) or inspissated pulmonary secretions.

Fiberoptic Airway Intubation

Fiberoptic airway intubation can be accomplished either orally or nasally and is usually performed when a difficult airway is anticipated or encountered (Table 6). Patients in whom a difficult airway might be anticipated and therefore fiberoptic intubation pursued include those with obvious anatomic abnormality (maxillofacial, pharyngeal, or laryngeal); unstable cervical spines secondary to trauma or to rheumatoid arthritis; temporomandibular joint dysfunction or trismus; micrognathia; and morbid obesity.

TABLE 6. *Indications for fiberoptic intubation*

Compromised airway
Disease involving head, neck, oral cavity, and larynx (e.g., tumor, cyst, supraglottic mass)
Infection
Facial trauma
Anatomic abnormalities (e.g., acromegaly, micrognathia)
Need to avoid neck extension
Spinal injury
Cervical degenerative disease
Vertebrobasilar insufficiency
Difficult airway suggested by the following:
Short, thick neck
Protruding upper incisors
Narrow mouth opening
Large tongue
Recessed mandible

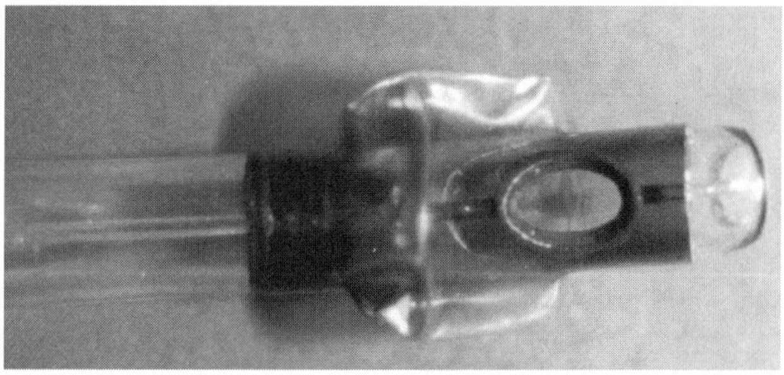

FIG. 6. Distal portion of a right-sided, double-lumen endobronchial tube (Mallinckrodt Inc., Glens Falls, New York) showing the slot provided to allow ventilation of the right upper lobe. From: Hanowell LH, Junod FL (eds). *Pulmonary care of the surgical patient.* Armonk, New York: Futura Publishing Co.; 1994:62, with permission.

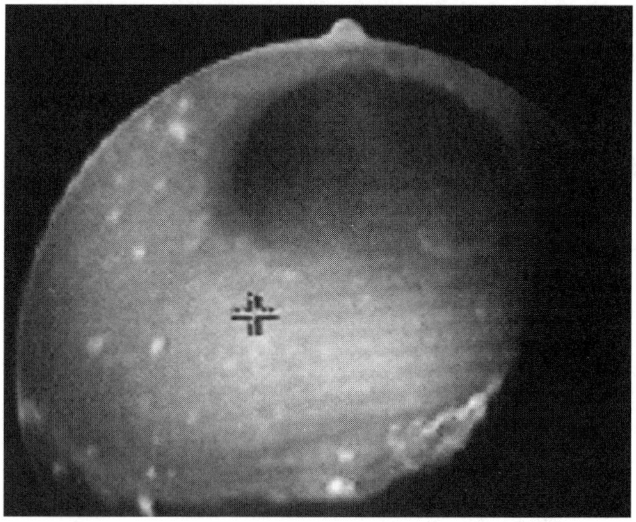

FIG. 7. View of right upper lobe orifice through the ventilation slot provided on a right-sided, double-lumen endobronchial tube.

Placement of Double-Lumen Tubes and Bronchial Blockers

Double-lumen endobronchial tubes are used for a variety of thoracic surgeries requiring intraoperative unilateral lung ventilation to enhance surgical exposure of the thorax. Such procedures include thoracoscopy, pneumonectomy, upper lobectomy, esophageal resection, repair of the thoracic aorta, and correction of thoracic scoliosis or other spinal disorders. Nonsurgically, these tubes are used to separate one lung from the other to prevent contamination of or spillage to the uninvolved lung (e.g., massive hemorrhage), to achieve selective ventilation (e.g., bronchopleural fistula or giant unilateral bulla), and to allow unilateral pulmonary lavage.

Ehrenwerth (4) and others (5,6) advocated the technique of bronchoscopy for correct positioning of double-lumen endobronchial tubes. The alternative to bronchoscopy is auscultation to determine the correct position of the endobronchial tube; alternately clamping the conduits leading to the tracheal or bronchial lumen results in loss of breath sounds on the clamped side (7).

Figure 6 is a photograph of the distal portion of a right-sided, double-lumen endobronchial tube. The side port of this tube permits ventilation of the right upper lobe bronchus (Fig. 7). Correct positioning of right-sided, double-lumen tubes is critical because of potential occlusion of the right upper lobe. Consequently, left-sided endobronchial tubes, which are less likely to cause left upper lobar collapse, are more commonly used than right-sided endobronchial tubes for one-lung anesthesia. With proper training, bronchoscopists can correctly place left- and right-sided double-lumen endobronchial tubes (8). Figure 8

A–C

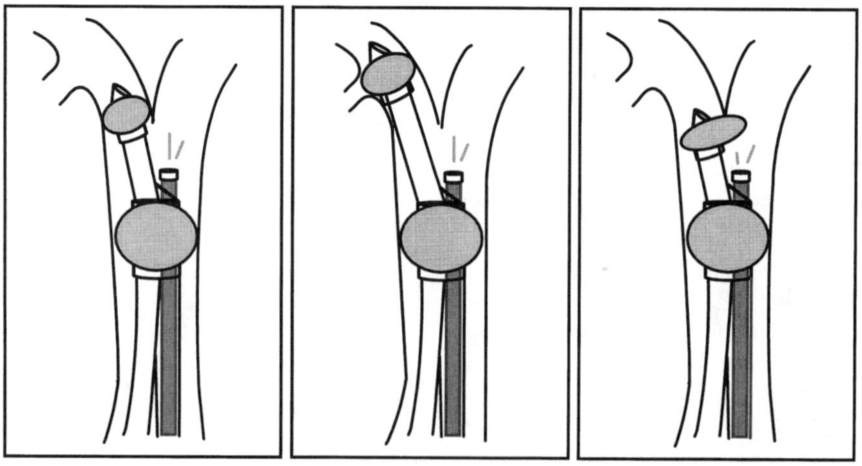

FIG. 8. This diagram demonstrates correct and incorrect positioning of the left double lumen endotracheal tube. Note correct **(A),** too distal **(B),** and too proximal **(C)** placement of this device in the airway. (From ref. 4.) (Computer graphics by Leland H. Hanowell.)

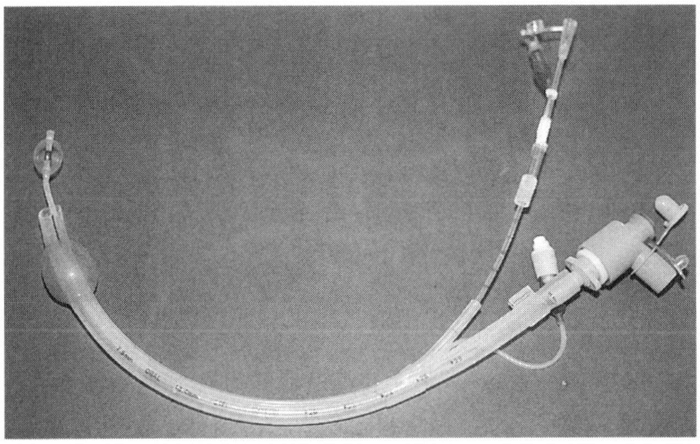

FIG. 9. An endotracheal tube with a built-in bronchial blocking balloon. The endobronchial blocking balloon is best positioned under fiberoptic guidance. From: Hanowell LH, Junod FL (eds). *Pulmonary care of the surgical patient.* Armonk, New York: Futura Publishing Co.; 1994:135, with permission.

demonstrates correct and incorrect placement of left-sided double lumen endotracheal tubes.

Newer bronchial blocking tubes (e.g., Univent, Fuji Systems Corporation, Tokyo, Japan) require the passage of a bronchial blocking balloon into the lumen of the bronchus of the lung that is to be isolated from ventilation (Fig. 9). Bronchoscopy is required to confirm correct placement of the endobronchial blocking balloon and is also recommended for correct placement of other airway dividers. Technical aspects of placement are discussed by Benumof et al. (9), who have evaluated balloon inflation pressures that safely and effectively seal the airway to isolate the lung. Figure 10A demonstrates positioning of the blocking balloon in the right main bronchus via the bronchoscope. Figure 10B–D shows bronchial balloon inflation to achieve adequate bronchial occlusion without overdistention.

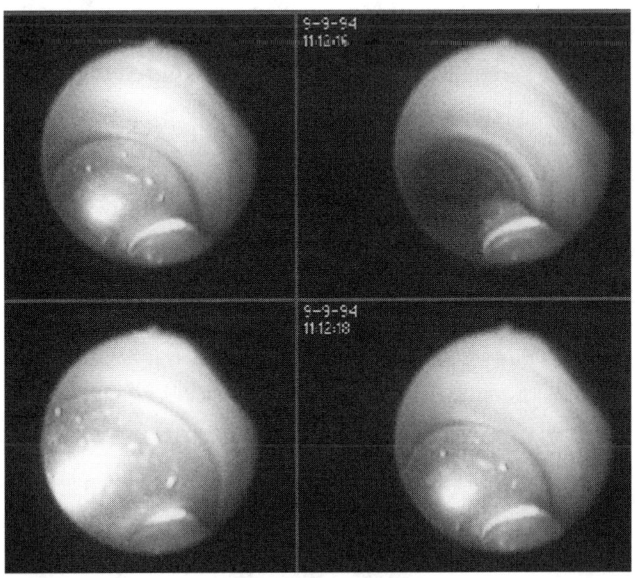

A B C D

FIG. 10. A–D: These images, acquired with a computer and video-enhanced bronchoscope, demonstrate the correct positioning and proper inflation of a bronchial blocking balloon in a model of the human airway.

Use of the Laryngeal Mask Airway As an Aid to Bronchoscopy

Benumof (10) recently reviewed the utility of the laryngeal mask airway (LMA), previously described by Brain (11) in 1983, for intraoperative airway management. The LMA (Fig. 11) is a device that is placed above the vocal cords to provide an airway during general anesthesia. It has also been used to manage the difficult airway and is an effective guide for oral fiberoptic intubation. When the device is correctly positioned in the supraglottic airway, a small ETT can be passed through the ventilation lumen of the device (Fig. 11). A bronchoscope is then inserted down the ETT in the ventilating conduit. The vocal cords are generally readily visualized through the central ventilation port (Fig. 11). Figure 12 demonstrates the bronchoscopic view of the ventilation ports of the LMA. Figure 13 illustrates the view of the cords seen through the LMA, here demonstrated in a model for clarity. The ETT can now be correctly positioned using the bronchoscope. With careful technique, it is possible to remove the LMA over the ETT, leaving the ETT in the correct position. A size 5 LMA, now available in the United States as well as abroad, can allow the placement of an ETT up to a size of 7.0 mm (Table 7).

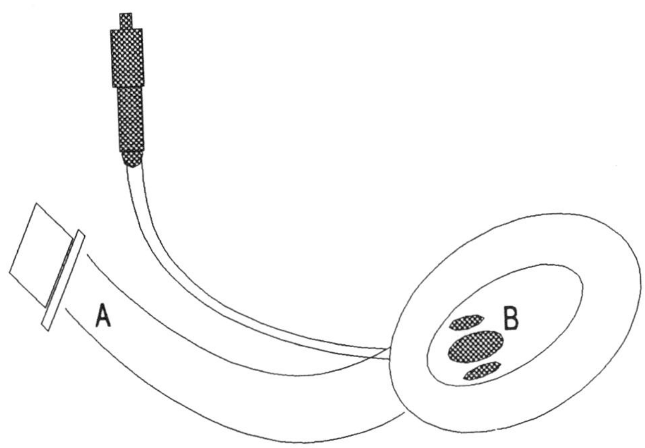

FIG. 11. A laryngeal mask airway. A bronchoscope can be passed through the conduit *(A)* to view the cords through the ventilation ports of the laryngeal mask airway *(B)*. From: Waldron RJ, Hanowell LH, Grande CM. Blunt airway trauma. In: *Seminars in Anesthesia*. Philadelphia: W.B. Saunders; 1994:13:138, with permission.

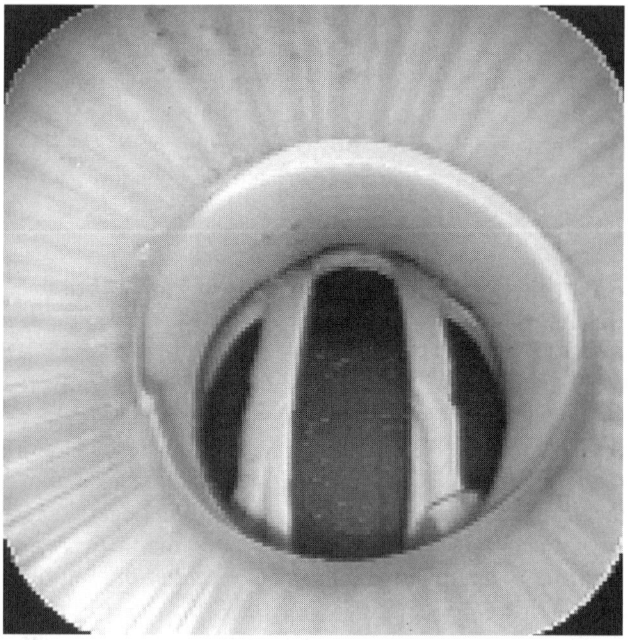

FIG. 12. Bronchoscopic view of the ventilation ports of a laryngeal mask airway. From: Waldron RJ, Hanowell LH, Grande CM. Blunt airway trauma. In: *Seminars in Anesthesia.* Philadelphia: W.B. Saunders; 1994:13:138, with permission.

Therapeutic Bronchoscopy and Pulmonary Hygiene

Bronchoscopy is commonly required after trauma or during postoperative care to alleviate lobar collapse of the lung. The lateral decubitus position commonly predisposes to drainage of secretions into the dependent lung. An intraoperative right lateral decubitus position, for example, in patients with copious pulmonary secretions may lead to right upper lobe obstruction by clotted blood (trauma) or pulmonary secretions.

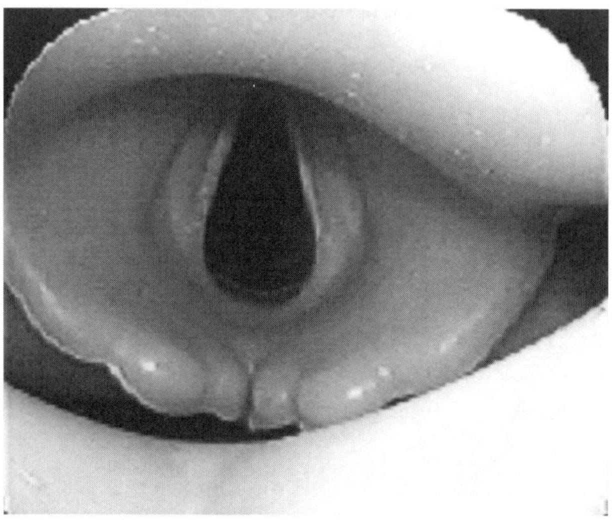

FIG. 13. Vocal cords of a human model imaged by a bronchoscope passed through a laryngeal mask airway to assist in orotracheal fiberoptic intubation. From: Waldron RJ, Hanowell LH, Grande CM. Blunt airway trauma. In: *Seminars in Anesthesia.* Philadelphia: W.B. Saunders; 1994:13:138, with permission.

TABLE 7. *Largest endotracheal tube passable through varying sizes of laryngeal mask airway*

LMA size	ETT size
1	3.5
2	5.0 uncuffed
2.5	6.0 uncuffed
3	6.0 cuffed
4	6.0 cuffed
5	7.0 cuffed

ETT, endotracheal tube; LMA, laryngeal mask airway.

To expedite postoperative bronchoscopy, should it be anticipated, the installation of an ETT with the largest diameter appropriate for the patient is recommended. This permits the use of a correspondingly large bronchoscope with an efficient suction channel. Smaller-gauge bronchoscopes that are accommodated by smaller-diameter tubes have smaller and thus less effective suction channels.

Suctioning bronchoscopes can be inserted into variously sized ETTs, including pediatric ETTs with an internal diameter of 5.5 mm; however, smaller ETTs may severely compromise the extent to which the patient can be effectively suctioned. Wood (12) noted that the narrow suction channels of pediatric bronchoscopes (one commercially available 3.5-mm pediatric bronchoscope has a 1.2-mm-diameter suction channel) can be obstructed by thick secretions. Suctioning of the airway with a catheter is advised prior to insertion of the bronchoscope when there are copious, thick secretions. Increased viscosity of secretions, decreased suction channel radius, inadequate vacuum suction, and increasing length of the bronchoscope are factors that promote inefficient removal of secretions through the bronchoscope suction channel.

Advances in bronchoscope design have permitted the manufacture of very small bronchoscopes that can be used to perform endoscopic examination and intubation even in neonates. Bronchoscopes as small as 2.2 mm in diameter have been recently described for intubation and inspection of the airway in infants (13).

PROCEDURAL ASPECTS OF BRONCHOSCOPY

Technologic advances in bronchoscopic airway imaging and computer graphic data storage have augmented pulmonary care of the surgical patient. Additionally, these advances can be utilized to enhance instruction in the techniques of bronchoscopy. For example, with such devices, bronchoscopic images can be magnified, transferred to computer tutorials, and/or recorded on videotape. These systems can be modified to teach bronchoscopic anatomy of the upper airway and bronchial tree. Regardless of the reason for utilizing a bronchoscope, an understanding of airway anatomy is essential to effective and safe handling of the bronchoscope (Figs. 14 and 15). When performing a fiberoptic intubation, familiarity with the anatomy of the pharynx and larynx is also very important to expedite the procedure. (Chapter 1 further describes the anatomy of these structures.)

Physiologic Responses to Awake Fiberoptic Bronchoscopy

Fiberoptic bronchoscopy (FOB) is tolerated in obtunded and intubated patients, including the critically ill, with adequate sedation alone (14). However, for the awake and nonintubated patient, numerous systemic and local responses to fiberoptic intubation must be recognized and controlled (15,16).

The physiologic responses to FOB should be well understood by practitioners involved with basic airway management. Briefly, cardiovascular effects include hypertension, tachycardia, and reflex bradycardia. At the level of the airway, laryngospasm and bronchospasm may occur. FOB may provoke movement through gagging, retching, or coughing responses, which may directly or indirectly result in airway trauma or hemorrhage. Finally, the process of FOB can provoke profound salivation and accumulation of oropharyngeal secretions, which can interfere with ventilation or completion of the procedure.

Adequate use of local anesthesia may control many of these untoward and undesired reflexes (17). Whether topical or more invasive techniques are employed, it is important to remain vigilant about patient selection, preparation, and local anesthetic use.

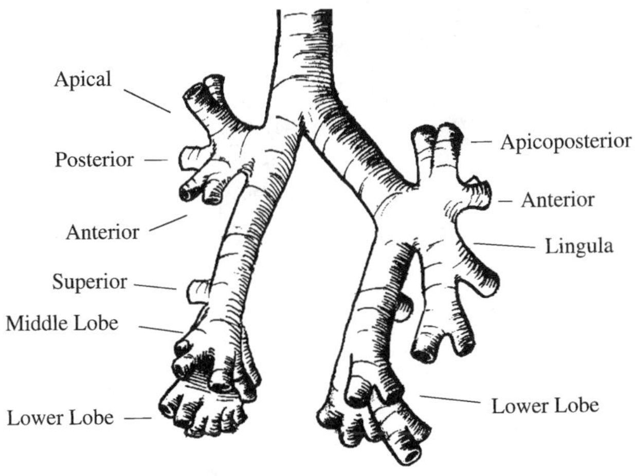

FIG. 14. The bronchial tree with (in a clockwise manner) *(a)* apicoposterior and anterior segments of the left upper lobe, *(b)* lingula, *(c)* left lower lobe, *(d)* right lower lobe, *(e)* right middle lobe, *(f)* superior segment of the right lower lobe, and *(g)* anterior, posterior, and apical segments of the right upper lobe. (Drawings by Jesse Hanowell, and computer graphics by Leland H. Hanowell.)

Evaluation of the Patient

Local anesthetic use must be tempered by patient conditions. Invasive blocks are relatively contraindicated if the patient has distorted anatomy, a coagulopathy, or an infection over the site of injection. Topical application entails recognition of the systemic absorption of the local anesthetic and knowledge of the patient factors that modify the maximum acceptable dose (18–24) (Table 8). For example, when local anesthetic is applied to compromised epithelium, the absorption can be greater than when it is applied to intact mucosal surfaces. In addition, patients with congestive heart failure, liver disease, and acquired or congenital cholinesterase deficiency may have impaired metabolism of local anesthetics and excessively high blood levels following topical application or injection (Table 9).

Preparation of the Patient

Consideration must be given to adequate preparation of the patient. The use of an antisialogogue and vagolytic is useful but must be balanced against the patient's underlying medical problems. For example, potential complications include producing undesirable tachycardia in the patient with ischemic heart disease and thickened secretions or mucous plugging in the patient with obstructive airway disease. Positioning of the patient may improve comfort. Most blocks and topical applications are better tolerated in the sitting position. Sedation can be accomplished with a combination of benzodiazepine, major tranquilizer, and/or short-acting narcotic in small doses (Table 10). In addition to providing sedation and amnesia, a combination of narcotics and benzodiazepines helps to suppress the cough reflex. The drugs midazolam and diazepam have the advantages of amnesic and anticonvulsant properties, making them slightly favored. As a rule, ketamine would be an agent with limited usage in FOB, because of its tendency to induce salivation and its sympathomimetic properties.

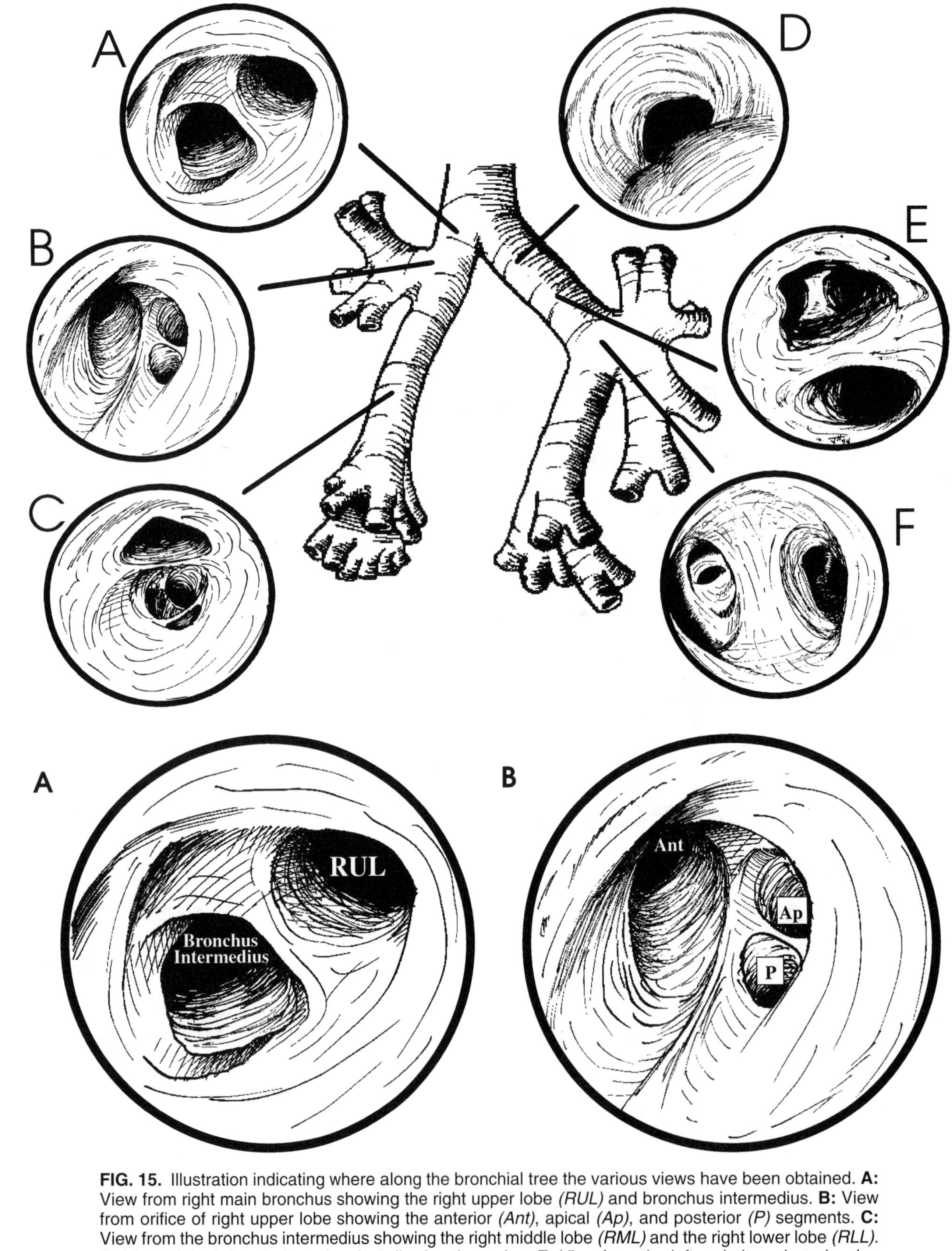

FIG. 15. Illustration indicating where along the bronchial tree the various views have been obtained. **A:** View from right main bronchus showing the right upper lobe *(RUL)* and bronchus intermedius. **B:** View from orifice of right upper lobe showing the anterior *(Ant)*, apical *(Ap)*, and posterior *(P)* segments. **C:** View from the bronchus intermedius showing the right middle lobe *(RML)* and the right lower lobe *(RLL)*. **D:** View of the left main bronchus just distal to the carina. **E:** View from the left main bronchus showing the upper division *(UD)* of the left upper lobe, the lingula, and the left lower lobe *(LLL)*. **F:** View from the orifice of the left upper lobe showing the upper division *(UD)* and the lingula. (Drawings by Jesse Hanowell, and computer graphics by Leland H. Hanowell.)

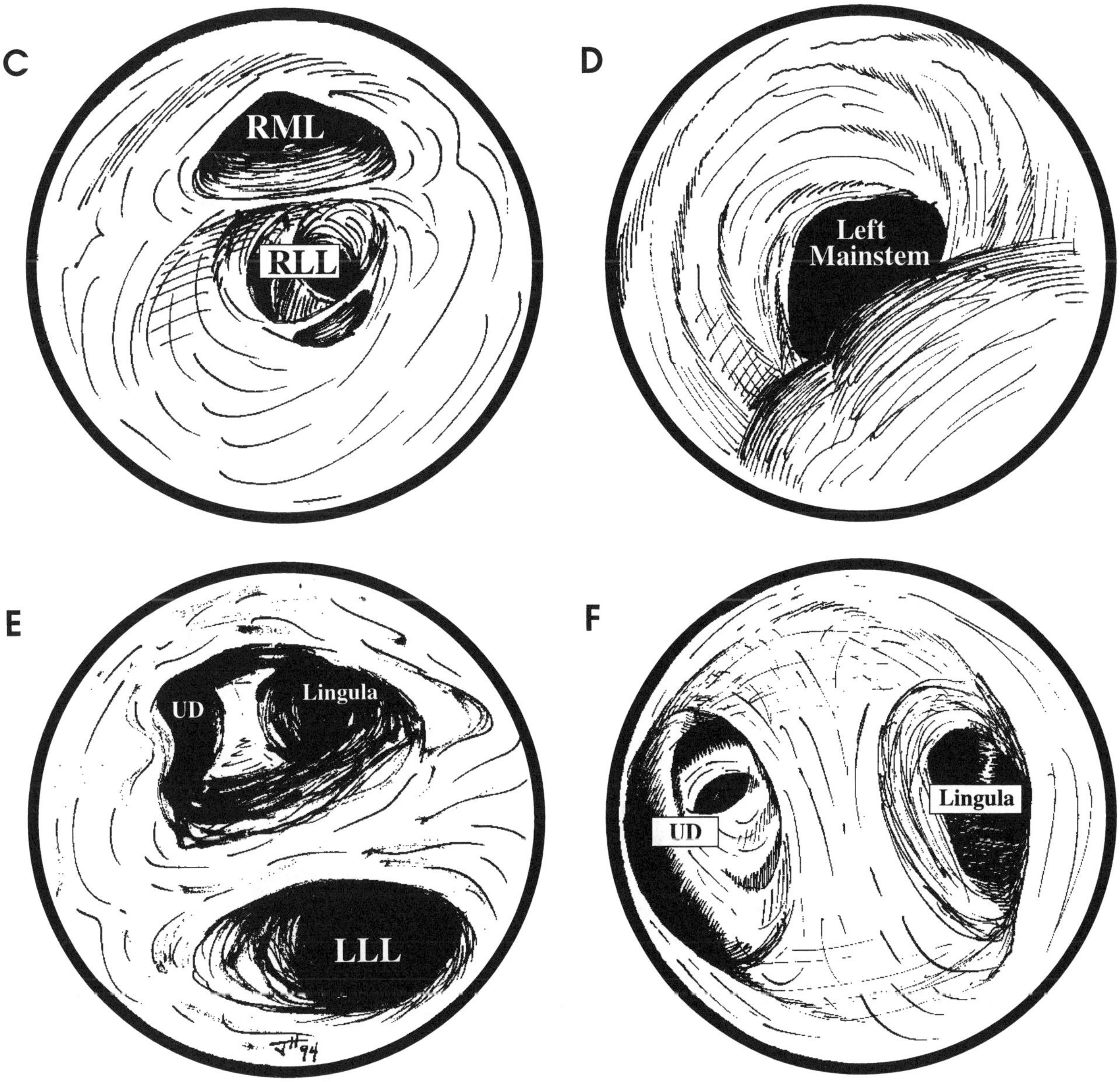

FIG. 15. *Continued.*

TABLE 8. *Maximum recommended drug dosages*

Adult dosing (average 70-kg patient)	
Lidocaine	300 mg
Dyclonine	200 mg
Benzonatate	200 mg
Benzocaine	200 mg
Pediatric dosing	
Lidocaine	3–4 mg/kg
Tetracaine	1 mg/kg
Cocaine	1 mg/kg

TABLE 9. *Factors associated with elevated blood levels of local anesthetic*

Total dose used
Method of application
Site of application
Spray > gel or viscous formulation
Tracheal/bronchial application > supraglottic application
Application to damaged or diseased epithelium > application to intact mucosa
Liver disease
Congestive heart failure (passive congestion of the liver)
Deficiency of cholinesterase (ester anesthetics)

TABLE 10. *Sedatives and analgesics for fiberoptic bronchoscopy*

Class	Uses	Drug	Dose[a]	Onset	Half-life	Side effects
Narcotics	Analgesic Sedative	Morphine Meperidine Fentanyl	1–10 mg 12.5–50 mg 25–250 μg	IV 5–15 min IV 5 min IV 2 min	2–4 h 1–4 h 4 h	Respiratory depression Tachycardia Laryngeal reflex depression
Benzodiazepines	Sedative Antegrade amnesia Antiepileptic	Diazepam Midazolam	1–10 mg 0.5–5 mg	IV 15 min IV 1–3 min	7–10 h 1–4 h	Painful on injection
Butyrophenone	Sedative Antiemetic	Droperidol	0.625–10 mg	IV 5–8 min		Extrapyramidal effects, inner anxiety

[a]Actual doses given vary with each patient and should therefore be given in small, incremental doses.

TOPICAL ANESTHESIA FOR AWAKE FIBEROPTIC BRONCHOSCOPY

Local Anesthetic Formulations

Many different forms of local anesthetics are available. These range from powders to solutions. Gel preparations, as a rule, are better tolerated.

Lidocaine

Lidocaine is formulated as simple solutions (1% to 10%), viscous solutions (2%), and gelatin (2%). Its effectiveness is widely accepted, and it is supported by the literature as a relatively safe and effective choice for topical anesthesia. Aerosol preparations appear to work as well with 2% as with 4% solutions and should be used to reduce the total drug administered. Peak blood levels depend on the formulation used; they are less with gel than with sprayed solutions. The gel is less irritating to the mucosa and apparently better tolerated by the patient.

Maximum doses of lidocaine are usually recommended not to exceed 300 mg (25). However, numerous articles indicate that higher doses have been tolerated by patients without neurologic complications, despite blood levels that approach the toxic range (26). For children, lidocaine in doses as high as 3–4 mg/kg appears safe, as long as the total dose does not exceed 175 mg/m^2 (27).

Recently, lidocaine has been formulated with prilocaine in a eutectic mixture (a mixture of two solids that results in a new, lower melting point) known as EMLA (Astra USA, Inc., Westborough, Massachusetts). EMLA has not been shown to be superior to lidocaine gel for topical application in the nose (28). Note that EMLA is not sterile and does not contain preservatives. Care should be exercised in administration to children less than 6 months of age and patients with a tendency to methemoglobin.

Benzocaine

Benzocaine is commonly used as a 20% spray to the airway. It has a rapid onset but is relatively short-acting. It is found in many over-the-counter preparations and is generally tolerated well. Cetacaine (Ceylite Industries, Inc., Pennsauken, New Jersey) is a combination of benzocaine 14% and tetracaine 2%. The recommended dose is a 1-second spray representing about 200 mg of benzocaine. The duration of action of benzocaine is about 10 minutes (29).

Tetracaine

Tetracaine is limited by its toxicity and slow onset, but has the advantage of producing a longer duration of topical effect than either benzocaine or lidocaine. The maximum recommended dose is 1 mg/kg. Current formulations offer the drug in a 1% to 2% concentration.

Cocaine

Cocaine is available as a solution or as a powder (30). The solutions should not exceed 4% concentration; the powder has little use clinically. The use of cocaine mud, which is prepared by mixing cocaine powder with epinephrine, is strongly discouraged. The intrinsic vasoconstrictor properties of cocaine do not require a supplemental alpha agonist. In addition, arrhythmias are a potential complication when epinephrine is used in conjunction with cocaine. A number of reports suggest that lidocaine and phenylephrine mixtures substitute adequately for cocaine (31–33). When cocaine is used, the absorbed dose should not exceed 1 mg/kg; peak blood levels may be delayed for 30 to 60 minutes, because of the vasoconstricting action of cocaine.

Dyclonine

Dyclonine is the active ingredient in Sucrets (SmithKline Beecham, Philadephia, Pennsylvania). It is a ketone rather than an amide or ester local anesthetic, and it is available as a 0.5% solution. It has typical local anesthetic toxicity, and most information suggests limiting the dose to 200 mg.

Benzonatate

Benzonatate is an unusual source of local anesthesia for the airway. It is the active ingredient of Tessalon Perles (Forest Pharmaceuticals, Inc., St. Louis, Missouri), a cough suppressant that produces numbness of the mouth if the gelatin capsules are chewed. One report describes using 200 mg to provide topical anesthesia (34). The capsules are punctured and chewed by the patient. It is recommended to limit the dose to 200 mg (two 100-mg capsules).

Adverse Effects of Local Anesthetic Agents

Local anesthetics, especially of the ester type, or their preservatives or vehicles can provoke hypersensitivity reactions ranging from dermatitis to anaphylaxis. The more common systemic effects of local anesthetics are well described and include central nervous system (sedation, agitation, confusion, and seizures) and cardiovascular (hypotension, arrhythmias, and myocardial depression) events (Table 11).

Topical application may have direct adverse effects. Pulmonary function tests reveal that there is a measurable (10%) decrease in forced expiratory volume (FEV_1) and forced vital capacity (FVC) following administration of lidocaine aerosol that lasts at least 20 minutes (35). Bronchospasm has been reported in asthmatic patients after inhalation of lidocaine solution (36). Hypoxemia has been variably reported.

APPLICATION OF LOCAL ANESTHETICS TO THE AIRWAY

Any consideration of local anesthesia use should be prefaced by a discussion of the innervation of the sites involved. Therefore, for each region of the airway, the appropriate anatomy is reviewed and various anesthetic options presented (Tables 12 and 13).

TABLE 11. *Signs and symptoms of local anesthetic toxicity*

Metallic taste	Tachycardia
Tinnitus	Bradycardia
Light-headedness	Hypertension
Anxiety	Hypotension
Restlessness	Cardiac arrest
Loss of consciousness	Tachypnea
Seizures	

TABLE 12. *Local anesthetic blocks for airway anesthesia*

Transtracheal injection
Superior laryngeal nerve block
Sphenopalatine and anterior ethmoid nerve block
Glossopharyngeal and pharyngeal plexus nerve block

Nose

The nasopharyngeal mucosa has afferent innervation primarily through the ophthalmic and maxillary branches of the trigeminal nerve (cranial nerve V). The ophthalmic nerve gives rise to the nasociliary nerve, which branches to form the anterior ethmoid nerve. The anterior ethmoid nerve approaches the nasal cavity just anterior to the cribriform plate and provides sensation to the anterior nasal mucosa medially and laterally. The maxillary division of cranial nerve V produces branches that form the posterior nasal nerves and the nasopalatine nerve. These nerves pass through the sphenopalatine ganglion, which rests submucosally at the posterior aspect of the middle turbinate in the sphenopalatine recess.

These nerves can be anesthetized by a number of techniques. Cotton packing strips soaked with local anesthetic can be layered into the nasal cavity using a bayonet forceps and nasal speculum. Cotton-tipped swabs can be placed high in the nasal cavity to block the anterior ethmoid nerve and posteriorly at the end of the middle turbinate to anesthetize the sphenopalatine ganglion. More simply, the nasal cavity can be sprayed with local anesthetic, with or without a vasoconstrictor such as phenylephrine, or gel formulations of local anesthetic can be introduced into the nose and sniffed by the patient. Cocaine has no pre-eminence in this regard, as its has been shown that other local anesthetic preparations are equally useful (37).

TABLE 13. *Devices and methods used to topicalize the airway*

1. Oxygen-driven respiratory-therapy nebulizers filled with local anesthetic can produce topical anesthesia as the patient inspires quietly.
2. Bulb atomizers
   a. can produce topical anesthesia when local anesthetic is sprayed while the patient is actively inspiring.
   b. with the bulb removed and connected to 4- to 6-L/min oxygen source can produce an oxygen-enriched spray. As in 2a, the patient should inspire deeply as the local anesthetic is sprayed.
3. Nebulizers can be connected to intubating airways and provide topical anesthesia such that one can advance the airway as topical anesthesia develops.
4. The Jackson laryngeal applicator forceps can be used to place local anesthetic-soaked pledgets in the pyriform sinuses to topicalize this area.
5. Fingertip-controlled syringes are useful whenever aspiration is important to safe block performance.

Oral Cavity and Pharynx

Sensation in the anterior tongue is provided by the lingual branch of cranial nerve V. The posterior third of the tongue is innervated by the glossopharyngeal (cranial nerve IX) and vagus (cranial nerve X) nerves via the pharyngeal plexus. Deeper in the oral pharynx (including the superior surface of the epiglottis), sensation is provided diffusely by the pharyngeal plexus.

The oral cavity can be topically anesthetized with sprays or gargles of local anesthetic solutions. Options include 0.5% dyclonine HCl, lidocaine 2% to 4%, benzocaine sprays, or combination formulations such as Cetacaine spray. One unusual technique involves having the patient chew or dissolve in his mouth Tessalon Perles, as noted above.

Alternatively, the glossopharyngeal nerve can be classically blocked by injecting local anesthetic at a site 0.5 cm behind the midpoint of the posterior tonsillar pillars (palatopharyngeal fold) (38). The tip of a depth-control needle (bent end or beaded shaft) is inserted laterally and slightly posteriorly at this spot, which represents a point between the superior and middle constrictors at the lateral pharyngeal wall. After aspiration to avoid injection into the carotid artery, local anesthetic (2 to 3 mL) is injected submucosally with a fingertip-controlled syringe. A variation of the technique has been reported that involves locating the anterior tonsillar pillar and noting the bridge of tissue from the tongue to the lateral pharyngeal wall as the tongue is retracted to one side of the mouth (39). This palatoglossal arch is punctured 0.5 cm from the root of the tongue and 2 mL of lidocaine injected after aspiration. Injection in this loose submucosal tissue results in spread to the ninth cranial nerve. If injection occurs too anteriorly, the hypoglossal nerve may be blocked and motor function to the tongue impaired.

Larynx

The inferior (laryngeal) aspect of the epiglottis, down to but not including the vocal cords, is innervated by the internal branch of the superior laryngeal nerve, a branch of the vagus. This nerve passes from the vagus anteriorly and travels between the thyroid cartilage and the hyoid bone until it pierces the thyrohyoid membrane and ramifies submucosally at the level of the pyriform recesses.

Anesthesia in this area can be accomplished by blocking the superior laryngeal nerve. The placement of local anesthetic-soaked pledgets in the pyriform sinuses, using Jackson laryngeal forceps (Jackson cross-action forceps), under direct visualization may accomplish this topically. As with other sites, this area can be anesthetized topically by diffuse application of an agent (aerosol sprayed through the bronchoscope under direct visualization).

These nerves can also be blocked using an external approach (40). To accomplish this block, the skin of the neck is cleansed with an antiseptic solution at the level of the lateral aspect of the hyoid bone. The superior cornu of the thyroid cartilage is located and the thyrohyoid membrane palpated. The carotid sheath rests under the finger at this point and can be retracted laterally. A 25- or 27-gauge needle on a syringe containing 2% lidocaine is inserted until the membrane is felt. An injection of 2 mL of local anesthetic is made at a level just superficial to the membrane. Alternatively, the needle can be advanced through the membrane until air is aspirated, then withdrawn submucosally. In this area of the neck, intravascular injections remain a possibility.

Proximal and Distal Trachea

Below the vocal cords, the mucosa of the trachea is innervated by the recurrent laryngeal nerve. This nerve originates from the vagus in the chest and runs cephalad in a groove between the esophagus and trachea. More distally, the trachea is innervated directly from the vagus.

Topically, anesthesia to the lower airway can be delivered by aerosol or spray if the droplet size is favorable. The size of droplets generated determines the distribution of the local anesthetic. Droplets larger than 100 μm are cleared in the mouth, nose, and pharynx. Aerosol droplets of 60 to 100 μm are deposited in the trachea and carina. Droplets of 30 to 60 μm pass into the medium-sized bronchi. Droplets of 10 to 30 μm are distributed to the

TABLE 14. *Anesthesia for awake fiberoptic intubation*

1. Glycopyrrolate 0.2 mg is given intravenously or subcutaneously. (If subcutaneously administered, onset of action may be delayed approximately 20 minutes.)
2. Lidocaine gel or viscous lidocaine 2%, 5 to 10 mL, is sniffed into the nose or spread in the mouth (on the back of the tongue) with a tongue blade. Alternatively, viscous lidocaine can be gargled by the patient.
3. Phenylephrine nasal spray is applied or a diluted solution of 1% phenylephrine is instilled in both nares.
4. Nasal airways lubricated with lidocaine gel are introduced into one naris in progressively larger sizes. For an oral approach, a similarly lubricated intubating airway or bite block is introduced into the mouth after the mouth is first sprayed with 2% lidocaine (step 5).
5. Lidocaine in an atomizer or aerosol is sprayed sufficiently into the nose or mouth to provoke coughing. The dose should be limited to 5 to 10 mL of 2% lidocaine applied over 5 minutes if sprayed, and as little as 3 mL of 2% xylocaine given as a nebulized treatment usually suffices to provide topical anesthesia. Caution should be taken to avoid excessively high doses that produce systemic toxicity, as the drug is readily absorbed from the tracheal and bronchial mucosa.
6. If additional tracheal anesthesia is required,
   a. inject 2 to 5 mL 2% lidocaine with a 22- to 25-gauge needle or catheter transtracheally.
   b. spray supplemental local anesthetic through the bronchoscope as needed under direct visualization.

small bronchi, and smaller particles pass out to the alveoli, where they rapidly enter the blood stream (29).

This area can also be anesthetized by transtracheal injection of local anesthetic. This is easily accomplished by palpating the cricothyroid membrane. By puncturing this membrane aseptically with a 20- to 22-gauge needle or catheter and demonstrating aspiration of air, one can easily introduce 4 mL of 2% lidocaine into the trachea. When done at maximum exhalation, loss of local anesthetic through cough is minimized (41). Although this is a simple technique, hemorrhage and death have been reported after laceration of a small artery in the cricothyroid membrane during transtracheal injection. As with all invasive blocks, it should be approached with caution in patients on anticoagulant therapy.

Comparisons of various anesthetic techniques have been done, but no clear consensus has been reached (42, 43,44). A simple protocol for anesthesia for awake fiberoptic intubation is given in Table 14.

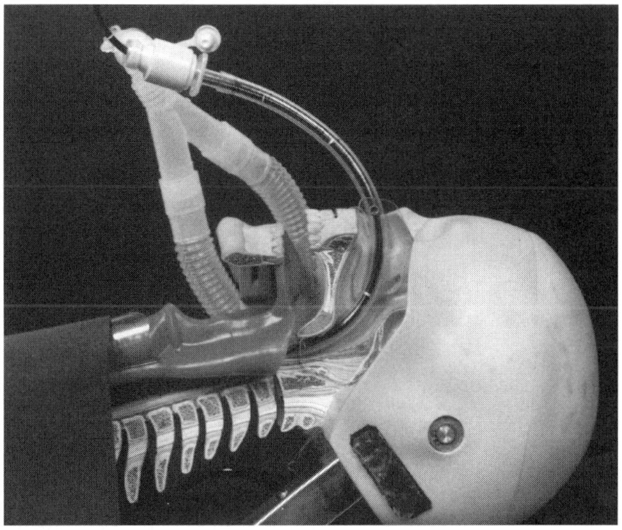

FIG. 17. Nasal fiberoptic intubation via a self-sealing diaphragm on an endotracheal tube inserted into the nasal passage distal to the turbinates.

FIBEROPTIC AIRWAY INTUBATION

Fiberoptic oral intubation of the airway requires preparation of equipment, including the bronchoscope, light source, and ETTs. Topical local anesthetic is applied to the nasopharynx and oropharynx, and then intravenous sedation is administered to provide amnesia and cough suppression. Generally, topicalization should occur prior to sedation if the patient's cooperation is required (e.g., gargling with viscous lidocaine). A bite block or airway should be used to avoid damage to the fiberoptic bundle of the bronchoscope. A drying agent such as glycopyrrolate may be administered in preparation for the procedure to minimize oral secretions that can impair visualization through the bronchoscope.

Suctioning of the pharynx is performed before inserting the bronchoscope, and to direct the bronchoscope in correct anatomic alignment, an intubating airway is placed in the oropharynx. An ETT is partially advanced through the airway, and the fiberoptic bronchoscope is inserted through the ETT (Fig. 16). The bronchoscope is advanced through the vocal cords, and the tube is then advanced over the bronchoscope into the trachea. The tube is positioned appropriately above the carina. Fiberoptic nasal intubation requires sedation and application of a substantial quantity of local anesthetic to the nasal passage; the ETT is inserted in a similar fashion after careful passage of the tube beyond the turbinates (Fig. 17).

If the intubation is unexpectedly difficult, an LMA may provide a means to oxygenate and ventilate the patient as well as act as a guide for fiberoptic intubation.

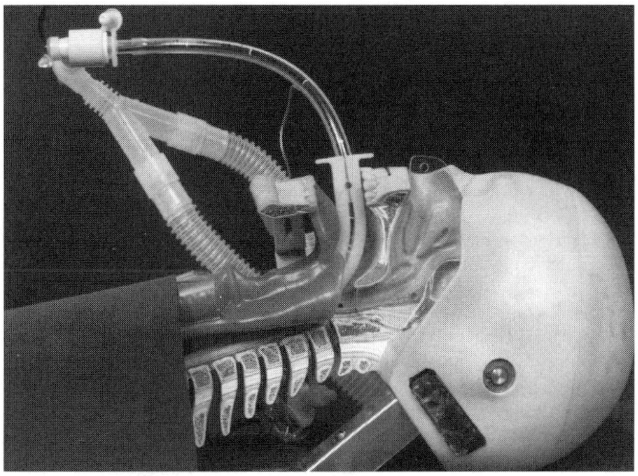

FIG. 16. Oral fiberoptic intubation via a self-sealing diaphragm on an endotracheal tube inserted into a break-away oral airway.

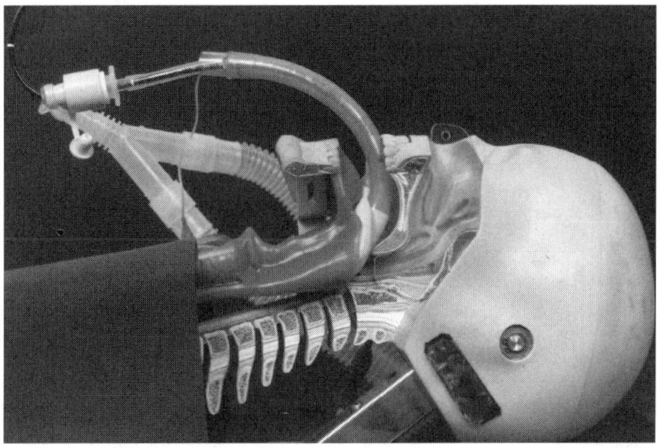

FIG. 18. Oral fiberoptic intubation via a self-sealing diaphragm on an endotracheal tube inserted into a laryngeal mask airway.

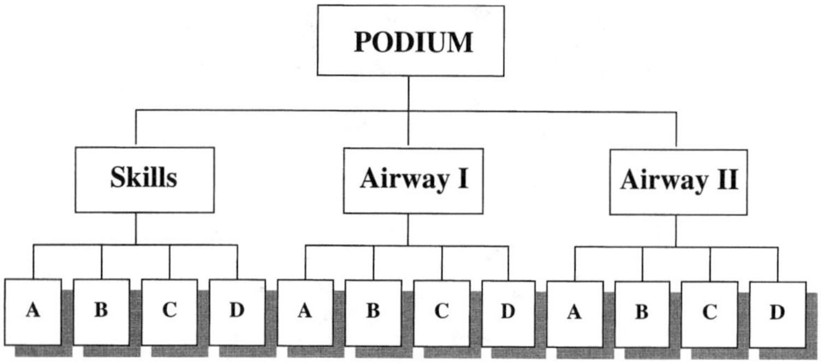

FIG. 19. Organization of a fiberoptic bronchoscopy course. Various stations are directed from a podium. Each station teaches various aspects of fiberoptic bronchoscopy and may utilize computer tutorials, (synthetic) human airway models, bronchoscopes, and video displays. From: Waldron RJ, Hanowell LH, Grande CM. Blunt airway trauma. In: *Seminars in Anesthesia.* Philadelphia: W.B. Saunders; 1994:13:140, with permission.

The small ETT is inserted into the ventilating conduit, and then a bronchoscope is inserted into the ETT. The bronchoscope is advanced through the vocal cords, and the ETT is then advanced over the bronchoscope into the trachea (Fig. 18). The LMA can be carefully removed if 1) the ETT circuit connector is first removed and 2) the ETT *in situ* is "lengthened" with a smaller ETT inserted into the proximal end.

Reed (15) reviewed the preparation of patients for awake flexible fiberoptic bronchoscopy. Obstruction of the airway, hypoxemia, cardiac arrhythmias, adverse drug reactions, and oversedation were cited as potential complications during such procedures. Reed emphasized the importance of monitoring oxygen saturation via a pulse oximeter and the need for administering supplemental oxygen during such procedures (Table 15). Those performing fiberoptic bronchoscopy in awake patients should provide sufficient sedation, analgesic drugs, and topical pharyngeal and laryngeal anesthesia to prevent pain and reflex sympathetic responses during insertion of the bronchoscope (45,46). Failure to do so results in hemodynamic instability (hypertension and tachycardia) and potential coughing, agitation, laryngospasm, and other adverse patient responses. These aspects of sedation, with respect to hemodynamic lability, are particularly important to assure optimal care of critically ill patients who require bronchoscopy during mechanical ventilation (47).

SUMMARY

Guidelines of the American Society of Anesthesiologists (ASA) cite the utilization of fiberoptic ETT placement as a method for management of the difficult airway (48). Additionally, perioperative bronchoscopy is essential in many circumstances during optimal perioperative pulmonary care, as discussed above. Airway trauma is one condition that mandates thorough familiarity with advanced airway management, including the use of the fiberoptic bronchoscope. University training programs, as well as those of other clinical departments of anesthesiology, should plan and define methods of training and updating anesthesia personnel in the techniques of perioperative bronchoscopy. Figure 19 illustrates diagramatically one possible organizational framework for a course in bronchoscopy. Such workshops can be guided from a podium and consist of various stations at which computer tutorials, human airway models, bronchoscopes, and video displays illustrate and teach appropriate techniques. Training protocols are in the best interest of optimal perioperative pulmonary care and are of vital importance to the optimal management of trauma victims with airway injury and other conditions that may require bronchoscopy.

TABLE 15. *Monitoring used during bronchoscopy*

Pulse oximetry
Noninvasive measurement of blood pressure
Electrocardiogram (for rate and rhythm)
Measurement of respiratory rate

REFERENCES

1. American Thoracic Society. Medical Section of the American Lung Association. Guidelines for fiberoptic bronchoscopy in adults. *Am Rev Respir Dis* 1987;136:1066.
2. Wedzicha JA, Pearson MC. Management of massive hemoptysis. *Respir Med* 1990;84:9–12.
3. Kirkpatrick MB, Smith JR, Hoffman PJ, Middleton RM. Bronchoscope damage and repair costs: results of a regional postal survey. *Respir Care* 1992;37:1256–1259.
4. Ehrenwerth J. Pro: proper positioning of a double-lumen endobronchial tube can only be accomplished with endoscopy. *J Cardiothorac Anesth* 1988;2:101–104.
5. Alliaume B, Coddens J, Deloof T. Reliability of auscultation in positioning of double-lumen endobronchial tubes. *Can J Anaesth* 1992; 39:687–690.
6. Hurford WE, Alfille PH. A quality improvement study of the placement and complications of double-lumen endobronchial tubes. *J Cardiothorac Vasc Surg* 1993;7:517–520.
7. Brodsky JA. Con: proper positioning of a double-lumen endobronchial tube can only be accomplished with endoscopy. *J Cardiothorac Anesth* 1988;2:105–109.
8. Slinger PD. Fiberoptic positioning of double-lumen tubes. *J Cardiothorac Anesth* 1989;3:486–496.
9. Benumof JL, Gaughan SD, Ozaki G. The relationship among bronchial blocker cuff inflation volume, proximal airway pressure, and seal of the bronchial blocker cuff. *J Cardiothorac Vasc Surg* 1992;6:404–408.
10. Benumof JL. Laryngeal mask airway: indications and contraindications [editorial]. *Anesthesiology* 1992;77:843–846.

11. Brain A. The laryngeal mask—a new concept in airway management. *Br J Anaesth* 1983;55:801–805.
12. Wood RE. Pitfalls in the use of the flexible bronchoscope in pediatric patients. *Chest* 1990;97:199–203.
13. Finer NN, Muzyka D. Flexible endoscopic intubation of the neonate. *Pediatr Pulmonol* 1992;12:48–51.
14. Trouillet J, et al. Fiberoptic bronchoscopy in ventilated patients. *Chest* 1990;97:927–933.
15. Reed AP. Preparation of the patient for awake flexible fiberoptic bronchoscopy. *Chest* 1992;101:244–253.
16. Ovassapian A, Yelick SJ, Dykes MHM, Brunner EE. Blood pressure and heart rate changes during awake fiberoptic nasotracheal intubation. *Anesth Analg* 1983;62:951–954.
17. Venus B, Polassani V, Pham CG. Effects of aerosolized lidocaine on circulatory responses to laryngoscopy and tracheal intubation. *Crit Care Med* 1984;12:391–394.
18. Rosenberg PH, Heinonen J, Takasaki M. Lidocaine concentration in blood after topical anesthesia of the upper respiratory tract. *Acta Anaesthesiol Scand* 1980;24:125–128.
19. Smith RB. Uptake of lidocaine from the trachea [letter]. *Anesthesiology* 1976;44:269.
20. Viegas O, Stoelting RK. Lidocaine in arterial blood after laryngotracheal administration. *Anesthesiology* 1975;43:491–493.
21. Scott DB, Littlewood DG, Covino BG, Drummond GB. Plasma lidocaine concentrations following endotracheal spraying with an aerosol. *Br J Anaesth* 1976;48:899–901.
22. Chu SS, Rah KH, Brannan MD, Cohen JL. Plasma concentration of lidocaine after endotracheal spray. *Anesth Analg* 1975;54:438–441.
23. Pelton DA, Daly M, Cooper PD, Conn AW. Plasma lidocaine concentrations following topical aerosol application to the trachea and bronchi. *Can Anaesth Soc J* 1970;17:250–255.
24. Campbell D, Adriani J. Absorption of local anesthetics. *JAMA* 1958;168:871–877.
25. Wu F. Seizure after lidocaine for bronchoscopy. *Pharmacotherapy* 1993;13:72–78.
26. Ameer B, et al. Systemic absorption of topical lidocaine in elderly and young adults undergoing bronchosocpy. *Pharmacotherapy* 1989;9:74–81.
27. Amitai Y, et al. Serum lidocaine concentrations in children during bronchoscopy with topical anesthesia. *Chest* 1990;98:1370–1373.
28. Randell T, et al. Topical anesthesia of the nasal mucosa for fiberoptic airway endoscopy. *Br J Anaesth* 1992;68:164–167.
29. Adriani J, et al. Topical anesthetics: use and misuse. *South Med J* 1985;78:1224–1229.
30. Verlander JM, Johns ME. The clinical use of cocaine. *Otolaryngol Clin North Am* 1981,14:521–531.
31. Goodell J, et al. Reducing cocaine solution use by promoting the use of a lidocaine-phenylephrine solution. *Am J Hosp Pharm* 1988;45:2510–2513.
32. Katz RI, Hovagim AR, Findelstein HS, et al. A comparison of cocaine, lidocaine with epinephrine and oxymetazoline for prevention of epistaxis on nasotracheal intubation. *J Clin Anesth* 1990;2:16–20.
33. Gross JB, Hartigan ML, Schaffer DW. A suitable substitute for 4% cocaine for blind nasotracheal intubation, 3% lidocaine-0.5% phenylephrine nasal spray. *Anesth Analg* 1984;63:915–918.
34. Morgan PD, et al. Rapid oral anesthesia for awake intubation. *J Clin Anesth* 1992;4:101–105.
35. Peacock A, et al. Effect of fiberoptic bronchoscopy on pulmonary function. *Thorax* 1990;45:38–41.
36. McAlpine I, et al. Lidocaine-induced bronchoconstriction in asthmatic patients. *Chest* 1989;96:1012–1015.
37. Middleton RM, et al. Topical nasal anesthesia for flexible bronchoscopy. *Chest* 1991;99:1093–1096.
38. Barton S, et al. Glossopharyngeal nerve block. *Arch Otolaryngol* 1971;93:186–188.
39. Woods A. Ablation of gagging and the hemodynamic response to awake laryngoscopy. *Anesthesiology* 1987;67:A220.
40. Gaskill J. Local anesthesia for peroral endoscopy. *Arch Otolaryngol* 1966;84:654–657.
41. Gotta A, et al. Anesthesia of the upper airway using topical and superior laryngeal nerve block. *Br J Anaesth* 1981;53:1055–1057.
42. Isaac PA, Barry JE, Vaughan RS, Rosen M. A jet nebuliser for delivery of topical anaesthesia to the respiratory tract. A Comparison with cricothyroid puncture and direct spraying for fibreoptic bronchoscopy. *Anaesthesia* 1990;45:46–48.
43. Kortilla K, Tarkkanen J, Tarkkanen L. Comparison of laryngotracheal and ultrasonic nebulizer administration of lidocaine in local anesthesia for bronchoscopy. *Acta Anaesthesiol Scand* 1981;25:161–165.
44. Graham DR, Hay JG, Clague J, Nisar M, Earis JE. Comparison of three different methods used to achieve local anesthesia for fiberoptic bronchoscopy. *Chest* 1992;102:704–707.
45. Fry WA. Techniques of topical anesthesia for bronchoscopy. *Chest* 1978;73:694–696.
46. Rees PJ, Hay JG, Webb JRL. Premedication for fiberoptic bronchoscopy. *Thorax* 1983;38:624–627.
47. Hawkyard SJ, Morrison A, Doyle LA, Croton RS, Wake PN. Attenuating the hypertensive response to laryngoscopy and endotracheal intubation using awake fiberoptic intubation. *Acta Anaesthesiol Scand* 1992;36:1–4.
48. American Society of Anesthesiologists Task Force on Management of the Difficult Airway. Practice guidelines for management of the difficult airway. *Anesthesiology* 1993;78:597–602.

Airway Management, edited by
L.H. Hanowell, M.D. and R.J. Waldron, M.D.,
Lippincott-Raven Publishers, Philadelphia © 1996.

CHAPTER 17

Retrograde Intubation and Transtracheal Jet Ventilation

Debra E. Morrison, Antonio Sanchez, and Ahmed Ghouri

INTRODUCTION

It has been generally accepted that the majority of deaths during the administration of anesthesia occur due to the failure to oxygenate and ventilate patients. Historically, incidence of failure in the operating room to ensure gas exchange by mask or endotracheal intubation resulting in brain damage or death has been estimated as 0.01–2.0 per 10,000 patients (1). The incidence of airway difficulty (grades II–IV by laryngoscopy) in the general surgical population is estimated at 1% to 18% (1). The operating room constitutes a relatively controlled environment in which skilled personnel may act according to the American Society of Anesthesiologists (ASA) algorithm (2) to maintain airway patency and ensure gas exchange using accepted techniques that are discussed elsewhere in this volume. Airway management out of the operating room in potentially uncontrolled and possibly more urgent circumstances (in the field, emergency room, intensive care units, or hospital wards) implies far higher risk of death, brain injury, organ injury, and airway trauma. The clinician in any circumstance must be skilled and prepared to utilize multiple techniques for intubation and ventilation. Among the techniques cited in the practice guidelines of ASA (2), retrograde intubation (RI) and transtracheal jet ventilation (TTJV) are invasive techniques for accessing the airway via the cricothyroid membrane (CTM). These techniques require special equipment that can be assembled in advance and maintained in a portable storage unit for difficult airway management. Both require prior knowledge and understanding of the anatomy and physiology of the airway and should be learned in the elective setting.

ANATOMY

Basic anatomic knowledge of the cricoid cartilage (Fig. 1) and the structures above and below it is required in order to minimize complication and failure when performing RI or TTJV. Indeed, regardless of the intubation technique planned, the cricoid cartilage and CTM should be identified preoperatively in every patient (3). Cartilage and membrane, vasculature, and the thyroid gland are relevant anatomy.

D.E. Morrison, A. Sanchez, and A. Ghouri: Department of Anesthesiology, University of California, Irvine Medical Center, Orange, California 92668.

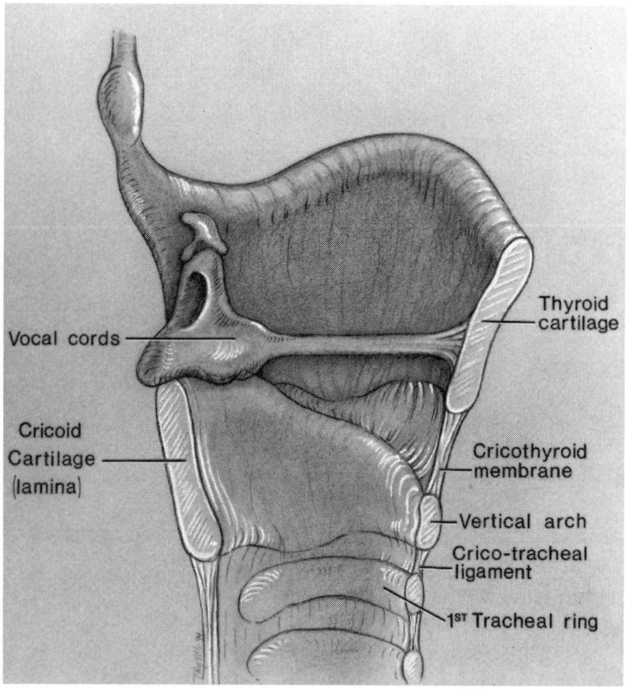

FIG. 1. Anatomy of the cricoid cartilage. From UCI Department of Anesthesia, with permission.

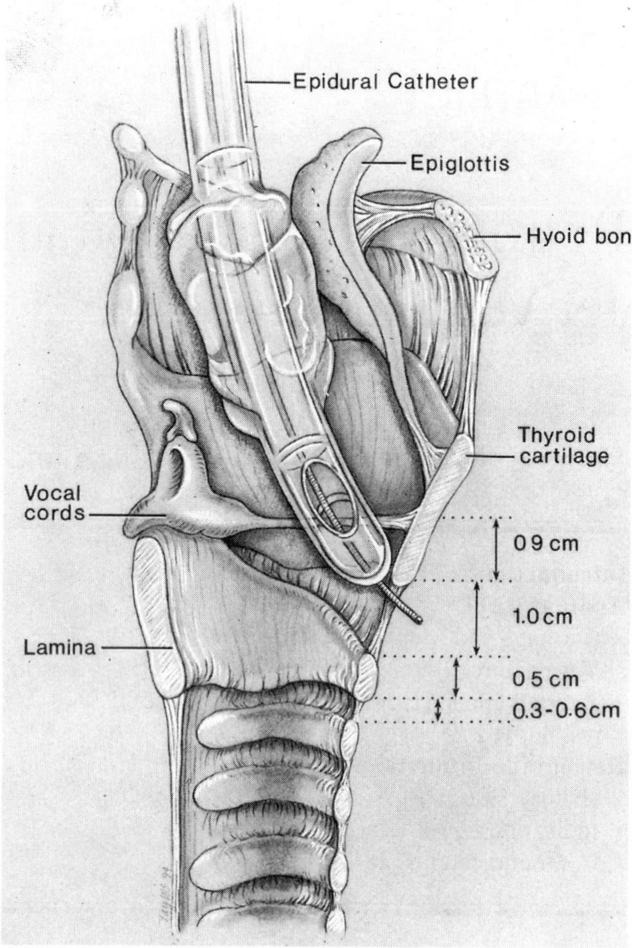

FIG. 2. Mid-sagittal view of the larynx and trachea showing the distance between the vocal cords and the upper border of the first tracheal ring. Note that only a small portion of the endotracheal tube Murphy eye is below the vocal cords. From UCI Department of Anesthesia, with permission.

Cartilage and Membrane

The signet ring-shaped cricoid cartilage (Fig. 1) consists of a broad, flat plate posteriorly called the *lamina* and a narrow, convex structure anteriorly called the *arch* (4,5). The vertical height of the arch (Fig. 2) is 0.5–0.7 cm (4). The CTM connects the superior border of the arch to the inferior border of the thyroid cartilage and measures approximately 1 cm in height (5). The cricotracheal ligament, measuring 0.3–0.6 cm in height, connects the inferior border of the arch to the upper border of the first tracheal ring (6). The distance between the inferior border of the thyroid cartilage and the vocal cords is approximately 0.9 cm, but varies with gender (7).

Vasculature

There are paired major blood vessels above and below the cricoid cartilage: the cricothyroid artery and the superior thyroid artery (Fig. 3). The cricothyroid artery (4, 7–9), a branch of the superior thyroid artery, runs along the anterior surface of the CTM, usually close to the inferior border of the thyroid cartilage. The cricothyroid arteries may anastomose in the midline and give rise to a descending branch that feeds the pyramidal lobe of the thyroid gland when it is present. One of the authors (AS) has found in cadaver dissections that the cricothyroid artery becomes insignificant in size as it approaches the midline. No mention of a major midline venous plexus could be found in the literature: AS finds no evidence of any in his dissections.

The bilateral anterior branches of the superior thyroid artery (4,7–9) run along the upper border of the thyroid isthmus and anastomose in the midline. The inferior thyroid artery anastomoses with the anterior branch of the superior thyroid artery at the level of the isthmus. The arteries are remarkable for their large size and frequent anastomoses. In less than 10% of the population, an unpaired thyroidea ima artery will ascend ventral to the trachea (from either the aortic arch or brachiocephalic artery) to anastomose at the level of the isthmus. Though normally small, it may be very large. A rich venous plexus is formed in and around the isthmus.

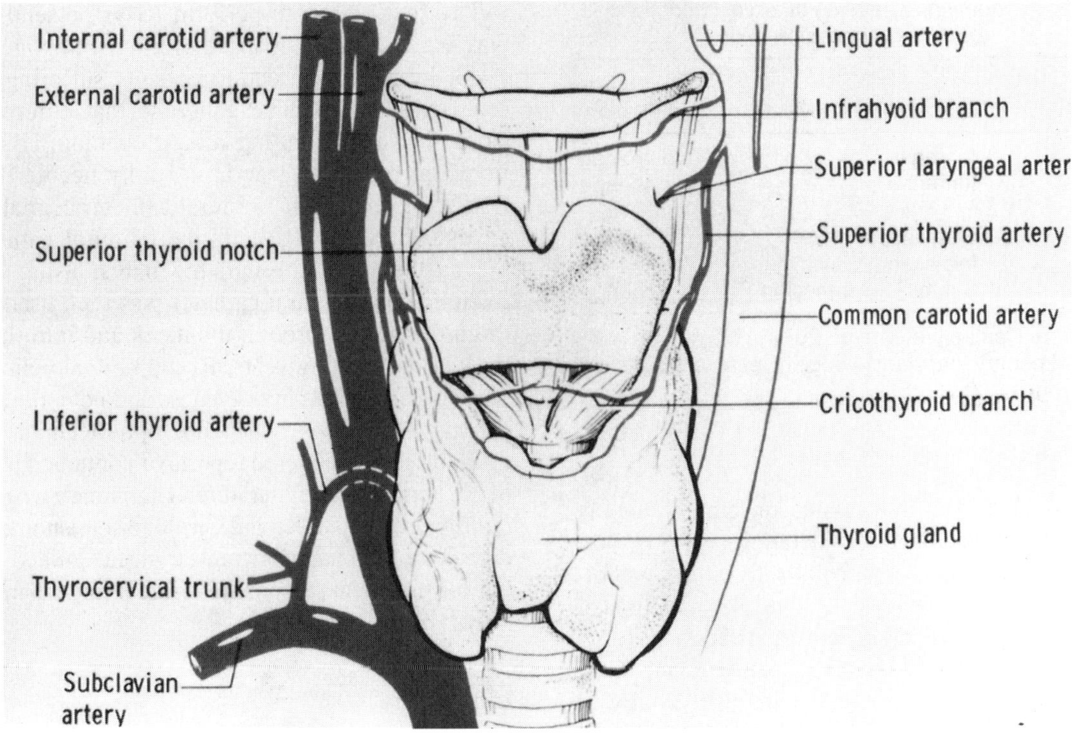

FIG. 3. Vascular anatomy above and below the cricoid cartilage. From Naumann, ref. 7, with permission.

Thyroid Gland (Isthmus, Pyramidal Lobe)

The isthmus of the thyroid gland (Fig. 3) is rarely absent and generally overlies anterior to the trachea between the first and fourth tracheal rings. Both vertical height and depth average 1.25 cm. Extending from the isthmus, the highly vascular pyramidal lobe (Fig. 4) is well developed in one-third of the population. It is found more frequently on the left of the midline and may extend into a thyromuscular continuation up to the hyoid bone. (4–6,8,9).

PHYSIOLOGY

Sympathetic stress response (increased heart rate, blood pressure, intraocular pressure, intracranial pressure, and elevated catecholamine levels) has been reported with laryngoscopy, endotracheal intubation, coughing, translaryngeal local anesthesia, laryngotracheal anesthesia, and fiberoptic intubation. Therefore, concern is appropriate when performing any airway maneuver in patients with coronary artery disease, elevated intraocular pressure, or elevated intracranial pressure (10–12). It is reasonable to argue, however, that RI, performed skillfully, need not be more stimulating than any other technique for managing the airway. The same statement can be made regarding elective use of TTJV, and in circumstances requiring

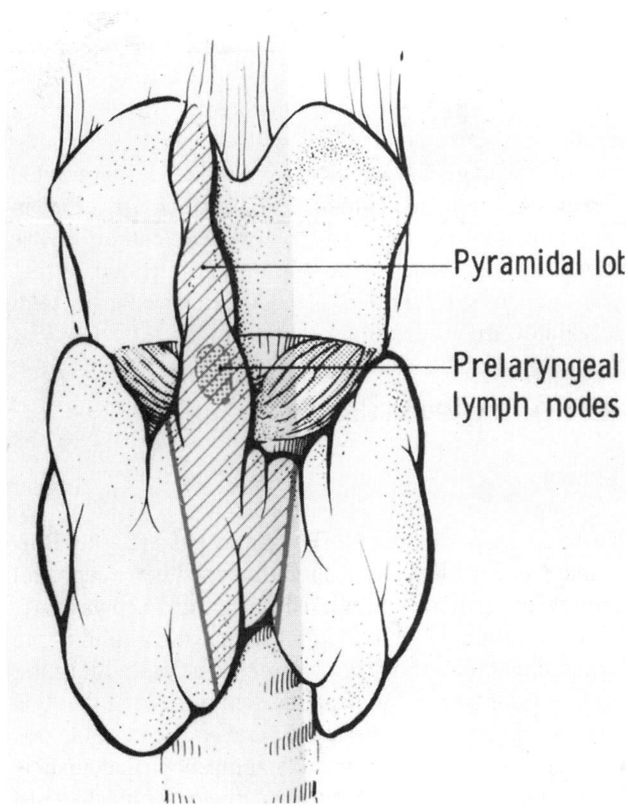

FIG. 4. Pyramidal lobe of the isthmus. From Naumann, ref. 7, with permission.

TABLE 1. *Hemodynamic effects of laryngoscopy vs. retrograde intubation*

Parameter	Laryngoscopy	Retrograde intubation
Heart rate	Increase	No change
Mean arterial pressure	Increase	No change
Cardiac index	Decrease	No change
PCWP	Increase	No change
ECG	3 mm ST depression	No change

Modified from Casthely et al., ref. 20.
PCWP, pulmonary capillary wedge pressure; ECG, ST segment changes in lead V5.

emergent use of TTJV, immediate concern for airway management overrides other considerations.

In multiple case reports of patients with cardiac pathology who underwent RI, neither those awake with topical anesthesia nor those under general anesthesia (13–23) had significant changes in hemodynamics noted. Casthely et al. (20) reported 25 patients with difficult airway secondary to rheumatoid arthritis who came for open heart surgery (coronary artery bypass graft and valvular replacement). Comparison of hemodynamic responses to rigid laryngoscopy (MacIntosh and Miller blades) and RI demonstrated no significant difference (Table 1). One patient underwent RI awake after topical anesthesia with no significant hemodynamic response. Two case reports (24,25) document patients with previous history of difficult airway and intracranial pathology (pseudotumor cerebri and intracranial tumor with elevated intracranial pressure) who underwent elective, awake RI after topical anesthesia with no evidence of further increase in intracranial pressure. Transtracheal jet ventilation has been used clinically in the appropriate elective setting (26) and can be performed, using topical anesthesia, with little untoward stimulation.

RETROGRADE INTUBATION

History

The first reported case of RI was in 1960 (27) by Butler and Cirillo, who passed a red rubber catheter cephalad through the patient's previously existing tracheostomy. Once the catheter exited the oral cavity, it was tied to the endotracheal tube (ET), allowing it to be pulled into the trachea. (Our surgical colleagues note in passing that this is not always possible, since the cutaneous end of the tracheocutaneous fistula is usually more cephalad than is the tracheal end, and the rubber catheter would have to make a 180° turn in order to go up the trachea.)

The first person to perform RI as presently practiced was Waters, a British anesthesiologist in Nigeria (28). In 1963, he reported treating patients suffering from cancrum oris, an invasive gangrene that deforms the oral cavity, severely limiting mouth opening. His technique involved passing a standard Tuohy needle through the CTM and feeding an epidural catheter cephalad into the nasopharynx. He "fished" the epidural catheter out of the nasopharynx through the nares, using a hook he devised. The epidural catheter was then used as a stylet to guide the ET through the nares and into the trachea.

Over the ensuing years, RI did not gain clinical acceptance because of its invasiveness and potential for complications. After 1964, when fiberoptic technology became available, only scattered reports of continued performance of RI appear in the literature. The name *retrograde intubation*, used by Butler and Cirillo, is a misnomer (29). The technique is actually a translaryngeal guided intubation, but for historical reasons we will continue using the name *retrograde intubation*.

Indications

Historically, RI has been used under the following circumstances: (1) following failed attempts at laryngos-

TABLE 2. *Pathology associated with retrograde intubations in 383 patients*

Pathology	No. patients
Oral cavity	
Cancrum oris	27
Mandibular/maxillary fracture	31
Perimandibular abscess	1
Ankylosis of temporomandibular joint	5
Microstomia	1
Macroglossia	1
Cancer of the tongue	8
Oral myxoma	1
Cervical	
Spinal cord injury	66
Ankylosing spondylitis	11
Rheumatoid arthritis	32
Pharynx and larynx	
Laryngeal cancer	70
Pharyngeal abscess	1
Epiglottitis	1
Pharyngeal edema	1
Laryngeal edema postburn	2
Others	
Pediatric anomalies	24
Obesity	11
Coronary artery bypass graft operations (failure to intubate)	28
Tracheostomy stoma	16
Trauma (failure to intubate)	33
Pathology not specified (failure to intubate)	12

From UCI Department of Anesthesia, with permission.

TABLE 3. *Experience with retrograde intubations*

Item	Data
Number of adult patients	357
Number of pediatric patients	26
Age range	1 day to 84 years
Average time for technique (range)	2.5 min (0.5–15 min)
Elective cases	113 patients
Failed attempts using RI	5 patients

From UCI Department of Anesthesia, with permission.

TABLE 4. *Contraindications to retrograde intubation (examples)*

Unfavorable anatomy
Lack of access to CTM (severe flexion deformity of the neck)
Poor anatomical landmarks (obesity)
Pretracheal mass (thyroid goiter)
Laryngotracheal pathology
Malignancy
Stenosis
Coagulopathy
Infection (pretracheal abscess)

From UCI Department of Anesthesia, with permission.

copy and/or fiberoptic intubation; (2) for the emergent establishment of an airway where visualization of the vocal cords is prevented by blood, secretions, or anatomical derangement; and (3) electively, when clinically deemed necessary, e.g., unstable cervical spine, mandibular fracture, or anatomical anomaly.

The RI technique has been used both in the hospital setting and in the field (prehospital mobile units) (30,31). It has been employed with the anticipated (28,30) and unanticipated (28,30) difficult airway, following failure to intubate using conventional means [direct laryngoscopy (13,20), blind nasal intubation (32), and Bougie (33) and fiberoptic laryngoscopy (14,34)]. It has been employed in both humans and animals (35,36). Data on approximately 500 retrograde intubations (383 patients and 117 cadavers), combined from the literature and from the experience of one of the authors (AS), have been evaluated.

Airway pathology necessitating RI has been of a wide variety (Table 2). RI has been used in patients with limited range of motion of the neck (153 trauma victims with potential cervical spine injury) and in patients with facial trauma. It has been employed in both the adult and pediatric population with success (Table 3).

Not all reported cases describe the amount of time required to perform the technique, but in one study using training mannequins the average time was 71 seconds (37). Barriot and Riou (30) described 13 patients with maxillofacial trauma who could not be intubated in the field using direct laryngoscopy (averaging 6 attempts over 18 min). The patients were subsequently intubated on the first RI attempt in an average time of less than 5 min. When RI was attempted in an additional 6 patients without prior direct laryngoscopy, intubation took less than 5 min.

Contraindications

Contraindications to RI have been cited, often anecdotally (Table 4). Most are relative contraindications and can be divided into four categories: (1) unfavorable anatomy; (2) laryngotracheal pathology; (3) coagulopathy; and (4) infection.

Unfavorable Anatomy

Since in most cases retrograde intubation is performed above or below the cricoid cartilage, the absolute lack of access to this region—as in severe flexion deformity of the neck—is a contraindication. For the same reason, the patient with nonpalpable landmarks (38), obesity (39), overlying malignancy (40), or large thyroid goiter (40) should be approached cautiously. Shantha (41) reported a case of RI in a patient with a large thyroid goiter. After failure of conventional intubating methods (including fiberoptic), the surgeons dissected down to the CTM and subsequently passed the catheter cephalad. A total of 11 cases of RI have been reported in the obese without major complications (39,42,43).

Laryngotracheal Pathology

Theoretically, laryngotracheal stenosis may contraindicate RI, since narrowing of the trachea or larynx could be made worse by either the needle puncture or the catheter (44). However, RI has been used in patients with laryngeal cancer (45), epiglottitis (16), and laryngeal edema secondary to burn injuries (46,47). It should not be used when there is laryngeal/tracheal stenosis directly under the intended puncture site.

Coagulopathy

Preexisting bleeding diathesis should be considered a relative contraindication. Though there is a potential for bleeding, the CTM is considered a relatively avascular plane (see section on anatomy). A small, self-limited hematoma (20) was reported in a patient who underwent coronary artery bypass graft with intraoperative heparin and postoperative disseminated intravascular coagulation (DIC) (40,44,48–54).

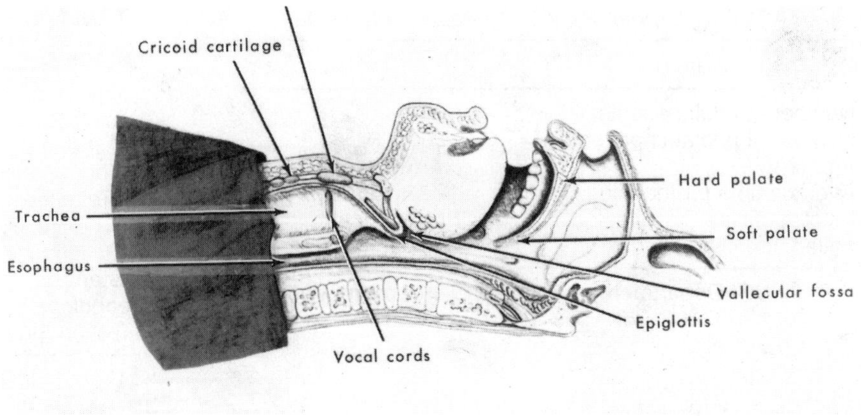

FIG. 5. A: Mid-sagittal view of the head and neck.

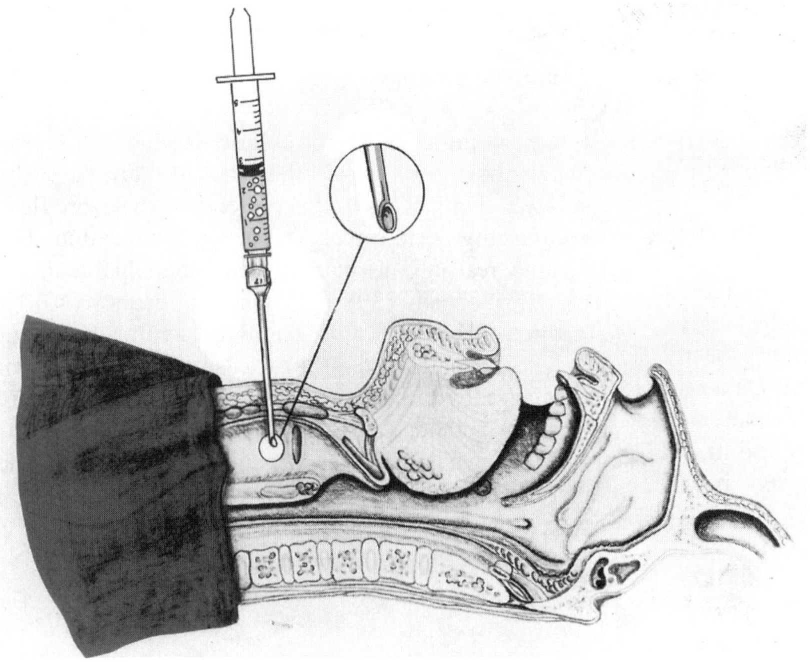

FIG. 5. B: Standard #17 Tuohy needle (with saline-filled syringe) is advanced (with bevel pointing sideways) through the cricothyroid membrane (CTM) at a 90° angle (trying to stay as close as possible to the upper border of the cricoid cartilage). Entrance into the trachea is verified by aspiration of air.

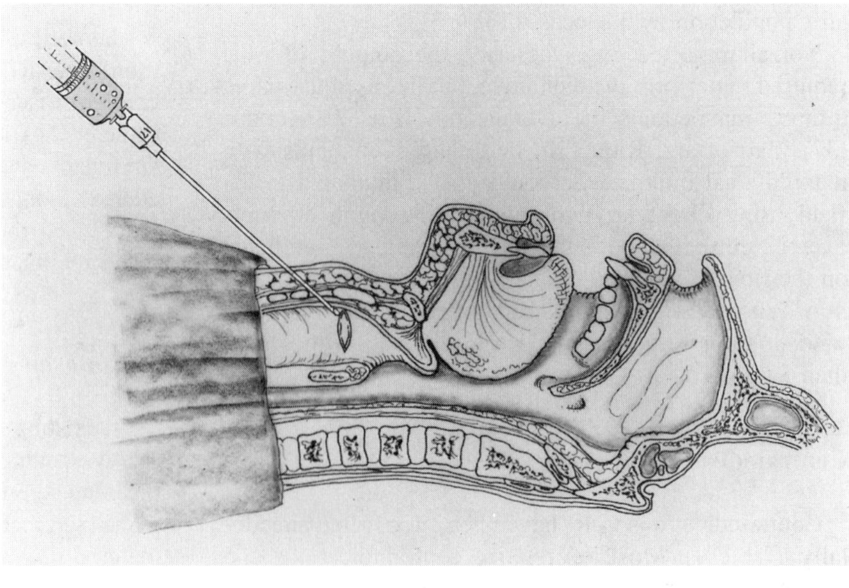

FIG. 5. C: Tuohy angle is changed to 45° with bevel pointing cephalad. (Again verifying position by aspirating air.)

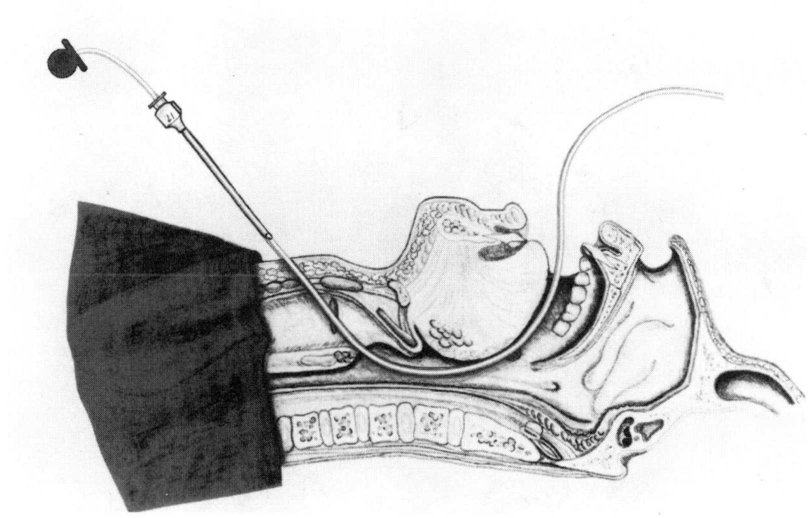

FIG. 5. D: Epidural catheter is advanced through the vocal cords and into the pharynx. During this time the patient is asked to stick tongue out or tongue can be pulled out manually. Most of the time the epidural catheter (EC) will come out of the mouth on its own. Tuohy is then withdrawn to hang at caudal end of the EC.

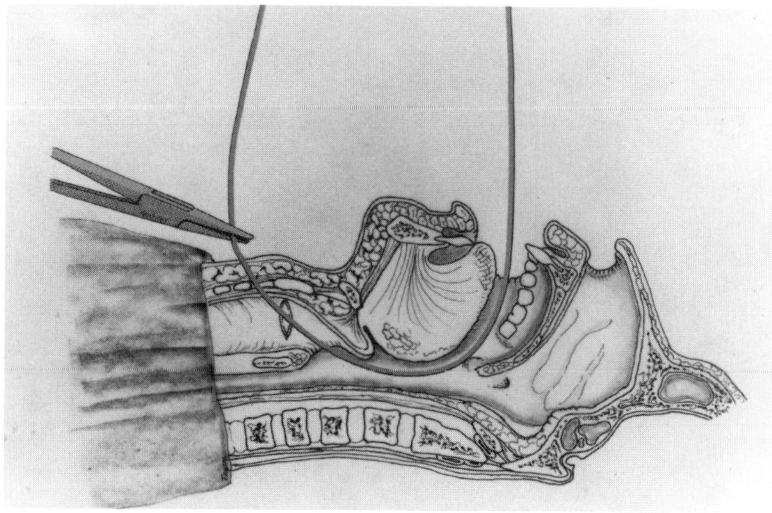

FIG. 5. E: Pull the EC out of the mouth to an appropriate length, then clamp a hemostat flush with the skin.

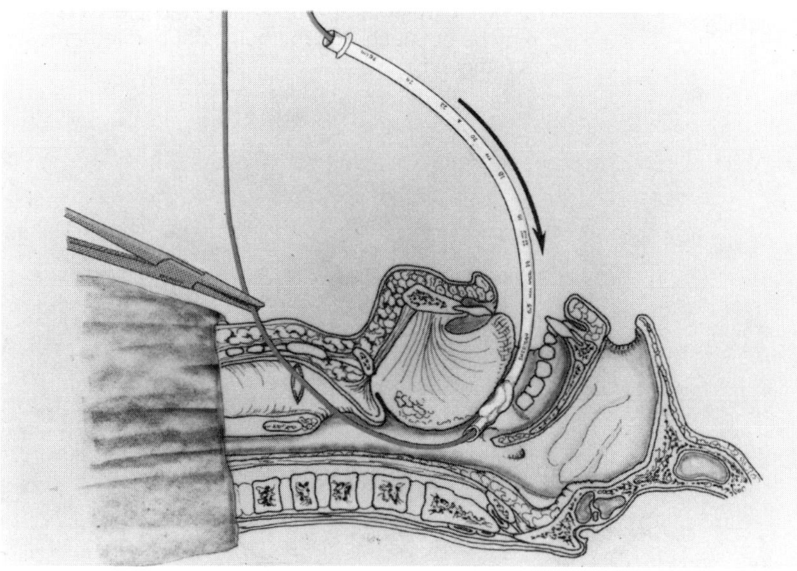

FIG. 5. F: Thread a well-lubricated endotracheal tube (ET) over the EC. Maintain a moderate amount of tension on the EC as the ET is advanced forward *(arrow)*: a small click can be felt as the ET travels through the vocal cords.

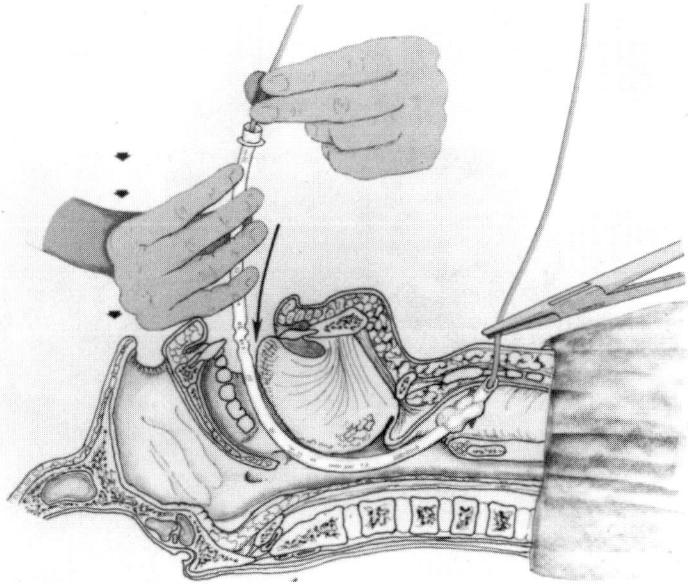

FIG. 5. G: When the ET reaches the CTM, it is important to maintain pressure *(small arrows)*, forcing the ET into the oropharynx *(large arrow)* to cause continuing pressure against the CTM with the tip of the ET. (Note: Moderate tension is still being maintained on the EC.)

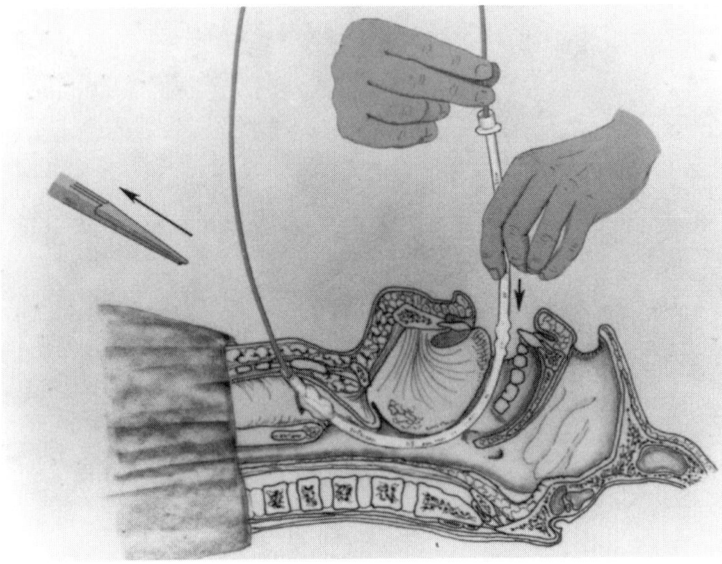

FIG. 5. H: An assistant should remove hemostat *(large arrow)* while pressure is maintained *(small arrow)* to push the ET up against the CTM. (The EC may be cut flush with the hemostat before hemostat is removed.)

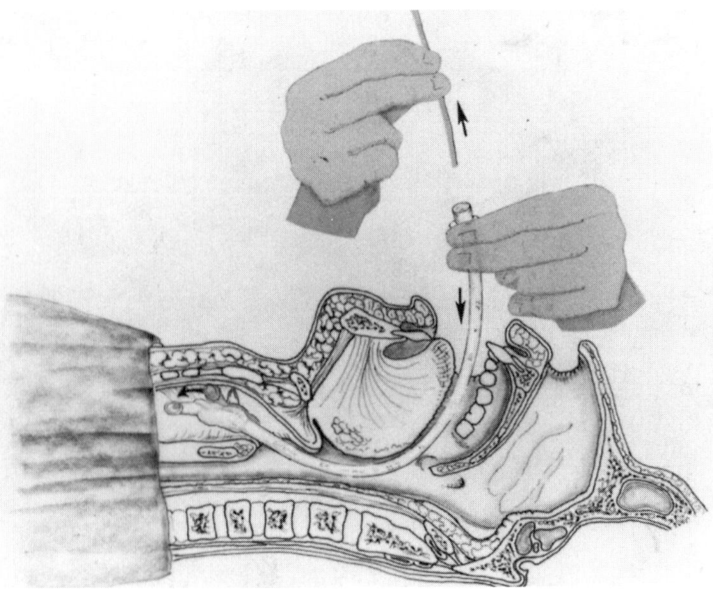

FIG. 5. I: Simultaneously *(straight arrows)* remove EC as the ET is advanced. The tip of the ET will drop from its position up against the CTM to midtrachea *(curved arrow)*. Advance ET to desired depth.

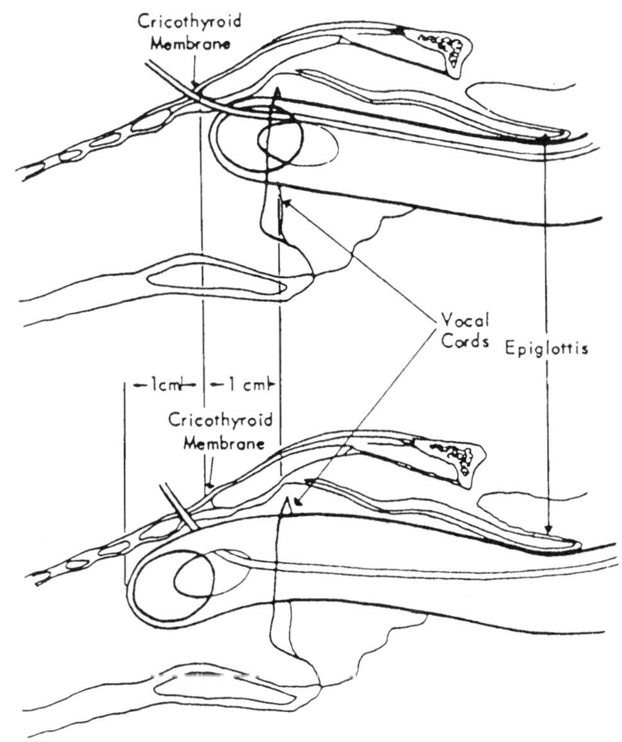

FIG. 5. J: Cross-section of larynx and trachea, with ET and catheter guide passing through the CTM. Catheter passes through end of ET, and 1 cm of ET passes the cords *(top)*. Catheter exits the side hole, allowing 2 cm of ET to pass beyond the vocal cords *(bottom)*. From UCI Department of Anesthesia and Bourke and Levesque, ref. 63, with permission.

Infection

Retrograde intubation in the presence of preexisting infection over the puncture site or in the path of the puncture—as in pretracheal abscess—could result in transmission of bacterial flora into the trachea and should be avoided. This, again, should be considered a relative contraindication, since transtracheal aspiration is performed for sputum sample in patients with pneumonia in spite of the possibility of pretracheal abscess (see section on complications) (40,44,48,52,55–57).

Techniques

Preparation

Although most documented retrograde intubations have not been elective, every effort should be made to perform RI using aseptic technique. An appropriate antisialagogue may be indicated, especially if the fiberoptic bronchoscope is to be employed (see section on fiberoptic technique). If time permits, the airway should be anesthetized to prevent sympathetic stimulation, laryngospasm, and discomfort. According to Sanchez (3), an awake RI with oral intubation can be performed with translaryngeal anesthesia (4 ml 2% lidocaine injected through the CTM) supplemented with topicalization (nebulized or sprayed local anesthetics) of the pharynx and hypopharynx. A 10% lidocaine metered-dose spray (Astra) is available and is quick and very effective for topicalization.

If the fiberoptic bronchoscope is to be employed as part of the technique (see section on fiberoptic technique), and an oral airway, (Ovassapian or Williams) is used, the gag reflex can be minimized by use of 10% lidocaine metered-dose spray (Astra). The gag reflex can also be ablated by injection of 2 ml 1% lidocaine bilaterally into the anterior tonsillar pillars where they join the base of the tongue, blocking the lingual branch of the glossopharyngeal nerve, which supplies sensory innervation to the posterior third of the tongue, the pharynx, and tonsils. To accomplish the block, retract the tongue anterolaterally with a blade (tongue or laryngoscope), thus placing the tonsillar pillar under tension and allowing visualization. A 25-gauge spinal needle is then inserted into the anterior tonsillar pillar, perpendicular to the palatoglossal fold (1). After aspirating for blood or air, inject 2 ml, which will cause a slight swelling. Bilateral blocks will allow the patient to accept an airway without gagging but will relax pharyngeal muscles and tongue base and can cause airway obstruction.

Further topicalization can be accomplished with 10% lidocaine via the airway once the gag is ablated. The cutaneous branches of the superior laryngeal nerve, which supplies the inferior aspect of the epiglottis and upper larynx (but not the vocal cords), can be effectively and quickly blocked topically.

The translaryngeal block provides anesthesia for the vocal cords, lower larynx, and trachea. Special caution should be exercised when performing translaryngeal anesthesia since coughing, grunting, sneezing, or swallowing causes the cricoid cartilage to travel cephalad, with the potential for breaking the needle in the trachea (52,58,59). To perform the block, identify the CTM and, if appropriate, make a small skin wheal. Insert a 20-gauge angiocatheter perpendicular to the trachea, with bevel pointing cranially. Confirm position in the trachea by aspiration of air, advance the catheter over the needle into the tracheal lumen, then remove the needle and aspirate for air before injecting the local anesthetic (4 ml 2% lidocaine) at the end of inspiration.

If nasal intubation is planned (see section on silk technique), the nasal mucosa should be anesthetized and vasoconstricted: 4% cocaine or 4% lidocaine with 0.5% to 1.0% phenylephrine are commonly applied with cotton-tipped applicators or pledgets over 5–10 min. Most failures result from insufficient time allowed for the drugs to work. Following adequate anesthesia and vasoconstriction of the nasopharynx, the nasal passage should be dilated with increasing sizes of soft rubber nasal airways lubricated with 2% lidocaine gel.

The ideal position for RI is in the supine sniffing position with the neck hyperextended (60). As a result, the cricoid cartilage and the structures above and below it are easier to palpate. Retrograde intubation can also be performed with the patient in a sitting position (3), which may be the only position that allows some patients to breathe comfortably. Potential cervical spine injury and/or limited range of motion of the cervical spine may necessitate RI with the neck in a neutral position, which is a well-documented practice (Table 2).

The transtracheal puncture site for RI can be made either above or below the cricoid cartilage. The CTM is relatively avascular and has less potential for bleeding (see section on anatomy). The disadvantage of the CTM is that initially only 1 cm of ET is actually placed below the vocal cords, and the angle of entry of the ET into the trachea is more acute. A cricotracheal ligament puncture site allows a longer initial length of ET below the vocal cords. The disadvantage is that this site has more potential for bleeding (though none has been reported). Both entry sites have been used successfully. In cadaver studies (61,62), the success rate for RI was higher with less vocal cord trauma when the cricotracheal ligament rather than the CTM was used. Vocal cord trauma has not been reported in the clinical setting.

Classical Technique

The classical RI is simple and is performed percutaneously using a standard 17-gauge Tuohy needle and epidural catheter (EC) (Figs. 5A–J). After preparation and anesthesia, a right-handed person should stand on the right side of a supine patient. The left hand is used to stabilize the trachea by placing the thumb and third digit on either side of the thyroid cartilage. The index finger of the left hand is used to identify the midline of the CTM as well as the upper border of the cricoid cartilage.

Since the Tuohy needle is blunt, a small incision through the skin and subcutaneous tissue with a #11 scalpel blade is recommended. Because of the significant force required to perforate the skin and the CTM, there is a risk of perforating the posterior tracheal wall as well. This has been verified in cadaver studies using a fiberoptic bronchoscope (FOB) (39).

The right hand then grasps the Tuohy needle (attached to a partially filled syringe) like a pencil, with the fifth digit used to brace the right hand on the patient's lower neck. The CTM is punctured, and aspiration of air confirms placement in the tracheal lumen, since the esophagus collapses under negative pressure.

Once the Tuohy needle is in place, the EC is advanced into the trachea. When advancing the EC, it is important to have the tongue pulled anteriorly to prevent the EC from coiling up in the oropharynx. The EC will usually exit on its own from either the oral or nasal cavity. If the EC has to be retrieved from the oropharynx, one of the authors (AS) recommends using a nerve hook (V. Mueller #NL2490, Baxter, Deerfield, Illinois). Magill forceps have been used, but these were designed to grasp large structures like the ET. Magill forceps may not grip the EC securely, since the distal tips do not completely occlude and may traumatize the pharynx.

Originally, the EC was threaded through the main distal lumen (beveled portion) of the ET. Bourke modified the technique by threading the EC through the Murphy eye (63) (Fig. 5J), reasoning that this would allow an additional 1 cm of ET to pass through the cords. Lleu, in cadaver studies, showed that using the cricotracheal ligament (61,62) as the puncture site in combination with threading the EC through the Murphy eye enhanced success over the original technique.

When advancing the ET over the EC, a moderate amount of tension should be employed (33,54). Excessive tension pulls the ET anteriorly, making it more likely to get caught up against the epiglottis, vallecula, or anterior commissure of the vocal cords. If there is difficulty in passing the opening of the glottis, the ET can be rotated 90° counter-clockwise (1,39) or exchanged for a smaller tube (39).

Guide Wire Technique

The modified technique (Figs. 6A–K) using a guide wire (14,29) developed because the flexible EC is prone to kinking (34,47). Equipment consists of an 18-gauge angiocatheter, a J-tip guide wire (GW) (0.038 inch outer diameter and 110–120 cm length), and a guide catheter (GC) (Fig. 6A). Use of a GW offers the following advantages: (1) the J-tip tends to be less traumatic to the airway (47,53); (2) retrieval of the GW from the oral or nasal cavity is easier (38,64); (3) the GW is less prone to kinking (65); (4) the GW can be used with the FOB (see section on fiberoptic technique); (5) the GW is easy to handle (66); and (6) the technique takes less time to perform than does the classical technique (38). Discrepancy between the external diameter of the GW and the internal diameter of the ET allows a railroading effect to occur, with the tip of the ET catching peripherally on the arytenoideae or vocal cords instead of passing straight through the cords. [Here, the term *railroading* implies that the endotracheal tube tip has the freedom to move laterally, anteriorly, or posteriorly with respect to the guidewire.] Sliding the GC over the GW from above (antegrade) once it has exited the mouth or nose increases the external diameter of the guide apparatus (1), and use of the GC in combination with a smaller-

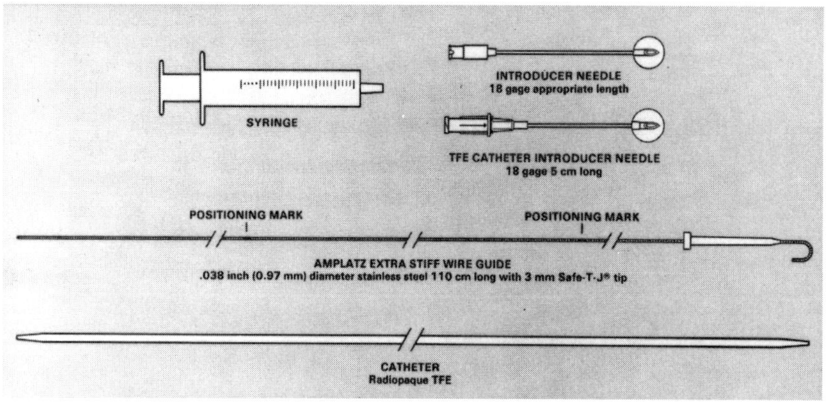

FIG. 6. A: Retrograde kit. From: Cook® Critical Care, Ellettsville, Indiana, with permission.

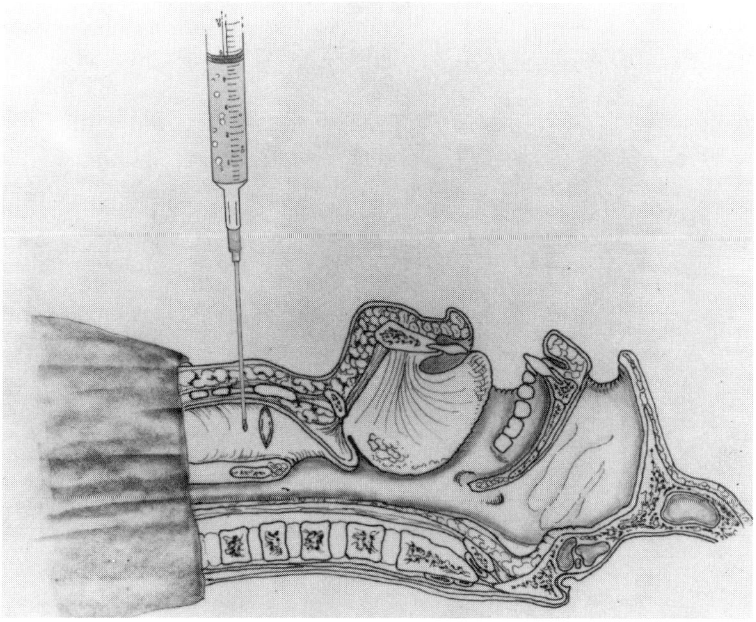

FIG. 6. B: 18-gauge angiocatheter placed at 90° to the cricothyroid membrane (CTM), aspirating for air to confirm position.

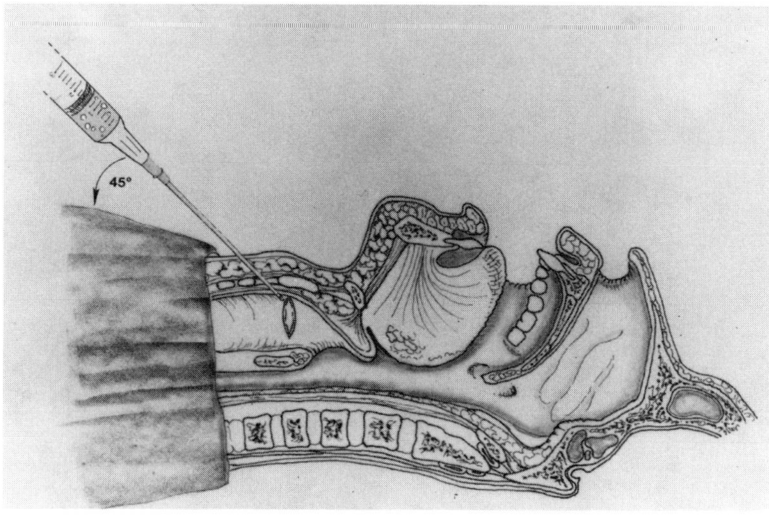

FIG. 6. C: Angle is changed to 45° (again aspirating air to confirm position).

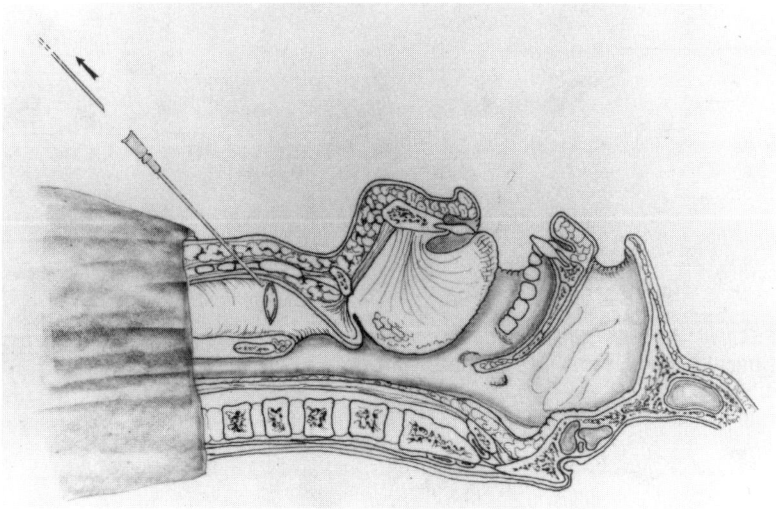

FIG. 6. D: Advance sheath of angiocatheter cephalad and remove needle.

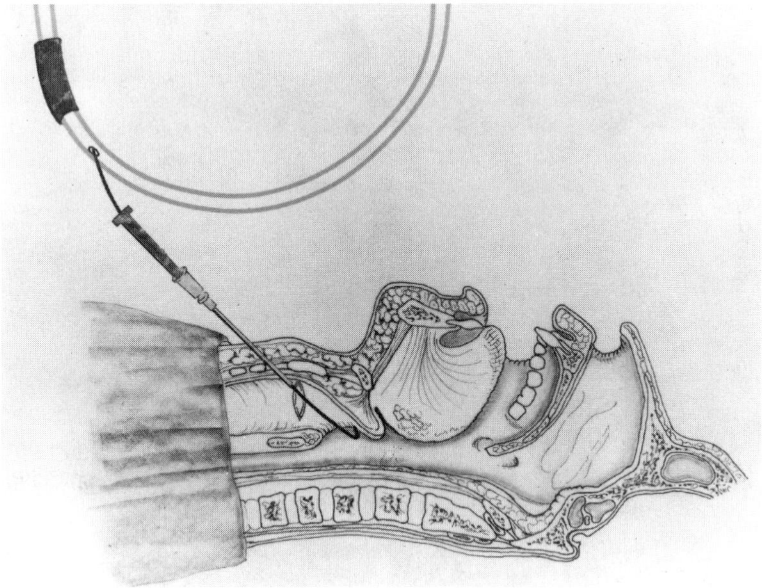

FIG. 6. E: Advance J-tip guide wire through angiocatheter sheath.

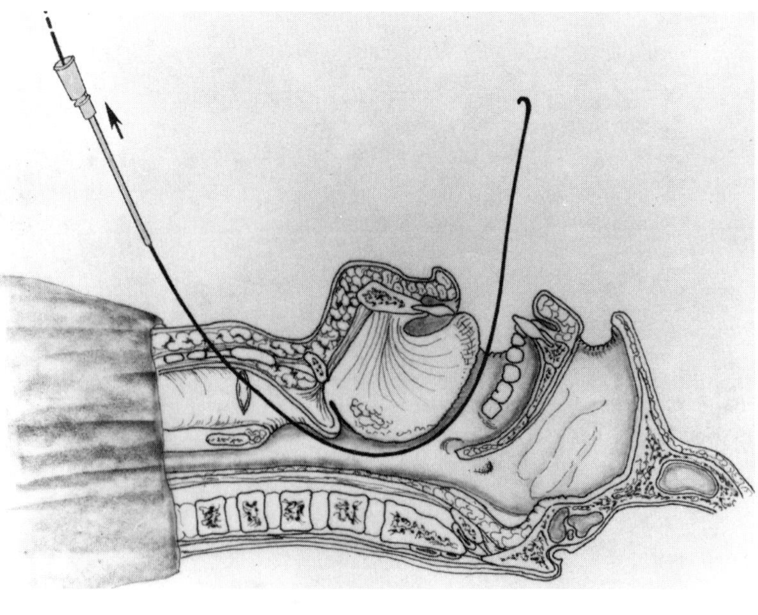

FIG. 6. F: Retrieve end of guide wire from mouth as in classical technique. Remove angiocatheter *(arrow)*.

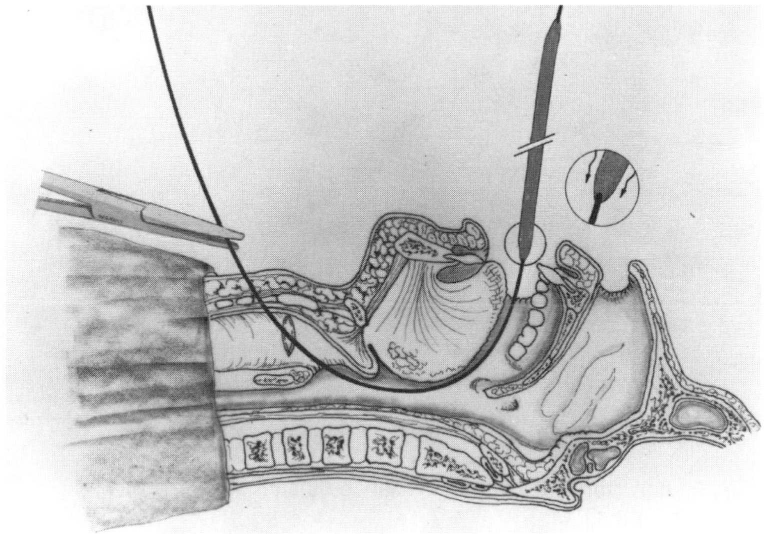

FIG. 6. G: Clamp hemostat flush with skin, and advance tapered tip of guide catheter *(insert)* over guide wire into mouth.

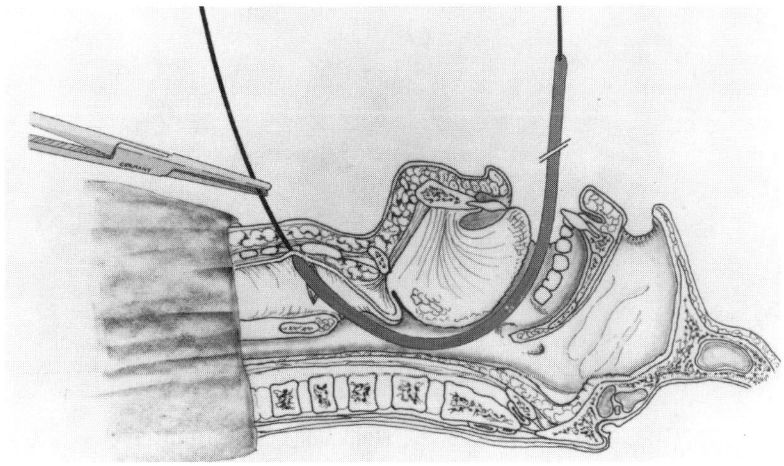

FIG. 6. H: Advance guide catheter to CTM.

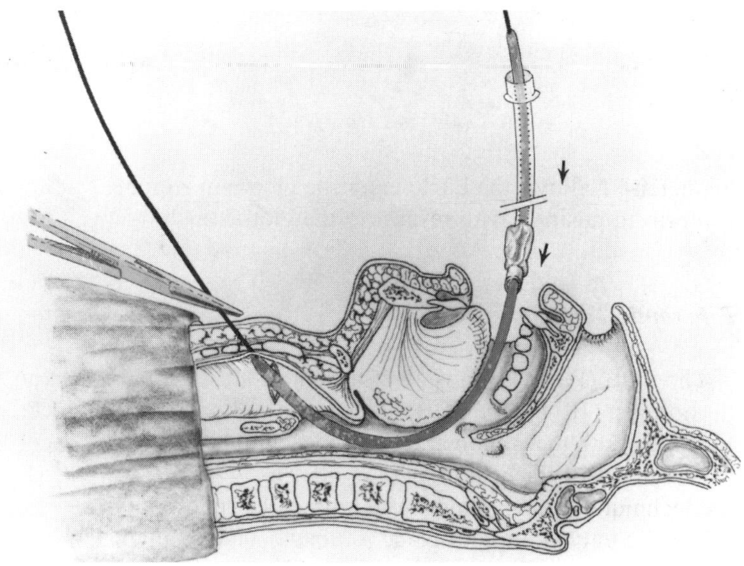

FIG. 6. I: Advance endotracheal tube (ET) over entire structure *(arrows)*. Use an ET that is 6.0–7.0 mm internal diameter. Size of the ET is dictated by the external diameter of the guide catheter.

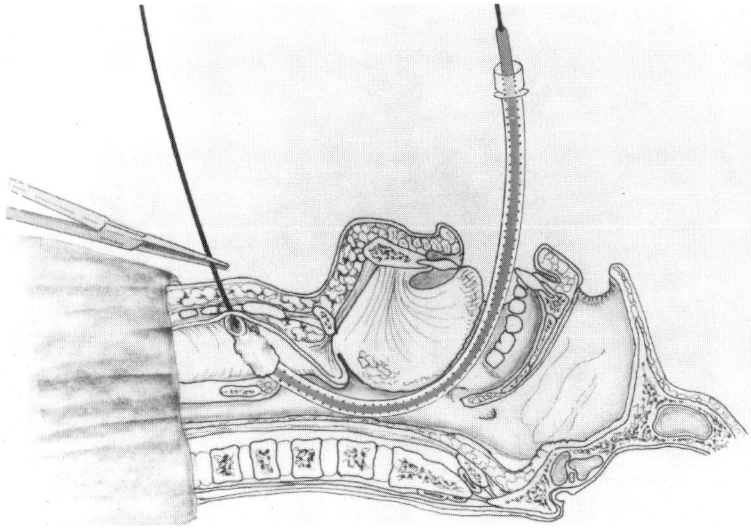

FIG. 6. J: Advance ET through vocal cords and up against the CTM.

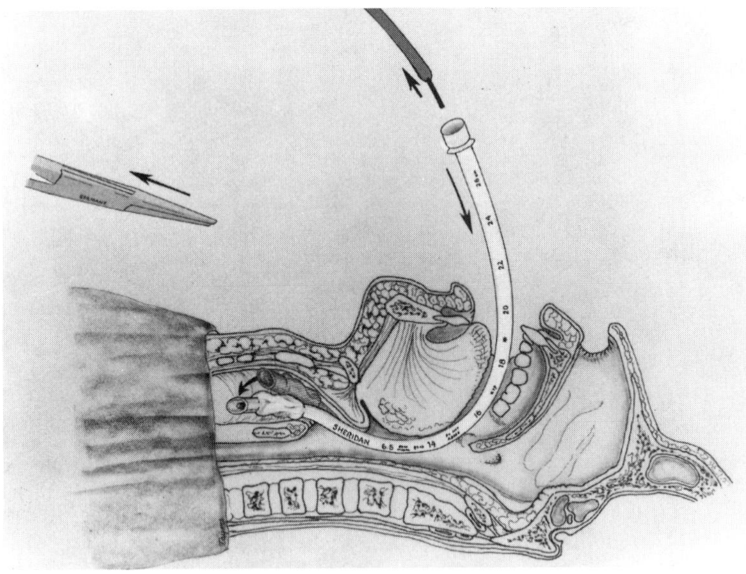

FIG. 6. K: Removal of wire and catheter as in classical technique, except that the guide wire and guide catheter are removed simultaneously. From UCI Department of Anesthesia and Cook Inc., Bloomington, IN, with permission.

diameter ET allows the ET to enter the glottis in a more centralized position with respect to the glottic opening.

Fiberoptic Technique

The FOB (Figs. 7A–I) is a versatile tool for the anesthesiologist (10) but the FOB, like RI, has its limitations. In some cases, the combination of two techniques allows achievement of tracheal intubation after a single or serial techniques (e.g., blind nasal, direct laryngoscopy, fiberoptic intubation, retrograde intubation) have failed. For example, the combination of RI with direct laryngoscopy (16) and RI using FOB (21) can improve the chance of successful intubation. The advantages of passing an FOB antegrade over a GW placed by RI are: (1) the outer diameter of the GW and the internal diameter of the suction port of the FOB form a tight fit, preventing railroading between both structures and allowing the FOB to follow a straight path through the vocal cords without getting caught on anatomical structures; (2) the FOB acts as a large GC (see section on guide wire technique) and prevents railroading of the ET; (3) once the FOB has passed over the GW through the vocal cords, it can be advanced freely beyond the puncture site to the carina, eliminating the problem of distance between cords and puncture site; (4) use of the FOB allows placement of the ET under direct vision; (5) the FOB can be utilized by the less-experienced operator; and (6) oxygen can be delivered continuously through the FOB with the GW still in place (see section on pediatrics). Preparation of the FOB should be completed before RI is initiated. The rubber casing from the proximal portion of the suction port must be removed (to allow the GW to exit from the handle), and the FOB should be armed with the appropriate ET. The RI is performed using the guide

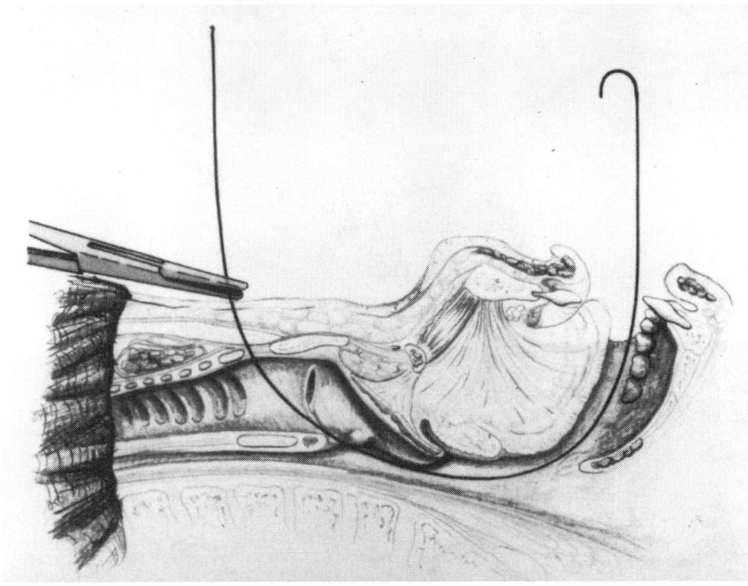

A

FIG. 7. **A:** Guide wire placed as in guide wire technique and pulled out to appropriate length in order to accommodate fiberoptic bronchoscope (FOB) (hemostat in place). **B:** J-tip of guide wire and distal tip of FOB. **C:** J-tip being fed into suction port of FOB.

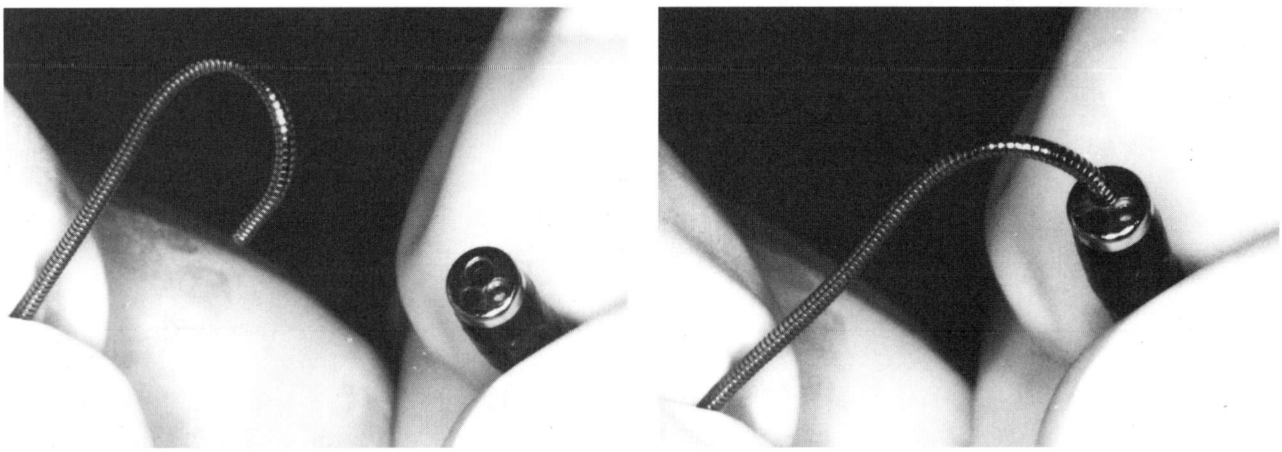

B C

wire technique, and the FOB then passed antegrade over the GW like a GC. Once the tip of the FOB abuts the CTM, there are three options:

1. Remove the GW distally (Fig. 7H) or proximally (through the fiberoptic handle) and, after advancing under direct vision to the carina, intubate. Removal distally is less likely to dislodge the FOB from the trachea, but anecdote suggests that removal proximally should decrease the incidence of infection from oral contaminants (1).
2. Instead of removing the GW, allow it to relax caudad into the trachea, advance the FOB below the cricoid cartilage, then remove the GW. This allows for a greater length of the FOB in the trachea before the GW is removed.
3. Remove the GW proximally only until it is seen through the FOB to have slipped out of the CTM and into the trachea, then advance it through the FOB to the carina. The FOB can then be advanced over the GW to the carina. This option is probably preferable.

Silk Technique

Various pull-through techniques have been described using epidural catheters (53,67), CVP catheters (23), monofilament sutures (68), and Fogarty catheters (69) (Figs. 8A–I). The silk technique is also a pull-through technique (3,39,43). The basic principle involves advancing the EC retrograde as in the classical technique—attaching it to the tip of the ET and using the EC to pull the ET into the trachea. The silk technique offers the following advantages: (1) equipment is readily available in the operating room; (2) the silk is intimately attached to the ET, eliminating railroading; (3) multiple attempts at intubation are allowed; (4) oxygen can be delivered via the ET using a standard anesthesia circle system, and in-line capnography can be used to verify placement of the ET; and (5) if necessary, postoperative reintubation can be accomplished using the silk, which is left in place until time of discharge from the recovery room. This technique employs the principles and equipment of the classical

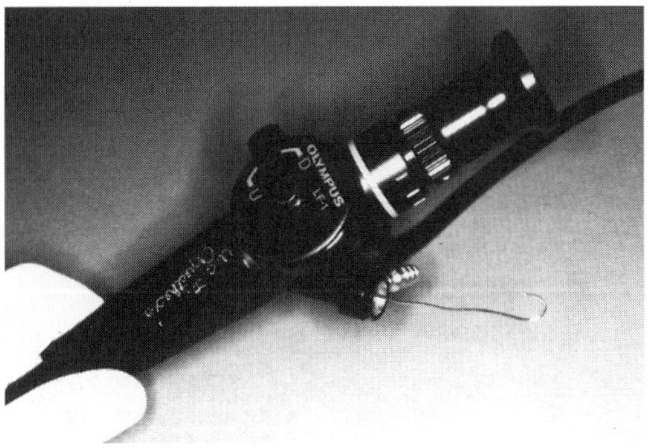
D

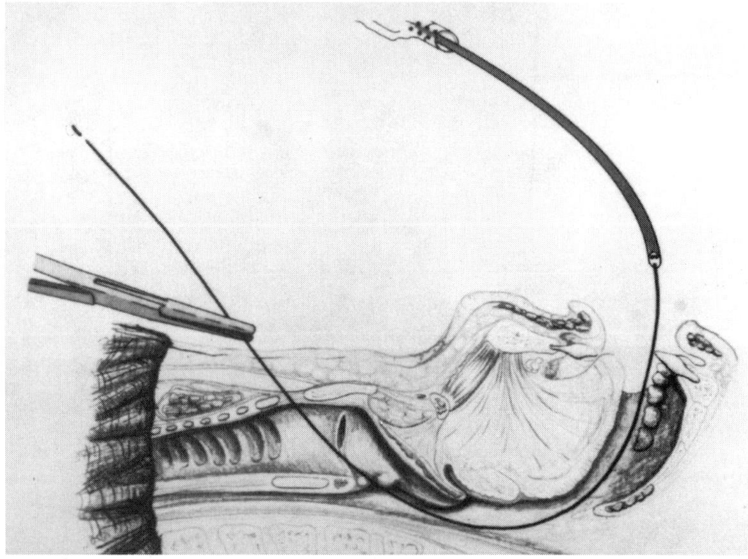
E

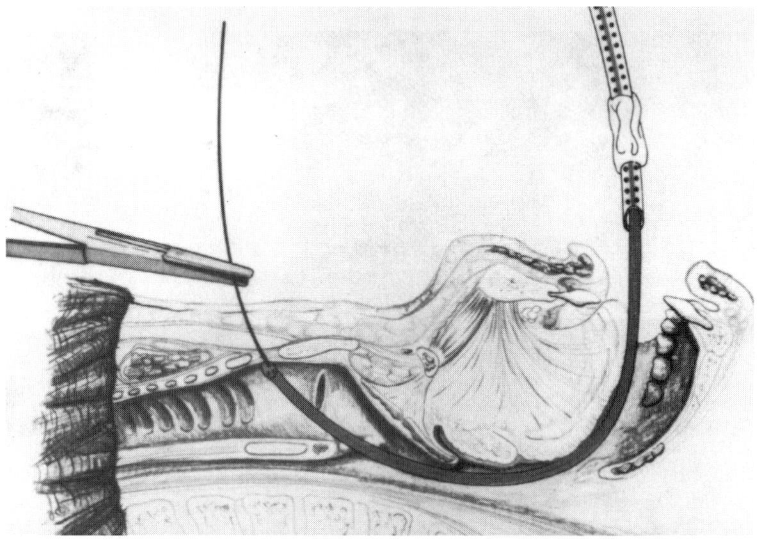
F

FIG. 7. *Continued.* **D:** J-tip exiting from FOB handle. **E:** Begin advancing the FOB [armed with the endotracheal tube (ET)] over the guide wire. **F:** Advance FOB to the CTM.

technique, with the addition of a length of silk suture (3-0 nylon monofilament may also be used). Once the EC (which is used only to place the silk) is out of the oral or nasal cavity, the silk suture is tied to the cephalad end of the EC and the silk is pulled antegrade through the CTM. The EC is cut off and discarded, and the cephalad end of the silk is tied to the Murphy eye. The silk suture is then used to pull the ET into the trachea. There is an adjunct to the silk technique: When a floppy epiglottis causes obstruction, one can deliberately intubate the esophagus. As the ET is being gently withdrawn from the esophagus, tension—applied simultaneously to the distal end of the silk—will pop the tip of the ET anteriorly, lift up the epiglottis, and allow the ET to enter the larynx. If a nasal intubation is required, a urological catheter (UC) can be advanced through a naris into the posterior oropharynx. It is then attached to the EC, which is exiting through the oral cavity. As the UC is withdrawn from the nare, the EC follows, now exiting the nasal rather than the oral cavity (Figs. 8F–I). The silk technique is easy, and because the silk can be left in place for the duration of the anesthetic and after extubation with no discomfort, emergent reintubation can be accomplished. One of the authors (AS) has used this technique to reintubate two patients in the recovery room: both had suffered maxillofacial trauma, were initially intubated awake using retrograde silk technique, and had arch bars placed in the operating room.

Pediatrics

The medical literature on the subject of RI in the pediatric population is not extensive (13,16,28,32,39,46,54,60,64,66,70–72). Retrograde intubation has been used in both the anticipated and the unanticipated difficult airway, primarily after failure of conventional intubating techniques (blind nasal intubation, direct laryngoscopy, fiberoptic intubation). The technique used is the same as

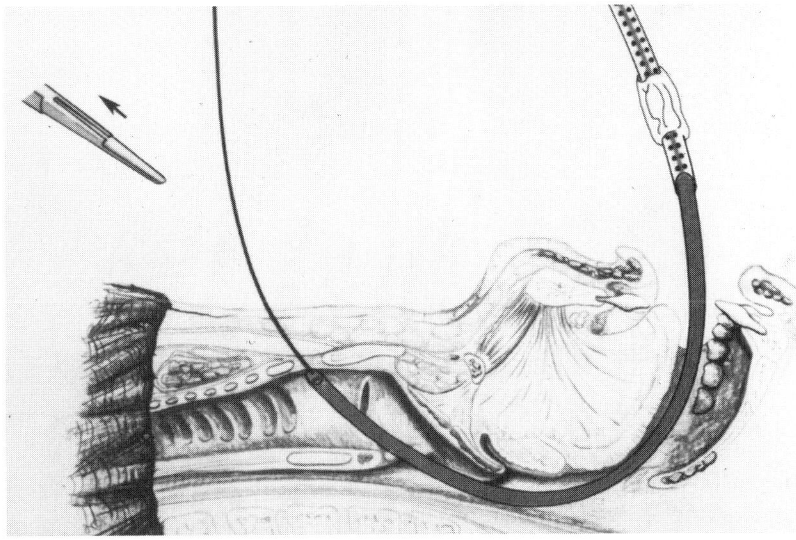

FIG. 7. G: Have assistant remove hemostat.

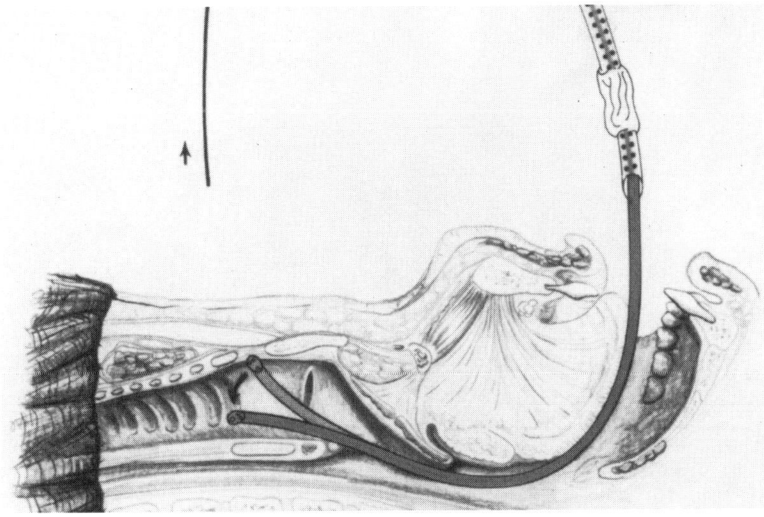

FIG. 7. H: Remove guide wire from the CTM *(straight arrow)*. The tip of the FOB will then drop into mid-tracheal position *(curved arrow)*.

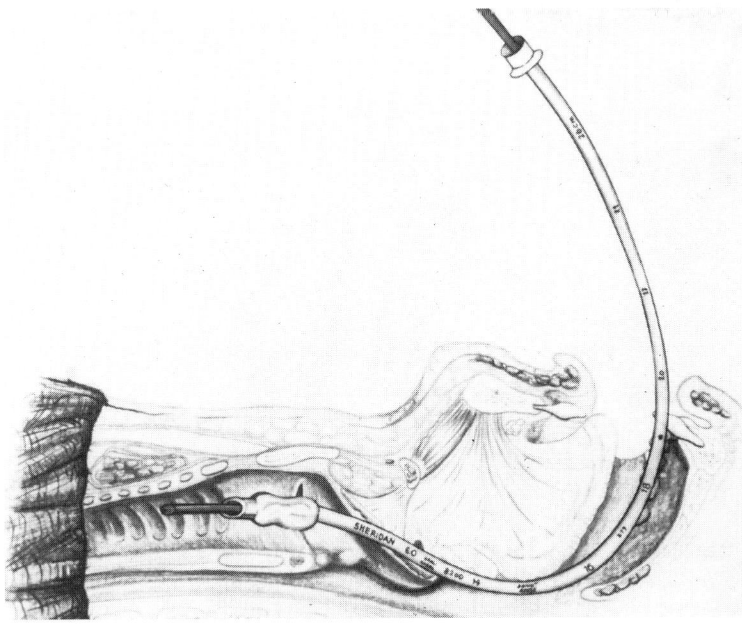

FIG. 7. I: Continue as you would in a standard fiberoptic intubation. From UCI Department of Anesthesia, with permission.

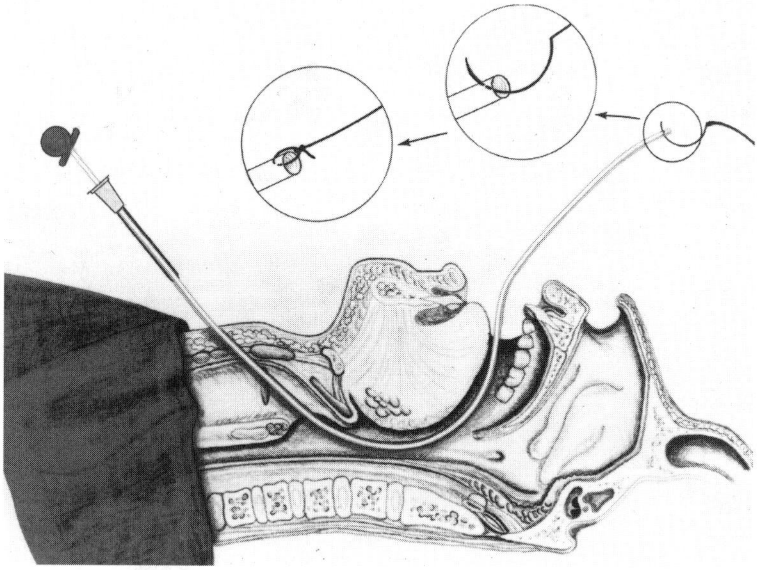

FIG. 8. A: After proceeding as in classical technique as the epidural catheter (EC) has exited the oral cavity, using a 3.0 non-cutting silk suture (30-in length), tie the suture to the EC as shown *(inserts)*.

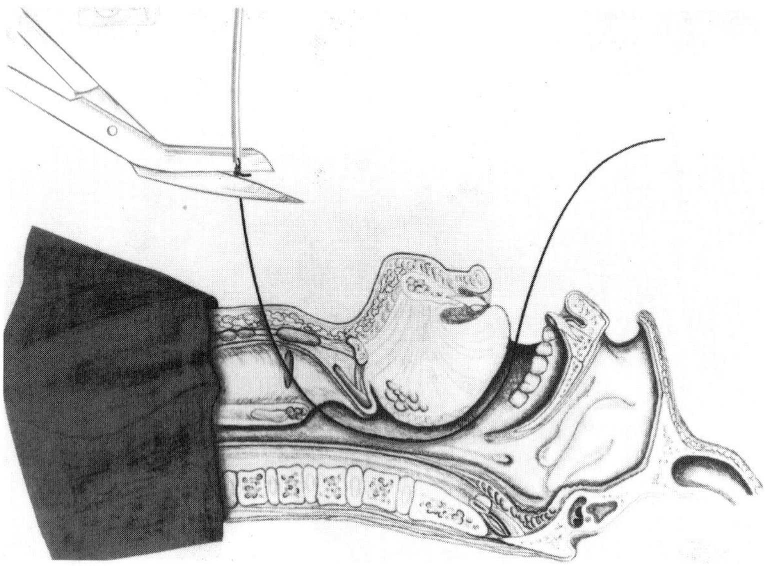

FIG. 8. B: Pull the EC caudad until the silk suture exits the skin above the cricothyroid membrane (CTM), then cut the EC off.

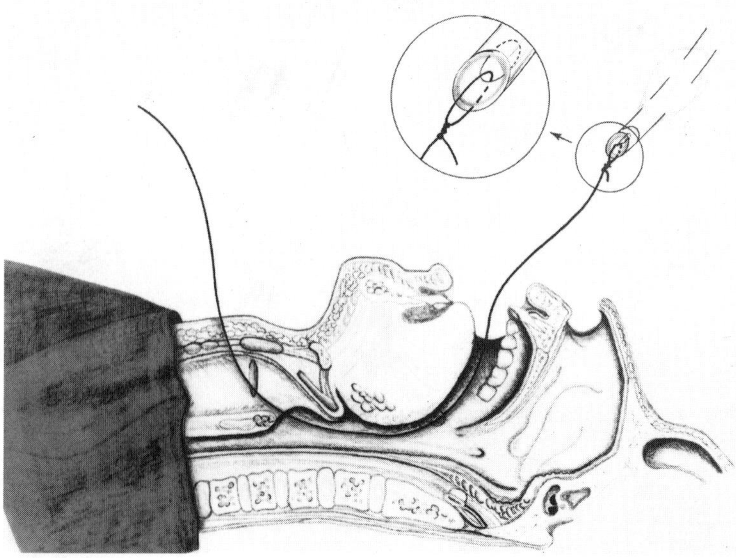

FIG. 8. C: Tie the suture to the Murphy eye as shown *(inserts)*. Have assistant pull patient's tongue forward. Begin pulling the suture with one hand while the opposite hand holds the endotracheal tube (ET) steady and in midline. At all times maintain tension on the suture while advancing the ET.

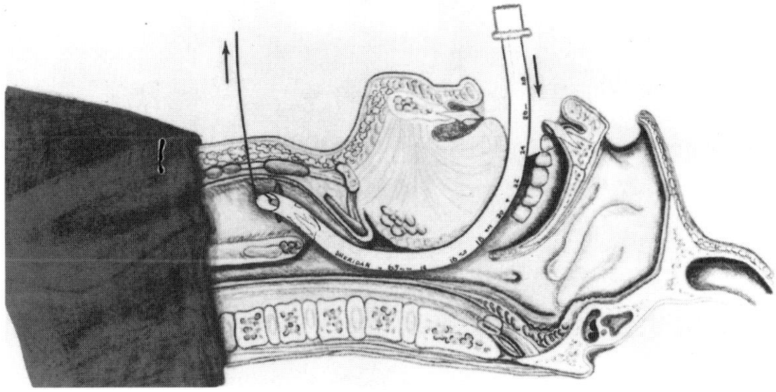

FIG. 8. D: Advance *(arrows)* ET to the CTM.

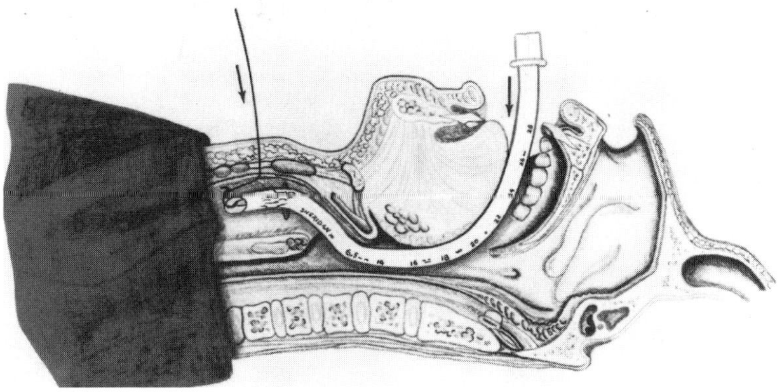

FIG. 8. E: Release the suture and with the opposite hand advance the ET to desired depth. The suture will partially retract into the trachea as the ET is advanced past the CTM. The remaining suture is secured to the neck with Op-Site® (a sterile, clear adhesive dressing). On extubation the silk is left in place as a precaution, should reintubation be required. The suture is removed in the recovery room upon discharge by cutting it flush with the skin and pulling it out of the oral cavity.

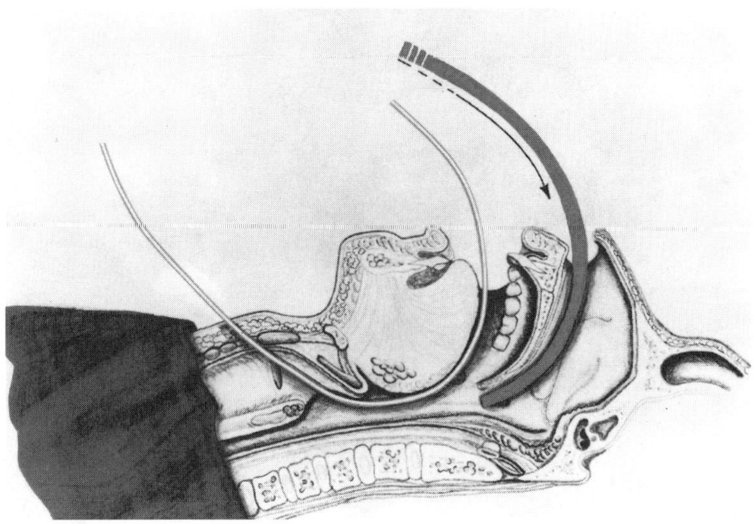

FIG. 8. F: With the EC already in place, a 16-Fr. red rubber urological catheter (UC) is advanced *(arrow)* through the nose.

in the adult, but a higher incidence of difficulties has been reported, including problems in cannulating the ET and/or inability to pass the ET through the glottic opening (66). In some cases, combined techniques have offered more success than has blind RI. In one case report of a 16-year-old with acute epiglottitis, intubation was accomplished only by RI combined with rigid laryngoscopy: The retrograde catheter marked a path through an otherwise completely distorted anatomy (16). The largest pediatric series with the highest success rate was reported by Audernaut (66), in which RI was performed on 20 pediatric patients, ages 1 day to 17 years, with airway difficulties primarily due to congenital anomalies. Their preferred approach, a combination of fiberoptic with retrograde guide wire, offered: (1) higher success rate; (2) faster intubation; (3) the ability to insufflate oxygen through the suction port of the FOB with the guide wire in place; (4) easy passage of the ET through the glottis; (5) minimal reliance on anatomical landmarks to guide the FOB into the trachea; and (6) less experience required

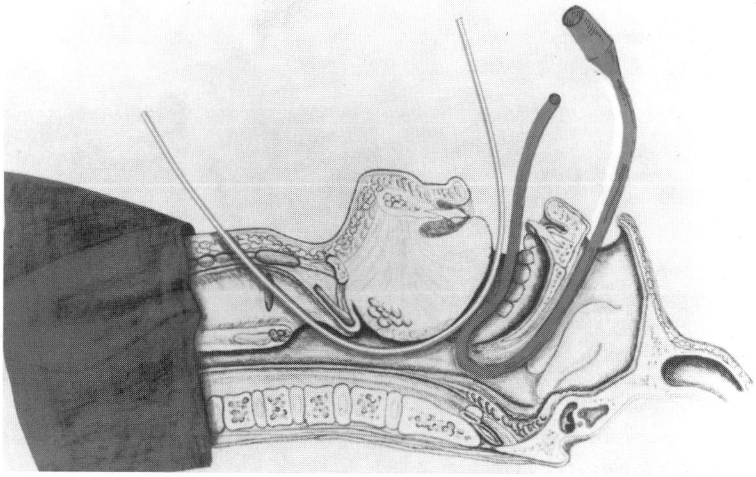

FIG. 8. G: The tip of the UC is retrieved from the oral cavity.

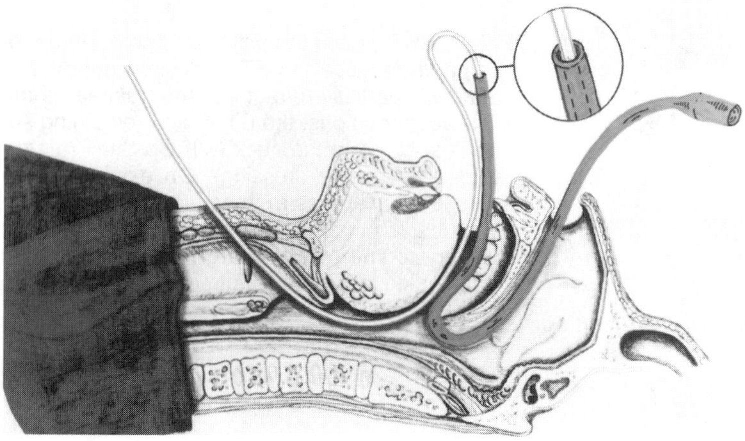

FIG. 8. H: The EC is fed into the UC *(insert)*.

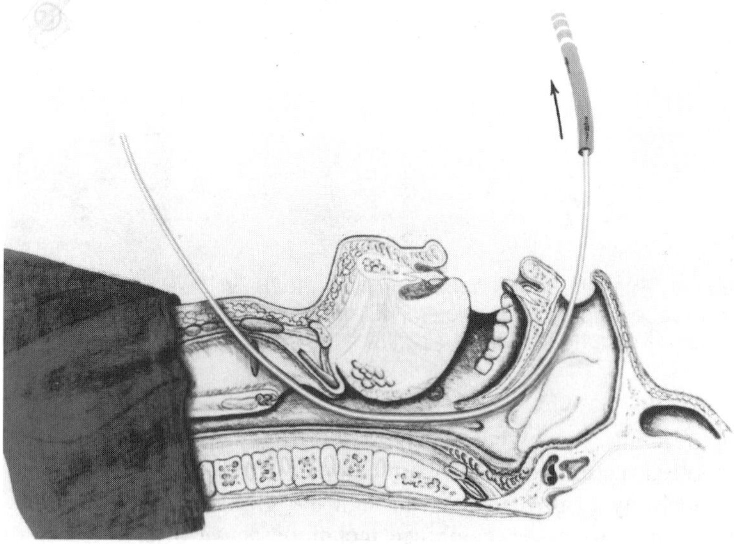

FIG. 8. I: UC is removed *(arrow)*, with the EC now exiting the nose. From UCI Department of Anesthesia, with permission.

TABLE 5. *Translaryngeal anesthesia complications in 17,500 reported cases*

Item	No.
Broken needles	2
Laryngospasms	2
Soft tissue infections	4

Modified from Gold and Buechel, ref. 52.

to manage the FOB. No major complications were reported, and the technique was considered a valuable addition to pediatric airway management.

Complications and Cautions

Although it has been demonstrated that transtracheal needle puncture is safe and associated with only minor complications (Table 5), numerous potential complications of RI have been suggested in the literature (Table 6). Actual documented complications are relatively few, and most were self-limited (Table 7). The most common complications were bleeding (20,30,31,44,45,53,54,65) and subcutaneous emphysema (31,65,70).

Bleeding

In RI, insignificant bleeding (4–5 drops) can be expected with CTM puncture (54,65). Even a patient who was heparinized intraoperatively and had postoperative DIC had only a small, self-limited hematoma (20). Controversy exists with respect to making the puncture below the cricoid cartilage because of a greater potential for bleeding (28,53,62). Three studies (31,53,70) with a total of 57 patients who underwent RI with punctures at the cricotracheal ligament or between the second and third tracheal rings showed no evidence of major bleeding. There are, however, scattered reports of severe hemoptysis following transtracheal needle puncture with resultant hypoxia, cardiorespiratory arrest, dysrhythmia, and death (48,50,73–75). Two patients suffered epistaxis (36,54) after nasal intubation (with no vasoconstricting agent used). The following measures have been suggested to decrease the potential for bleeding: (1) avoid RI in patients with bleeding diathesis; (2) apply pressure to the puncture site for 5 min; (3) apply a pressure dressing to the puncture site for 24 hours; and (4) maintain the patient in the supine position for 3–4 hours after puncture.

TABLE 6. *Potential complications of retrograde intubation*

Esophageal perforation
Hemoptysis
Intratracheal submucosal hematoma with distal obstruction
Laryngeal edema
Laryngospasm
Pretracheal infection
Tracheal fistula
Tracheitis
Vocal cord damage

From UCI Department of Anesthesia, with permission.

TABLE 7. *Reported complications of retrograde intubation*

Item	No.
Self-limited	
Bleeding	
Puncture site	8
Peritracheal hematoma	1
Epistaxis	2
Sub-cutaneous emphysema	4
Pneumomediastinum	1
Breath holding	1
Catheter traveling caudad[a]	2
Not self-limited	
Trigeminal n. trauma	1
Pneumothorax	1
Loss of hook[b]	2

From UCI Department of Anesthesia, with permission and Waters, ref. 28.

[a]Catheter traveling in a caudad direction toward the lungs instead of cephalad toward the oral cavity.

[b]Waters technique of retrieving catheter from nasopharynx using a self made hook.

Subcutaneous Emphysema

Subcutaneous emphysema (31,49,51,59,65,70,75–79), localized to the area of a transtracheal needle puncture site, is common but self-limited. In severe cases, air may track through the fascial planes of the neck leading to tracheal compression with airway compromise, pneumomediastinum, and pneumothorax (48,49,51,58,70,77,78). Accumulation of air occurs gradually (49,77) over 1–6 hours after a transtracheal puncture. Severe subcutaneous emphysema has been attributed to: (1) use of a large bore needle and (2) exposure of the puncture site to persistent elevated intratracheal pressure (coughing, grunting, sneezing).

Other Complications

Other reported self-limited complications were breath-holding (54) and the catheter (a straight, flexible guide wire) traveling caudally (70) (this is also likely to occur when the catheter is inserted through a tracheostomy stoma). Complications that were not self-limited included: (1) trigeminal nerve trauma (42), which may have been related to multiple laryngoscopies; (2) guide wire fracture, in which the wire had to be surgically removed (19); (3) loss of hook (the type that was originally used by Waters and is no longer used) (28,54,72); and (4) pneumothorax, requiring a chest tube (49).

TRANSTRACHEAL JET VENTILATION

History

Although TTJV has become the subject of great interest during the past decade, Hooke (84) first described an account of preserving life in animals by insufflating gases through percutaneous tracheal cannulae almost 300 years ago. In the mid-1950s, Reed (85), Jacoby (86), and their co-investigators reported using TTJV for resuscitating patients. Until the early 1970s, the work of these groups was viewed primarily as an experimental curiosity: Surgical tracheostomy or cricothyroidotomy were considered the only effective options when ventilation became impossible. These procedures, when performed emergently, required considerable skill and were associated with numerous complications. Transtracheal jet ventilation was discussed as an effective alternative to emergent tracheal incision by Spoerel et al. in 1971 (87) and by Jacobs in 1972 (88). Following these initial reports, various investigators have elucidated the potential of TTJV in emergent as well as elective management of the difficult airway, during cardiopulmonary resuscitation, and in instances of complete airway obstruction. In addition, others have now delineated the physical requirements for an efficacious system and addressed limitations of the technique.

Efficacy of TTJV Systems

Transtracheal jet ventilation requires that oxygen sufficient to sustain life be administered to a patient's lungs via a catheter placed through the trachea and that alveolar ventilation be ensured to prevent acidosis. With conventional ventilation through a cuffed endotracheal tube, the relationship between ventilator settings and alveolar (lung) ventilation are straightforward. However, TTJV is an open system, and there are several important differences when compared to conventional endotracheal ventilation using a cuffed tube. Insufflation of oxygen through a transtracheal cannula should provide for gas exchange in the lungs via two mechanisms: flow of oxygen through the catheter and entrainment of room air into the lungs (Venturi effect). The amount of entrainment is a function of the patency of the glottis during insufflation, and entrainment could increase the total gas flow to the lungs by as much as 40% over the amount delivered through the catheter (87). While entrainment of less than 100% oxygen will decrease the FIO_2, it should provide additional flow of gas to the alveoli. The glottis is usually not completely patent, however, and may actually close during insufflation due to negative pressure generated cephalad to the catheter. Experimental data in animals suggest that entrainment usually does not occur, and these findings have been accurately extrapolated to humans (89). There are two requirements for an effective TTJV system: adequate oxygenation and adequate ventilation. The average oxygen consumption of a resting, nonstressed, 70-kg adult is approximately 250 ml/min. A ventilation technique that supplies this amount of oxygen to the alveoli can, therefore, maintain arterial oxygen saturation at a level close to normal and, thus, sustain life. Similarly, an approximate alveolar ventilation of 5 L/min is required to maintain normocarbia, preventing a potentially lethal respiratory acidosis. In 1953, Reed and colleagues demonstrated that a compressed oxygen source of at least 50 psi and a 16-gauge or larger cannula for TTJV are required to ensure adequate oxygenation and ventilation (85). This critical finding has been confirmed by several other investigators. However, numerous other papers subsequently appeared that served to foster misconceptions about TTJV, and the principal confusion has resulted from a failure to distinguish adequate oxygenation from adequate ventilation. Some authors, for example, have advocated using an 18-gauge catheter connected to a continuous-flow source [a continuous positive airway pressure- (CPAP-) like system], a bag-valve apparatus (Ambu bag), or an oxygen flush valve connected to the catheter using corrugated tubing (90,91). While it has been shown that low-pressure oxygen (corresponding to flows of 4–8 L/min) can be used to maintain adequate oxygenation, these systems are incapable of providing ventilation sufficient to prevent acidosis, and no controlled trials have demonstrated that these systems can reverse existing hypoxia. In addition, manual ventilation of the lungs by squeezing a self-inflating reservoir bag will rapidly fatigue even the most vigorous rescuer (50 psi is the recommended minimum driving pressure for adequate TTJV; 70 cm H_2O = 1 psi). Finally, the use of corrugated tubing (as used in most breathing circuits) precludes adequate ventilation, regardless of sufficient driving pressure at the oxygen source. Yealy and Stewart (92) have shown that even a 12 gauge transtracheal catheter could not ensure adequate ventilation when a demand-valve mechanism of only 60 cm H_2O (less than 1 psi) driving pressure served as the oxygen source. In fact, the only way a bag valve or demand valve system could provide satisfactory ventilation was when a 4.0-mm internal diameter or larger tracheal cannula was used. In summary, a TTJV system that provides both adequate oxygenation and ventilation in an adult requires, at a minimum: (1) a high-pressure oxygen source (50 psi); (2) a stiff (noncompliant) circuit from the oxygen source to the catheter; (3) a transtracheal catheter of at least 16-gauge diameter; and (4) the absence of obstruction to exhalation through the glottis.

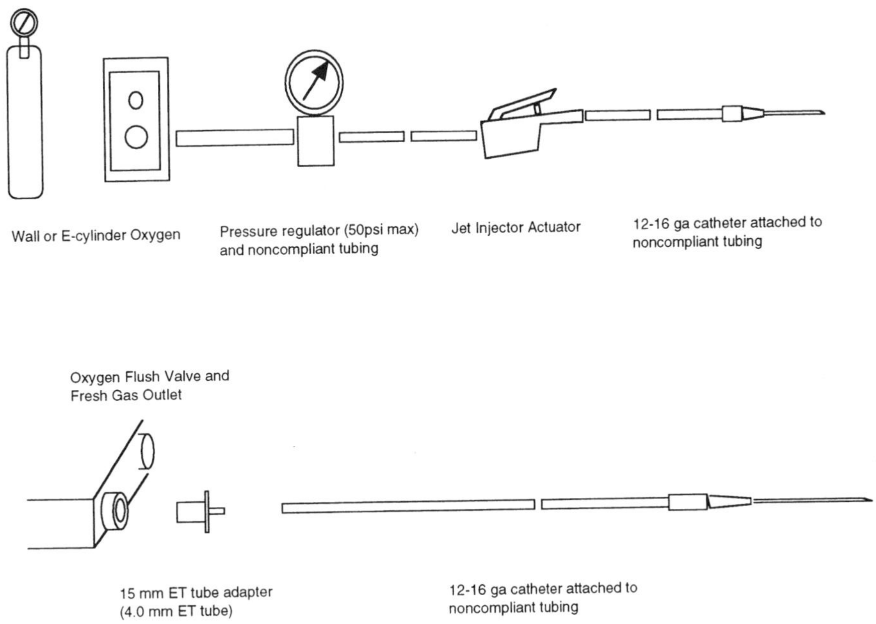

FIG. 9. A: Two acceptable transtracheal jet ventilation systems.

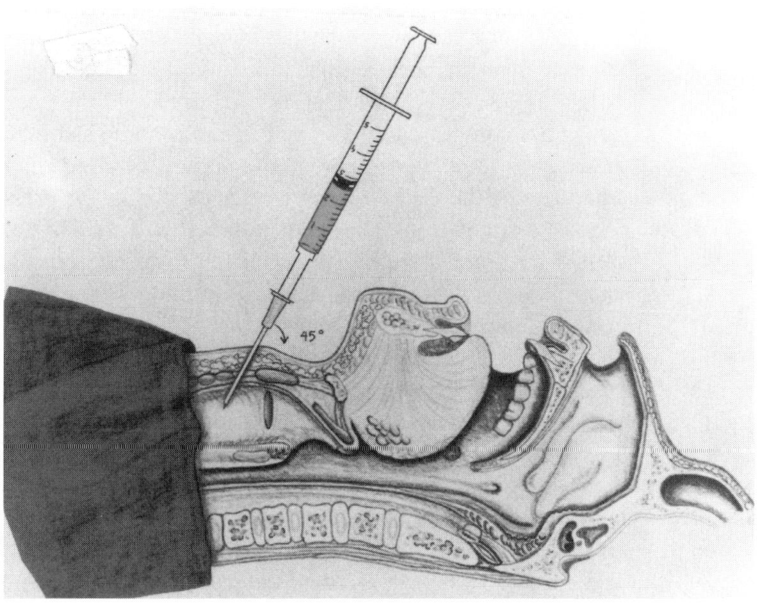

FIG. 9. B: Identification and puncture of the cricothyroid membrane with an angiocatheter, aspirating for air.

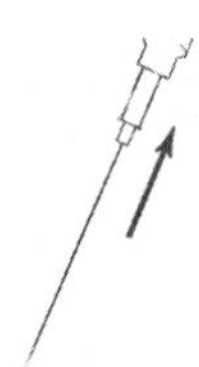

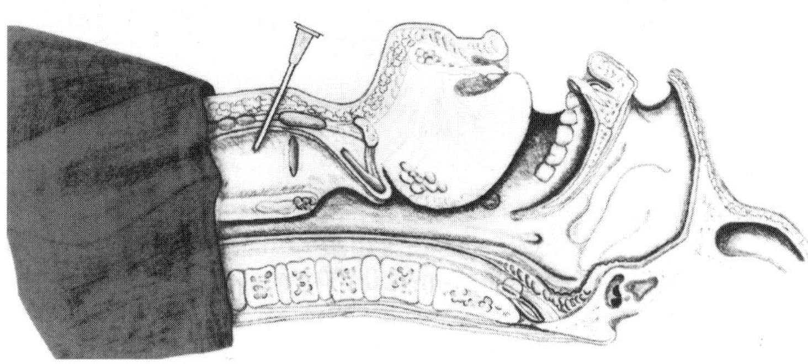

FIG. 9. C: Advancement of the catheter into the trachea in a caudad direction while removing the needle. From UCI Department of Anesthesia, with permission.

In order to meet these requirements, Benumof and Scheller (26) have outlined three acceptable TTJV systems and have provided a detailed description of each component, including part numbers and manufacturers. All three systems are relatively inexpensive (less than $150 at 1989 prices) and are, in order of preference: (1) a jet injector powered by a regulated (50 psi) wall or tank oxygen pressure; (2) a jet injector powered by unregulated wall or tank oxygen pressure; and (3) a jet injector connected directly to the anesthesia machine fresh gas outlet and activated by the oxygen flush valve.

It should be emphasized that all systems require noncompliant tubing from the oxygen source to the patient. Any other construction is less than ideal and cannot be relied on to ensure adequate oxygenation and ventilation during TTJV. Two examples of acceptable TTJV systems are shown in Fig. 9A. Jet injectors powered by wall oxygen pressure should have a wall O_2 disconnect/hose barb component compatible with hospital wall outlets. While all other systems are discouraged, they may provide some degree of oxygenation that is unquestionably desirable when the alternative is death. However, according to Benumof and Scheller (26), "If one is suddenly confronted with a cannot-ventilate–cannot-intubate situation, it will take significant extra time and hands to find the parts for these connections, for what is in the end analysis, not the best transtracheal ventilation system." Succinctly, it is best to be prepared with an adequate TTJV system at the outset.

In summary, if an acceptable TTJV system is used, oxygenation and ventilation can be provided for hours, if necessary, allowing one to secure a permanent airway (including formal tracheostomy) without duress. This has been demonstrated both experimentally in animals and in clinical case reports in humans. It appears that when using a 16-gauge (or larger) transtracheal catheter in conjunction with a 50-psi oxygen source, the peak airway pressures remain between 20 and 50 cm H_2O, provided the respiratory rate is low (approximately 20 breaths/min) and the I:E ratio is approximately 1:2 (87). Factors that determine the overall effectiveness of TTJV are summarized in Table 8 (93).

TABLE 8. *Determinants of TTJV efficacy*

Mechanical
Driving pressure of oxygen source
Compliance of TTJV system and tubing
Length and diameter of transtracheal catheter
Patient
Cross-sectional area of trachea
Compliance of lungs and thorax
Degree of obstruction to exhalation
Entrainment of room air (Venturi effect)
CO_2 production
Oxygen consumption
Preexisting hypercarbia, hypoxia
Oxygenation/ventilation parameters
F_{IO_2} of oxygen source
Respiratory frequency
Duty cycle (I:E ratio)

From UCI Department of Anesthesia, with permission.
TTJV, transtracheal jet ventilation.

Clinical Applications of TTJV

Description of the Preferred Technique

The administration of TTJV is simple and requires minimal training. Once the decision has been made to proceed with TTJV, the technique is as follows:

1. The patient's CTM is identified (if TTJV ventilation is being used in a patient with an anticipated difficult airway, this landmark should be routinely identified prior to the administration of anesthesia).

2. A right-handed rescuer should stand on the patient's left side near the neck region.

3. The rescuer's right hand is used to extend the neck (when not contraindicated). The left hand should stabilize the trachea. A lower puncture site should be used only when use of the CTM is contraindicated (as in the presence of a friable tumor immediately below the CTM). It should be understood that a lower puncture site constitutes a more difficult and hazardous route because of greater possibility of bleeding (see section on anatomy) and because a lower puncture site may interfere with the establishment of a surgical airway.

4. A 12- or 14-gauge angiocatheter is attached to a 20-ml syringe. Holding the catheter assembly like a pencil in the right hand, stabilizing the hand on the jaw, and stabilizing the trachea with the left hand, the CTM is punctured at a caudad angle of approximately 45° (Fig. 9B). The catheter must be directed caudally for TTJV to be effective. Puncture is identified by a characteristic "pop" or slight loss of resistance once the needle has penetrated the membrane.

5. Aspiration of air confirms proper location (Fig. 9B). A 20-ml syringe will allow aspiration of air from the trachea but should collapse the esophagus. A 20-ml syringe is strongly encouraged, as larger syringes are cumbersome and smaller syringes allow generation of sufficient negative pressure to produce a false positive aspiration of air. The catheter is then advanced, with the left hand, over the needle and into the trachea (Fig. 9C), and aspiration of air is reconfirmed. If, as a result of false positive aspiration, the catheter is advanced subcutaneously instead of transtracheally, the result will be tissue emphysema, absence of ventilation, and death. Some authors advocate simultaneous aspiration during puncture of the CTM. This may be satisfactory in most instances; how-

ever, experience has shown that holding the needle in the same fashion as a pencil allows better control.

6. Holding the catheter firmly in place with the left hand, the oxygen tubing is attached with the right hand using a Luer-lock mechanism. Assuming that a driving pressure of 50 psi of 100% oxygen is available (for adults), ventilation is started. Using either a jet injector valve or oxygen flush valve (Fig. 9A), approximately 20 breaths per min are administered, with 1 full sec for inspiration, followed by 2 sec of expiration. The rescuer should audibly count inspiration and expiration and witness the rise of the chest wall with each breath.

It should be noted here that kits for establishing transtracheal access for ventilation are being developed commercially. The authors have not had the occasion to use them clinically, but encourage clinicians to be familiar with them.

In the case of emergent TTJV, once the transtracheal catheter has been successfully placed, the rescuer has four absolute obligations:

1. To manually maintain the transtracheal catheter in proper position. The catheter cannot be relied upon to remain in place by suture, tape, or any other means.
2. To watch the chest rise with each inspiration. Failure of the chest to rise demands immediate reassessment of catheter placement and TTJV apparatus functioning.
3. To listen for exhalation of air through the patient's mouth during expiration. The absence of exhalation may imply a complete obstruction to exhalation (see discussion below), in which case immediate surgical tracheostomy should be undertaken to prevent barotrauma and subsequent total inability to ventilate.
4. Never to cease ventilation, under any circumstances, until a definitive airway has been achieved (either successful endotracheal intubation or surgical tracheostomy). The catheter should not be removed to allow for a surgical tracheostomy, which is to be performed in a location distal to and away from the CTM (usually between the second and third tracheal rings). If there are other problems during emergent TTJV, such as hemodynamic instability, the rescuer should instruct an assistant to monitor vital signs and/or administer medications. At no time should the rescuer leave the patient's airway.

The Unanticipated Difficult Airway

Failure to intubate a hypoxic patient who cannot be ventilated by mask is a daunting prospect for any rescuer. While surgical tracheostomy is a viable option to secure an airway emergently, a surgeon may not be immediately available, and the rescuer may be inadequately trained to perform the procedure. Transtracheal jet ventilation has been successfully used in nearly every emergency scenario, including: (1) upper airway obstruction; (2) anatomic anomaly; (3) laryngeal edema; (4) supraglottic and glottic tumors; (5) subglottic and airway edema; (6) infectious processes; (7) obstruction by foreign body; and (8) refractory laryngospasm (26,94–96). In each case report, given the circumstances under which TTJV was instituted, it is highly likely that TTJV was lifesaving. The clinician who is apt to be the first to be called when airway difficulties arise is likely to encounter this problem several times during the course of a career and should realistically be prepared either to perform a surgical tracheostomy or to institute TTJV.

The Completely Obstructed Airway

Complete or near-total airway obstruction, in combination with the inability to mask ventilate or intubate, is a rare but dire emergency. The role of TTJV in this setting is the subject of controversy and continuing investigations. While it is known that adequate ventilation and oxygenation are possible with TTJV using a 16-gauge or larger needle in conjunction with a 50-psi oxygen source, this technique poses several problems in the case of an obstructed airway. The most important concern is the severe increase of tracheal pressure with resultant barotrauma. The use of low-pressure oxygen via a bag-valve apparatus instead of a 50-psi driving source could conceivably provide a life-sustaining level of oxygenation (not ventilation) without inflicting barotrauma on the lungs. Alternatively, the use of a high-pressure oxygen driving source with very short insufflation times might also minimize barotrauma (97). This has not been rigorously evaluated, but Neff et al. (98) and Goldman et al. (99) have demonstrated in animals that a critical transtracheal orifice of 2.4 mm (internal diameter) is mandatory to assist or control ventilation during complete airway obstruction. The standard 14-gauge catheter used in TTJV has an internal diameter of only 1.47 mm and, thus, is inadequate. The concept of using a second catheter for exhalation alongside the insufflating catheter has been proposed but not adequately evaluated, and its use is not, therefore, recommended. In the case of complete upper airway obstruction to exhalation, all TTJV systems should be converted immediately to a formal tracheostomy or large-bore cricothyroidotomy tube (greater than 3 mm inner diameter). It should be understood that the inability to mask ventilate does not imply an obstruction to exhalation. In fact, many (if not most cases) of airway obstruction are inspiratory, and TTJV will work well under these circumstances.

Elective Uses of TTJV

There are two circumstances in which TTJV can be used electively: (1) to facilitate intubation of the trachea by other means (such as fiberoptic bronchoscopy) and thereby prevent the cannot-ventilate–cannot-intubate scenario; and (2) to allow for maximal exposure for surgical operations involving the airway. Experience has shown that TTJV catheters can be placed under local anesthesia in conscious patients without difficulty (100). Elective placement of a TTJV catheter through the CTM has been demonstrated not to interfere with nasotracheal, orotracheal, or fiberoptic–assisted intubation. Formal tracheostomy during TTJV is also practical, in both emergent and nonemergent situations. Numerous case reports demonstrate the efficacy of elective TTJV in nearly every situation in which a difficult airway has been anticipated (94–96,101–105). Additionally, TTJV has been advocated, in conjunction with high-frequency jet ventilation, as a mechanism to prevent aspiration by causing a continuous gas flow outward through the larynx (106). The CTM lies below the true vocal cords; therefore, TTJV allows accessibility to the entire upper airway. Interest in using TTJV as an alternative to a ventilating bronchoscope in airway operations began in the early 1970s, following the work of Spoerel and colleagues (87). Subsequently, nearly every type of airway operation has been described in conjunction with TTJV (94,96).

Pediatric Uses of TTJV

The use of TTJV in pediatrics is poorly described in the literature, and whether or not TTJV is indicated in the pediatric population remains controversial. Although barotrauma, tissue emphysema, and loss of anatomical landmarks can result from attempts at TTJV, there are arguably no absolute contraindications to TTJV when it is used emergently and with success. Indeed, when one is confronted with the cannot-ventilate–cannot-intubate scenario, conventional techniques have failed, and the alternative is death; if the site of airway obstruction is above the CTM, TTJV should be considered. We suggest using a 20-gauge angiocatheter for a newborn, an 18-gauge angiocatheter for an infant or small child, and a 16-gauge angiocatheter for a larger child. It is prudent to start ventilation at approximately 5 psi driving pressure (as compared to 50 psi in the adult) and to increase pressure gradually until the chest wall is observed to rise adequately and oxygenation is maintained. The lowest effective driving pressure should be used.

Role of TTJV in Cardiopulmonary Resuscitation

Rapid establishment of an airway is the first imperative of cardiopulmonary resuscitation (CPR). Without adequate oxygenation, chest compressions and pharmacotherapy are futile. Classically, endotracheal intubation has been the recommended technique for ensuring continued ventilation during CPR. However, the cannot-ventilate–cannot-intubate scenario is potentially encountered more frequently during CPR than during anesthesia, since CPR is often performed in the field where persons skilled in airway management may not be available. Historically, emergency medical services personnel have not performed tracheostomy in the field. The esophageal obturator airway (EOA) was proposed as a "moderate" approach to a failed endotracheal intubation when mask ventilation was not possible (107). Its effectiveness over a standard mask and oral airway, however, has not been convincingly demonstrated, and its use has been abandoned by many emergency medical services (108). Transtracheal jet ventilation is an easily learned, relatively safe, and effective technique that requires considerably less skill than does performing a tracheostomy and may be a viable option for nonphysician rescuers performing CPR. Swartzman (109) studied 83 emergency medical technicians (EMTs) and found that TTJV was a feasible alternative to conventional methods of ventilation during CPR, even in the hands of those inexperienced in airway management. Although medical, legal, and logistic issues involved in training nonphysicians to use TTJV during CPR are complex and no consensus has been reached to date, TTJV represents a promising modality that may help reduce morbidity and mortality during CPR in the future (100).

Complications

The frequency of complications, principally cervical subcutaneous and mediastinal emphysema, associated with TTJV is surprisingly low when it is used electively. Benumof and Scheller (26) cite two clinical series of elective TTJV in which the incidence of tissue emphysema ranged from 2% to 10% (26). However, other authors have described more frequent complications when TTJV was used emergently, including arterial injury and bleeding, problems related to exhalation, esophageal tear, and pneumothorax (26,101). In the setting of TTJV, therefore, tachycardia or bradycardia, in

TABLE 9. *Complications reported with TTJV*

Arterial injury (hemoptysis, hematoma)
Dislodgement of catheter
Emphysema, cervical subcutaneous
Emphysema, mediastinal
Esophageal perforation
Exhalation difficulty
Pneumothorax
Subglottic stenosis
Tracheal mucosal ulceration
Tracheomalacia
Vocal cord changes

From UCI Department of Anesthesia, with permission.
TTJV, transtracheal jet ventilation.

association with hypotension or unequal breath sounds, should be assumed to represent a pneumothorax. Tracheal mucosal ulceration following TTJV in animals has also been described, which implies risk of subsequent tracheal stenosis, but long-term sequelae are unknown (26). A summary of complications reported with TTJV is provided in Table 9. Transtracheal jet ventilation, when performed emergently, is a lifesaving measure, and most complications resulting from TTJV can be treated successfully. In no clinical series have the complications associated with TTJV been lethal when ventilation was successful (111).

CONCLUSION

Interest in TTJV remained dormant for nearly three centuries following Hooke's first descriptions (84), but over the past two decades, efforts have been made to better describe its role in both elective and emergent clinical situations. Although further investigation is certainly warranted, it has been convincingly demonstrated that TTJV is an inexpensive, easily learned, and lifesaving technique that should be readily available to all clinicians. Retrograde intubation has been a particularly useful alternative in difficult intubations after multiple manipulations have caused bleeding, in facial injuries where bleeding is already present, and in patients with limited neck movement. The technique is easy to learn, requires little equipment, and in practiced hands is a rapid, safe, and effective method for intubating the trachea. In the vast majority of cases, the airway can be secured using conventional techniques, but in a small number of cases these techniques cannot be successfully applied to the clinical problem at hand. No method of airway management offers 100% success; therefore, it is wise to have multiple available options and to be facile with alternative techniques for intubation. Techniques allowing access to the airway via the CTM should be included as part of the armamentarium of clinicians involved in the care of seriously injured or ill patients.

ACKNOWLEDGMENTS

With special thanks to Tay McClellan for her outstanding medical illustration.

REFERENCES

1. Benumof JL. Management of the difficult adult airway. *Anesthesiology* 1991;75:1087–1110.
2. American Society of Anesthesiologists Task Force on Management of the Difficult Airway. Practice guidelines for management of the difficult airway. *Anesthesiology* 1993;78:597–602.
3. Sanchez AS. *ASA Airway safety video*, part II, 1992.
4. Clemente Carmine. *Gray's Anatomy*, 13th edition. Philadelphia: Lea Febiger, 1985;1366–1368.
5. Caparosa RJ, Zavatsky AR. Practical aspects of the cricothyroid space. *Laryngoscope* 1957;67:577–591.
6. Shantha TR. Retrograde intubation using the subcricoid region. *Br J Anaesth* 1992;68:109–112.
7. Naumann H, ed. *Head Neck*, vol 4. Philadelphia: WB Saunders, 1984; 162–181.
8. Bergman R, Thompson S. In: Bergman R, Thompson S. *Compendium of Human Anatomic Variation* (Text, Atlas, and World Literature). Baltimore/Munich: Urban & Schwarzenberg. 1988,65–116,175–190.
9. Anson BJ. In: Anson BJ, ed. *Human Anatomy: A Complete System Treatise*, 12th ed. New York: McGraw-Hill, 1966;674–702,1545–1551.
10. Ovassapian A. Topical anesthesia (Ch. 4), Fiberoptic tracheal intubation (Ch. 5). *Fiberoptic Airway Endoscopy in Anesthesia and Critical Care*. New York: Raven Press, 1990;45–79.
11. Stone DJ, Gal TJ, Wedel DJ, Brown DL, Shapiro HM. (Ch. 39) Airway management (Ch. 46), Nerve blocks (Ch. 54). In: Miller RD, ed. *Neurosurgical Anesthesia and Intracranial Hypertension*, vol 2, 3rd ed. New York: Churchill Livingstone, 1990;1265–1292;1407–1437; 1737–1789.
12. Cuchiara RF, Black S, Steinkeler JA, Stehling SC. Anesthesia for intracranial procedures (Ch. 31), Management of the airway (Ch. 20). In: Barash PG, Cullen BF, Stoelting RK, eds. *Clinical Anesthesia*. Philadelphia: J.B. Lippincott Co., 1989;543–561,849–876.
13. Cooper CM, Murray-Wilson A. Retrograde intubation: management of a 4.8 kg 5-month infant. *Anaesthesia* 1987;42:1197–1200.
14. Lechman MJ, Donahoo JS, Macvaugh H. Endotracheal intubation using percutaneous retrograde guidewire insertion followed by antegrade fiberoptic bronchoscopy. *Crit Care Med* 1986;14:589–590.
15. Pintanel T, Font M, Aguilar JL , et al. Intubation orotracheal retrograde (cartas al director). *Rev Esp Anestesiol Reanim* 1988;35:344–345.
16. Heslet L, Christensen KS, Sanchez R, et al. Facilitated blind intubation using a transtracheal guide wire. *Dan Med Bull* 1985;32:275–277.
17. Lee YW, Lee YS, Kim JR. Retrograde tracheal intubation, *Yonsei Med J* 1987;28:3.
18. Schmidt SI, Hasewinkel JV. Retrograde catheter-guided direct laryngoscopy. *Anesthesiol Rev* 1989;16:49–50.
19. Contrucci RB, Gottlieb JS. A complication of retrograde endotracheal intubation. *Ear Nose Throat J* 1989;69:11,776–778.
20. Casthely FA, Landesman S, Fyman PN, et al. Retrograde intubation in patients undergoing open heart surgery. *Can J Anaesth* 1985;32:6, 661–664.
21. Carlson CA, Perkins HM. Solving a difficult intubation. *Anesthesiology* 1986;64:4,537.
22. Maestro CM, Andujar MJJ, Sancho CJ, et al. Intubacion retrograda en un paciente con una malformacion epiglotica (cartas al director). *Rev Esp Anestesiol Reanim* 1988;35:344–345.
23. Raza S, Levinsky L, Lajos TZ. Transtracheal intubation: useful adjunct in cardiac surgical anesthesia. *J Thorac Cardiovasc Surg* 1978;76:721–7222.
24. Gupta B, McDonald JS, Brooks HJ, et al. Oral fiberoptic intubation over a retrograde guidewire. *Anesth Analg* 1989;68:517–519.
25. Amanor-Boadu SD. Translaryngeal guided intubation in a patient with raised intracranial pressure. *Afr J Med Med Sci* 1992;21(1): 65–66.
26. Benumof JL, Scheller MS. The importance of transtracheal jet ventilation in the management of the difficult airway. *Anesthesiology* 1989;71:769–778.
27. Butler FS, Cirillo AA. Retrograde tracheal intubation. *Anesth Analg* 1960;39:333–338.
28. Waters DJ. Guided blind endotracheal intubation: for patients with deformities of the upper airway. *Anaesthesia* 1963;18:158–162.
29. King HK, Wang LF, Wooten DJ. Endotracheal intubation using translaryngeal guided intubation vs percutaneous retrograde guidewire insertion (letter). *Crit Care Med* 1987;15:183.
30. Barriot P, Riou B. Retrograde technique for tracheal intubation in trauma patients. *Crit Care Med* 1988;16:712–713.
31. Mahiou, Bouvet FR, Korach JM, et al. Intubation retrograde. [Abst R26] *XXXI Congres De Intubacion Tracheal* 1983, 107
32. Borland LM, Swan DM, Leff S. Difficult pediatric endotracheal intubation: a new approach to the retrograde technique. *Anesthesiology* 1981;55:577–578.
33. Freund PR, Rooke A, Schwid H. Retrograde intubation with a modified Eschmann stylet. [Letter] *Anesth Analg* 1988;67:596–606.

34. Heller EM, Schneider K, Saven B. Percutaneous retrograde intubation. *Laryngoscope* 1989;99:555–556.
35. Sanchez AS. *Retrograde Intubation in the Llama*. American Association of Zoological Veterinarians Annual Meeting St. Louis, 1993.
36. Corleta O, Habazettl H, Kreimeier U, et al. Modified retrograde orotracheal intubation technique for airway access in rabbits. *Eur Surg Res* 1992;24:129–132.
37. Van Stralen DW, Rogers M, Perkin RM, Fea S. *Retrograde intubation training using mannequins*. [Abst] Eighth Annual Conference, National Association of EMS Physicians, June 16, 1992
38. Stern Y, Spitzer T. Retrograde intubation of the trachea. *J Laryngol Otol* 1991;105:746–747.
39. Sanchez AS. *International Symposium on the Difficult Airway*. Newport Beach, CA: 1993
40. McNamara RM. Retrograde intubation of the trachea. *Ann Emerg Med* 1987;16:6:115–117.
41. Shantha TR. Retrograde intubation using the subcricoid region. [Letter] *Br J Anaesth* 1983;55:855.
42. Faithfull NS. Injury to terminal branches of the trigeminal nerve following tracheal intubation. *Br J Anaesth* 1985;57:535–537.
43. Sanchez AS. *American Society of Anesthesiologists Annual Meeting*. Las Vegas, 1990.
44. Guggenberger H, Lenz G. Training in retrograde intubation. [Letter] *Anesthesiology* 1988;69:292.
45. Guggenberger H, Lenz G, Heumann H. Success rate and complications of a modified guided blind technique for intubation in 36 patients. *Anaesthesist* 1987;36:703–707.
46. Manchester GH, Mani MM, Master FW. A simple method for emergency orotracheal intubation. *Plast Reconstr Surg* 1972;49:312.
47. Hines MH, Meredith JW. Modified retrograde intubation technique for rapid airway access. *Am J Surg* 1990;159:597–599.
48. Ries K, Levison ME, Kaye D, et al. Transtracheal aspiration in pulmonary infection. *Arch Intern Med* 1974;133:453–458.
49. Poon YK. Case history number 89: a life-threatening complication of cricothyroid membrane puncture. *Anesth Analg* 1976;55: 298–301.
50. Unger KM, Moser KM. Fatal complication of transtracheal aspiration: a report of two cases. *Arch Intern Med* 1974;132:437–439.
51. Kalinske RW, Parker RH, Brandt D, et al. Diagnostic usefulness and safety of transtracheal aspiration. *N Engl J Med* 1967;276: 604–608.
52. Gold MI, Buechel, DR. Translaryngeal anesthesia: a review. *Anesthesiology* 1959;20:181–185.
53. Abou-Madi MN, Trop D. Pulling versus guiding: a modification of retrograde guided intubation. *Can J Anaesth* 1989;36:3:336–339.
54. Akinyemi OO. Complications of guided blind endotracheal intubation. *Anaesthesia* 1979;34:590–592.
55. Green DC, Strait GB. A complication of transtracheal anesthesia: Nocardia cellulitis. *Ann Thorac Surg* 1969;8:561–563.
56. Yoshikawa TT, Chow AW, Montgomerie JZ, et al. Paratracheal abscess: an unusual complication of transtracheal aspiration. *Chest* 1974;65:105–106.
57. Deresinski SC, Stevens DA. Anterior cervical infections: complications of transtracheal aspirations. *Am Rev Respir Dis* 1974;110:354–356.
58. Wilson JKV. Cricothyroid bronchography with a polyethylene catheter. Description of a new technique. *Am J Roentgenology* 1959; 81:305–311.
59. Newman J, Schiltz S. Bronchography by cricothyroid catheterization. *Laryngoscope* 1965;75:774–782.
60. France NK, Beste DJ, Gregory GA. Anesthesia for pediatric ear, nose and throat surgery (Ch. 16), Induction of anesthesia (Ch. 31). In: Gregory GA, ed. *Pediatric Anesthesia*, 2nd ed. Churchill Livingstone, 1989;1127–28,557–558.
61. Lleu JC, Forrler M, Forrler C, et al. L'intubation oro-tracheale par void retrograde. *Ann Fr Anesth Reanim* 1989;8:632–635.
62. Lleu JC, Forrler M, Pottecher T, et al. Retrograde intubation using the subcricoid region. [Letter] *Br J Anaesth* 1983;55:855.
63. Bourke D, Levesque PR. Modification of retrograde guide for endotracheal intubation. *Anesth Analg* 1974;53:1013–1014.
64. Thomas P. Retrograde intubation. In: Daily RD, Simon B, et al, eds. *The Airway Emergency Management*. St. Louis: Mosby Year Book, 1992;107–113.
65. Powell WF, Ozdil T. A translaryngeal guide for tracheal intubation. *Anesth Analg* 1967;46:231–234.
66. Audernaut SM, Montgomery CL, Stone B, et al. Retrograde-assisted fiberoptic tracheal intubation in children with difficult airways. *Anesth Analg* 1991;73:660–664.
67. Kubo K, Takahashi S, Oka M. A modified technique of guided blind intubation in oral surgery. *J Maxillofac Surg* 1980;8:135–137.
68. Harrison CA, Wise CC. Retrograde intubation. [Letter] *Anaesthesia* 1988;43:609.
69. Carlson RC, Sadove MS. Guided non-visualized nasal endotracheal intubation using a transtracheal Fogarty catheter. *Illinois Medical Journal* 1973;143(4):364–365.
70. VanNiekerk JV, Smalhout B. Retrograde endotracheal intubation using a catheter. *Ned Tijdschr Geneeskd* 1987;131:1663–1667.
71. Levin RM. Anesthesia for cleft lip and cleft palate. *Anesthesiol Rev* 1979;6:25–30.
72. Akinyemi OO, John A. A complication of guided blind intubation. *Anesthesia* 1974;29:733–735.
73. Spencer CD, Beaty HN. Complications of transtracheal aspiration. *N Engl J Med* 1972;286:304–306.
74. Schillaci RF, Iacovoni VE, Conte RS, et al. Transtracheal aspiration complicated by fatal endotracheal hemorrhage. *N Eng J Med* 1976; 295(9):4884–4890.
75. Hemley SD, Arida EJ, Diggs AM, et al. Percutaneous cricothyroid membrane bronchography. *Radiology* 1961;76:763–769.
76. Hahn HH, Beaty HN. Transtracheal aspiration in the evaluation of patients with pneumonia. *Ann Intern Med* 1970;72:183–187.
77. Massey JY. Complications of transtracheal aspiration—a case report. *J Arkansas Med Soc* 1971;67(8):254–256.
78. Won KH, Rowland DW, et al. Massive subcutaneous emphysema complicating transcricothyroid bronchography. *Am J Roentgenol Radium Ther Nucl Med* 1967;101:953–956.
79. Radigan LR, King RD. A technique for the prevention of post-operative atelectasis. *Surgery* 1960;47:184.
80. Keenan RL, Boyan CP. Cardiac arrests due to anesthesia. *JAMA* 1985;253:2373–2377.
81. Taylor G, Larson CP, Presthwich R. Unexpected cardiac arrest during anesthesia and surgery. An environmental study. *JAMA* 1976;236: 2758–2760.
82. Bolander FM. Deaths associated with anesthesia. *Br J Anaesth* 1975; 47:36–40.
83. Harrison GG. Death attributable to anesthesia. *Br J Anaesth* 1978;50: 1041–1046.
84. Hooke R. Account of an experiment made by R Hooke, of preserving animals alive by blowing through their lungs with bellows. *Philos Trans R Soc Lond* 1667;2:539.
85. Reed JP, Kemph JP, Hamelberg W, et al. Studies with transtracheal artificial respiration. *Anesthesiology* 1954;15:28–41.
86. Jacoby JJ, Hamelberg W, Ziegler CH, et al. Transtracheal resuscitation. *JAMA* 1956;162:625–628.
87. Spoerel WE, Narayanan PS, Singh NP. Transtracheal ventilation. *Br J Anaesth* 1971;43:932–939.
88. Jacobs HB. Emergency percutaneous transtracheal jet ventilation. *J Trauma* 1972;12:50–55.
89. Klain M, Smith RB. High frequency percutaneous transtracheal jet ventilation. *Crit Care Med* 1977;5:280–287.
90. Attia RR, Battit GE, Murphy JD. Transtracheal ventilation. *JAMA* 1975;234:1152–1153.
91. Stinson TW. A simple connector for transtracheal ventilation. *Anesthesiology* 1977;47:232.
92. Yealy DM, Stewart RD, et al. Myths and pitfalls in emergency translaryngeal ventilation: correcting misimpressions. *Ann Emerg Med* 1988;17:690–692.
93. Abbrecht PH, Bryant HJ, et al. Determinants of alveolar ventilation during high frequency transtracheal jet ventilation in dogs. *Crit Care Med* 1986;14:563–569.
94. Layman PR. Bypassing a problem airway. *Anaesthesia* 1983;38:478–480.
95. Wagner DJ, Coomb DW, Doyle SC. Percutaneous transtracheal ventilation for emergency dental appliance removal. *Anesthesiology* 1985;62:664–666.
96. Weymuller EA, Paugh D, Pavlin EG, Cummings CW. Management

of difficult airway problems with percutaneous transtracheal ventilation. *Ann Otol Rhinol Laryngol* 1987;96:34–37.
97. Stother JC, Stout MJ, Lewis LM, et al. High pressure transtracheal ventilation: the use of large gauge intravenous type catheters in the totally obstructed airway. *J Emerg Med* 1990;8:184–189.
98. Neff CC, Pfister RC, Van Sonnenberg E. Percutaneous transtracheal ventilation—experimental and practical aspects. *J Trauma* 1983;23: 84–90.
99. Goldman E, McDonald JS, Peters SS, et al. Transtracheal ventilation with oscillatory pressure for complete upper airway obstruction. *J Trauma* 1988;28:611–614.
100. Klain M, Keszlar J, Brader E. High frequency jet ventilation in CPR. *Crit Care Med* 1981;9:421–422.
101. Craft TM, Chambers PH, Ward ME, et al. Two cases of barotrauma associated with transtracheal jet ventilation. *Br J Anaesth* 1990;64: 524–527.
102. Boucek CD, Gunnerson HB, Tullock WC. Percutaneous transtracheal high-frequency jet ventilation as an aid to fiberoptic intubation. *Anesthesiology* 1987;67:247–249.
103. Baraka A. Transtracheal jet ventilation during fiberoptic intubation under general anesthesia. *Anesth Analg* 1986;65:1091–1092.
104. McAlpine G, Williams RT. Fiberoptic assisted tracheal intubation under general anesthesia with IPPV. *Anesthesiology* 1987;66:853.
105. Todesco JM, Williams RT. Percutaneous transtracheal high-frequency jet ventilation as an aid to fiberoptic intubation. *Anesthesiology* 1987;68:298.
106. Klain M, Keszlar H, Stool S. Transtracheal high frequency jet ventilation prevents aspiration. *Crit Care Med* 1983;11:170–172.
107. Don Michael TA. The esophageal obturator airway. *JAMA* 1981;246: 1098.
108. Bryson TK, Benumof JL, Ward CF. The esophageal obturator airway, a clinical comparison to ventilation with a mask and oropharyngeal airway. *Chest* 1978;74:537.
109. Swartzman S, Wilson MA, Hoff BH, et al. Percutaneous transtracheal jet ventilation for cardiopulmonary resuscitation: evaluation of a new jet ventilator. *Crit Care Med* 1984;12:8–13.
110. Morgan GE, Mikhail MS. Cardiopulmonary resuscitation. In: *Clinical Anesthesiology*. Norwalk: Appleton & Lange, 1992; 663–667.
111. Thomas T, Zornow M, Scheller MS, Unger R. The efficacy of three different modes of trans-tracheal ventilation in hypoxic hypercarbic swine. *Can J Anaesth* 1988;35:S61.

Airway Management, edited by
L.H. Hanowell, M.D. and R.J. Waldron, M.D.,
Lippincott-Raven Publishers, Philadelphia © 1996.

CHAPTER 18

Surgical Airways

James E. Morrison and Felix D. Battistella

HISTORY

Early evidence of surgical access to the airway is found in the Rigeda, a Hindu book written circa 2000 B.C., and in ancient Egyptian manuscripts (1). Technical descriptions of tracheostomy date back to the Classical Ages, when the Greek surgeon, Asclepiades of Bithynia (circa 120–170 B.C.), is credited with performing the procedure for airway obstruction (2). Formal references in the medical literature first begin to appear in the sixteenth century. Lorenz Heister introduced the term *tracheostomy* in the 1700s. However, prior to 1825, medical literature documents only 28 successful tracheostomies (3).

Prior to the turn of the century, tracheostomy was advocated as a last resort measure to be performed only in emergency situations. In 1909, Chevalier Jackson recommended establishing surgical airways electively prior to the progression of airway obstruction (4). Thus, in the early 1900s, airway compromise due to diphtheria became a common indication for tracheostomy. Shortly thereafter, a controversy arose as to the best method of establishing a surgical airway. The pros and cons of tracheostomy versus cricothyroidotomy are still debated today (5).

J. E. Morrison and F. D. Battistella: Department of Surgery, University of California, Davis School of Medicine and Medical Center, Sacramento, California 95817.

Tracheostomy Versus Cricothyroidotomy

Jackson's first paper was followed 14 years later by an article entitled "High Tracheotomy and Other Errors; the Chief Cause of Chronic Laryngeal Stenosis." In this classic paper, he warned against the use of cricothyroidotomy (what he referred to as a "high tracheostomy"), based on the increased incidence of subglottic stenosis. He called for surgical texts to be rewritten to correctly describe the procedure (6). Jackson attributed the high incidence of stenosis following cricothyroidotomy to hasty operative technique, performance of the operation under general anesthetic with loss of normal airway protective mechanisms, division of the cricoid cartilage, sewing up the wound, improper postoperative care, poor wound hygiene, and the effects of a poorly fitted cannula.

Prior to the polio epidemics of the 1950s, tracheostomy was used primarily in cases of airway obstruction; however, with the need for prolonged mechanical ventilation, tracheostomy was used increasingly for airway management and pulmonary hygiene. For years, elective cricothyroidotomy was avoided. However, in 1976, Brantigan and Grow (7) reported the use of elective cricothyroidotomy in cardiothoracic patients. They preferred this operation due to the higher location of the tube away from the median sternotomy incision. In contrast to Jackson's experience, Brantigan and Grow reported complications in only 6% of

655 patients studied. The differences in their results were attributed to improved surgical techniques, antibiotics, and performing the procedure in the absence of inflammation—most of Jackson's patients had diphtheria.

Since then, numerous articles have been written comparing and contrasting tracheostomy and cricothyroidotomy. Careful review of the literature shows neither procedure to be without complication (8–13). In spite of the controversy, both tracheostomy and cricothyroidotomy continue to be useful techniques in airway management and are used routinely. Each technique has advantages over the other, depending on the setting and circumstances.

Cricothyroidotomy is a fast and simple procedure that can be performed in less than 1 min; and it requires very few instruments. For these reasons, it has become the procedure of choice in the emergency setting where rapid airway management is crucial. It may be performed at the roadside, in an ambulance, in the emergency room, or in the operating room, and can be performed by properly trained emergency medical technicians (EMTs), nurses, emergency physicians, surgeons, or anesthesiologists (14,15).

Tracheostomy is a slightly more complex procedure associated with fewer long-term complications and is the procedure of choice in an elective setting.

SURGICAL AIRWAYS

When urgent access to the airway is needed, several options other than cricothyroidotomy and/or tracheostomy are available, including retrograde intubation and needle cricothyroidotomy. Retrograde intubation requires passing a wire through the cricothyroid membrane and out the mouth. This is then used as a guide to direct the endotracheal tube into the trachea. Patients can also be ventilated through a needle cricothyroidotomy placed percutaneously through the cricothyroid membrane, using high-pressure, 50-psi oxygen. This method of ventilation is analogous to transtracheal jet ventilation. These techniques are described in more detail in Chapter 17.

Commercial kits, designed to cannulate the trachea by percutaneous puncture, have been available since the mid-1980s. Some of these involve direct puncture with a large trocar; others use sequential dilators that culminate with placement of the airway. To date, these techniques have been used primarily to establish elective airways in critically ill patients in an intensive care unit (ICU) setting (16).

While the procedures described above require certain surgical skills and a thorough understanding of the neck's anatomy, for the purpose of this chapter, we will limit our definition of surgical airway to the standard cricothyroidotomy and tracheostomy.

TABLE 1. *Indications for urgent surgical airway*

Airway obstruction
Failed translaryngeal intubation
Maxillofacial trauma inhibiting endotracheal intubation
Excessive oropharyngeal hemorrhage
Cervical spine injury with vocal cords difficult to visualize

Indications for Urgent Surgical Airway

Indications for establishing an urgent surgical airway are listed in Table 1. These include severe maxillofacial trauma where injuries make the airway inaccessible for translaryngeal intubation; severe hemorrhage or emesis obscuring the necessary landmarks for successful endotracheal intubation; and clenched teeth or airway obstruction prohibiting translaryngeal intubation. In a setting where the spine is potentially unstable and visualization of the airway is not successful, cricothyroidotomy is the fastest and safest method to secure the airway (7). Finally, when attempts at orotracheal and nasotracheal intubation have failed, obtaining a surgical airway should not be delayed in an unventilated patient.

While cricothyroidotomy is generally the procedure of choice in emergency situations, tracheostomy also can be performed urgently. Tracheostomy is the procedure of choice in children requiring an urgent surgical airway or in patients with severe tracheal/laryngeal trauma.

Indications for Elective Surgical Airway

Indications for elective tracheostomy are summarized in Table 2.

Prolonged Ventilator Dependence

Neither cricothyroidotomy nor tracheostomy are without risk, and for this reason there is a tendency to prolong the period of translaryngeal intubation (18). However, Rodriquez et al. (19) showed that patients undergoing early tracheostomy fared significantly better, with fewer ICU days and fewer ventilator days. This approach has been supported by others (15), who recommend early tracheostomy (within 3 days) if prolonged ventilator dependence (more than 7 days) is expected.

TABLE 2. *Indications for elective surgical airway*

Partially obstructing lesions
Sleep apnea
Facial trauma
Inability to protect airway
Chronic ventilator dependency

We concur with Heffner's (20) recommendation that the decision be made case by case. Patients clearly needing intubation for more than 21 days should undergo early tracheostomy. Those who are likely to be extubated within 10 days should remain intubated orally or nasally. The remaining group should be reevaluated daily, with a final decision made on day 7. Patients who will require mechanical ventilation for an additional week or longer should have a tracheostomy. However, tracheostomy should be delayed in patients requiring high ventilatory pressures until their peak airway pressures are below 35 cm H_2O.

Obstructing Lesions

Obstructing lesions include traumatic airway injuries, soft tissue swelling, foreign bodies, and head and neck tumors. Elective tracheostomy often precedes many operations in the head and neck where progressively obstructing lesions are present. Tumors requiring resection of the larynx mandate permanent tracheostomy. Children with cystic hygromas or large hemangiomas may also require tracheostomy. Subglottic stenosis from previous orotracheal intubation or as a complication of cricothyroidotomy may require tracheostomy. Ludwig's angina, which involves progressive swelling of the floor of the mouth due to infection, usually requires a surgical airway. Patients with severe facial burns associated with progressive, oropharyngeal swelling and airway edema may benefit from early tracheostomy if prolonged mechanical ventilation is required.

Sleep Apnea

Sleep apnea syndrome is a disorder in which patients have episodes of apnea during sleep. An apneic episode is defined as cessation of breathing for a period of at least 15 sec—less if associated with bradycardia. Patients may have hundreds of such episodes each night. The etiology may be obstructive mechanical, central (no message from the respiratory center), or mixed. The patient's spouse will often note severe snoring or violent movements. Such patients often complain of morning headaches, and daytime somnolence may affect their productivity. Other complications include cardiac arrhythmias during the apneic episodes and pulmonary hypertension. Nonsurgical therapies include weight loss and the use of nerve stimulators. Surgical treatment for obstructive apnea involves tracheostomy (21).

Facial Trauma

Gunshot wounds or crush injuries can result in massive facial trauma. Such injuries may be associated with profuse bleeding, extensive lacerations, or hematomas of the tongue or floor of the mouth. Associated spine injuries may further complicate attempts at endotracheal intubation. These patients often require an immediate surgical airway.

Some trauma victims with severe maxillofacial injuries may initially present with a stable airway; however, postinjury or postoperative edema and swelling may compromise their ventilation. If this is anticipated, tracheostomy should be performed electively at the time the facial injuries are repaired.

Airway Protection

Patients with severe head injuries and coma are often unable to protect their airways. They have diminished gag and cough reflexes and may be unable to swallow or control their own secretions. Tracheostomy is helpful both in maintaining the airway and in providing pulmonary hygiene. Infants with respiratory distress syndrome, bronchopulmonary dysplasia, or prematurity may also fall into the category of needing airway protection (22).

Respiratory Failure

Prolonged translaryngeal intubation may cause airway injury. Factors associated with injury include the number of days of intubation, size of endotracheal tube relative to the larynx, and tube movement. In addition to reducing the complications associated with prolonged translaryngeal intubation, tracheostomy facilitates the process of weaning mechanical ventilation in patients requiring prolonged support. Tracheostomy permits patients to breath spontaneously without incurring the risks and trauma associated with reintubation, should they need further mechanical ventilatory support. Tracheostomy reduces dead space ventilation, thus decreasing the work of breathing, compared to nasotracheal or orotracheal intubation, which increase work of breathing. Pulmonary hygiene and management of tracheobronchial secretions are also facilitated in patients with tracheostomies.

Children

Indications for a surgical airway in children include acquired subglottic stenosis, bilateral vocal cord paralysis, congenital airway malformations, tumor, and chronic pulmonary insufficiency. Less common indications include head injury, bilateral diaphragmatic paralysis, and Ondine's curse syndrome.

The decision to perform tracheostomy in children should take into account the fact that surgical airways are associated with a high incidence of complications (23,

24). Cricothyroidotomy should be avoided in the child as the cricoid cartilage is the narrowest part of their airway.

TRACHEOSTOMY—OPERATIVE PROCEDURE

Anesthesia

Tracheostomy is easiest to perform under general anesthesia if translaryngeal intubation is possible. However, in the patient with a tenuous airway and a marginal ventilatory status, tracheostomy can be performed with local anesthesia.

Patient Positioning and Preparation

The anesthetized patient is placed in the supine position. A rolled sheet or towel is placed under the shoulders to hyperextend the neck as long as a cervical injury does not preclude this. The neck and upper chest are prepped and draped in a standard way.

The patient with an imminent airway obstruction undergoing awake, urgent tracheostomy should be left in a semiupright position to avoid further compromise of the airway.

Operative Technique

Landmarks such as the thyroid cartilage (Adam's apple), the sternal notch, and the cricoid cartilage are carefully identified. A transverse incision is made approximately half the distance from the sternal notch to the thyroid cartilage, approximately two finger breadths above the sternal notch (Fig. 1). The length of the incision required is variable depending on the anatomy; however, in most cases it should equal the diameter of the trachea. This incision allows for some superior or inferior variance in the location of the trachea. Best cosmetic results are achieved if the incision is hidden in an existing skin fold.

The skin is incised sharply and the platysma is divided using electrocautery. The exposed strap muscles are separated in the midline where they meet at the median raphe. They can then be displaced laterally with a self-retaining retractor. The anterior jugular veins can be retracted laterally or ligated and divided as needed to achieve adequate exposure.

With the muscles retracted laterally, the thyroid isthmus should be visible in the center of the field. While some authors suggest dividing the isthmus, we recommend retracting it superiorly. The inferior thyroid veins are ligated and divided, and the attachments of the thyroid isthmus to the underlying trachea are freed bluntly

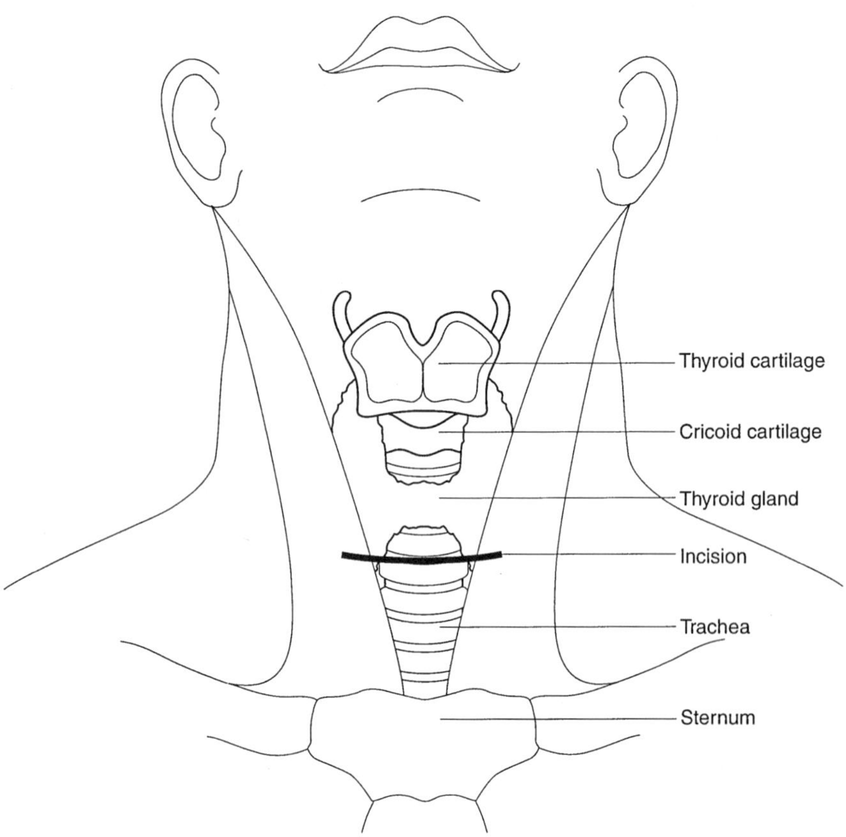

FIG. 1. Anatomy of the neck and location of tracheostomy incision.

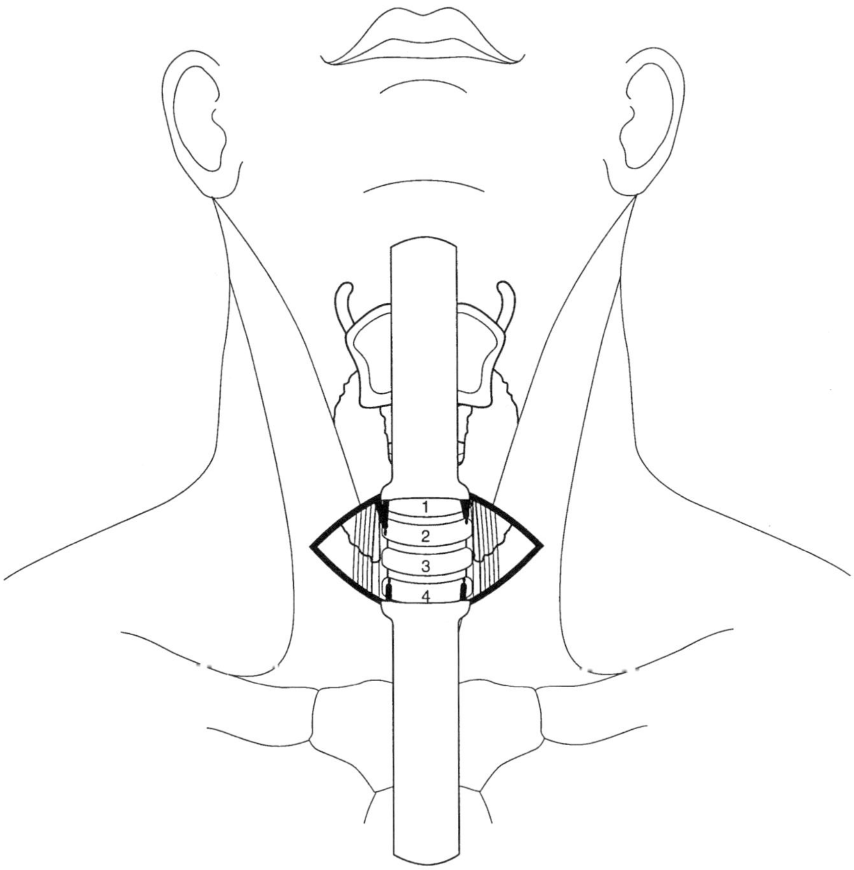

FIG. 2. Exposure of trachea with thyroid isthmus retracted cephalad. Tracheal rings (1–4) are exposed.

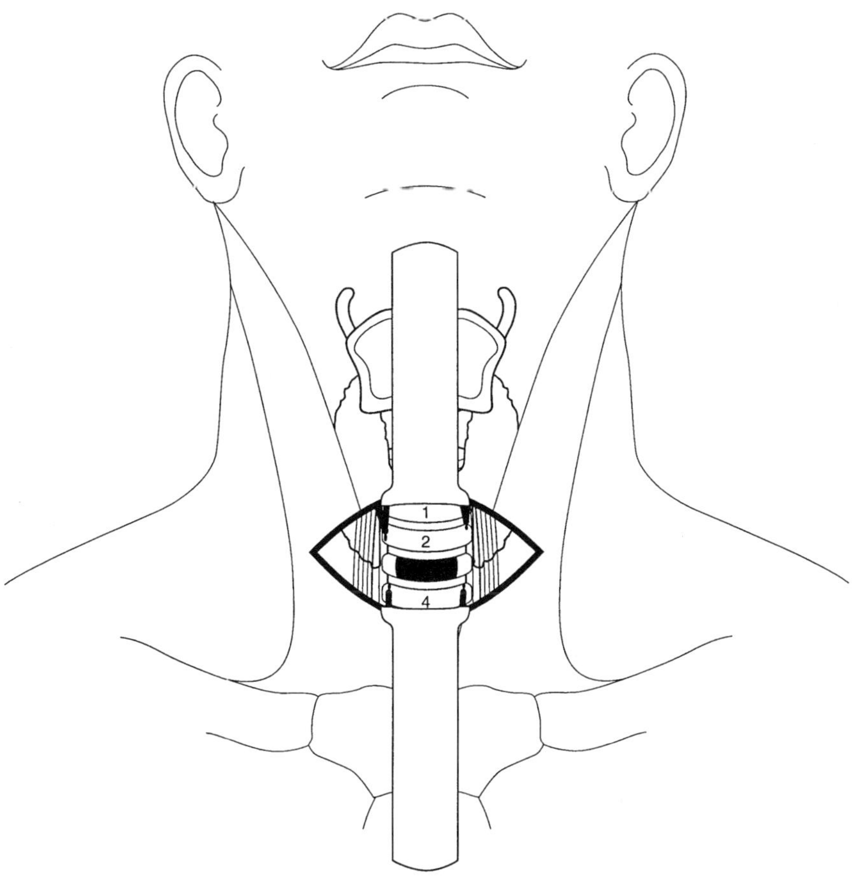

FIG. 3. Tracheostomy with partial excision of third tracheal ring.

using a clamp. This will allow the isthmus to be retracted superiorly, exposing the underlying tracheal rings (Fig. 2). Palpation of the cricothyroid cartilage allows identification of the second and third tracheal rings. Care should be taken not to place the tracheostomy at the first tracheal ring as this may lead to an increased incidence of tracheal stenosis. Use of the second ring is acceptable, though the third is preferred. Placing the tracheostomy below the third tracheal ring increases the risk of tracheoinnominate artery fistula.

Stay sutures can be placed around the second tracheal ring anterolaterally to help retract the trachea cephalad. These sutures can be left in place for several days until the tracheostomy tract is well formed. The interspaces between the second and third, and third and fourth tracheal rings are incised using the electrocautery. If the patient has an endotracheal tube in place, care should be taken not to puncture the cuff. Once the cuff is deflated, it becomes difficult to ventilate the patient, and the tracheostomy should be completed as quickly as possible. A small portion approximately one-fourth of the circumference of the third tracheal ring is excised in order to facilitate insertion of the tracheostomy tube (Fig. 3).

A tracheal hook can be used to retract the superior portion of the trachea in a cephalad direction to help expose the tracheal opening. Excessive traction on the trachea may stimulate the vagus nerve and precipitate severe bradycardia. If the tracheal opening is not large enough to allow passage of the tracheostomy tube, a Trousseau dilator may be helpful in enlarging the opening.

In the mechanically ventilated patient, the endotracheal tube is withdrawn under direct vision until the tip is just above the stoma. The tracheostomy tube is then inserted and the cuff inflated. Care should be taken while inserting the tracheostomy tube to avoid creating a false passage parallel to the trachea. Once the tracheostomy is inserted, ventilation to both lungs should be confirmed. The tube should be secured in place and a dressing applied underneath the base of the tracheostomy. A postoperative chest x-ray should be obtained to confirm the absence of pneumothorax.

Patients with tracheostomies should have their air supplies humidified, as the upper airway that normally provides this function is bypassed.

CRICOTHYROIDOTOMY—OPERATIVE PROCEDURE

Anesthesia

Cricothyroidotomy is most commonly performed in an emergency setting in the patient without an airway. Often, the patient is unresponsive; in such cases, no anes-

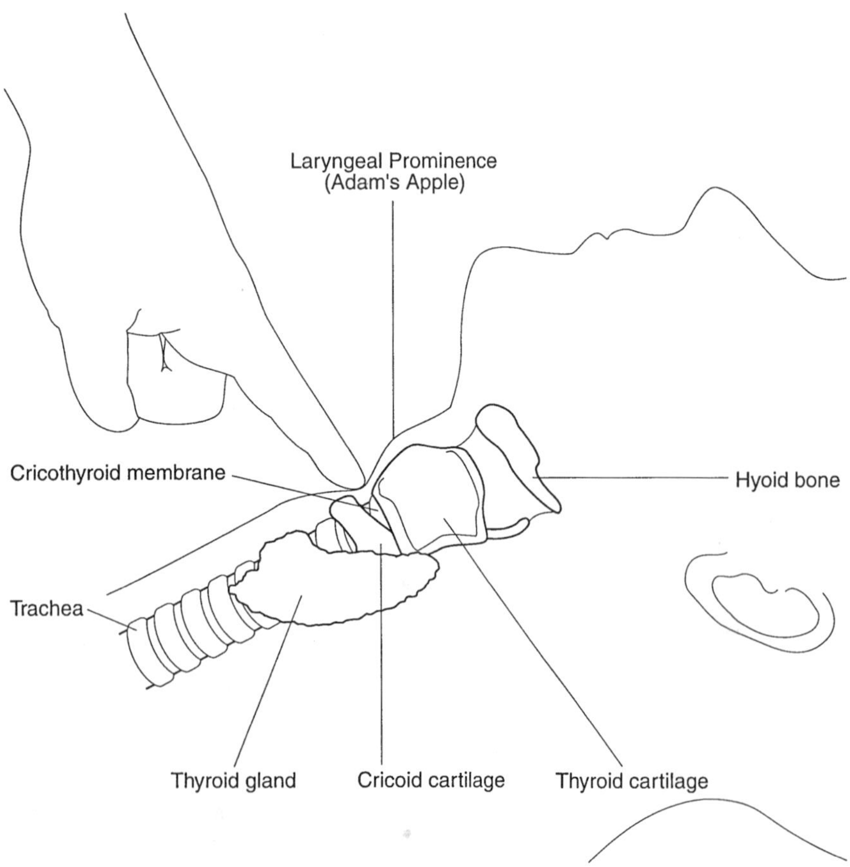

FIG. 4. Identifying cricothyroid membrane using external landmarks.

thetic is indicated. In the awake patient, if the situation permits, a local anesthetic may be used.

Patient Positioning and Preparation

The patient should be in the supine position. In the trauma patient, potential cervical injury will preclude hyperextension of the neck. Most often there is no time for a formal preparation of the field.

Operative Technique

Cricothyroidotomy can be performed using a standard surgical approach or percutaneous devices. The percutaneous devices incorporate a Seldinger technique by placing a needle through the cricothyroid membrane and passing a series of dilators over a wire to enlarge the tract. Both methods can be performed successfully in the field; however, the standard surgical approach is faster and requires few instruments and less equipment (25). In brief, performing a cricothyroidotomy involves identifying the cricothyroid membrane, incising the membrane, dilating the opening, and placing an artificial airway into the trachea.

The procedure is best performed by standing on the side of the patient that corresponds to the surgeon's dominant hand. The thyroid cartilage is easily identified by running a finger down the midline of the neck (Fig. 4). The thyroid cartilage is the major prominence encountered. The cricothyroid membrane is palpable as a slight indentation or notch just below the thyroid cartilage. Once the cricothyroid membrane is identified, the thyroid cartilage can be stabilized by placing traction on the skin with the nondominant hand. A scalpel is used to make a horizontal incision in the skin overlying the cricothyroid membrane (Fig. 5). A stab incision is made in the membrane to enter the airway. While many hospitals have cricothyroidotomy kits with different hooks and dilators, it is quickest to simply insert the scalpel handle into the incision and rotate it 90°. This will dilate the opening (Fig. 6). A cannula, such as a small trache-

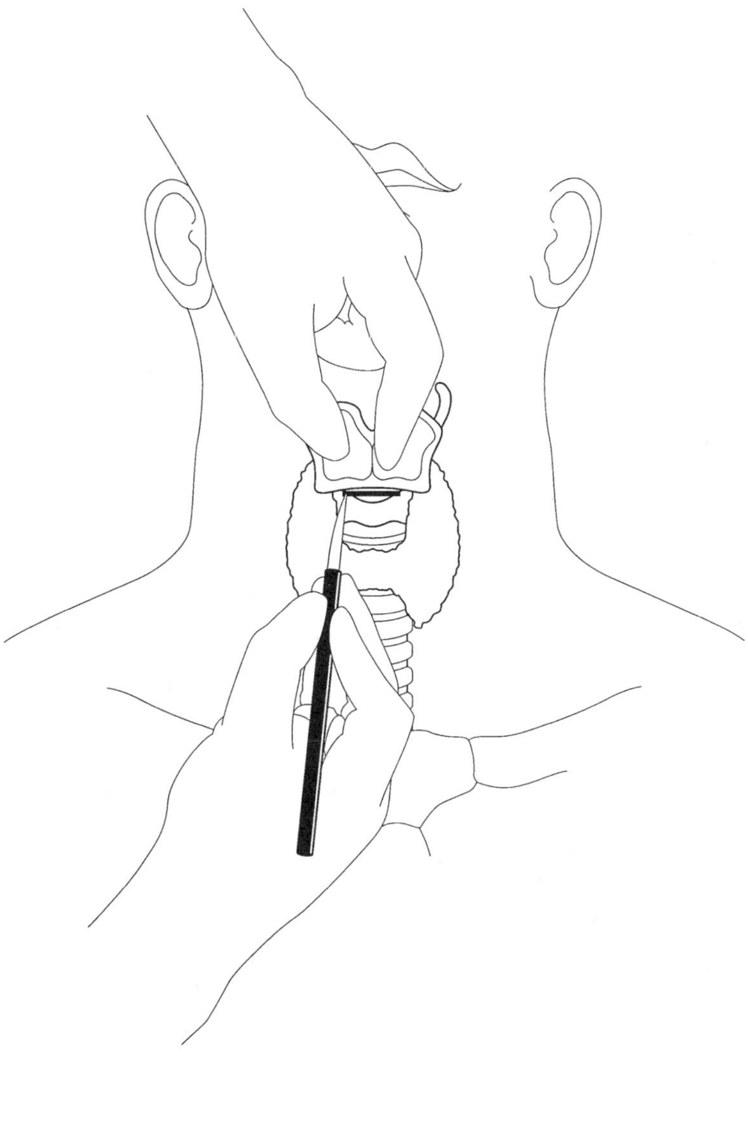

FIG. 5. Cricothyroidotomy incision. Nondominant hand used to stabilize thyroid cartilage.

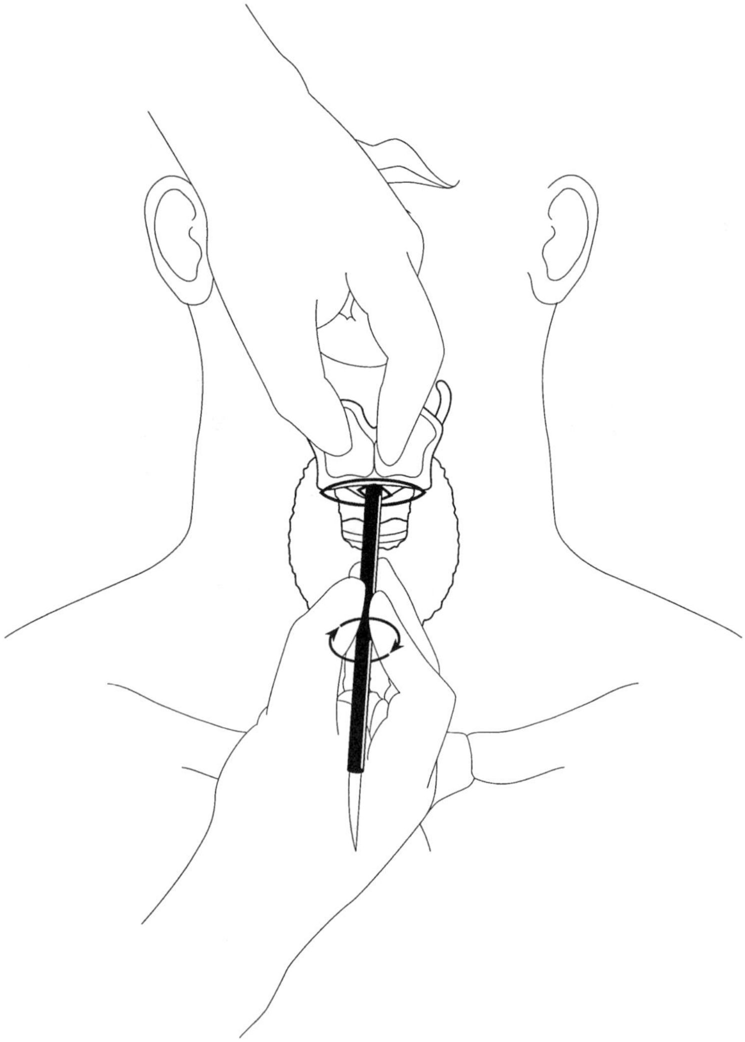

FIG. 6. Dilating cricothyroidotomy using handle of scalpel.

ostomy tube or whatever is available (i.e., a small endotracheal tube), is inserted into the opening to secure the airway.

COMPLICATIONS OF SURGICAL AIRWAYS

As with any surgical procedure, surgical airways are not without risk. The complication rate for urgent cricothyroidotomy is often clouded by the fact that most of the patients in whom it is performed are trauma victims with an associated high morbidity and mortality due to their injuries.

Intraoperative Complications

The intraoperative complications of tracheostomy and cricothyroidotomy (Table 3) are primarily related to technical difficulties.

Hemorrhage

The most common sources of bleeding encountered while establishing a surgical airway are the anterior jugular veins or the thyroid vessels. Venous bleeders can be identified and controlled with direct pressure and ligation. Bleeding associated with urgent cricothyroidotomy is usually self-limited and can be controlled simply by inserting the cannula through the tract. The tube applies pressure to the area, causing the bleeding to tamponade. Arterial hemorrhage is rare, but may originate from the thyroid gland or the thyroid ima artery. Arterial bleeding should be controlled as it is identified.

Extensive lateral dissection may lead to injuries to the carotid artery or jugular vein. Although rare, injuries to large arteries or veins are best treated by obtaining proximal and distal control and performing a careful repair. Care should be taken to prevent air embolization whenever large venous injuries are encountered.

TABLE 3. *Intraoperative complications of surgical airways*

Hemorrhage
Vagal nerve stimulation
Misplacement of tube
Injury to recurrent laryngeal nerve
Injury to posterior tracheal wall
Injury to esophagus
Pneumothorax
Hypoxia/obstruction
Death

Vagal Nerve Stimulation

Vigorous traction on the trachea, particularly with the tracheal hook, may stimulate the vagus nerve. This can cause marked bradycardia, hypotension, and even cardiac arrest. Close monitoring by the anesthesiologist will alert the surgeon when this occurs. Traction on the airway should be released if the patient develops bradycardia during the procedure.

Misplacement of Tube

As most cricothyroidotomies are performed urgently in suboptimal conditions, misplacement of the tube into the mediastinum or esophagus may occur. This may also occur during tracheostomy if careful attention is not paid to placing the tube under direct vision. Accurate placement of the tube is facilitated by good exposure and a hemostatic surgical field.

Other complications resulting from tube misplacement include injury to the recurrent laryngeal nerve, injury to the vocal cords, and laceration of the posterior tracheal wall (26).

Pneumothorax

Injury to the pleura and pneumothorax is rare and occurs following extensive dissection at the base of the neck. A routine chest x-ray should be performed after the procedure to exclude pneumothorax. This complication occurs far more frequently in children, where the structures of the neck and chest are in closer proximity (24).

Hypoxia

In the patient without an airway, significant hypoxia may result from delay in establishing an adequate airway or from intraoperative aspiration. Similar complications can occur during an elective tracheostomy if preoperative preparation or operative technique is inadequate.

TABLE 4. *Early postoperative complications of surgical airways*

Obstruction/atelectasis
Hemorrhage
Mediastinal emphysema
Infection
Aspiration
Accidental extubation
Voice change

Postoperative Complications

Some intraoperative complications may not become evident until the postoperative period. These account for most of the early postoperative complications (Table 4).

Hemorrhage

Postoperative bleeding is most often due to inadequate hemostasis at time of surgery. A thrombus that provided intraoperative hemostasis may become dislodged, leading to postoperative hemorrhage. For this reason, meticulous intraoperative hemostasis is recommended. Direct pressure usually controls the bleeding, and a return to the operating room for exploration and hemostasis is rarely needed.

Mediastinal Emphysema

Subcutaneous or mediastinal emphysema may arise in the patient in whom the tracheal tube is too small or in patients with uncuffed tubes. Violent coughing often contributes to the problem.

Obstruction/Atelectasis

Atelectasis is a common complication following general anesthesia. It results from hypoventilation of portions of the lung and may be more pronounced in patients undergoing tracheostomy if the patient is subjected to a prolonged period of hypoventilation during the procedure. Obstruction of the airway from pooled secretions or bleeding may contribute to the problem. These secretions can become thick and tenacious, making them increasingly difficult to clear if the inspired air is not adequately humidified. These problems are easily corrected with aggressive pulmonary hygiene and by keeping the inhaled air humidified. If the airway dries out, tracheitis sicca will develop.

Infection

Infection may occur in the wound or within the tracheobronchial tree. Soft tissue infections include local wound infections, mediastinitis, and sternal wound infections. Common pathogens include normal oropharyngeal or skin flora. Severe necrotizing infections occur rarely. Airway and pulmonary infections include tracheitis, tracheobronchitis, and pneumonia (13,27). It remains unclear to what degree tracheostomy contributes to the development of these infections.

Accidental Extubation

Accidental extubation early in the postoperative course is dangerous in that the tracheal stoma and tract are not well formed. If the tube comes out prematurely, the tract may close and the airway may be lost. This problem can be further compounded by the creation of a false passage along the trachea during attempts to replace the tube. If the initial attempt to replace the tracheostomy is unsuccessful, an orotracheal airway should be established until reinsertion of the tracheostomy tube can be facilitated.

Voice Changes

Patients often complain of voice changes following intubation of the airway and, particularly, after cricothyroidotomy. These changes include loss of voice intensity, fatigue, deeper voice, or narrowed vocal range. The incidence of voice change is reported to be as high as 50% to 75% (28); however, the changes are often self-limited. Often, the damage is caused by laryngeal fracture, injury to the vocal cords, damage to the cricothyroid muscle, recurrent laryngeal nerve injury, and formation of scar tissue that restricts movement of the cartilage (29).

Late Complications

Complications occurring in patients with chronic tracheostomies are related to erosion into adjacent structures, airway stenosis, or persistent stoma (Table 5).

Tracheoinnominate Artery Fistula

The innominate artery runs between the trachea and the sternum. Long-standing tracheostomy tubes or their cuffs may erode through the trachea into the innominate artery. This is a rare complication, occurring more frequently when the tracheostomy is placed low in the trachea (26). Uncontrolled hemorrhage from the artery is usually preceded by a small herald bleed. When bleeding is massive, patients die due to exsanguination into the airway.

Rapid intervention is critical, and the first step should be to establish and protect the airway by placing a translaryngeal endotracheal tube, with its cuff beyond the site of bleeding. With the tracheostomy tube removed, a finger can then be inserted through the stoma into the pretracheal space. This will permit direct compression of the innominate artery against the sternum. With the airway secured and the bleeding controlled, the patient is then taken immediately to the operating room for ligation of the artery via a median sternotomy.

TABLE 5. *Long-term complications of surgical airways*

Tracheoinnominate artery fistula
Tracheoesophageal fistula
Stenosis
Persistent stoma
Poor cosmetic result

Tracheoesophageal Fistula

Tracheoesophageal fistulas occur when high cuff pressures cause ischemic necrosis of the posterior tracheal wall and esophagus. Local infection may contribute to the development of ischemia and subsequent fistula formation (3). Diagnosis is usually suggested by increased tracheobronchial secretions, particularly when these are bilious or when tube feed is noted in the tracheal aspirate. Patients with suspected tracheoesophageal fistulas should undergo endoscopy and bronchoscopy to diagnose and locate the fistula. Infusion of methylene blue into the esophagus may facilitate locating the anomalous connection. Treatment of these fistulas involves repairing both the tracheal and esophageal perforations and interposing a muscle flap. The tracheal balloon should be moved away from the site of injury, and feedings should be provided through a gastrostomy to protect the esophageal wound. In patients too ill to undergo primary repair, the esophagus should be diverted in the neck, and the stomach should be decompressed with a gastrostomy. Formal repair of the esophagus can be undertaken once the patient has recovered.

Stenosis

Cannulation of the airway by any means can be complicated by tracheal stenosis. This can occur due to cricoid cartilage injury, local inflammation and scarring, or tracheal cartilage reabsorption with subsequent collapse of the airway. Cricothyroidotomies and high tracheostomies can lead to the development of subglottic stenosis. Because of this, elective cricothyroidotomy is discouraged. Stenosis at the cuff site is usually due to the pressure of the cuff, leading to local ischemia. This can be minimized by using low-pressure cuffs and by monitoring the pressures. Excessive traction from the ventilator tubing can contribute to narrowing at the stoma site (26,30).

Airway stenosis can manifest immediately after extubation or later in the patient's course, when increased activity leads to exertional dyspnea. Evaluation of the patient with suspected tracheal stenosis requires laryngoscopy and bronchoscopy. Current treatment recommendations include steroid injection, laser therapy, dilatation, and segmental tracheal resection.

Persistent Stoma

Once the tracheal tube is removed, the stomal tract will usually close spontaneously. However, in rare cases, it may remain open indefinitely if the tract is well epithelized. The risk of persistent stoma is directly proportional to the duration of cannulation. Surgical closure is indicated if the stoma remains open longer than 2 months. Closure requires excision of the skin tract and reapproximation of the trachea, strap muscles, platysma, and skin in layers. For large openings in the trachea, it may be necessary to cover the defect with a perichondrial flap taken from the thyroid cartilage (31).

CONCLUSION

All methods of airway access result in some damage to the airway itself. Translaryngeal intubation is almost always the best initial option. In an emergency setting, if translaryngeal intubation is not possible, cricothyroidotomy is the procedure of choice. Cricothyroidotomy may not be possible in patients with significant laryngeal injury, and they may require urgent tracheostomy. Although cricothyroidotomy can be left in place long term, it is best converted electively to a tracheostomy.

Tracheostomy is the procedure of choice in patients requiring a surgical airway in an elective setting, such as slowly progressing airway obstruction or a history of prolonged intubation.

REFERENCES

1. Stock CR. What is past is prologue: a short history of the development of tracheostomy. *Ear Nose Throat J* 1987;66:166–190.
2. Lyons AS, Petrucelli RJ. *Medicine, an Illustrated History*. New York: Harry N. Abrams, Inc., 1987;232.
3. Stemmer EA, Oliver C, Carey JP, Connolly JE. Fatal complications of tracheostomy. *Am J Surg* 1976;131:288.
4. Jackson C. Tracheostomy. *Laryngoscope* 1909;18:285.
5. Deans J. Emergency cricothyroidotomy. [Letter] *J Laryngol Otol* 1992;106:470.
6. Jackson C. High tracheotomy and other errors the chief causes of chronic laryngeal stenosis. *Surg Gynecol Obstet* 1923;32:392.
7. Brantigan CO, Grow JB. Cricothyroidotomy: elective use in respiratory problems requiring tracheotomy. *J Thorac Cardiovasc Surg* 1976;71:72–81.
8. DeLaurier G, Hawkins M, Treat RC, Mansberger AR. Acute airway management: role of cricothyroidotomy. *Am Surg* Jan 1990;56:12.
9. McGill J, Clinton J, Ruiz E. Cricothyrotomy in the emergency department. *Ann Emerg Med* 1982;11:361.
10. Boyd AD, Romita MC, Conlan AA, Fink SD, Spencer FC. A clinical evaluation of cricothyroidotomy. *Surg Gynecol Obstet* 1979;149: 365–358.
11. Sise MJ, Shackford SR, Cruickshank JC, Murphy G, Fridlund PH. Cricothyrotomy for long term tracheal access: a prospective analysis of morbidity and mortality in 76 patients. *Ann Surg* 1984;200:13.
12. Weymuller EA, Cummings CW. Cricothyroidotomy: the impact of antecedent endotracheal intubation. *Ann Otol Rhinol Laryngol* 1982; 91:437.
13. Miller JD, Kapp JP. Complications of tracheostomies in neurosurgical patients. *Surg Neurol* 1985;22:186.
14. Miklus RM, Elliott C, Snow N. Surgical cricothyrotomy in the field: experience of a helicopter transport team. *J Trauma* 1989;29:506.
15. Mulder DS, Marelli D. The 1991 Fraser Gurd lecture: evolution of airway control in the management of injured patients. *J Trauma* 1992; 33:856.
16. Anderson HL, Bartlett RH. Elective tracheotomy for mechanical ventilation by the percutaneous technique. *Clin Chest Med* 1991;12:555.
17. Salvino C, Dries D, Gamelli R, Murphy-Cacabobby M, Marshall W. Emergency cricothyroidotomy in trauma victims. *J Trauma* 1993;34: 503.
18. Berlauk JF. Prolonged endotracheal intubation versus tracheostomy. *Crit Care Med* 1986;14:742.
19. Rodriquez JL, Steinberg SM, Luchetti FA. Early tracheostomy for primary airway management in a surgical critical care setting. *Surgery* 1990;108:655.
20. Heffner J. Timing of tracheotomy in ventilator dependent patients. *Clin Chest Med* 1991;12:611.
21. Weinberger S. *Principles of Pulmonary Medicine*. Philadelphia: WB Saunders, 1986;213.
22. Nyhus L, Baker R. *Mastery of Surgery*. Boston: Little, Brown and Co., 1992;151,166,249–273.
23. Puhakka HJ, Kero P, Valli P, Iisalo E. Tracheostomy in pediatric patients. *Acta Paediatr* 1992;81:231.
24. Simma B, Spehler D, Burger R, Uehlinger J, Ghelfi D, Dangel P, et al. Tracheostomy in children. *Eur J Pediatr* 1994;153:291.
25. Johnson D, Dunlap A, McFeeley P, Gaffney J, Busick B. Cricothyrotomy performed by prehospital personnel: a comparison of two techniques in a human cadaver model. *Am J Emerg Med* 1993;11:207.
26. Kenan PD. Complications associated with tracheostomy: prevention and treatment. *Otolaryngol Clin North Am* 1979;12:807.
27. Esses BA, Jafek BW. Cricothyroidotomy: a decade of experience in Denver. *Ann Otol Rhinol Laryngol* 1987;96:519.
28. Gleeson MJ, Pearson RC, Armistead S, Yates AK. Voice changes following cricothyroidotomy. *J Laryngol Otol* 1984;98:1015.
29. Holst M, Hertegard S, Perrsson A. Vocal dysfunction following cricothyrotomy: a prospective study. *Laryngoscope* 1990;100:749.
30. Grillo HC, Cooper JD, Geffin B, Pontoppidan H. Low pressure cuff for tracheostomy tubes to minimize tracheal injury: a comparative clinical trial. *J Thorac Cardiovasc Surg* 1971;62:898.
31. Fisher S. Closure of tracheocutaneous fistula with perichondrial flap following cricothyroidotomy. *Laryngoscope* 1991;101:684.

PART V

Specialized Areas

Airway Management, edited by
L.H. Hanowell, M.D. and R.J. Waldron, M.D.,
Lippincott-Raven Publishers, Philadelphia © 1996.

CHAPTER 19

Pediatric Airway Management

Mark R. Ezekiel and Jalil Riazi

INTRODUCTION

Pediatric patients can present challenging problems in airway management. Newborns and infants differ in many respects from older children and adults. Not only do they differ physiologically and in their pharmacologic response to drugs, but also anatomically, with features that make their airway more difficult to manage (1). Additionally, pediatric patients may present with various congenital anomalies that can adversely affect the airway. Some of these difficult airways are easily recognized, while others may be encountered during induction of anesthesia.

Respiratory mishaps represent the highest single cause of poor outcome in pediatric patients (2–5). Difficulty in achieving adequate ventilation or inability to intubate the trachea are major reasons for the increased adverse outcome. Differences in airway anatomy and physiology make such events more common in children than in adults. It is important to understand the distinguishing anatomic features of the pediatric airway and to be familiar with some of the congenital defects that are suggestive of a difficult airway. Early recognition of such problem patients can allow appropriate preparation for their successful management.

PEDIATRIC AIRWAY ANATOMY

Anatomic Differences

Nasopharynx

The pediatric nasopharynx is relatively narrow (6). Resistance to air flow in the nasal passages accounts for

M. R. Ezekiel and J. Riazi: Department of Anesthesiology, University of California, Irvine Medical Center, Orange, California 92668.

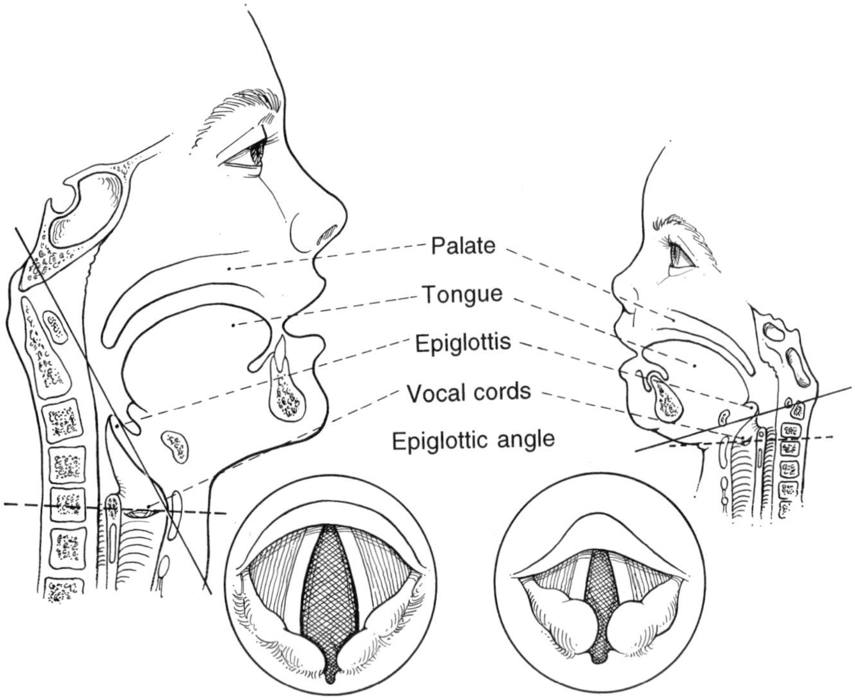

FIG. 1. Comparison between the adult and infant airway. The *stippled horizontal lines* show the relative position of the glottis to the cervical spine. The *solid lines* depict the angle created between the body of the epiglottis and the glottis, which in the infant is more acute than in the adult.

about 25% of the total resistance to air flow in a neonate, as compared with 60% in an adult (7–9) (Fig. 1). This decreased resistance results in the nasal passages being the path of least resistance. Blood, swelling, congestion, anatomic deformities, or a nasogastric tube may significantly increase nasal airway resistance and compromise the infant's ability to breathe (10–12).

Occiput

Compared with the adult patient, the pediatric patient up to the age of 3 years has a relatively large occiput. The large head and occiput may influence how the pediatric patient should be positioned to optimize visualization of the glottis during direct laryngoscopy. The use of a towel under the head in order to bring the oral, pharyngeal, and laryngeal axes in line is usually not necessary in children below the age of 9 years, and may actually result in air flow obstruction. The large occiput in the infant sometimes results in excessive neck flexion, in which case head extension and/or placement of a small towel under the shoulders improves air flow and axial alignment.

Larynx

In the normal adult, the inferior border of the cricoid cartilage lies at the level of C6-7. In the full-term infant, the larynx is at the level of C-4, and in the premature infant it is at the level of C-3. The rima glottidis is higher by one or two vertebrae. The more rostral or superior location of the larynx creates difficulty visualizing laryngeal structures because of the more acute angulation between the base of the tongue and the laryngeal inlet. Thus, the infant's larynx may appear to be in a more anterior location than that of the adult. The result is a more difficult laryngoscopic examination and intubation. This high position also changes the relationship of the axes of the oral cavity, pharynx, and larynx, which must be aligned for visualization of the glottic opening. Utilization of a straight laryngoscope blade facilitates visualization of an infant's larynx.

The most significant difference between the adult and the infant larynx is the overall diameter of the airway (Fig. 2). The diameter of the adult airway is approximately 8 mm or greater, whereas an infant's is typically 3 to 4 mm in diameter. In the neonate, a 1-mm reduction in this diameter reduces the overall cross-sectional area of the airway by at least 50%. By comparison, in the adult airway, 1 mm of circumferential edema leaves an airway with a diameter of at least 6 mm, at most a 25% reduction.

Tongue

The pediatric patient's tongue is relatively large in proportion to the rest of the oral cavity. The cephalad location of the larynx forces the tongue to lie entirely within the oral cavity, thus more easily obstructing the airway, especially in a neonate. The relatively large tongue is also more difficult to manipulate and stabilize with the laryngoscope blade.

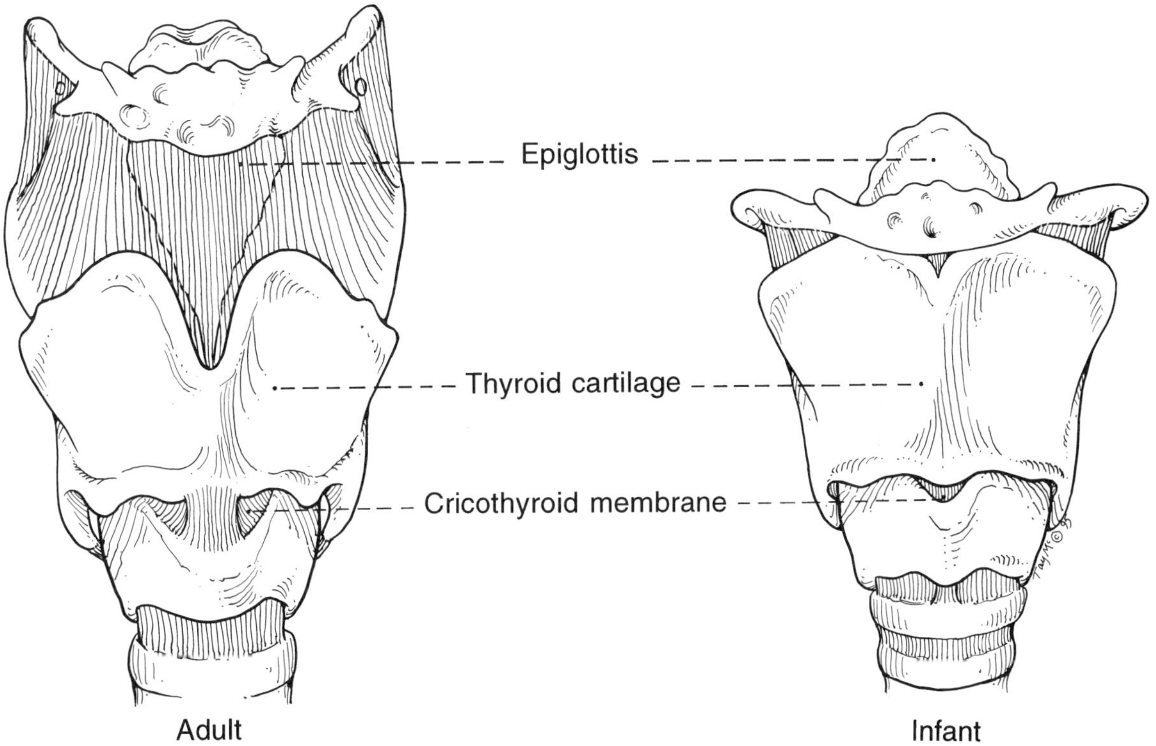

FIG. 2. Anterior view of the adult and infant larynx, showing the smaller dimensions of the thyrohyoid and the cricothyroid ligaments in the infant.

Epiglottis

The epiglottis in the infant is relatively floppy, narrow, short, and angled in a more posterior direction over the glottic opening (i.e., away from the axis of the trachea). Attachment of the epiglottis at the base of the tongue creates a shallow vallecular notch. The shape of the epiglottis reaches adult configuration around 3 years of age. In the normal adult, the epiglottis is at the level of C-3. In the infant less than 5 months of age, the epiglottis is at the level of C-1.

Vocal Cords

The pediatric vocal cords are inclined so that the anterior attachments are more caudad than the posterior connections. In comparison, in the normal adult airway, the axis of the vocal cords is perpendicular to the trachea. In the infant, the arytenoids are large compared with the glottic opening.

Subglottic Region

In the pediatric patient, there is progressive reduction in size from the hyoid to the cricoid, so that the larynx and its support have a conic shape (Fig. 3). The cricoid is contiguous with the trachea and represents the narrowest part of the larynx, as opposed to the glottic opening in the adult. The pediatric airway, at the level of the cricoid cartilage, is lined with pseudostratified, ciliated epithelium that is loosely bound to areolar tissue. A tight-fitting endotracheal tube that compresses the tracheal mucosa may cause edema within the subglottic structures, significantly reducing the lumen and greatly increasing the resistance to air flow. Even a small amount of circumferential edema of the subglottic region of an infant is more compromising than in an adult (13). Resistance to air flow is increased by a factor inversely proportional to the radius of the lumen to the fourth power for laminar flow, and to the fifth power for turbulent flow (14).

Airway Physiology

Respiratory Mechanics

The chest wall of the newborn and premature infant is more compliant than that of the adult. On the other hand, the infant lung is relatively stiff and noncompliant. The combination of a compliant chest wall and stiff lungs contributes to the low passive functional residual capacity (FRC) seen in infants. Passive FRC, the point at which the inward (lung recoil) and outward (chest wall) forces

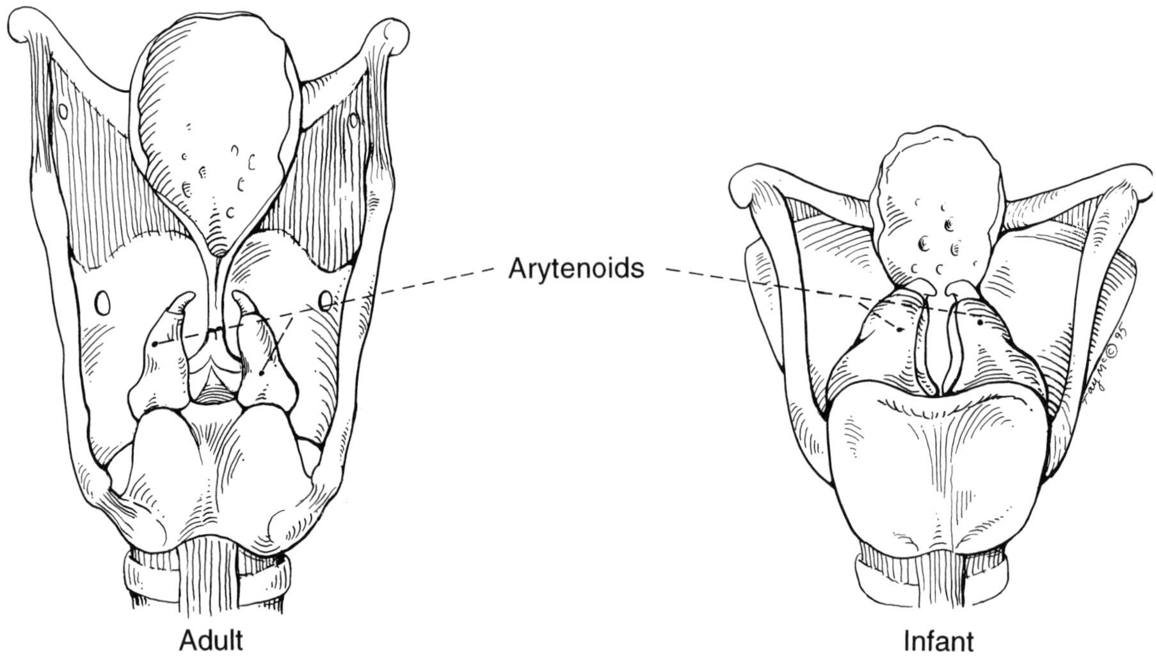

FIG. 3. Posterior view of the adult and infant larynx. Note the prominence of the arytenoids and the conic shape of the larynx in the infant.

balance each other, results in a resting lung volume near residual volume, or at about 15% of total lung capacity (TLC). In the adult, the resting point results in a lung volume of about 30% of TLC (15,16).

The infant compensates for low passive FRC in two primary ways. First, inspiration is started before passive exhalation is completed and before lung volume has fallen close to residual volume. Second, the respiratory rate in infants is high. The accelerated respiratory rate prevents the infant from reaching passive FRC by limiting the volume of air expelled during passive exhalation. As a result of these two factors, measured FRC during active tidal volume breathing in infants is approximately 35% of TLC.

Ventilation in the awake patient is accomplished by coordinated contraction of three inspiratory muscle groups: the diaphragm, the external intercostal muscles, and the muscles of the neck and upper airway. In the pediatric patient, ventilation is primarily diaphragmatic. Diaphragmatic excursion can be hampered by bulky abdominal viscera, as may be seen if the stomach or bowel is distended.

Obligate Nasal Breathing

The newborn is generally described as an obligate nasal breather. The immaturity of oropharyngeal motor output and sensory input result in lack of coordination between mouth breathing and swallowing efforts. In addition, with the larynx more rostral in the infant neck, the distances between the tongue, hyoid bone, epiglottis, and roof of the mouth are shorter than in an older child or adult. This makes mouth breathing difficult but enables the infant to breathe and swallow simultaneously (17,18). Being obligate nasal breathers, infants with obstruction of the nasal passages (e.g., children with bilateral choanal atresia) can experience total airway obstruction. As the infant develops over the first 3 to 5 months of life, the ability to coordinate respiratory and oral function develops, the larynx enlarges and moves lower in the neck, and the infant begins to breathe orally.

Work of Breathing

Resistance to laminar air flow is inversely proportional to the radius of the lumen to the fourth power and resistance to turbulent airflow is inversely proportional to the radius of the lumen to the fifth power. In neonates and infants, the most resistance occurs in the bronchial and small airways, whereas in the adult the greatest resistance to air flow occurs in the nasal passages (7,19–21). The nasal passages account for 60% of the total resistance to air flow in the adult, compared with 25% in the neonate (22). The tracheal and bronchial structures of the neonate are immature, elastic, and highly compliant. Consequently, they are susceptible to mechanical compression and dynamic airway collapse, leading to functional airway closure with every breath (23,24). Both agitation and

TABLE 1. *Pediatric vs. adult respiratory physiology*

Respiratory parameter	Neonate	Adult
Tidal volume, mL/kg	6	6
Dead space, mL/kg	2	2
FRC, mL/kg	28	30–35
Oxygen consumption, mL/kg	4–6	2–3
Alveolar ventilation, mL/kg	100–150	50–60
VA:FRC	4.5:1	1.5:1
Closing volume	Increased	

FRC, functional residual capacity; VA, alveolar ventilation.

airway edema can have a profound effect on air flow through an already narrowed airway.

The total oxygen consumption (per kilogram of body weight) of a neonate is two to three times that of an adult (25,26) (Table 1). However, the work of breathing for each kilogram of body weight is similar in infants and children. The oxygen consumption of the respiratory muscles of a premature infant is three times that in adults (6% vs. 2% of total oxygen consumption). In the adult, if the work of breathing is increased by a factor of two or three, total oxygen consumption increases minimally (from 2% to between 4% and 6%). In contrast, because breathing constitutes a larger portion of total oxygen consumption in the infant, an increase of twofold or threefold in work of breathing produces an increase in oxygen consumption that the infant may not tolerate (an increase from 6% to between 12% and 18%) (27).

Differences in muscle fiber composition of the diaphragm and intercostal muscles of premature and full-term infants may predispose them to early respiratory fatigue as compared with older children. Type 1 muscle fibers (fatigue-resistant, highly oxidative) in the diaphragm and intercostal muscles are proportionately reduced in children under the age of 2 years: 10% of the diaphragm in the premature neonate and 25% in the full-term neonate as compared with 55% in the adult (28–30).

EVALUATION OF THE PEDIATRIC AIRWAY

Accurate prediction of the difficult airway is paramount in allowing a safe, calculated approach to securing the airway. Recognizing a difficult airway requires availability of predictive tests and adequate patient cooperation to allow precise evaluation to take place. The first step in evaluating the pediatric airway is a thorough history and physical examination.

A history of difficulty managing the airway should be taken seriously and may be the only clue to potential difficulty in an otherwise normal-appearing airway. The history should emphasize prior airway difficulties during administration of anesthesia, as well as congenital, inflammatory, traumatic, or other acquired problems that may adversely affect the airway. History may also reveal problems with respiratory infections and feedings that have led to severe coughing and cyanosis. Any history of snoring or noisy breathing, recurrent croup, stridor, hoarse voice, reactive airway disease, prior surgery (tracheotomy or operations on the palate or larynx), or prior radiation treatments should alert the anesthesiologist to the possibility of an abnormal airway. Medical records should be examined in detail, including antenatal workup, surgical records, and previous anesthetic records, for details of both successful and unsuccessful techniques employed.

The physical examination should focus on the airway and the respiratory and cardiovascular systems. The examination should include observation of the color of the mucous membranes; mouth breathing; evidence of respiratory distress (retractions, tracheal tug, stridor, anxiety, nasal flaring); respiratory rate; absent, loose, or chipped teeth; and neck mobility. The size and shape of the mandible; the size and configuration of the tongue, tonsillar pillars, uvula, soft palate; and the distance between the ramus of the mandible and the thyroid cartilage should also be examined. A narrow, high-arched palate may increase the difficulty of intubation, as may a narrow lower jaw. Uvular visibility is of less significance than the amount of potential space for soft tissue displacement.

Physical examination may reveal gross abnormalities, such as a hypoplastic mandible, or a short or webbed neck, that may fit a recognizable syndrome. Where there is one congenital malformation, there may be another less obvious, such as cardiac or renal abnormalities. If the child in fact has a syndrome, or a syndrome is suspected, specific anesthetic implications must be considered.

Clinical evaluation of the airway in the infant or small child may be hindered by lack of patient cooperation and difficulty in interpretation. As a result, the anesthesiologist is often faced with the prospect of inducing anesthesia with less objective airway information available than may be necessary to predict a difficult airway accurately. This places the anesthesiologist at a disadvantage in confronting an unexpectedly difficult airway, and highlights the added significance of airway history, when available.

Routine evaluation of the airway usually requires only a thorough history and physical examination. However, if airway disease is revealed, radiologic and biochemical studies may be invaluable to evaluate and clarify a disorder further. Roentgenograms of the lateral neck and chest, tomograms, xerograms, and computed tomography provide detailed information of airway anatomy. Blood gas analysis or noninvasive pulse oximetry may help in assessing the degree of physiologic compromise. Pulmonary function tests (and flow-volume loops) are effective in evaluating the nature and degree of pulmonary dysfunction.

PEDIATRIC AIRWAY EQUIPMENT

Oropharyngeal Airways

Indications for the use of an oropharyngeal airway consist of an obstructed upper airway in an unconscious infant or child. An oral airway can also be used as a bite block to protect an endotracheal tube and as an adjunct for oropharyngeal suctioning. An oral airway should not be used in a conscious or lightly anesthetized child because it may induce vomiting.

Oral airways are easy to use and are available for pediatric patients of all ages. It is important to select an oral airway of appropriate size in order to provide a clear, unobstructed airway. An improperly sized oral airway may fail to keep the tongue separated from the back of the pharynx and may, in some cases, actually worsen airway obstruction. A small airway may push the base of the tongue posteriorly, causing airway obstruction, while a large airway may obstruct the glottic opening by pushing the epiglottis down. A properly sized oral airway is one that extends from the corner of the mouth and ends just cephalad to the angle of the mandible. The airway may be placed next to the face to evaluate the size. Insertion of an oral airway can be facilitated with a tongue blade.

Complications associated with oral airways are uncommon. Malposition can traumatize the teeth, tongue, and pharynx. In addition, as noted previously, improper placement can aggravate airway obstruction.

Nasopharyngeal Airways

Nasopharyngeal airways are trumpeted, soft rubber or polyvinyl chloride tubes that may be used in awake, semicomatose, or lightly anesthetized patients. This alternative airway device provides a conduit for gas flow between the tongue and the posterior pharyngeal wall. Measurement of the tube size is based on its outer diameter and circumference; tubes are available in sizes 12F to 36F (French).

The more patent naris should be selected for insertion. The nasal trumpet should be well lubricated and inserted in a posterior direction perpendicularly to the coronal plane and passed along the floor of the nasopharynx. A local vasoconstrictor like phenylephrine should be applied prior to insertion to minimize bleeding. The proper length of insertion is estimated by measuring the distance from the tip of the nose to the tragus of the ear.

Contraindications to nasal airways include nasal airway occlusion, nasal fractures, markedly deviated septum, suspected or proven basilar skull fractures, coagulopathy, prior transsphenoidal hypophysectomy, cerebrospinal rhinorrhea, and adenoid hypertrophy (relative) (31).

Nasal airway complications include damage to adenoid tissue or mucosa, epistaxis, and laryngospasm. Small-diameter nasal airways may easily become obstructed with mucus, blood, vomitus, or adenoid tissue and require frequent suctioning, making them unreliable for long-term use.

Masks

The ideal pediatric mask should provide an airtight seal between the mask and the patient's face without excessive pressure on the eyes. It should accommodate an oropharyngeal or nasopharyngeal airway during spontaneous, assisted, or controlled ventilation. When a mask is held, care should be taken to avoid digital pressure in the region of the submental triangle, which can push the tongue up to the roof of the mouth and aggravate any airway obstruction.

The three most common types of pediatric face masks are the Ohio anatomic mask, the transparent cushioned disposable mask, and the Rendell-Baker-Soucek mask. The Ohio anatomic mask and the Rendell-Baker-Soucek masks both have low dead space and lack a cushioned rim. The transparent cushioned disposable mask has an air cushion attached to the rim, which helps attain a good mask seal. The primary disadvantage of this mask is the increase in dead space, although it appears to be of little clinical consequence.

A poor mask fit can result in gas leaks that lead to a waste of gas and contamination of the operating room air, inability to maintain positive pressure, and potentially compromised ventilation and oxygenation. Other complications associated with using a face mask include pressure from an incorrectly positioned mask or a seal that is too tight, resulting in skin, nerve, or eye injury. Reactions to the residue from the sterilization process and allergies to the mask material, while rare, have been reported.

Laryngoscope Blades

Two general types of laryngoscope blades are used in pediatric anesthesia, the curved blade and the straight blade. All other blades are variations of these. The straight blade is usually used for laryngoscopy in neonates, infants, and young children. The curved blade is more commonly used in older children.

Straight blades commonly have a straight tip (Jackson-Wisconsin blade) or a curved tip (Miller blade). The straight blade is designed to be placed under the epiglottis and relies on direct upward pressure on the epiglottis to expose the vocal cords. The most commonly used straight blades are the Miller blades. A modification of the Jackson-Wisconsin blade, the Wisconsin-Hipple (Wis-Hipple 1.5) blade, is especially designed for infants ages 9 months to 2 years.

The Macintosh curved blade is designed to lift the epiglottis out of the way by indirect vallecular traction when

TABLE 2. *Laryngoscope blade selection for pediatric patients*

	Size		
Age	Miller	Wis-Hippel	Macintosh
Premature	0		
Neonate	0 or 1		
1 mo–2 y	1	1.5	
2–6 y		1.5	2
6–12 y	2		2 or 3
> 12 y	2 or 3		3

its tip is inserted into the vallecula anterior to the epiglottis. A guide to the laryngoscope blades commonly used in pediatric anesthesia can be found in Table 2.

Endotracheal Tubes

Endotracheal tubes are constructed from many different materials: polyvinyl chloride (PVC), medical-grade silicone rubber, red rubber, nylon, or Teflon plastic (32). The only size requirement for manufacturers is that they standardize the internal diameter (ID) of an endotracheal tube. The external diameter varies depending on the manufacturer and tube construction. The most commonly used endotracheal tube in pediatric care today is the PVC tube.

Because of the many chemicals used in constructing endotracheal tubes, extensive testing has been done to ensure patient safety. Manufacturers test for tissue toxicity and irritant properties by either implant testing in a rabbit psoas muscle or by an *in vitro* implant testing method involving mouse fibroblast culture. Endotracheal tubes that have been implant-tested are stamped "I.T."; tubes tested by an *in vitro* method are stamped with the designation "Z-79" (Z-79 Committee of the American National Standards Institute).

Endotracheal tubes are calibrated according to internal diameter (millimeters), external diameter (millimeters), and length (centimeters). Oral endotracheal tubes are beveled approximately 45° in relation to their long axis. The bevel opening faces left in oral tubes and aids tube insertion through the vocal cords. Most endotracheal tubes are equipped with a side port (Murphy eye) to allow ventilation when the main port is occluded by secretions, blood clot, or tracheal wall.

There are numerous methods for estimating correct endotracheal tube size, including the patient's age, height, weight, and diameter of the external nares and smallest finger (33–37). Keep and Manford (33) have shown that calculations of endotracheal tube size based on patient height are more accurate than those based on either age or weight. By passing progressively larger tubes until they found the largest tube that could be gently passed into the trachea, Chodoff and Helrich (37a) discovered that the best correlation with tube size was age rather than height, weight, or body surface area. Although no formula or table guarantees selection of the appropriate endotracheal tube, the most common method is based on age (Table 3). Several formulas based on age have been proposed (38). Single-formula methods have been shown to lead frequently to inappropriate endotracheal tube selection (39,40). Penlington (41) suggested two formulas to estimate endotracheal tube size based on age. For a child younger than 6 years of age, endotracheal tube size can be estimated by the following formula:

$$\text{ETT Size (mm ID)} = \text{Age (y)}/3 + 3.75$$

For a child older than 6 years of age, endotracheal tube size can be estimated by the formula:

$$\text{Tube Size (mm ID)} = \text{Age (y)}/4 + 4.5$$

TABLE 3. *Endotracheal tube selection for pediatric patients*

	Size (mm ID)
Weight	
< 1500 g	2.5
1500–2500 g	3.0
> 2500 g	3.5
Age	
3–6 mo	3.5
6–12 mo	3.5–4.0
1–6 y	Age (y)/3 + 3.75
> 6 y	Age (y)/4 + 4.5

ID, internal diameter.

For premature and full-term infants during the first year of life, endotracheal tube size is typically selected on the basis of weight. The rapid growth during this period makes formulas based on age alone invalid. Suggested endotracheal tube size for premature infants weighing less than 1500 g is 2.5 mm; for neonates weighing 1500 to 5000 g, 3.0 to 3.5 mm; for infants 3 to 6 months, 3.5 mm; for infants 6 to 12 months, 3.5 to 4.0 mm. Because these are estimates, one should always have immediately at hand endotracheal tubes half a size smaller and larger than the one selected to allow for individual variability.

In general, uncuffed endotracheal tubes are selected in pediatric patients younger than 8 to 10 years. In addition, a higher incidence of postoperative sore throat, laryngeal damage, and tracheal stenosis occurs when a tube that is too large is used.

A properly sized uncuffed endotracheal tube allows a leak between 20 and 30 cm H_2O peak inflation pressure. The leak is easily assessed by slowly inflating the reservoir bag while listening over the mouth or larynx for an audible leak. The pressure at which the leak is audible approximates the pressure against the tracheal wall (42). If the leak occurs at less than 10 cm H_2O, the tube should be replaced with the next larger size. If a cuffed endotracheal tube is used, an endotracheal tube with a smaller internal diameter should be selected to compensate for the endotracheal tube cuff. Once the cuff is inflated, there should be an air leak between 20 and 30 cm H_2O peak inflation pressure. During general anesthesia with nitrous oxide, intracuff pressure increases because of diffusion of nitrous oxide into the cuff (43–45). Periodic re-evaluation of the air leak may protect against tracheal damage.

After intubation, the proper insertion distance must be established. In neonates and children up to 1 year of age, the length of the trachea (vocal cords to carina) varies from 5 to 9 cm. An approximation of length of insertion from the lips is 7 to 10 cm for premature and term infants, 10 cm for infants up to 3 months of age, 11 cm for infants up to 6 months of age, and 12 cm for infants 6 to 12 months of age. For children over the age of 1 year, the correct length of tube insertion (oral) can be approximated by formulas based on age or weight (35,46,47):

$$\text{Tube length (cm)} = \text{age (y)}/2 + 12$$

$$\text{Tube length (cm)} = \text{weight (kg)}/5 + 12$$

These formulas provide only a guideline. Endotracheal tube insertion length must be confirmed by auscultation for equality of breath sounds, observation of symmetric chest expansion, and clinical judgment. For nasally placed endotracheal tubes, 3 cm should be added to the oral formula (48).

Specialized Endotracheal Tubes

The RAE Tube

Preformed or RAE tubes (named after its inventors, Drs. Ring, Adair, and Elwyn) are available in all sizes (2.5- to 11.0-mm ID) in both oral and nasal forms. These are PVC tubes that are angled to allow a low facial profile to minimize kinking in patients having oromaxillofacial surgery. A major limitation of these tubes is their availability in only one length for each internal diameter. Should a patient require a tube larger than usual for age, the tube may be too long, increasing the risk of kinking or endobronchial intubation.

The Endotrol Tube

The Endotrol or guidable tube is a PVC tube with a built-in stylet system to facilitate its guidance into the larynx. When the trigger at the proximal end is pulled, traction is applied to the tip of the tube, causing it to antevert.

The Armored/Anode/Reinforced Tube

The armored/anode/reinforced tube has a stainless steel reinforcing or nylon filament embedded in the tube wall. This design provides resistance to collapse or kinking. Increased flexibility necessitates the use of a stylet during intubation. This tube can be inserted orally, nasally, or through a tracheotomy or laryngectomy stoma.

The Laser Tube

The laser tube is designed to decrease the risk for airway fire and release of toxic by-products (49–51). All endotracheal tubes not made of metal are capable of combustion. Endotracheal tubes (usually red rubber) can be protected with metallic tape to decease the risk for penetration and ignition. Another effective method of protecting conventional endotracheal tube shafts is with Laser-Guard (America Corporation, Mystic, Connecticut) (52). Laser-Guard consists of a layer of silver foil covered with a thin, absorbent sponge layer that acts as a heat sink when moistened.

There are several other endotracheal tubes specifically designed for laser surgery. The Xomed Laser tube (Xomed, Jacksonville, Florida) is a silicone tube with metal particles covering the main shaft and cuff. The Laser-Flex tube (Mallinckrodt, Glen Falls, New York) is a double-cuffed, silicone-coated metal tube that is impervious to laser radiation. The Norton endotracheal tube (A.V. Mueller, Niles, Illinois) is constructed of spirally wound stainless steel with no cuff and is the only commercially available, completely nonflammable endotracheal tube (53).

One problem with all cuffed laser tubes is the vulnerability of the cuff to laser beam penetration. Filling the cuff with water or saline solution instead of air is a commonly practiced safety precaution. The fluid acts as a heat sink, which in cases of rupture may help in dousing the fire (54). Methylene blue can be added to the cuff as a visual indicator of cuff rupture (55).

The Double-Lumen Endobroncheal Tube

Double-lumen tubes are used whenever it is desirable to ventilate or isolate one lung selectively. They consist of two tubes attached together, side by side, with one side longer than the other and with the tip curved to the longer side. Double-lumen tubes are designed for insertion into the left or right main bronchus.

Various double-lumen tubes are available (Carlens tube, White tube, Bryce Smith tube, and Robertshaw tube). The left-sided double-lumen endobronchial tube is more commonly used because it is easily placed and has a greater margin of safety.

TECHNIQUES OF TRACHEAL INTUBATION

Direct Laryngoscopy

Head and Neck Position

The optimal position for pediatric intubation is the classic "sniffing" position—cervical flexion with head extension (56). This position results in proper alignment of the oral, laryngeal, and pharyngeal axes for more direct visualization of the laryngeal structures and improved hypopharyngeal patency (57). In older children and adults, this position can be achieved by placement of padding beneath the occiput of the head, resulting in anterior displacement of the cervical spine and extension of the head at the atlanto-occipital joint. The prominent occiput in infants can cause the head to flex on the cervical spine, making it unnecessary to elevate the occiput. Simple extension of the head or padding below the shoulders allows head extension and cervical flexion. Incorrect positioning of the head and neck is the most common cause of difficult intubation.

Cricoid Pressure

Application of cricoid pressure, or "Selleck's maneuver," is commonly used in patients at risk for aspiration (58). The cricoid cartilage is the only tracheal ring that is complete. Pressure directed posteriorly on this cartilage compresses and occludes the esophagus against the C-6 vertebra. Properly applied cricoid pressure requires a force of 44 newtons ($kg \cdot m/s^2$) to prevent regurgitation of gastric contents (59). This maneuver helps prevent passive regurgitation of gastric contents into the larynx and pharynx and limits gastric inflation during mask ventilation. It does not prevent active vomiting.

Stylets

The stylet is a thin, malleable introducer commonly made of metal or plastic. When inserted into the lumen of an endotracheal tube, the stylet can be bent into a "hockey stick" shape to facilitate intubation of an anteriorly positioned larynx. The stylet should be well lubricated to ease placement and withdrawal. Since most intubations can be performed safely without a stylet, they should not be used routinely, except in small (< 4.0 mm) endotracheal tubes. Stylets should be reserved for rapid-sequence induction, emergency intubation, or cases in which a difficult airway is anticipated. To avoid trauma and possible perforation of the larynx, trachea, or esophagus, the stylet should not extend through the Murphy eye or beyond the tip of the endotracheal tube.

Light-Wand Intubation

The light wand or lighted stylet is a reusable malleable stylet with a small, battery-powered light source or fiberoptic beam at its distal end. It is a useful adjunct in managing the difficult airway in both awake and anesthetized patients whose glottic opening cannot be completely visualized by direct laryngoscopy (60–62). This technique is useful in patients with suspected neck injury, because minimal movement of the neck is required.

Prior to insertion, the light wand is preformed into a "hockey stick" to facilitate entry into the glottic opening. The light wand is lubricated and inserted into an appropriately sized endotracheal tube. The tube and stylet are then orally inserted, while the neck is observed for transillumination. Turning off the room lights aids in identification of translaryngeal illumination. A well-defined, bright, cherry red glow at the level of the cricothyroid ensures proper position of the stylet. A diffuse or a laterally displaced light indicates the stylet is not in the correct position. Once properly positioned, the endotracheal tube is passed over the light wand into the trachea.

A major disadvantage of the light wand is that it entails a blind technique. However, for the same reason, blood and secretions in the oropharynx that would obscure direct vision with conventional laryngoscopy or fiberoptic bronchoscopy do not pose much of a problem with the light wand.

Tactile Tracheal Intubation

The tactile method of intubation, one of the first methods of endotracheal intubation, was developed in 1880 as a simple method without the need for instruments (63–65). Tactile intubation can be performed on awake, topically anesthetized patients; patients under general anesthesia; or deeply comatose patients (66). One advantage is that the technique can be accomplished with minimal movement of the head and neck.

The technique of tactile intubation consists of palpating the epiglottis with the middle and index fingers of the left hand, palm side down. The left hand retracts the tongue forward. The right hand introduces the curved endotracheal tube into the mouth and pharynx. The index finger of the left hand directs the tube under the epiglottis as the tongue and jaw are lifted. At this point, the endotracheal tube can be slipped through the vocal cords.

Anterior Commissure Laryngoscope with Optic Stylet

The use of the anterior commissure laryngoscope with optic stylet (or optic telescope) can improve the visualization of the larynx in children with mandibular hypoplasia and/or macroglossia. An endotracheal tube placed over the optic stylet can be advanced through the anterior commissure laryngoscope and into the trachea under direct visualization. For a neonate, a 9-mm laryngoscope with a small telescope allows intubation with a 3.0-mm endotracheal tube.

Flexible Fiberoptic Laryngoscopy

The primary reasons for the use of the flexible fiberoptic bronchoscope is to facilitate tracheal intubation and assess location of the tip of the endotracheal tube within the airway (67,68). There are numerous other diagnostic and therapeutic indications for its use. The only absolute contraindication to flexible fiberoptic bronchoscopy is patient refusal. Successful fiberoptic intubation requires a relatively secretion-free environment and space that can be seen through. The presence of copious secretions or blood in the airway, as in trauma, makes fiberoptic work difficult. Fiberoptic bronchoscopy is a learned skill, and it requires considerable time to achieve proficiency (69).

Pediatric flexible fiberoptic bronchoscopes are available in various sizes (1.8, 2.2, 2.7, and 3.5 mm). These numbers represent outer diameter, in contrast to rigid bronchoscopes, for which the size numbers indicate internal diameter. The major advantage of the 3.5-mm flexible fiberoptic bronchoscope is the presence of the suction channel. Its drawback for pediatric use is its size: the smallest endotracheal tube it can pass through is the 4.5-mm tube. On the other hand, the ultrathin pediatric flexible fiberoptic bronchoscope (2.2 mm) can be accommodated by a 2.5-mm-ID endotracheal tube (70). If an ultrathin pediatric flexible fiberoptic bronchoscope is not available or the endotracheal tube is smaller than the available endoscope, a guide wire can be passed into the trachea through the suction port of the endoscope (71, 72). After the guide wire is passed and the endoscope is removed, the endotracheal tube can be threaded over the wire into the trachea. The retrograde-assisted fiberoptic intubation is another possible method of tracheal intubation for patients whose vocal cords are difficult to visualize with the fiberoptic bronchoscope. The laryngeal mask airway is useful to guide the flexible fiberoptic bronchoscope to the glottis in both awake patients with topical anesthesia and patients with general anesthesia who are breathing spontaneously (73–79).

Fiberoptic bronchoscopy can be performed in awake patients, using appropriate topical and regional anesthesia, and in anesthetized patients. If flexible fiberoptic bronchoscopy is being performed because of a difficult airway, then allowing the patient to breathe spontaneously under deep inhalation anesthesia is preferable. The possibility of laryngospasm and airway obstruction and a plan for its treatment should be kept in mind. Alternatively, some patients with a difficult airway may be anesthetized, relaxed, and intermittently ventilated during flexible fiberoptic bronchoscopy if they have a history of being easy to ventilate.

In the awake, sedated patient, placing the patient partly head up (in a semiseated position) may facilitate bronchoscopy by displacing the tongue and soft tissue more caudad and out of the way of the bronchoscope. In the anesthetized patient, the supine position is maintained.

Complications from flexible fiberoptic bronchoscopy are rare when it is performed in a well-controlled setting with appropriate patient monitoring and skilled personnel. Potential complications include injury to the nasopharynx, mechanical injury, pneumothorax, hypoventilation and hypoxia (from the presence of a bronchoscope within a small-diameter lumen, or from oversedation or aspiration), and iatrogenic pulmonary infection. Newborns and infants are more susceptible to bradycardia from vagal stimulation.

Retrograde Intubation

The retrograde wire intubation technique is an alternative to intubation when other methods have been unsuccessful (80). The technique in a child is similar to that for the adult. The cricothyroid membrane is identified and punctured in the midline with a 20-gauge IV catheter, and its intratracheal position is confirmed by aspiration of air. A 0.021-cm guide wire is threaded through this needle and directed cephalad through the trachea, larynx, and pharynx and retrieved through the mouth. An endotracheal tube is passed over the wire and advanced beyond the vocal cords by using the wire as a guide.

Laryngeal Mask Airway

The laryngeal mask airway (LMA) was first described in the early 1980s and made commercially available in the United States in 1991 (81). The LMA consists of a silicone rubber shaft connected to a distal elliptical mask-like device with an inflatable rim. The LMA is available in five sizes, both adult and pediatric, and is reusable (Table 4). The LMA is designed to be positioned blindly in the pharynx, forming a low-pressure seal around the subglottic area. It is relatively simple to insert and has been successfully used in pediatric patients in whom tracheal intubation was difficult or even impossible (82,83).

The LMA is inserted with the patient in the sniffing position (84,85). The posterior aspect of the LMA should be lubricated with a water-soluble lubricant after the cuff is fully deflated. Holding the LMA like a pencil, the operator inserts it through the mouth blindly in the midline with the concavity forward, while pressing on the anterior shaft with the tip of the index finger toward the hard

TABLE 4. *Laryngeal mask airway selection*

Size	Patient	Cuff volume (mL)
1	Infant < 6.5 kg	2–4
2	Infant 6.5–20 kg	10
2.5	Children 20–30 kg	15
3	Children > 30 kg and small adults	20
4	Average and large adults	30

palate and guiding it toward the pharynx. When the upper esophageal sphincter is reached, a characteristic resistance is felt. The cuff is then inflated with air (normally the cuff should be inflated without holding the tube to enable the expanding cuff to find its correct position in the pharynx). When correctly placed, the black vertical line on the posterior aspect of the tube should always face directly backward, toward the head of the patient. The LMA should be left in place until the patient can open his or her mouth on command. During emergence, the patient should not be stimulated (i.e., suctioned) and the cuff should not be deflated (until the patient can open his or her mouth on command).

This device should be used only as an adjunct to airway management and not as a substitute for endotracheal intubation. The LMA does not form an airtight seal around the larynx, and airway pressures exceeding 15 to 20 cm H_2O may predispose to gastric insufflation and regurgitation/aspiration (86). Other patients for whom the LMA is considered unsuitable include those with low pulmonary compliance or high airway resistance, residual airway reflexes, inability to extend the neck, and pharyngeal disease or trauma.

Complications associated with the LMA are rare and include the possibility of regurgitation of gastric contents and pulmonary aspiration, oral and pharyngeal mucosal injury during insertion, laryngeal spasm and coughing (which may occur if the LMA is inserted in a lightly anesthetized patient), and negative-pressure pulmonary edema after improper placement in a spontaneously breathing patient (87–89).

Bullard Laryngoscope

The Bullard laryngoscope, functioning as an indirect fiberoptic laryngoscope, provides direct visualization of the vocal cords (90,91). It is available in both adult and pediatric sizes. The advantage of this laryngoscope is that it can be introduced into the oropharynx with minimal mouth opening (oral opening of 0.64 cm required). Preloading the intubating stylet involves lubricating the stylet and positioning the endotracheal tube so that the distal end of the stylet projects through the Murphy eye of the endotracheal tube. The blade is then inserted into the mouth with the handle in the horizontal plane and rotated into the vertical plane, allowing it to slide around the midline of the tongue and into the posterior pharynx. Gentle traction is applied against the posterior surface of the tongue to obtain visualization of the glottic aperture. With the stylet pointed directly at the glottic opening, the endotracheal tube is advanced under direct vision into the trachea. As with other retraction blades, a considerable amount of practice is required to become skilled with its use.

SURGICAL AIRWAYS

Cricothyroidotomy

The pediatric cricothyroid membrane is of small width (approximately 1 mm in the infant) and can be easily damaged during attempts at cricothyroidotomy. This procedure generally is reserved for airway emergencies (92–94).

Cricothyroidotomy involves placing a large IV catheter through the cricothyroid membrane into the trachea. After placement is confirmed by aspiration of air, oxygen can be administered by connecting the breathing circuit directly to the IV catheter with the use of a 3-mm adapter from a pediatric endotracheal tube. Oxygenation, but not ventilation, can be achieved through the catheter at rates of 10 to 12 L/min (95,96). This is a temporary measure and is contraindicated in patients with complete upper airway obstruction. Some ventilation can be achieved when the catheter is connected to some form of jet ventilation (97–99). The jet source must include a regulator to adjust the pressure. However, this technique must be used with extreme caution in infants and children (100). Massive subcutaneous emphysema or tension pneumothorax may occur with the use of percutaneous jet ventilation.

Complications of emergency needle cricothyroidotomy include perforation of the esophagus, breakage or bending of the needle, subcutaneous emphysema, pneumothorax, pneumomediastinum, pneumopericardium, hypoventilation with hypercapnia, bleeding, and infection.

Tracheostomy

Elective tracheostomy with local anesthesia should be considered for infants and children who have severe upper airway obstruction. Emergency tracheostomy in the pediatric patient is fraught with potential hazards of esophageal perforation, uncontrolled bleeding, and technical difficulty. Not only are structures smaller and more difficult to expose, but general anesthesia is almost always required. Emergency tracheostomy should be considered only in extreme situations when intubation is technically impossible.

MANAGEMENT OF SPECIFIC DISEASE STATES

Cystic Hygroma

Cystic hygroma is a benign congenital tumor of lymphatic origin (101,102). It is a multiloculated, fluid-containing lesion that most commonly occurs in the neck and tongue but can also be found in other locations, including the mediastinum. The lesion may involve the tongue sufficiently to fill the oral cavity, often protruding outside the mouth. Involvement of the upper airway may include the tongue, lips, floor of the mouth, styloid process, larynx, epiglottis, and aryepiglottic folds. The lesion may be present at birth but usually occurs during the first year of life. Although growth of the lesion is unpredictable, spontaneous regression rarely occurs.

The majority of cystic hygromas are asymptomatic and present as soft, fluid-filled masses in the subcutaneous tissue. Lesions involving the tongue, pharynx, or larynx may be symptomatic and life-threatening. Mediastinal cystic hygromas also may result in respiratory distress, chylothorax, and chylopericardium.

Treatment is surgical excision when the diagnosis is made. Delay is unwarranted because of the hazards of infection, progressive growth with extension into previously uninvolved areas, and dysphagia or airway obstruction.

The extent of the tumor should be defined by computed axial tomography (CAT) or magnetic resonance imaging (MRI) before surgery. In addition, all patients should receive a chest x-ray. If the tumor involves the tongue, tracheostomy under local anesthesia is the safest way to establishing the airway (103). An alternative to tracheostomy is fiberoptic bronchoscopy (104). Needle aspiration of the cysts may be carried out as a temporizing emergency procedure.

Cervical Spinal Injury

Pediatric spinal cord injuries account for only 5% of all spinal cord injuries; however, they carry a high mortality rate (105–108). Although spinal cord injuries are rare in the pediatric population, all children with an injury above the clavicle should be treated as though they have a cervical spinal injury.

The type of cervical spinal injury varies according to age (106,109–114). Injuries in infants and young children occur chiefly at the atlanto-occipital, atlantoaxial, and C2-3 levels and are ligamentous in nature. Older children display an adult-type injury pattern characterized by fractures anywhere along the length of the cervical spine, particularly in the lower cervical levels. Children under 4 years of age are at increased risk for upper cervical spinal injury when placed in forward-facing car seats (115,116). Children with Down syndrome are also reported to be at greater risk for cervical spinal injury following trauma (117,118).

Children with spinal cord injury or disruption of the spinal cord commonly present in respiratory distress, often in cardiopulmonary arrest (119). Impaired respiratory function and respiratory failure are the major cause of morbidity and mortality following an isolated cervical spinal injury (107). The level of injury determines the degree of impairment. Lesions involving the phrenic nerve (C3-5) usually result in apnea. Lesions at C-5 leave partial diaphragmatic innervation but impair abdominal and intercostal accessory muscles. Lesions between C-6 and T-7 leave diaphragmatic innervation intact, but cause diminished accessory muscular function.

Airway management in patients with known cervical injuries is controversial. Orotracheal and nasotracheal intubation, and tracheotomy can be performed successfully without spinal cord damage as long as the neck is adequately immobilized (108,120–122). Outcome data indicate that there is no difference in terms of incidence of neurologic deficit between awake intubation (orotracheal or nasotracheal) and intubation under general anesthesia as long as the head is not moved (i.e., in-line cervical stabilization is used) (106). In-line cervical stabilization means immobilization and not traction.

Orotracheal intubation facilitated by rapid-sequence intravenous induction and axial in-line stabilization is the technique of choice for intubating the trachea of spinal cord-injured patients. Induction of anesthesia and muscle relaxation in these patients are associated with some disadvantages. The success of orotracheal intubation diminishes when cervical spinal injuries preclude positioning of the head and neck in the sniffing position. Subsequent multiple attempts at endotracheal intubation may predispose the patient with abolished airway reflexes to aspiration and airway obstruction. Application of cricoid pressure may cause further displacement of vertebral fragments, particularly because cervical fractures/dislocations occur frequently at C-5 and C-6, the area at which the pressure is applied (123).

An awake intubation, either blind nasal, fiberoptic, or surgical, is recommended by some authors so that neurologic status can be verified after intubation. The most frequently emphasized disadvantages of this protocol are the risks for nasal bleeding and endotracheal tube entry into the cranial vault when co-existing head and/or facial injuries have caused cranial base fractures.

Maxillary and Mandibular Disorders

Maxillary or midfacial disorders affecting airway management include hypoplasia, trauma, and mass lesions. Maxillary hypoplasia results from premature synostosis of facial and cranial sutures and generally represents one of multiple facial dysmorphic features found in certain forms of craniosynostosis, such as Apert, Pfeiffer, and Crouzon syndromes. These syndromes include characteristic head and facial dysmorphic features and can have associated anomalies of the central nervous system, head, and extremities (124). Both the upper and lower airway may be adversely affected in these patients (125). Maxillary retrusion may be associated with choanal stenosis, reduction in nasopharyngeal size, and palatal deformity (126). Together, such features can result in upper airway obstruction and influence adequacy of mask fit (127). In certain forms of craniosynostosis, the cervical spine and lower airway may also be abnormal (128). Patients with Apert and Crouzon syndromes may have cervical spinal fusion, tracheomalacia, bronchomalacia, solid cartilaginous trachea, and tracheal stenosis (129,130).

Mandibular hypoplasia or micrognathia is a finding in a number of syndromes (131). Pierre Robin syndrome, Goldenhar syndrome, Nager syndrome, and Treacher Collins syndrome are just a few examples (Fig. 4). Micrognathia is often associated with other anomalies adversely affecting the airway. Patients with Pierre Robin syndrome have glossoptosis and cleft palate in addition to micrognathia. A reduced mandibular size causes posterior regression of the tongue and reduced hyomental space. Such patients often present with airway obstruction during infancy resulting from contact between the tongue and the hypopharynx, requiring interventions such as nasopharyngeal tube placement, anterior suturing of the tongue, or tracheostomy. If tracheal intubation is required, visualization of the glottis may be difficult or impossible owing to reduced anterior space for displacement of the tongue. It should be noted that micrognathia may also hamper placement of a tight-fitting mask.

Airway management in these patients requires a complete history and physical examination. Events such as snoring, airway obstruction, and previous anesthetic difficulties encountered in managing the airway and associated features such as choanal stenosis, upper airway obstruction, tracheomalacia, and cervical spinal fusion must be sought out. There should be a detailed examination of the airway, evaluating the extent of mouth opening, tongue size, hyomandibular distance, and head and neck mobility. In small or uncooperative pediatric patients, complete examination may be hampered. Based on the evaluation, a primary anesthetic plan and alternatives should be formulated. In children who are not easily separated from the parent, the use of premedication should be individualized. If the child has a history of significant airway obstruction or obstructive apnea, premedication is best avoided. If premedication is used, the child must be closely observed, and suction and airway equipment must be close at hand. Parental presence during induction of anesthesia as an alternative to premedication should be considered.

If the child's airway is assessed as difficult to manage, one of the various awake methods of tracheal intubation with adequate topical anesthesia is preferable (132–134). Inspection during awake direct laryngoscopy may provide information regarding the ability to visualize the glottis following general anesthesia. In small children, awake tracheal intubation may be difficult, and sedation or general anesthesia may be necessary. Sedation in children with a difficult airway should be used with extreme caution and titrated in small increments. If general anesthesia is chosen, then inhalation induction with halothane and oxygen can be used. Placement of a laryngeal mask airway in the awake infant and its use for induction of inhalation anesthesia followed by tracheal intubation has been described (135). When the LMA is correctly positioned, it may be used with a flexible fiberoptic broncho-

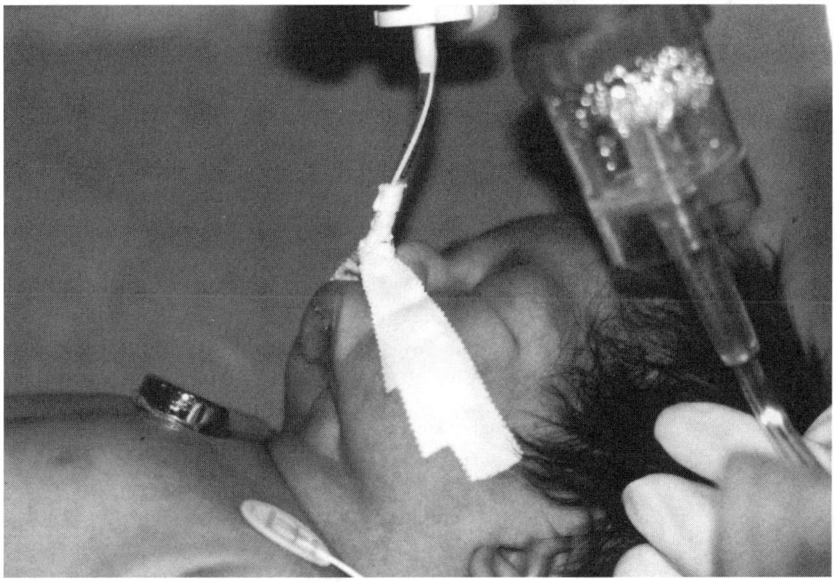

FIG. 4. Pierre Robin sequence. Note the marked mandibular hypoplasia, which in this infant contributed to airway obstruction following birth. A nasopharyngeal airway was necessary to maintain airway patency. This infant was tracheally intubated with an ultrathin flexible fiberoptic bronchoscope and required a tracheostomy.

scope to intubate the trachea, or it may be removed while tracheal intubation is accomplished by indirect techniques, as with the lighted stylet (135,76). Use of an anticholinergic agent in infants and young children helps avoid bradycardia during deep inhalation anesthesia and also helps diminish oral secretions. Allowing maintenance of spontaneous ventilation provides an added safety element should mask ventilation become difficult in these patients. In select patients who are easy to mask ventilate, muscle relaxants can be used to facilitate tracheal intubation following anesthesia. One must realize that face mask fit may not be ideal, and there must be alternate plans of intervention should airway obstruction occur during inhalation anesthesia. Continuous positive airway pressure (CPAP), optimal head and neck positioning, and oral or nasopharyngeal airways may be necessary to maintain a patent airway. If airway obstruction or laryngospasm persists despite these measures, the use of succinylcholine must be considered. Following deep inhalation anesthesia, direct laryngoscopy may be performed, but the number of attempts should be limited to avoid pharyngeal swelling and airway obstruction (136). Alternatively, one of several methods of indirect laryngeal visualization or "blind" techniques (e.g., lighted stylet) may be used to secure the airway.

Epiglottitis

Epiglottitis, also referred to as "supraglottitis," constitutes an airway emergency, as it can quickly progress to complete obstruction of the airway. Epiglottitis almost always results from bacterial infection, which causes inflammation and swelling of the epiglottis. In children, the bacterial etiology is most commonly *Haemophilus influenzae* type b (Hib). Since the introduction of Hib vaccine, epiglottitis caused by Hib, as well as the overall incidence of epiglottitis, is decreasing (137). The age group with the highest predilection is 2 to 6 years, although epiglottitis can occur in infants, older children, and adults (138–140). Recent studies seem to suggest the age range is increasing (138).

The signs and symptoms of epiglottitis in children differ from those in adults, both in nature and speed of onset (138). The child may complain of a sore throat and display dysphagia, drooling, muffled voice, respiratory distress, preference for the sitting position, high fever, and a toxic appearance (141). In the pediatric population, the disease is quickly progressive, often with only a few hours between onset of symptoms and complete airway obstruction (142,143). The younger the child, the more significant the respiratory distress and danger of airway compromise. Epiglottitis is generally diagnosed based on clinical findings. When the diagnosis of epiglottitis is suspected, it should be treated as an airway emergency with a systematic approach in management (144,145). Children should not have their oropharynx manipulated, nor should they be placed in the supine position (143, 146). If the diagnosis is questionable, and the patient condition permits, a lateral neck film can aid in the diagnosis by demonstrating a swollen enlarged epiglottis shadow and a distended hypopharynx (147–149). Radiologic studies must be carried out in the presence of a physician skilled in managing the pediatric airway. Definitive diagnosis is made following direct visualization of the epiglottis after general anesthesia (Fig. 5).

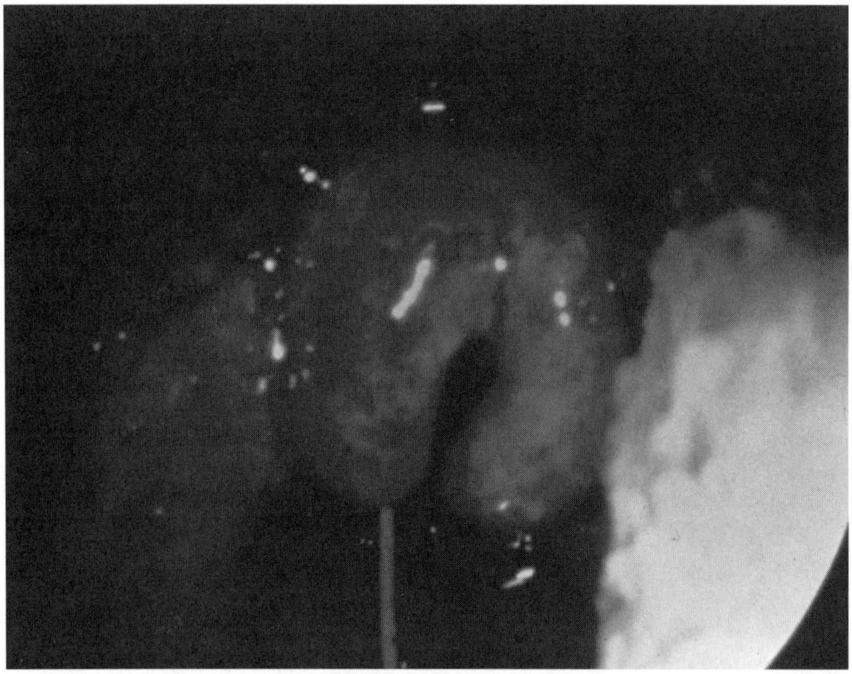

FIG. 5. Epiglottitis. This child's trachea was intubated following deep inhalation anesthesia. The epiglottis appears enlarged, erythematous, and friable.

Management of a child with epiglottitis involves prompt coordination of efforts between the anesthesiologist, otolaryngologist, and operating room staff (148). Because of the high risk for airway obstruction, children with epiglottitis should prophylactically have their airway secured in the operating room (148,150,151). It is important not to disturb the child with irritating procedures, such as attempts at intravenous placement and oral examination. These patients are at risk for acute laryngospasm (152). The child should be transported to an appropriately equipped operating room in the presence of a surgeon skilled in performing emergent tracheostomy in case the patient's airway becomes obstructed. If the child is stressed by parental separation, then one should consider taking a parent along to facilitate the induction of anesthesia. Sedating a child with epiglottitis may result in disastrous consequences.

Following gentle placement of minimally invasive monitors (pulse oximeter and precordial stethoscope), an inhalation induction is performed with the child in his/her preferred position, usually sitting. Oxygen and halothane are the preferred induction agents. If nitrous oxide is used to facilitate induction, it should be withdrawn as soon as possible. After the child is adequately anesthetized, he/she may be placed in a reclined position with the head slightly up, the remaining monitors attached, and an intravenous line secured. Atropine is recommended to maintain heart rate and to help dry oral secretions. The neck may be prepped for tracheostomy, should airway obstruction occur. Spontaneous ventilation should be preserved, although CPAP may be necessary to help maintain airway patency. After an adequate level of anesthesia has been established, which may require 10 to 15 minutes or more of breathing halothane, direct laryngoscopy is performed. The glottic opening will be reduced in size and sometimes may be difficult to appreciate. Gentle pressure on the child's chest may push out lung gas and reveal the glottic opening. A styletted, uncuffed, endotracheal tube, one or two sizes smaller than that normal for the child's age, should be inserted into the trachea and placement confirmed by auscultation and capnography. Some prefer to place an orotracheal tube initially and then change to a nasotracheal route for increased stability (149). If there is airway obstruction during induction of anesthesia or if tracheal intubation is unsuccessful, surgical airway tracheostomy or transtracheal jet ventilation should be accomplished.

After controlling the airway, appropriate cultures should be taken and antibiotics started. Patients are managed in the intensive care unit with adequate sedation and analgesia. Appropriate measures should be taken to ensure that the airway is not accidentally lost. After 24 to 48 hours of antibiotic therapy, the epiglottis is re-evaluated for possible controlled tracheal extubation, preferably in the operating room under anesthesia (153).

"Croup" is a term used to describe the clinical triad of barking cough, stridor, and hoarseness (154) (Fig. 6).

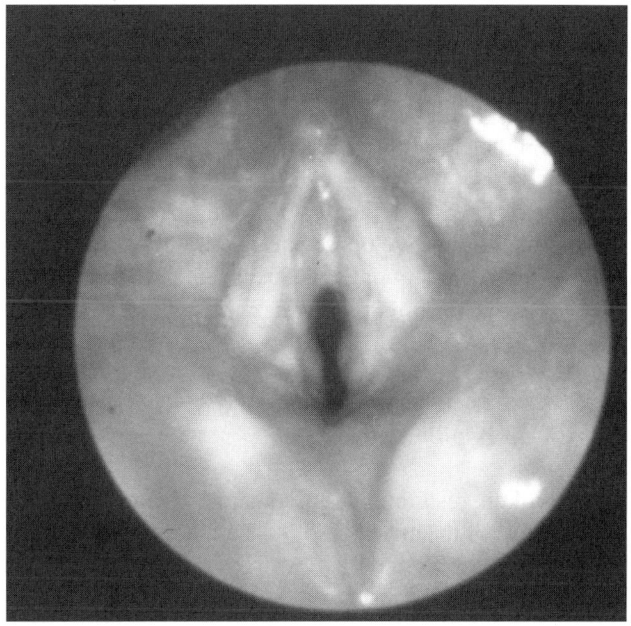

FIG. 6. Croup. This young child displays the subglottic edema consistent with laryngotracheobronchitis.

Although croup encompasses a group of disease states, it most commonly refers to laryngotracheobronchitis, a viral disease that afflicts children primarily between the ages of 1 and 3 years (155). The etiology is usually parainfluenza virus. Croup is a self-limited disease that generally begins as an upper respiratory infection progressing to a brassy cough, stridor, and hoarseness, with exacerbation of symptoms at night. Diagnosis is based on history and physical examination. An anterior-posterior neck x-ray may reveal a pencil or steeple sign, a nonspecific finding corresponding to a narrowing of the subglottic area

TABLE 5. *Comparison of epiglottitis and croup*

Factor	Epiglottitis	Croup
Age	2–6 y	6 mo–3 y
Sex	No. boys = No. girls	No. boys > No. girls
Etiology	Bacterial (*H. influenzae*)	Viral (Parainfluenza 3 virus)
Recurrence	Rare	Fairly common
Incidence	Uncommon	Common
Clinical features	Inspiratory stridor	Inspiratory stridor
	Sitting up/leaning forward	Lying down
	Dysphagia	Croupy cough
	Drooling	No drooling
	High fever	Low-grade fever
	Muffled voice	Hoarse voice
	Toxic appearance	Rhinorrhea
Lab/radiologic features	Neutrophilia	Lymphocytosis
	Swollen epiglottis	Narrowing of subglottic area
Onset	Sudden (hours)	Gradual (days)
Progression	Rapid	Slow, variable

(156). Treatment consists of adequate hydration, cool mist with possible need for supplemental oxygen, steroids, and racemic epinephrine. If children require supplemental oxygen or treatment with racemic epinephrine, they should be hospitalized for observation. Effectiveness of steroid therapy has long been the center of controversy, but it may have beneficial effects on spasmodic croup. Rarely, children develop severe respiratory distress despite medical treatment, requiring tracheal intubation (157). The features of epiglottitis and croup are compared in Table 5.

Laryngeal Papillomatosis

In children, respiratory papillomatosis is a severe recurrent disease of the airway (158). The disease is caused by the human papillomavirus, which is transmitted from affected mothers either by the intra-uterine or hematogenous route (159,160). Airway papillomatosis affects primarily the larynx, but it may extend to other structures of the airway, including the lung parenchyma. When the latter is involved, mortality is high. The disease afflicts mainly children ages 2 years and older, but it may occur in infancy, when the prognosis appears to be poor (161).

Airway disease relates to papilloma growth on the larynx and in the trachea, causing obstruction to air flow. Signs and symptoms include hoarse or altered voice, stridor, and respiratory distress. If left untreated, respiratory papillomatosis can lead to airway obstruction and death (Fig. 7). Although there are various medical treatment modalities, especially for severe forms of the disease, the major method of therapy remains laser surgical ablation (162–165). Children with aggressive papillomatosis may need laser therapy as frequently as every 1 to 2 weeks. These children come to the operating room with a mild to severe degree of airway obstruction and are at risk for complete airway occlusion, hypoventilation, and hypoxemia. In addition, the airway has to be shared with the surgeon, who must be provided with adequate access to the airway while adequate patient oxygenation and ventilation are ensured.

Sedation should be avoided in patients with severe obstruction and respiratory distress. If sedation is used, patients should be closely monitored, with personnel trained in airway management immediately available. Parental presence during induction of anesthesia is an alternative to premedication in selected patients.

Induction of anesthesia or muscle relaxation in the pediatric patient with airway papillomatosis can lead to a decrease in airway patency or result in complete airway obstruction. During induction of anesthesia, the child should be allowed to breathe spontaneously. Halothane and oxygen are ideal agents for inhalation induction. If nitrous oxide is used, it should be discontinued as soon as possible. CPAP may help maintain airway patency. An intravenous line should be secured and an anticholinergic agent may be administered. Direct laryngoscopy may be performed in order to evaluate the airway and its securability prior to muscle relaxation. Anesthesia may be maintained with intravenous medications, such as propofol, opioids, and benzodiazepines.

Alternative methods of ventilation and oxygenation during laser surgery include the jet Venturi system, the endo-

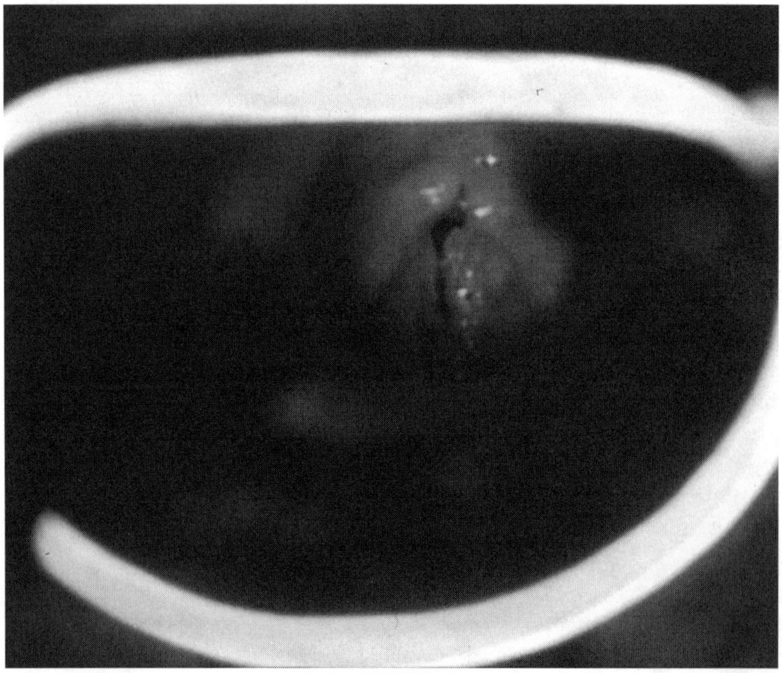

FIG. 7. Laryngeal papillomatosis. This photo of the glottis was taken with a suspension laryngoscope in place. The right vocal cord is the major site of papillomatous involvement in this child, who required frequent visits for laser therapy.

tracheal tube, or spontaneous ventilation (166). During jet ventilation or use of an endotracheal tube, patients may be relaxed with short- or intermediate-acting nondepolarizing muscle relaxants to improve chest wall compliance and immobilize the vocal cords during laser therapy.

Jet Venturi ventilation is established after induction of anesthesia and placement of a laryngoscope with a Luer-Lok attachment for connection to a wall oxygen source (167). An appropriate rate of jet ventilation is provided for the child's age. The jet Venturi system should be equipped with a pressure regulator to enable the anesthesiologist to use reduced pressures, adjusted to adequate chest movement for the child. This pressure varies with the size of the patient, lung and chest compliance, and accurate positioning of the tip of the jet ventilator system. The patient is best relaxed during this mode of ventilation. With correct use of the jet Venturi system, the patient can be adequately oxygenated and ventilated. The major advantage of this mode of ventilation is the surgeon's unhindered view of and access to the lesions. The disadvantages include potential complications of the high-pressure ventilation, such as barotrauma, hypoventilation, gastric distention, and potential distal displacement of resected tissue, viral particles, and blood (168,169).

A second method of providing anesthesia for airway papillomatosis is placement of an endotracheal tube following deep inhalation anesthesia. Maintenance anesthesia may be accomplished with any combination of intravenous or inhalation agents. Muscle relaxation facilitates the laser therapy. The surgeon may then alternate between removing the endotracheal tube during short periods of laser therapy and replacing it for oxygenation and ventilation. Alternatively, laser therapy may be possible with a laser-resistant endotracheal tube in place, although this may impede access to the lesion.

Another option is to allow the patient to breathe spontaneously during laryngoscopy and laser therapy (166). The potential advantage of this technique is the reduced chance of advancing resected tumor and viral particles into the distal airway. The disadvantages are the potential for laryngospasm and vocal cord movement during laser therapy.

Foreign Body Aspiration

Foreign body aspiration is a major cause of morbidity and mortality in children (170,171). Those between the ages of 1 and 2 years are the most frequently affected (172,173). The most common objects aspirated are food particles and toys, with many incidents of aspiration going unwitnessed, potentially delaying diagnosis (174, 175). The foreign body may be localized in any part of the airway, although most end up in the bronchial tree (Fig. 8). Airway manifestations of foreign body aspiration depend on the object's size relative to the airway, and the location and nature of the foreign body. The acute risk of foreign body aspiration is obstruction to air flow, affecting adequacy of ventilation and oxygenation. Long-term sequelae include atelectasis, pneumonia, bronchospasm, hemoptysis, lung abscess, and bronchiectasis. Patients with esophageal foreign bodies can present with symptoms and complications of airway obstruction (176,177).

Signs and symptoms of aspiration range from total acute airway obstruction to chronic manifestations of recurrent pneumonia and recurrent bronchospasm. Children who have aspirated may display stridor, voice change, cough, tachypnea, retractions, labored breathing, and cyanosis. The location of the foreign body within the airway can often be determined by a combination of auscultation and radiographic studies (178,179). MRI has been used to diagnose foreign body aspiration (180). Wheezing or decreased breath sounds may be detected on the affected side. Chest film may show a radiopaque object, atelectasis, mediastinal shift, or air trapping on the affected side when right and left decubitus films are compared. However, most chest films are negative in the first 24 hours following foreign body aspiration.

Removal of foreign body from the airway may need to be carried out as an emergency procedure or may be delayed after an appropriate period of nothing by mouth. Emergency management is required if the patient is in respiratory distress, if the foreign body is in a compromising location (e.g., larynx), or if the nature of the for-

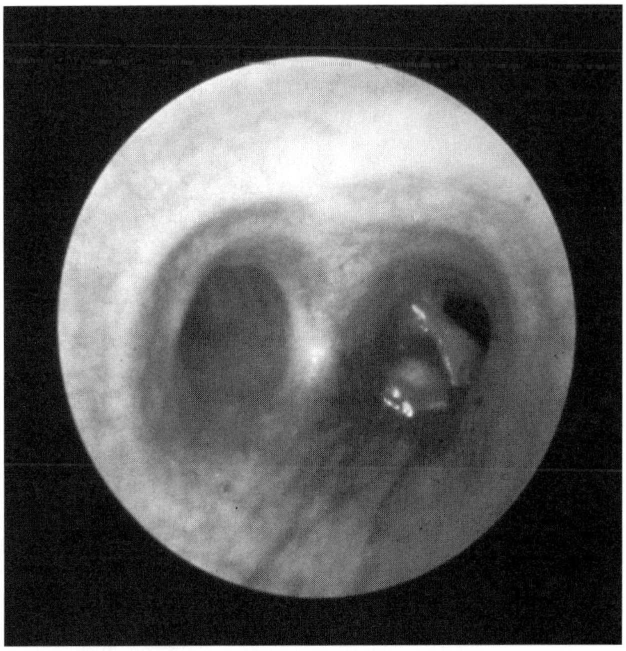

FIG. 8. Foreign body aspiration. The right main bronchus is visualized. A fragmented pecan is obstructing the bronchus and causing mucosal bleeding.

eign body merits removal as soon as possible (e.g., sharp objects or caustic agents, such as peanuts). Foreign bodies in place for a long period of time generally do not require emergency removal. Use of antibiotics and steroids before removal of foreign body may reduce complication rates (181).

Children with respiratory distress or a foreign body in a compromising location should not receive premedication. Agitation may be a sign of hypoxemia, which should be ruled out by oximetry. Parental presence to make the induction period less distressing should be considered. In anxious children with minimal respiratory distress, and in those with long-standing aspiration, premedication may be used when necessary. The premedicated child should be closely observed and appropriate suction and airway equipment kept at hand.

There are several controversial issues regarding the treatment of foreign body aspiration in pediatric patients. These include inhalation vs. intravenous induction, spontaneous vs. controlled ventilation, and the use of muscle relaxants, rapid-sequence induction, and cricoid pressure. Regardless of the controversies surrounding these issues, the important goals of management in these patients remain a smooth induction and an adequate depth of anesthesia to allow direct laryngoscopy without cough, laryngospasm, bronchospasm, or displacement of the foreign body. Inhalation induction allows titration of anesthetic depth and maintenance of spontaneous ventilation with minimal effect on moving the foreign body, although it does not protect against aspiration. One often may need to supplement the anesthetic with a muscle relaxant following insertion of the bronchoscope into the airway. Rapid-sequence induction with cricoid pressure is an alternative method of induction preferred by some (182,183). It has the advantage of protecting the airway from aspiration of stomach contents and allowing the use of muscle relaxants, which immobilize the vocal cords, eliminate coughing, and generally permit better lung ventilation and oxygenation. The potential disadvantages are inability to ventilate following muscle relaxation and the theoretical concern of displacing the foreign body into a more compromising position during positive-pressure ventilation and/or tracheal intubation. Rapid-sequence induction should not be done if it has been determined that ventilation and oxygenation may be difficult after muscle relaxation. Cricoid pressure is not recommended if the foreign body is in the larynx or can potentially cause a penetrating injury (e.g., an open safety pin). Other alternatives for retrieving a foreign body include tracheal incision for large or pointed objects with little chance of passing the glottis, elective use of transtracheal jet ventilation in cases with high risk for complete upper airway obstruction, and occasionally thoracotomy (184,185).

The otolaryngologist should be present in the operating room and ready to proceed at the start of anesthesia. Inhalation induction may be carried out with oxygen and halothane. Nitrous oxide is not recommended in patients with respiratory distress or hypoxemia, or in those at risk for complete airway obstruction. Once an appropriate depth of anesthesia has been achieved, an intravenous line may be started if not already in place. Administration of an anticholinergic agent helps reduce oral secretions and maintain heart rate under the deep levels of halothane anesthesia necessary to allow direct laryngoscopy. CPAP or gentle assisted ventilation may sometimes be necessary to keep the airway patent. It is best to use 100% oxygen during such procedures. Once the depth of anesthesia is sufficient, direct laryngoscopy is performed. Lidocaine can be injected at the vocal cords and into the trachea for added anesthesia and reduction of airway reflexes in response to bronchoscopy. A rigid bronchoscope equipped with a sidearm is then advanced into the airway under direct view to retrieve the foreign object. If the foreign body is not quickly retrieved, the patient may have to be ventilated actively and oxygenated through the sidearm of the rigid bronchoscope. If the leak around the bronchoscope is large, it may be difficult to ventilate the patient, and high oxygen flows or a larger size of bronchoscope may be necessary. The anesthetic may be continued with inhalation or intravenous agents. The patient may require muscle relaxation to prevent coughing and immobilize the vocal cords so as to facilitate removal of the foreign body and minimize trauma to the airway. Once the foreign body has been removed, the trachea can be intubated with an endotracheal tube and the patient allowed to emerge from anesthesia. If there is airway obstruction during inhalation induction, one must quickly differentiate between upper airway obstruction, laryngospasm, and foreign body. If airway obstrution occurs during bronchoscopy, then the foreign body is most likely in the larynx or at the level of the carina, from which it must be immediately removed or displaced into a main bronchus. In patients who may have residual gastric contents, the stomach should be aspirated by passing an orogastric tube before tracheal extubation.

Most children should be in a position to have their trachea extubated following foreign body removal. This depends on the degree of injury to the airway, the size of the child, and the suspected degree of airway swelling. Some children may display stridor and croupy cough, requiring humidification, racemic epinephrine, and steroids. Other complications associated with foreign body removal from the airway include bronchospasm, laryngospasm, airway obstruction, pneumothorax, bronchial rupture, fragmentation of the foreign body, and hemorrhage (186). The success rate for foreign body removal by bronchoscopy is 95% to 98%; the remainder of cases require surgical removal (tracheotomy, thoracotomy). A small percentage of children require a second bronchoscopy for removal of residual foreign body or granulation tissue.

Tongue Disease

The size of the tongue relative to the size of the mouth and submandibular space is a determinant of the success of direct laryngoscopy in allowing visualization of the glottis. In pediatric patients, tongue enlargement can result from various disorders. Beckwith-Wiedemann syndrome, Down syndrome, Hurler syndrome, and hypothyroidism are all associated with macroglossia (187). Vascular malformations of the tongue, such as hemangioma or lymphangioma, are rare occurrences that can result in massive enlargement of the tongue, sometimes resulting in its extension beyond the lip margins (188). The palate, epiglottis, and vallecula may also be involved, further complicating airway management. These children may require surgical resection of the tongue and tracheostomy. Tongue enlargement may also result from factors that cause swelling, such as prolonged surgical traction, burns, trauma, and infection. Macroglossia can result in airway obstruction and may make direct laryngoscopy difficult. Patients with chronic airway obstruction are at risk for cor pulmonale (189).

Airway management in patients with macroglossia must take into consideration the relative size of the tongue and degree of airway obstruction. In children with extensive enlargement of the tongue or severe airway obstruction, tracheal intubation should be accomplished by an awake technique, such as with a flexible fiberscope, retrograde technique, or lighted stylet. In children with mild enlargement of the tongue and minimal signs of airway obstruction, tracheal intubation may be attempted following administration of general anesthesia.

REFERENCES

1. Marchildon MB. Physiological considerations in the newborn surgical patient. *Surg Clin North Am* 1976;56:245.
2. Cheney FW, Posner KL, Caplan RA. Adverse respiratory events infrequently leading to malpractice suits. *Anesthesiology* 1991;75:932–939.
3. Caplan RA, Posner KL, Ward RJ, Cheney FW. Adverse respiratory events in anesthesia: a closed claims analysis. *Anesthesiology* 1990;72:828–833.
4. Geiduschek JM, Morray JP, Caplan RA, Ward RJ, Cheney FW. Review of closed malpractice claims in pediatric anesthesia. *Anesthesiology* 1989;71:A1174.
5. Morray JP, et al. A comparison of pediatric and adult anesthesia closed malpractice claims. *Anesthesiology* 1993;78:461–467.
6. Ferris BG, Mead J, Opie LH. Partitioning of respiratory flow resistance in man. *J Appl Physiol* 1964;19:653.
7. Polgar G. Airway resistance in the newborn infant. *J Pediatr* 1961;59:915–921.
8. Polgar G, Kong GP. The nasal resistance of newborn infants. *J Pediatr* 1965;67:556–567.
9. Eckenoff JE. Some anatomic considerations of the infant larynx influencing endotracheal anesthesia. *Anesthesiology* 1951;12:401.
10. Maniglia AJ, Goodwin WJ Jr. Congenital choanal atresia. *Otolaryngol Clin North Am* 1981;14:167–173.
11. Hobolth N, Buchmann G, Sandberg LE. Congenital choanal atresia. *Acta Paediatr Scand* 1967;56:286–294.
12. Passy V, Newcron S, Synder S. Rhinorrhea with airway obstruction. *Laryngoscope* 1975;85:888–895.
13. Fearon B, Whalen JS. Tracheal dimensions in the living infant. *Ann Otol Rhinol Laryngol* 1967;76:965–974.
14. Macintosh R, Mushin WW, Epstein HG. *Physics for the Anaesthetist*, 2nd ed. Oxford: Blackwell; 1958.
15. Mansell A, Bryan C, Levison H. Airway closure in children. *J Appl Physiol* 1972;33:711–714.
16. Harris TR. Physiological principles. In: Goldsmith JP, Karotkin EH, eds. *Assisted Ventilation of the Neonate*. Philadelphia: WB Saunders; 1988.
17. Bosma JF. Introduction to the symposium. In: Bosma JF, Showacre J, eds. *Symposium on Development of Upper Respiratory Anatomy and Function: Implications of Sudden Infant Death Syndrome*. Washington, D.C.: U.S. Government Printing Office; 1975:5–49.
18. Crelin ES. Development of the upper respiratory system. *Ciba Found Symp* 1976;28:3–30.
19. Sharp JT, Druz WS, Balagot RC, et al. Total respiratory compliance in infants and children. *J Appl Physiol* 1970;29:775–779.
20. Lacourt G, Polgar G. Interaction between nasal and pulmonary resistance in newborn infants. *J Appl Physiol* 1971;30:870–873.
21. Doershuk CF, Matthews LW. Airway resistance and lung volume in the newborn infant. *Pediatr Res* 1969;3:128–134.
22. Butler J. The work of breathing through the nose. *Clin Sci* 1960;19:55–62.
23. Anthonisen NR, Danson J, Robertson PC, et al. Airway closure as a function of age. *Respir Physiol* 1969;8:58–65.
24. Motoyama, EK. Airway function tests in infants and children. *Int Anesthesiol Clin* 1988;26:6–13.
25. Cross KW, Tizard JPM, Trythall DAH. The gaseous metabolism of the newborn infant. *Acta Paediatr Scand* 1957;46:265–285.
26. Thibeault DW, Clutario B, Auld PAM. The oxygen cost of breathing in the premature infant. *Pediatrics* 1966;37:954–959.
27. Epstein RA, Hyman AI. Ventilatory requirements of critically ill neonates. *Anesthesiology* 1980;53:379–384.
28. Keens TG, Bryan AC, Levison H, et al. Developmental pattern of muscle fibers in human ventilatory muscles. *J Appl Physiol* 1978;44:909–913.
29. Keens TG, Lanuzzo CD. Development of fatigue-resistant muscle fibers in human ventilatory muscles. *Am Rev Respir Dis* 1979; 2 (Suppl 119):139–141.
30. Keens TG, Chen V, Patel P, et al. Cellular adaptations of the ventilatory muscles to a chronic increased respiratory load. *J Appl Physiol* 1978;44:905–908.
31. Stauffer JL, Silvestri RL. Complications of endotracheal intubation, tracheostomy, and artificial airways. *Respir Care* 1982;27:417–422.
32. Caldwell SL, Sullivan KN. Artificial airways. In: Burton GG, Hodgkin JF, eds. *Respiratory Care: a Guide to Clinical Practice*. Philadelphia: JB Lippincott; 1984.
33. Keep PJ, Manford ML. Endotracheal tube sizes for children. *Anaesthesia* 1974;29:181.
34. Corfield HMC. Orotracheal tubes and the metric system. *Br J Anaesth* 1963;34.
35. Cole F. Pediatric formulas for the anesthesiologist. *Am J Dis Child* 1957;94:672–673.
36. Mayer BW. *Pediatric Anesthesia: a Guide to Its Administration*. Philadelphia: JB Lippincott; 1981.
37. Slater HM, Sheridan CA, Ferguson RH. Endotracheal tube size: a statistical analysis. *Anesthesiology* 1967;28:779.

37a. Chodoff P, Helrich M. Factors affecting pediatric endotracheal tube size: a statistical analysis. *Anesthesiology* 1967;28:779–782.

38. Levin RM. *Pediatric Anesthesia Handbook*. New York: Medical Examination Publishing Company; 1980.
39. Lee KW, Templeton JJ, Douglas R. Tracheal tube size and post-operative croup in children. *Anesthesiology* 1980;53:S325(abst).
40. Mostafa SM. Variation in subglottic size in children. *Proc R Soc Med* 1976;69:793.
41. Penlington GN. Endotracheal tube sizes for children. *Anesthesia* 1974;29:494.
42. Finholt DA, Henry DB, Raphaely RC. Factors affecting leak around tracheal tubes in children. *Can Anaesth Soc J* 1985;32:326.
43. Stanley TH, Kawamura R, Graves C. Effects of nitrous oxide on volume and pressure of endotracheal tube cuffs. *Anesthesiology* 1974;41:256.
44. Stanley TH. Effects of anesthetic gases on endotracheal tube cuff gas volumes. *Anesth Analg* 1974;53:480.
45. Stanley TH. Nitrous oxide and pressures and volumes of high and low pressure endotracheal tube cuffs in intubated patients. *Anesthesiology* 1974;42d:637.

46. Morgan GAR, Steward DJ. Linear airway dimensions in children: including those with cleft palate. *Can Anaesth Soc J* 1982;29:1–8.
47. Morgan GAR, Steward DJ. A preformed paediatric orotracheal tube design based on anatomical measurements. *Can Anaesth Soc J* 1982; 29:9–11.
48. Finucane BT, Santora AH. *Principles of Airway Management*. Philadelphia: Davis; 1988.
49. Cozine K, Rosenbaum LM, Askanazi J, et al. Laser-induced endotracheal tube fire. *Anesthesiology* 1981;55:583.
50. Keon TP. Anesthetic considerations for laser surgery. *Int Anesthesiol Clin* 1988;26:50.
51. Snow JC, Norton ML, Saluja TS, et al. Fire hazard during CO_2 laser microsurgery on the larynx and trachea. *Anesth Analg* 1976;55:146.
52. Sosis MB, Dillon F, Heller S. Prevention of CO_2 laser-induced endotracheal tube fires with the Laser-Guard protective coating. *Can J Anaesth* 1989;36:S88.
53. Norton ML, DeVos P. New endotracheal tube for laser surgery of the larynx. *Ann Otol* 1978;87:554.
54. LeJeune FE, Guice C, Letard F, et al. Heat sink protection against lasering endotracheal cuffs. *Ann Otol Rhinol Laryngol* 1982;91:606.
55. Sosis MB, Dillon F, Heller S. Saline-filled cuffs help prevent laser-induced polyvinylchloride endotracheal tube fires. *Can J Anaesth* 1989;36:S152.
56. Vandam LD. Functional anatomy of the larynx. *Weekly Anesthesiology Update* 1977;1:2–6.
57. Morikawa S, Safar P, DeCarlo J. Influence of the head-jaw position upon upper airway patency. *Anesthesiology* 1961;22:265–279.
58. Sellick BA. Cricoid pressure to control regurgitation of stomach contents during induction of anaesthesia. *Lancet* 1961;2:404.
59. Wright WJ, Chamney AR, Howells TH. The determination of an effective cricoid pressure. *Anaesthesia* 1983;38:461.
60. Holzman RS, Nargozian CD, Florence FB. Lightwand intubation in children with abnormal upper airways. *Anesthesiology* 1988;69:784–787.
61. Ellis DG, Jakymec A, Kaplan RM, et al. Guided orotracheal intubation in the operating room using a lighted stylet: a comparison with direct laryngoscopic technique. *Anesthesiology* 1986;64:823–826.
62. Weis FR, Hatton MN. Intubation by the use of the light wand: experience with 253 patients. *J Oral Maxillofac Surg* 1989;47:577.
63. Macewen W. Clinical observations on the introduction of tracheal tubes by the mouth instead of performing tracheotomy or laryngotomy. *Br Med J* 1880;2:122.
64. Sykes WS. Oral endotracheal intubation without laryngoscopy: a plea for simplicity. *Anesth Analg* 1937;16:133.
65. Siddal WJW. Tactile orotracheal intubation. *Anaesthesia* 1966;21: 221.
66. Stewart R. Tactile method of oral intubation in comatose trauma patients. *Ann Emerg Med* 1984;13:175.
67. Wood RE, Sherman JM. Pediatric flexible bronchoscopy. *Ann Otol Rhino Laryngol* 1980;89:414.
68. Nussbaum E. Flexible fiberoptic bronchoscopy and laryngoscopy in infants and children. *Laryngoscope* 1983;93:1073.
69. Ovassapian A, Yelich SJ, Dykes MHM, et al. Learning fiberoptic intubation: use of simulators vs. traditional teaching. *Br J Anaesth* 1988;61:217.
70. Fan LL, Sparks LM, Dulinski JP. Applications of an ultrathin flexible bronchoscope for neonatal and pediatric airway problems. *Chest* 1986;89:673.
71. Stiles CM. A flexible fiberoptic bronchoscope for endotracheal intubation in infants. *Anesth Analg* 1974;53:1017.
72. Berthelsen P, Prytz S, Jacobsen E. Two-stage fiberoptic nasotracheal intubation in infants: a new approach to difficult pediatric intubation. *Anesthesiology* 1985;63:457.
73. Brimacombe J, Newell S, Swainston R, et al. A potential new technique for awake fiberoptic bronchoscopy—use of the laryngeal mask airway. *Med J Aust* 1992;156:876–877.
74. Walker RWM, Murrell D. Yet another use for the laryngeal mask airway [Letter]. *Anaesthesia* 1991;46:591.
75. Maekawa N, Mikawa K, Tanaka O, Goto R, Obara H. The laryngeal mask may be a useful device for fiberoptic airway endoscopy in pediatric anesthesia [Letter]. *Anesthesiology* 1991;75:169–170.
76. Benumof JL. Use of the laryngeal mask airway to facilitate fiberoptic-aided tracheal intubation [Letter]. *Anesth Analg* 1992;74:313.
77. Smith JE, Sherwood NA. Combined use of laryngeal mask airway and fiberoptic laryngoscope in difficult intubation [Letter]. *Anaesth Intensive Care* 1991;19:472.
78. McNamee CJ, Meyns B, Pagliero KM. Flexible bronchoscopy via the laryngeal mask: a new technique. *Thorax* 1991;46:141.
79. Silk JM, Hill HM, Calder I. Difficult intubation and the laryngeal mask. *Eur J Anaesthesiol Suppl* 1991;4:47.
80. Borland LM, Swan DM, Leff S. Difficult pediatric intubation. A new approach to the retrograde technique. *Anesthesiology* 1981;55:577.
81. Brain AIJ. The laryngeal mask—a new concept in airway management. *Br J Anaesth* 1983;55:801–805.
82. Brain AIJ. Three cases of difficult intubation overcome by the laryngeal mask airway. *Anaesthesia* 1985;40:353–355.
83. Pennant JH, White PF. The laryngeal mask airway. Its uses in anesthesiology. *Anesthesiology* 1993;79:144–163.
84. Brain AIJ. *The Intravent Laryngeal Mask Instruction Manual*, 2nd ed. Henley-on-Thames, England: Intravent International; 1991.
85. Brain AIJ. Proper technique for insertion of the laryngeal mask [Letter]. *Anesthesiology* 1990;73:1053–1054.
86. Nanji GM, Maltby JR. Vomiting and aspiration pneumonitis with the laryngeal mask airway. *Can J Anaesth* 1992;39:69–70.
87. Wittmann PH, Wittmann FW. Laryngeal mask and gastric dilatation [Letter]. *Anaesthesia* 1991;46:1083.
88. Lee JJ. Laryngeal mask and trauma to uvula [Letter]. *Anaesthesia* 1989;44:1014.
89. Dasey N, Mansour N. Coughing and laryngospasm with the laryngeal mask [Letter]. *Anaesthesia* 1989;44:865.
90. Saunders PA, Geisecke AH. Clinical assessment of the adult Bullard laryngoscope. *Can J Anaesth* 1989;36:5118–5119.
91. Borland LM, Casselbrandt M. The Bullard laryngoscope: a new indirect oral laryngoscope (pediatric version). *Anesth Analg* 1990;70: 105–108.
92. Smith RB, Schaer WB, Pfaeffle H. Percutaneous transtracheal ventilation for anaesthesia and resuscitation: a review and report of complications. *Can Anaesth Soc J* 1975;22:607–612.
93. Stinson TW III. A simple connector for transtracheal ventilation. *Anesthesiology* 1977;47:232.
94. Cote CJ, Eavey RD, Todres ID, et al. Cricothyroid membrane puncture: oxygenation and ventilation in a dog model using an intravenous catheter. *Crit Care Med* 1988;16:615–619.
95. Frumin MJ, Epstein RM, Cohen G. Apneic oxygenation in man. *Anesthesiology* 1959;20:789–798.
96. Goldstein B, Shannon DC, Todres ID. Supercarbia in children: clinical course and outcome. *Crit Care Med* 1990;18:166–168.
97. Zornow MH, Thomas TC, Scheller MS. The efficacy of three different methods of transtracheal ventilation. *Can J Anaesth* 1989;36:624–628.
98. Bedrer RC Jr, Chang JL. A jet-stylet endotracheal catheter for difficult airway management. *Anesthesiology* 1987;66:221–223.
99. Benumof JL, Scheller MS. The importance of transtracheal jet ventilation in the management of difficult airway. *Anesthesiology* 1989;71: 769.
100. Steward DJ. Percutaneous transtracheal ventilation for laser endoscopic procedures in infants and children. *Can J Anaesth* 1987;34: 429–430.
101. MacDonald DJF. Cystic hygroma: an anesthetic and surgical problem. *Anaesthesia* 1978;49:433.
102. Harrington JF. Cystic hygroma. In: Stehling LC, ed. *Common Problems in Pediatric Anesthesia*. Chicago: Year Book; 1982:97.
103. Weller RM. Anaesthesia for cystic hygroma in a neonate. *Anaesthesia* 1974;29:588.
104. Ovassapian A, Dykes MHM. Difficult pediatric intubation—an indication for the fiberoptic bronchoscope. *Anesthesiology* 1982;56:412.
105. American College of Surgeons. *Advanced Trauma Life Support*. Chicago: American College of Surgeons; 1989.
106. Hadley MN, Zabramski JM, Browner CM, et al. Pediatric spinal trauma: review of 122 cases of spinal cord and vertebral column injuries. *J Neurosurg* 1988;68:18–24.
107. Hamilton MG, Myles ST. Pediatric spinal injury: review of 61 deaths. *J Neurosurg* 1992;77:705–708.
108. Stellin GP, Barker S, Murdock KM, et al. Oral-tracheal intubation in trauma patients with cervical fractures. *Crit Care Med* 1989;17:534.
109. Bohn D, Armstrong D, Becker L, Humphreys R. Cervical spine injury in children. *J Trauma* 1990;30:463.
110. Hill SA, et al. Pediatric neck injuries. *J Neurosurg* 1984;60:700–706.

111. Huelke DF, O'Day J, Mendelsohn RA. Cervical injuries suffered in automobile crashes. *J Neurosurg* 1981;54:316–322.
112. Pang D, Pollack IF. Spinal cord injury without radiographic abnormality in children: the SCIWORA syndrome. *J Trauma* 1989;29:654–664.
113. Ruge JR, et al. Pediatric spinal injury: the very young. *J Neurosurg* 1988;68:25–30.
114. Stauffer ES, Mazur JM. Cervical spine injuries in children. *Pediatr Ann* 1982;11:502–511.
115. Diekema DS, Allen DB. Odontoid fracture in a child occupying a child restraint seat. *Pediatrics* 1988;82:117–119.
116. Fuchs S, et al. Cervical spine fractures sustained by young children in forward-facing car seats. *Pediatrics* 1989;84:348–354.
117. Pueschel SM, Scola FH. Atlantoaxial instability in individuals with Down syndrome: epidemiologic, radiographic, and clinical studies. *Pediatrics* 1987;80:555–560.
118. Davidson RG. Atlantoaxial instability in individuals with Down syndrome: a fresh look at the evidence. *Pediatrics* 1988;81:857–865.
119. Bohn D, et al. High cervical spine injuries associated with severe head injury in children: an unrecognized cause of cardio-respiratory arrest. *Crit Care Med* 1989;17:S117.
120. Grande CM, Barton CR, Stene JK. Appropriate techniques for airway management of emergency patients with suspected spinal cord injury. *Anesth Analg* 1988;67:714–715.
121. Yealy DM, et al. Emergency airway management in trauma patients with suspected cervical spine injury. *Anesth Analg* 1989;68:413–414.
122. Chekan EM, Weber S. Intubation with or without neuromuscular blockade in trauma patients with cervical spine injury. *Anesth Analg* 1990;70:S54.
123. Bunegin L, Hung TK, Chang GL. Biomechanics of spinal cord injury. *Crit Care Clin* 1987;3:453.
124. Marsh JL, Galic M, Vannier MW. The craniofacial anatomy of Apert syndrome. *Clin Plast Surg* 1991;18:237–249.
125. Cohen MM Jr, Kreiborg S. Upper and lower airway compromise in the Apert syndrome. *Am J Med Genet* 1992;44:90–93.
126. McGill T. Otolaryngologic aspects of Apert syndrome. *Clin Plast Surg* 1991;18:309–313.
127. Mixter RC, David DJ, Perloff WH, et al. Obstructive sleep apnea in Apert's and Pfeiffer's syndromes: more than a craniofacial abnormality. *Plast Reconstr Surg* 1990;86:457–463.
128. Kreiborg S, Barr M, Cohen MM Jr. Cervical spine in Apert syndrome. *Am J Med Genet* 1992;43:704–708.
129. Sagehashi N. An infant with Crouzon's syndrome with a cartilaginous trachea and a human tail. *J Craniomaxillofac Surg* 1992;20:21–23.
130. Stone P, Trevenen CL, Mitchell I, Rudd N. Congenital tracheal stenosis in Pfeiffer syndrome. *Clin Genet* 1990;38:145–148.
131. Jones KL, ed. *Smith's Recognizable Pattern of Human Malformation*. 4th edition. Philadelphia: WB Saunders; 1988:725.
132. Nargozian C. Apert syndrome: anesthetic management. *Clin Plast Surg* 1991;18:227–230.
133. Scheller JG, Schulman SR. Fiber-optic bronchoscopic guidance for intubating a neonate with Pierre-Robin syndrome. *J Clin Anesth* 1991;3:45–47.
134. Finer NN, Muzyka D. Flexible endoscopic intubation of the neonate. *Pediatr Pulmonol* 1992;12:48–51.
135. Markakis DA, Sayson SC, Schreiner MS. Insertion of the laryngeal mask airway in awake infants with Robin sequence. *Anesth Analg* 1992;75:822–824.
136. Benumof JL. Management of the difficult adult airway: with special emphasis on awake tracheal intubation. *Anesthesiology* 1990;75:1087–1110.
137. Gorelick MH, Baker MD. Epiglottitis in children, 1979 through 1992. Effects of Haemophilus influenzae type b immunization. *Arch Pediatr Adolesc Med* 1992;148:47–50.
138. Ryan M, Hunt M, Snowberger T. A changing pattern of epiglottitis. *Clin Pediatr* 1992;31:532–535.
139. Baxter JD. Acute epiglottitis in children. *Laryngoscope* 1967;77:1358.
140. Rowe LD. Advances and controversies in the management of supraglottitis and laryngotracheobronchitis. *Am J Otolaryngol* 1980;1:235–244.
141. Lazoritz S, Saunders BS, Bason WM. Management of acute epiglottitis. *Crit Care Med* 1979;7:285–290.
142. Bass JW, Steele RW, Wiebe RA. Acute epiglottitis: an acute surgical emergency. *JAMA* 1974;229:671–675.
143. Bass JW, Fahardo JE, Brian JH, et al. Sudden death due to epiglottitis. *Pediatr Infect Dis J* 1985;4:447–449.
144. Oh TH, Motoyama EK. Comparison of nasotracheal intubation and tracheostomy in management of acute epiglottitis. *Anesthesiology* 1977;46:214–216.
145. Hannallah R, Rosales JK. Acute epiglottitis: current management and review. *Can Anaesth Soc J* 1978;25:84–91.
146. Bates JR. Epiglottitis: diagnosis and treatment. *Pediatr Rev* 1979;1:173–176.
147. Rapkin RH. The diagnosis of epiglottitis: simplicity and reliability of radiographs of the neck in the differential diagnosis of the croup syndrome. *J Pediatr* 1972;80:96–98.
148. Podgore JK, Bass JW. The "thumb sign" and "little finger sign" in acute epiglottitis. *J Pediatr* 1976;88:154–155.
149. Gevin JL, Lee FA. Radiologic case of the month: acute epiglottitis. *Am J Dis Child* 1976;130:195–196.
150. Johnson GK, Sullivan JL, Bishop LA. Acute epiglottitis. *Arch Otolaryngol* 1974;100:333–337.
151. Battaglia JD, Lockhart CH. Management of acute epiglottitis by nasotracheal intubation. *Am J Dis Child* 1975;129:334–336.
152. Contrell RW, Bell RA, Morioka WF. Acute epiglottitis: intubation versus tracheostomy. *Laryngoscope* 1978;88:994–1005.
153. Henry RL, Bingham AL, Halliday JA. The management of epiglottitis in a small pediatric intensive care unit. *J Qual Clin Pract* 1994;14:17–21.
154. Baugh R, Gilmore BB Jr. Infectious croup: a critical review. *Otolaryngol Head Neck Surg* 1986;95:40–46.
155. Wald ER. Croup. In: Oski F, ed. *Pediatrics*, 2nd ed. Philadelphia: JB Lippincott; 1994:981–982.
156. Rapkin RH. The diagnosis of epiglottitis: simplicity and reliability of radiographs of the neck in differential diagnosis of the croup syndrome. *J Pediatr* 1972;80:96–98.
157. Lenney W, Milner AD. Treatment of acute viral croup. *Arch Dis Child* 1978;53:704–706.
158. Strong M, Vaughan C, Healy G, et al. Recurrent respiratory papillomatosis. *Ann Otol* 1976;85:508–516.
159. Sedlacek T, Lindheim S, Eder C, et al. Mechanism for human papillomavirus transmission at birth. *Am J Obstet Gynecol* 1989;161:55–59.
160. Tseng CJ, Lin CY, Wang RL, et al. Possible transplacental transmission of human papillomavirus. *Am J Obstet Gynecol* 1992;166:35–40.
161. Chipps BE, McClurg FL Jr, Freidman EM, Adams GL. Respiratory papillomas: presentation before six months. *Pediatr Pulmonol* 1990;9:125–130.
162. Lusk R, McCabe B, Mixon J. Three-year experience of treating recurrent respiratory papilloma with interferon. *Ann Otol Rhinol Laryngol* 1987;96:158–162.
163. Abramson A, Waner M, Brandsma J. The clinical treatment of laryngeal papillomas with hematoporphyrin therapy. *Arch Otolaryngol Head Neck Surg* 1988;114:795–800.
164. Shikowitz M. Comparison of pulsed and continuous wave light in photodynamic therapy of papillomas: an experimental study. *Laryngoscope* 1992;102:300–310.
165. Ossoff R, Werkhaven J, Dere H. Soft-tissue complications of laser surgery for recurrent respiratory papillomatosis. *Laryngoscope* 1991;101:1162–1166.
166. Hermens JM, Bennett MJ, Hirshman CA. Anesthesia for laser surgery. *Anesth Analg* 1983;62:218–229.
167. Scamman FL, McCabe BF. Supraglottic jet ventilation for laser surgery of the larynx in children. *Ann Otol Rhinol Laryngol* 1986;95:142–145.
168. O'Sullivan TJ, Healy GB. Complications of Venturi jet ventilation during microlaryngeal surgery. *Arch Otolaryngol* 1985;111:127–131.
169. Wegrzynowicz ES, Jensen NF, Pearson KS, et al. Airway fire during jet ventilation for laser excision of vocal cord papillomata. *Anesthesiology* 1992;76:468–469.
170. Eller WC, Haugen RK. Food asphyxiation. *N Engl J Med* 1973;289:81.
171. Cohen SR, Lewis GB Jr, Herbert WI, Geller KA. Foreign body in the airway: five-year retrospective study with special reference to management. *Ann Otol* 1980;89:437–442.
172. Menendez AA, Gotay CF, Seda FJ, et al. Foreign body aspiration: experience at the University Pediatric Hospital. *P R Health Sci J* 1991;10:127–133.

173. Mu L, He P, Sun D. Inhalation of foreign bodies in Chinese children: a review of 400 cases. *Laryngoscope* 1991;101:657–660.
174. Pasaoglu I, Dogan R, Demircin M, et al. Bronchoscopic removal of foreign bodies in children: retrospective analysis of 822 cases. *Thorac Cardiovasc Surg* 1991;39:95–98.
175. Baraka A. Bronchoscopic removal of inhaled foreign bodies in children. *Br J Anaesth* 1974;46:124–126.
176. Brady PG. Esophageal foreign bodies. *Gastroentrol Clin North Am* 1991;20:691–701.
177. Byard RW, Moore L, Bourne AJ. Sudden and unexpected death—a late effect of occult intraesophageal foreign body. *Pediatr Pathol* 1990;10:837–841.
178. Parsons DS, Kearns D. The two-headed stethoscope: its use for ruling out airway foreign bodies. *Int J Pediatr Otorhinolaryngol* 1991;22: 181–185.
179. Mu LC, Sun DQ, He P. Radiologic diagnosis of aspirated foreign bodies in children: review of 343 cases. *J Laryngol Otol* 1990;104: 778–782.
180. Kitinaka S, Mikami I, Tokumaru A, et al. Diagnosis of peanut inhalation by MRI. *Pediatr Radiol* 1992;22:300–301.
181. Steen KH, Zimmermann T. Tracheobronchial aspiration of foreign bodies in children: a study of 94 cases. *Laryngoscope* 1990;100:525–530.
182. Kain ZN, OConnor TZ, Berde CB. Management of tracheobronchial and esophageal foreign bodies in children: a survey study. *J Clin Anesth* 1994;6:28–32.
183. Keon TP. Bronchoscopy for a foreign body. In: Stehling L, ed. *Common Problems in Pediatric Anesthesia*, 2nd ed. St. Louis: Mosby-Year Book; 1992.
184. Ohkouchi Y, Inomoto Y, Suzuki C, et al. Bronchoscopy for airway foreign bodies: consideration based on an extraordinarily large one. *Fukushima J Med Sci* 1992;38:99–104.
185. Eyrich JE, Riopelle JM, Naraghi M. Elective transtracheal jet ventilation for bronchoscopic removal of tracheal foreign body. *South Med J* 1992;85:1017–1019.
186. Wilkinson KA, Beckett W, Brown TC. Pneumothorax secondary to foreign body inhalation in a 20-month-old child. *J Paediatr Child Health* 1992;28:67–68.
187. Weiss LS, White JA. Macroglossia: a review. *J La State Med Soc* 1990;142:13–16.
188. Balakrishnam A, Bailey CM. Lymphangioma of the tongue. A review of pathogensis, treatment and use of surface laser photocoagulation. *J Laryngol Otol* 1991;105:924–930.
189. Smith DF, Mihm FG, Flynn M. Chronic alveolar hypoventilation secondary to macroglossia in the Beckwith-Wiedemann syndrome. *Pediatrics* 1982;70:695–697.

Airway Management, edited by
L.H. Hanowell, M.D. and R.J. Waldron, M.D.,
Lippincott-Raven Publishers, Philadelphia © 1996.

CHAPTER 20

Obstetric Airway Management

Michael J. Paech

ANATOMIC AND PHYSIOLOGIC CHANGES: IMPLICATIONS FOR MANAGEMENT

The Upper Airway

The upper airway of the pregnant woman is affected by increased fat deposition in the head, neck, and breasts. Particularly in the obese woman, this deposition may restrict access for a laryngoscope and may limit neck extension. Increased abdominal contents raise the diaphragm and alter the normal anatomic alignment of the upper airway.

Increases in interstitial fluid and capillary engorgement result in increased vascularity and edema of mucous membranes in the nasal passages, larynx, and tongue. Pharyngolaryngeal edema (1) and severe swelling of the face or tongue are rare but well described complications that are most commonly associated with preeclampsia (gestational proteinuric hypertension), but may also be present with prolonged labor, straining, fluid overload, and respiratory tract infection. Voice changes or stridor are uncommon, yet unexpected acute airway obstruction requiring intubation may occur within an hour or two (2,3). When intubating severe preeclamptics, the induced hypertensive response may require attenuation.

Airway obstruction can present in the early postextubation period (4,5). If severe upper airway edema is noted at intubation, the decision to extubate should be based on repeated fiberoptic assessment and the ability to breathe around the tube with its cuff deflated and lumen occluded. Other pathology, for example, submandibular abscess (6) or acute thyroid enlargement (7), may also produce acute obstruction during pregnancy.

Management Implications

1. Attention to optimal patient positioning is crucial prior to attempting intubation.
2. Manipulations within the upper airway may cause mucosal trauma, and insertion of a nasal airway or of a nasogastric or nasotracheal tube may result in epistaxis.

M. J. Paech: Department of Anaesthesia, King Edward Memorial Hospital for Women, Perth, Western Australia, Australia.

3. Signs or symptoms of upper airway edema mandate early comprehensive airway assessment and continuous observation.
4. Tracheal tubes of 7–8 mm internal diameter are appropriate for most preeclamptic women; smaller tubes (6.0 mm or less) must be available.

The Respiratory System

Physiologic changes in lung volume and mechanics, resistance and compliance, and ventilation and gas exchange, many of which are further exaggerated during labor, have implications with respect to airway management (8,9). Arterial oxygen tension rises and carbon dioxide falls (range 28–34 mmHg) due to a first-trimester increase in alveolar ventilation, peaking at 70% by term. Hypoxemia and hypercarbia occur with frightening rapidity when airway obstruction or apnea occur, principally due to increased oxygen consumption and a reduction in functional residual capacity (and, thus, oxygen stores) in the second half of pregnancy. These changes are exaggerated when closing volume falls within tidal volume range, as it may with obesity or smoking; the supine, lithotomy, or Trendelenburg positions; or induction of general anesthesia (GA). In anesthetized, apneic pregnant women, arterial oxygen tension falls at almost 2½ times the rate of nonpregnant controls (10). Thus, only very short periods of apnea or hypoxia are tolerated, and the use of an increased inspired oxygen fraction helps to optimize fetomaternal condition during induction of GA, fetal compromise, maternal hypoventilation, apnea, or airway obstruction.

At term, physiologic dead space is reduced, probably due to increased cardiac output with favorable ventilation–perfusion matching, so that alveolar–arterial oxygen tension differences are minimal.

Management Implications

1. Supplemental oxygen therapy, including routine preoxygenation, increases maternal safety and may benefit the fetus and neonate.
2. Early oxygenation and ventilation by means other than tracheal intubation may be lifesaving when difficulty with laryngoscopy and intubation occurs.
3. Capnography, in addition to its primary role as a method of detection of esophageal intubation, is a valuable respiratory monitor.

The Gastrointestinal System

Gastrointestinal changes predispose to an increased risk of regurgitation and aspiration of gastric content, one of the two main causes of anesthetic-related maternal mortality. In the first trimester, elevated levels of progesterone may decrease lower esophageal sphincter pressure (LESP); later, the enlarging uterus increases intragastric pressure and decreases the normal oblique angle of the gastroesophageal junction (11,12). Although symptomatic reflux (regurgitation) peaks in late pregnancy, major reflux may be asymptomatic (13). Plasma motilin levels fall, and paracetamol (acetaminophen) absorption is delayed from early pregnancy, while a progressive rise in plasma gastrin levels may result in gastric hypersecretion (14–17).

Recent longitudinal studies during pregnancy and the puerperium, some using new, noninvasive methods of assessing solid and liquid phase emptying, indicate that pregnancy alone has no significant effect on the rate of gastric emptying (14,15,17–19). In contrast, established labor results in an unpredictable delay, which is markedly potentiated by opioids administered either parenterally or epidurally, the largest residual volumes being in those who have had pethidine (meperidine) (20–22). Ultrasound imaging demonstrates that many women in active labor have solid food present, independent of the time to last oral intake—some despite not having eaten for 8–24 hours (23). In the postpartum period, gastric pH and volume do not differ from nonpregnant controls. Gastric emptying remains impaired 2 hours after delivery but is rapid later on the first postpartum day; gastroesophageal reflux has decreased significantly by the second day (18,24,25).

It has been postulated that the purported poor outcome from aspiration in obstetric patients is related to increased permeability and interstitial water in the lung and to decreased colloid osmotic pressure and lymphatic clearance (26).

Management Implications

1. Opinions vary as to whether gastric aspiration precautions are needed in early pregnancy (16), though this should be considered in all pregnant women, depending on relevant medical and surgical factors. A history of heartburn is an indication. Most obstetric anesthetists practice routine prophylaxis and airway protection after about 20 weeks gestation, with continuation until 48 hours into the puerperium (27).
2. All pregnant women having emergency surgery or who have been in labor should be considered to have a full stomach, irrespective of the duration of fasting.

AIRWAY ASSESSMENT IN PREGNANCY

General

A history of relevant medical conditions (e.g., rheumatoid arthritis, temporomandibular joint dysfunction) or details of previous intubation may provide vital information, although many obstetric anesthetists have encountered women who had previously been intubated uneventfully but proved difficult to intubate when pregnant. Few of the methods of airway assessment have been validated in pregnancy, and none is ideal. Difficult cases may not be obvious even after careful, unhurried evaluation, since tongue size and mobility, for example, are not easily seen (28–31). Endler et al. (32) suggested that many airway problems may be avoided if all women were assessed antenatally or on admission. Although ideal, this is often not feasible, and occasionally evaluation may need to be repeated, since changes can occur during the course of labor (33). When urgent GA is imperative, airway history and examination may have to be extremely brief, but must never be omitted.

Predictive Tests

The classical factors predictive of difficult intubation are well detailed (see Chapter 4). Despite interest in simple, practical bedside tests, measurements, and scores; data from obstetric patients are limited. Samsoon and Young (29) reassessed seven failed obstetric intubations and found all—bar one—to have a modified Mallampati class IV airway, leading others to evaluate this test prospectively. Yeo et al. (34) found that a Mallampati III or IV view predicted a third of the difficult obstetric laryngoscopic views but was of no predictive value in gynecologic patients. Savva (35) studied 322 patients, of whom only 28 were obstetric, and supported other investigators' opinion that this test was insensitive and lacking in specificity, a class III or IV score being associated with difficult intubation in only 8% of cases.

Rocke et al. (36) used the modified Mallampati test to assess 1500 women having Cesarean section preoperatively, followed by stepwise multiple logistic regression analysis to determine other factors predictive of increased risk of difficult intubation. The latter were short neck (which was associated with obesity), with receding mandible and protruding maxillary incisors. A class IV score predicted only 6% of very difficult intubations and neither of the two failed intubations. A class I score was reassuring in that a problem was very unlikely, although difficult intubation still occurred (in 0.4% and 1.8% of class I or II, respectively). New measurements or combining tests may improve prediction (37,38). For example, Rocke et al. (36) noted that about 1 in 100 women had both a short neck and class IV score, this combination being associated with a 15% probability of difficult intubation. The predicted probability of difficulty in those with a class IV view, short neck, and receding mandible was over 60%.

Practical Recommendations

1. Airway history and examination, with preparation of a strategy for airway management, are essential to safe obstetric practice. Factors may be identified that allow appropriate expert assistance and special equipment to be obtained.
2. Airway assessment should be performed in the recumbent as well as sitting position, since repositioning of pillows and supports to elevate the shoulders, neck, and head may bring the anatomic axes into line and markedly reduce difficulty (see Figs. 6A,6B, Chapter 4). This is especially helpful in the airway management of the obese patient.
3. Even if no risk factors are apparent, unexpected difficulty with intubation may still occur. Preparation is, thus, essential in all cases, and a "difficult intubation trolley" should be readily available (preferably in the operating room) for all obstetric GAs.

ASPIRATION OF GASTRIC CONTENT IN OBSTETRICS: RISK, PREVENTION, AND MANAGEMENT

Risk

Regurgitation during emergency Cesarean section may occur in up to 1% of women (36). Gastric aspiration during pregnancy and the early puerperium may lead to either acute obstruction and hypoxia or late pneumonitis. In contrast to the 1:660 incidence reported in the classic paper by Mendelson (39), aspiration is now, fortunately, rare. Small, recent prospective series report no cases in 7452 GAs in an Australian (40) and two in 5908 anesthetics in a Canadian hospital over 5 years (41). This is consistent with the rate in general surgical populations (1.5–6 per 10,000 anesthetics) (42). A review of older maternal mortality data until the mid-1980s by Glassenberg (43) found that the fatality rate from aspiration had fallen over three decades, but at two deaths per million births (1 per 30,000 anesthetics), it was, nevertheless, seven times that of the nonobstetric surgical population.

Mortality after aspiration is about 5%, and in obstetric anesthesia it has remained one of the leading causes of anesthetic-related maternal mortality in all developed countries for several decades, despite various modifications to technique (e.g., the introduction of relaxant anesthesia and rapid sequence induction) or to pharmacologic prophylaxis (e.g., the change to nonparticulate antacids). In the triennial Confidential Enquiries into Maternal Death (CEMD) in England and Wales (more recently, the UK) (44), aspiration has been responsible for 35% of direct deaths in the four triennia between 1979 and 1990 and precipitated 10 of 44 deaths from adult respiratory distress syndrome in the 1988–1990 report. In the US, a review of 152 deaths from 1979 to 1990 found aspiration to be the equal leading cause (32 cases, 21% of total deaths) (45). Findings were similar in New Zealand between 1969 and 1986, aspiration accounting for 8 of 24 anesthesia-related maternal deaths, with mask anesthesia and obesity among the risk factors (46).

Despite the hazards introduced by tracheal intubation, which is now established in modern obstetric anesthesia (47), mask anesthesia appears a greater danger, as evidenced by the original report by Mendelson, the New Zealand data, and that from the state of Massachusetts for 1954–1985 (48), where 10 of 17 deaths in the first decade, 3 of 17 in the second, and none of only 3 in the third, were from aspiration during mask anesthesia. Serious nonfatal morbidity is also a leading cause of obstetric admission to intensive care (40).

A large percentage of fatal maternal aspirations are associated with very difficult intubation (43). Although most aspirations occur at induction of GA, especially for emergency Cesarean, deaths have also been reported at extubation, in the postoperative period, and in association with termination of pregnancy and complications of regional anesthesia.

Prevention and Management

Aspiration prophylaxis aims to limit gastric volume, reduce intragastric solid residue and acidity, prevent reflux and regurgitation, and protect the airway from vomited or regurgitated material (14,42,49). Prophylactic pharmacologic regimens, often involving routine drug administration at significant cost, vary widely between countries, hospitals, and individuals (50–52). Accurate data on the effect of various interventions on outcome are not available, and practice is, thus, based on experimental data describing numbers apparently at risk and clinical experience. It may be that greater awareness of the problem, increased use of regional blocks, and better experience or supervision of those conducting obstetric anesthesia has had the greatest impact on the apparent recent fall in deaths secondary to aspiration in the UK (53,54).

Management Principles

1. Safe obstetric airway management is centered not only on combination pharmacologic prophylaxis but also on multiple strategies aiming to avoid acid aspiration.

Fasting Policies

Despite argument to the contrary (55), the author contends that fasting policies are integral to safe management. The aspiration of solid residue is particularly serious in terms of both early obstructive hypoxic effects and of the subsequent severity of pneumonitis. Reduction in fasting interval for solids is not recommended in obstetric patients (56). Although studies have not been conducted in pregnant women, physiologic considerations and a postpartum study (57) suggest fluid fasting for elective surgery should be less restrictive.

Fasting Recommendations

1. Most units pursue a policy of no solids on the day of surgery or at the time of labor. Our policy is to permit free clear fluid until 3 hours prior to elective surgery.
2. In active labor, policies vary (58), but most units advocate nil per oris for women at high risk of operative delivery.

Reduction of Gastric Volume and Acidity; Prevention of Reflux

Outcome may be determined by both the volume and pH of aspirate. Animal models show low volumes of very acidic liquid cause serious lung pathology, as do larger volumes up to pH 4.5 (the level at which pepsin loses its activity) and very large volumes of neutral fluid (59–62). In obstetrics, pneumonitis after aspiration of content of pH 3.5 has been reported (63), but larger volumes of acidic aspirate than previously thought may be necessary to cause serious damage (64). The insertion of a nasogastric tube perioperatively in an attempt to reduce gastric volume is controversial and seldom practiced, in view of its limited efficacy and the potential for trauma or regurgitation (65,66). Instead, this is often attempted pharmacologically, either by promoting gastric emptying or by reducing gastric acid secretion.

Gastric emptying, including following opioid analgesia, is enhanced by the use of 10 mg of intravenous (IV) (but not intramuscular or oral) metoclopramide (67,68). Metoclopramide also increases LESP and may have an antiemetic effect (11,14,42). Although efficacy is limited, subtle psychomimetic and extrapyramidal reactions, serious cardiovascular complications, and fetal effects are rare. Cisapride (Propulsid) is a new prokinetic agent that increases LESP. Parenterally, it is more effective than metoclopramide in preventing morphine-induced delay in gastric emptying (69) but has yet to be evaluated in obstetric populations. Anticholinergics (atropine, glycopyrrolate) decrease gastric secretion, increase pH, and, in combination with antacid, reduce the number of women at risk (42) but have been superseded by the H_2-receptor antagonists, which are more effective and do not decrease LESP.

The regular administration of antacid during labor has been abandoned because protection is unreliable and because intragastric volume may be markedly increased. Ranitidine (Zantac) has a better side effect profile and longer duration of action than does cimetidine (Tagamet) and is widely used (52). Newer agents such as nizatidine (Axid) may be marginally more reliable in general surgical populations (70) but have not been studied in obstetrics. Omeprazole (Losec), the parietal cell proton pump inhibitor, reduces both volume and pH. Omeprazole (40 mg) orally administered the evening before and on the morning of surgery is more effective and reliable in increasing pH above 3.5 than are either higher single-dose therapy or oral ranitidine (71,72). Forty mg IV given at least 40 min before emergency GA Cesarean section reduces the number at risk to a minimum (73), but a ranitidine and sodium citrate combination is more cost-effective than is 12-hourly oral administration during labor (74).

Nonparticulate antacids like sodium citrate effectively alkalinize large volumes of acid but must be administered within 30 min of surgery, since the reliable duration of action is less than an hour (75,76). Particulate antacids should be avoided since they cause lung injury if aspirated (62,77,78). Appropriately timed regimens of ranitidine reduce acidity and volume to acceptable levels in all but a few patients per hundred, so subsequent administration of antacid is controversial. The author's approach is to also include antacid prior to GA and to all emergency surgery but to omit it for elective surgery conducted using central neuraxis block. Prior to emergency surgery, IV ranitidine is warranted, irrespective of preoperative timing, because it is likely to have significantly reduced acid aspiration risk at extubation. A combination of sodium citrate and IV ranitidine leaves less than 1% of women at risk at the end of Cesarean section (79).

Management Principles for Pharmacologic Prophylaxis

1. Recommended regimens of oral ranitidine include 150 mg on the evening before and at least 90–120 min prior to surgery (80) and IV ranitidine 50 mg, preferably given at least 30 min prior to surgery to confer protection at induction (79). Routine or selective administration 6 hourly during active labor is practiced in some units (81,82).
2. The routine use of (IV) metoclopramide has been recommended (14,54).
3. Since an empty stomach can never be guaranteed, neutralization of residual acidic content with a nonparticulate antacid such as sodium citrate (0.3 molar 30 ml) is mandatory before emergency surgery or where fasting status is in doubt.

Further Prevention and Treatment of Aspiration

Given the limitations of pharmacologic prophylaxis and the high likelihood of particulate intragastric residue in women having emergency surgery or in labor, protection is best achieved by avoiding GA or oversedation and routinely using well-conducted regional anesthesia. Nevertheless, it may be necessary to secure and protect the airway when GA is indicated or unavoidable, when unexpected perioperative complications arise (for example, high or unsatisfactory block requiring administration of sedatives or opioids, or a surgical complication necessitating intubation for controlled ventilation), and in nonsurgical obstetric emergencies (for example, eclampsia, a major complication of epidural analgesia in labor, major trauma, drug overdose, or cardiopulmonary resuscitation). Except in exceptional circumstances, airway protection is normally achieved by tracheal intubation after the application of cricoid pressure. The latter is then maintained until the trachea is intubated, the lungs ventilated, airway leak eliminated, and the position of the tube confirmed (by capnography in the surgical setting).

Treatment of aspiration pneumonitis is mainly supportive, involving oxygenation; positioning (right-lateral, head-down); suctioning, bronchoscopy, and removal of solid material; and continuous positive airway pressure or intermittent positive pressure ventilation as required. Treatment of infection and circulatory support may be required in severe cases. Pulmonary lavage, prophylactic antibiotics, and steroids are not of value (83).

Management Principles

1. Protection of the airway is the final and arguably the most crucial preventative measure. This is best afforded if the woman's own protective upper esophageal and laryngeal reflexes have not been obtunded by sedation or GA.

NORMAL AIRWAY MANAGEMENT DURING PREGNANCY

Introduction

Clinical experience indicates that the risk of aspiration during spontaneous breathing with mask anesthesia in early and midpregnancy is low (84), probably due to the function of the upper esophageal sphincter in preventing regurgitation in the absence of neuromuscular block (85). Nevertheless, fatal aspiration in this setting has been reported (44,86).

Later in pregnancy, a GA is normally managed by tracheal intubation after preoxygenation and a rapid sequence induction with cricoid pressure. Similarly, the airway should be protected from soiling at the earliest possible time, should consciousness be lost (e.g., during cardiopulmonary resuscitation or apnea from total spinal anesthesia), either by adoption of the lateral, head-down position (allowing gravity to direct gastric content away from the larynx and aspirate to affect only one lung) or by immediate application of cricoid pressure and rapid intubation.

Extubation is also a time of increased risk. The pharynx should be suctioned and extubation deferred until the woman has roused to a level of response to command and is in the lateral, head-down position.

Oxygen Therapy in the Pregnant Woman

This is advisable during regional anesthesia, when consciousness is impaired, the fetus compromised, or sometimes following the administration of opioids or sedatives. Oxygen delivery is equally effective using 8 L/min via a mask or 4 L/min via nasal prongs (87).

Preoxygenation prior to GA results in more rapid denitrogenation during pregnancy (88) and adequately performed results in mean oxygen tensions of 350 (maternal arterial), 34, and 18 (fetal umbilical venous and arterial) mm Hg, with 95% of women optimally oxygenated (89, 90). In cases of extreme urgency, the Gold technique of four vital capacity breaths in 30 sec using a circle-system has been validated in obstetric patients (89). Attention to detail is important (e.g., prefilling the reservoir bag with 100% oxygen and avoiding leaks), and if apnea is prolonged or a Magill circuit used, the four-breath technique may be less effective (90,91). The fetus responds rapidly to increased maternal oxygen tension and, provided exposure to increased inspired oxygen exceeds 3 min, equilibration is likely (92,93). Should maternal arterial oxygen tension fall below 100 mm Hg, fetal condition deteriorates (94). In contrast to obese nonpregnant women, the 45° sitting position during preoxygenation does not reduce the rate of desaturation (95).

Oxygen Therapy During Pregnancy

1. In conjunction with the avoidance of aortocaval compression, supplemental oxygen therapy is frequently indicated.
2. Preoxygenation (preferably with at least 5 L/min of 100% oxygen via a tight-fitting mask for a minimum of 2 min) is mandatory before GA.

Cricoid Pressure

Identification of the cricoid cartilage may be difficult (especially in the obese), and cricoid pressure is frequently poorly performed (96), due to poor training and the difficulty of simulating effective cricoid pressure without a suitable model. Anatomic distortions encountered include lateral displacement of the larynx (97) (corrected by realignment to the right when the woman is in left-lateral tilt) and obliteration of the glottic opening (due to excessive force or application above the cricoid). Inadequate force may allow regurgitation. Most obstetric anesthetists have experienced these problems (98), and the author's experience supports the view that the incorrect application of cricoid pressure is of greater etiologic importance in difficult intubation than are anatomic factors (99).

Although Sellick originally described single-handed cricoid pressure, various modifications have been suggested to ensure the head does not flex on the neck. Bimanual cricoid pressure with the second hand supporting the cervical vertebrae has been recommended (44, 100) but is not widely used (101). Effective cricoid pressure applied to an awake patient cannot be tolerated and may provoke coughing, with deaths from both aspiration and esophageal rupture reported (97,102,103). Since upper esophageal sphincter pressure begins to fall after induction of GA but prior to loss of consciousness (11), an ideal force of about 10–20 N (1–2 kg) should be applied to the awake patient, increasing to 3–4 kg with loss of consciousness (104). This is easily learned if training with a model and scale is available (97,105).

The Role of Cricoid Pressure During Pregnancy

1. The correct timing and application of cricoid pressure are of vital importance to safe airway management.
2. Attention to teaching and supervision of assistants is paramount.

Intravenous Anesthetic and Neuromuscular Blocking Drugs

Thiopentone (Pentothal) is still considered the induction agent of choice, although ketamine (Ketalar) and propofol (Diprovan) are appropriate alternatives in special circumstances (106). An adequate dose of succinylcholine (1–1.5 mg/kg) gives satisfactory relaxation within 50 sec and lasts 6 min (107,108), although Carmie (109) has demonstrated that junior anesthetists attempt to intubate far sooner when dealing with an obstetric case, often failing to allow sufficient time for adequate intubating conditions. The short duration of action is important, should difficulty with intubation occur. Measures to reduce succinylcholine-induced muscle pain are not necessary, since the incidence during pregnancy is low (110,111). When succinylcholine is contraindicated, the choice lies between awake intubation techniques or a modified rapid sequence induction using a nondepolarizing relaxant. Vecuronium (Norcuron) is suitable for the latter but this approach requires careful consideration because of its prolonged effect, should unexpected difficulty with intubation follow. Vecuronium lacks cardiovascular effects at generous intubating doses and acts more rapidly during pregnancy (112), although cricoid pressure needs to be maintained for 90 sec to achieve satisfactory intubating conditions, and recovery is slower (113,114). Thorough preoxygenation and the use of a peripheral nerve stimulator are advisable. Newer nondepolarizing relaxants have not as yet had their role defined in obstetrics, although rocuronium (Esmeren) has the potential to be a suitable substitute for vecuronium (115).

Mask ventilation is usually avoided until intubation, although if ventilation is easy, it is unlikely to cause gastric insufflation. Maintenance of neuromuscular block is achieved using short-acting relaxants. Succinylcholine infusion or repeat boluses, or small doses of nondepolarizing relaxant [vecuronium 0.05 mg/kg or atracurium (Tracrium) 0.1–0.25 mg/kg] provide readily reversible relaxation for 10–30 min and are alternatives, depending on the duration of surgery. Profound abdominal relaxation is not required during Cesarean section, and long-acting relaxants like pancuronium should be avoided, since postoperative hypoventilation due to inadequate reversal of block has accounted for several deaths (44).

Pharmacologic Recommendations for General Anesthesia

1. Induction of GA should be performed with a well-evaluated and rapidly acting agent such as thiopentone.
2. Succinylcholine remains the relaxant of choice for rapid sequence induction, and long-acting nondepolarizing relaxants are usually unnecessary.

AIRWAY PROBLEMS IN OBSTETRICS

Difficult and Failed Intubation: Risk, Outcome, and Management

Risk and Outcome

The reported incidence of difficult intubation depends on the criteria used (e.g., difficult laryngoscopic view, multiple attempts at intubation, failed intubation). The incidence of failed intubation also varies with the patient population studied, how early the anesthetist resorts to other means to establish satisfactory ventilation, and, most importantly, the anesthetist's experience. Very difficult intubation has been noted in about 2% of both obstetric and general surgical populations (34,36,38), with failed intubation occurring in approximately 1:300 to 1:2000 nonobstetric cases (31,38,116). Older data suggest a much higher rate of failed intubation in obstetric populations (43), but teaching hospitals in different countries have more recently reported incidences from 1:300 (117) to 1:750 (36) and 1:1900 (116).

The consequences of failed intubation in obstetrics may be profound, especially as it frequently occurs at induction of GA for emergency Cesarean section. Difficult intubation or unrecognized esophageal intubation (leading to hypoxic cardiac arrest and/or aspiration) are now the leading causes of anesthetic-related maternal mortality and accounted for 47% of such deaths in the CEMD 1976–1987, including 10 of 19 deaths in 1982–1984, 6 of 8 in 1985–1987, and 1 of 4 in 1988–1990. Other problems, such as equipment failure, disconnection, and tube obstruction accounted for 7% of deaths between 1967 and 1984. Although obesity is not a strong predictor of difficulty (36), many of these women were of short stature and obese; a detailed, single-center review of morbidly obese obstetric patients found that 6 of 17 were difficult to intubate (118). Similarly, failed intubation and other airway or ventilation problems accounted for 8 of 24 anesthetic-related maternal deaths in New Zealand (46). In the US, 38 of 152 deaths were secondary to induction/intubation problems or hypoventilation, these being the first-ranked causes (45).

Increased fetal mortality and neonatal and maternal morbidity have not been quantified. Complications of GA involving the airway (e.g., suspected aspiration, disconnection, and obstruction) are, however, the most common anesthetic-related reasons for obstetric admissions to intensive care (40,119). Intubation problems are the most common reasons for obstetric malpractice claims against anesthesiologists in North America (120).

A decline in the absolute number (and probably incidence) of anesthetic-related deaths in recent consecutive triennia in the UK may reflect improving safety standards due to the greater involvement of experienced anesthetists, better monitoring and recovery room facilities, and the trend to fewer GA Cesarean sections.

Management

If difficult intubation is anticipated, a decision must be made regarding the use of regional block, awake intubation, or GA (121). Any woman in whom difficulty was experienced should be counseled, given a letter of explanation, and, if appropriate, recommended to obtain a Medic Alert bracelet or something similar.

Airway Management Principles

1. After assessment, decide on a clear, practical plan for airway management (122–125).
2. In obstetrics, usually aim to use regional anesthesia.
3. It is a fundamental rule of anesthesia never to induce neuromuscular block if there is doubt about the ability to ventilate.

Esophageal Intubation

Unrecognized esophageal intubation is said to account for 22 deaths per million obstetric anesthetics, compared to 1.8 in the nonobstetric population (43). Familiarity with the methods of detection and their limitations is essential. It must be remembered that preoxygenation may delay for several minutes the onset of cyanosis after esophageal intubation. An exhaled CO_2 analyzer, indicating a sustained CO_2 trace over several breaths, is the only reliable means of excluding esophageal intubation.

Practical Implications

1. Always auscultate breath sounds in both axillae. Apply the maxim "when in doubt, take it out."
2. Capnography should be combined with pulse oximetry during GA in obstetrics.

Awake Intubation

Indications for awake intubation include the acutely compromised airway, known or expected difficulty with intubation, and failed intubation where the woman has been allowed to waken but surgery must proceed. Techniques for awake intubation are described in Part IV of this book and in a comprehensive review (126). In the emergency obstetric situation, some options may be more hazardous or difficult, and plans for a surgical approach to the airway should be made if awake intubation fails.

The pregnant woman poses several difficulties. Antisialagogues lower LESP and are, thus, often omitted. The oral route, using a split oral airway, is preferable for fiberoptic intubation. Rarely, massive tongue swelling, limited mouth opening, or other pathology may preclude this approach and mandate blind nasal or nasal fiberoptic intubation (6,127,128). Adequate topical nasal anesthesia and vasoconstriction is essential to minimize epistaxis if the nasal route is employed. Cocaine should be avoided if possible, because of its deleterious sympathomimetic effects in preeclampsia and its reduction of uterine blood flow (127). Ten-percent lidocaine spray with vasoconstrictors, such as ephedrine (Isofedrol) 1% or phenylephrine 0.125%, provide better hemodynamic stability, although the latter may also reduce uteroplacental perfusion.

Sedatives increase the potential for aspiration and have fetal effects, although small incremental doses of midazolam (Versed) or opioid are unlikely to produce significant neonatal depression (6,128). Supplemental oxygen should be administered via nasal cannulae or insufflated via the suction port of the fiberoptic scope.

Given that protective reflexes are blunted by topical anesthesia, increasing aspiration risk, it is reassuring that no such cases have been reported, despite experience in hundreds of both nonobstetric and obstetric patients (including the use of transtracheal injection for anesthesia below the cords) (43,129).

Recommendations for Obstetric Awake Intubation

1. Obtain expert help from a second anesthetist, use the semisitting position with left pelvic tilt, and, if possible, avoid sedation and cricothyroid injection for topical anesthesia below the vocal cords.

Unexpected Very Difficult Intubation

The unexpected very difficult intubation is every obstetric anesthetist's worst nightmare, and because it is likely to be encountered infrequently, the practice of regularly simulating a grade III laryngoscopic view on elective surgical patients not at risk of regurgitation has been recommended (28) and is being evaluated (116). The critical message was emphasized by Scott (47): "Patients do not die from a 'failure to intubate.' They die either from failure to stop trying to intubate or from undiagnosed esophageal intubation."

Management Principles

1. Take early decisive action, which usually means accepting failure and abandoning attempts to intubate in order to concentrate on oxygenation and ventilation by alternative means.
2. A "failed intubation drill" (130) and associated aspects of airway management should be learned early in postgraduate education programs and practiced in nonemergency situations. Safety is likely to be compromised by attempts to use unfamiliar techniques and equipment.

Failed Intubation Drill

Since Tunstall's (130) 1976 description of a "failed intubation drill" to achieve "oxygenation without aspiration," (131) many modifications have been suggested (Fig. 1). All "drills" (Table 1) are management guidelines, with provision for the clinician to exercise judgment. The benefit of the drills is as an algorithm, linking strategies with clear, logical progression. They are akin to, but less didactic than, algorithms for cardiopulmonary resuscitation. Hard copy of a simple drill should be readily available in every location where obstetric anesthesia is conducted. In addition, special equipment, as recommended in Part IV of this book and by Davies (125) and the ASA Guidelines (121) (especially a laryngeal mask airway or LMA and aids to intubation and ventilation), must be readily available on a portable trolley. Valuable examples include special laryngoscopes, such as the Kessel laryngoscope, in which the angle of the blade to the handle is opened by a further 20° (see Fig. 34, Chapter 15). Other laryngoscopes that may be helpful in air-

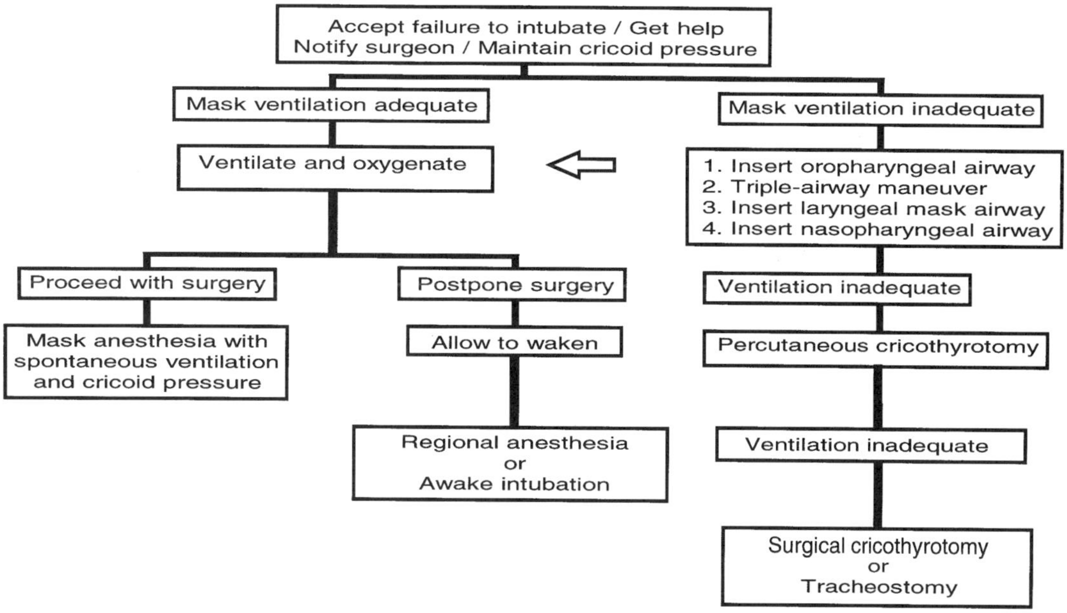

FIG. 1. Abbreviated "failed intubation drill."

way management under these circumstances are the Datta-Briwa short-handled laryngoscope (see Fig. 36, Chapter 15) and the Bellhouse laryngoscope with detachable prism (Avulunga Pty Ltd, New South Wales) (Fig. 11, Chapter 15). Another aid to intubation is a flexible bougie with sufficient rigidity to maintain curvature at its tip. This is positioned with the tip protruding 5 cm through a tracheal tube in such a way that it is a guide for intubation. If this is used in conjunction with an Oxford tube, which has an anterior bevel that is less likely to catch on the arytenoideae or cords, passage of the endotracheal tube over the bougie and through the glottis ("railroading") can be more readily achieved. The place of and controversies regarding the LMA in obstetric anesthesia have been well reviewed recently (132).

The vast majority of difficult intubations in obstetrics present with a grade III laryngoscopic view (32). In the rare case of an unexpected grade IV view, it may be wise to institute a failed intubation drill immediately, since the chances of successful blind oral intubation are remote. The number of attempts made to intubate when confronted with a grade III view will be determined by clinical circumstances. Rosen (133) suggests a maximum of two attempts of 1 min each, separated by 30 sec of ventilation (133). The view of the larynx may be improved by patient repositioning; adjustment of cricoid pressure; use of an alternative laryngoscope; or backward, upward, and rightward external pressure on the thyroid cartilage (134, 135). As a general rule, additional doses of IV anesthetic or muscle relaxant should not be given, since they delay the return of spontaneous ventilation. Tracheal intubation should be abandoned for face-mask ventilation, aided by an oropharyngeal airway or Safar's two-handed triple-airway maneuver (131) if necessary, while cricoid pressure is maintained.

If ventilation remains inadequate, the main alternatives are the modified esophageal gastric tube airway (EGTA) or combitube, the more readily available and familiar laryngeal mask airway (LMA), or turning to the left-lateral head-down position and retrying mask ventilation. If ventilation is possible though not completely satisfactory, spontaneous ventilation is returning, and the decision has been made to postpone surgery, it is safest to follow Tunstall's recommendation of turning the woman to the full left-lateral head-down position and continuing with a face mask, preferably releasing cricoid pressure only when she wakes and airway reflexes have returned. The EGTA was originally designed for CPR and for those inexperienced with intubation; it provides a vent for regurgitated material. It may improve mask ventilation by lifting the epiglottis and larynx anteriorly, away from the posterior pharyngeal wall, but it also has limitations and risks (124,131,136). A similar device, the esophageal tracheal combitube, has been used (137); but the recently designed esophageal vent laryngeal mask (138) has not. Deliberate esophageal intubation to act as an obturator, or leaving the tube *in situ* after accidental esophageal intubation, has its enthusiasts (139,140) but, like the LMA, this by no means guarantees that aspiration around the tube will not occur (141).

The insertion of an LMA is the author's preference when the woman is paralyzed, difficult to move, and initial attempts at mask ventilation are inadequate. Anecdotal evidence suggests that insertion is usually not a prob-

TABLE 1. *Detailed management strategy for failed intubation in obstetric patients*

1. Maintain cricoid pressure.
2. Call for anesthetic help.
3. Repeat laryngoscopy after
   - optimizing patient position,
   - realigning or reducing poorly applied cricoid pressure.
   - obtaining aids to intubation (smaller tube; different laryngoscope; malleable stylet; Oxford tube with bougie).
4. If still unsuccessful,
   - do not give further anesthetic or relaxant,
   - inform obstetrician and review fetal condition,
   - concentrate on ventilation with 100% O_2 by mask.

A. If ventilation is easy or adequate (SpO_2 > 90% on 100% O_2) *and* it is decided to postpone surgery,
   1. Maintain cricoid pressure.
   2. Ventilate with 100% O_2 via a face mask.
   3. Review fetal condition.
   4. Allow spontaneous ventilation to resume.
   5. Turn patient to left lateral with head-down tilt.
   6. Release cricoid pressure when awakening.
   7. Allow to waken.
   8. Decide on regional anesthesia or awake intubation (preferably fiberoptic) followed by general anesthesia.

B. If ventilation is easy *and* it is decided to proceed with surgery,
   1. Maintain cricoid pressure.
   2. Ventilate with 100% O_2 and volatile anesthetic via face mask.
   3. Increase depth of anesthesia with volatile and N_2O, maintaining SpO_2 > 95% while allowing spontaneous ventilation to resume.
   4. Ask obstetrician to expedite surgery and avoid compression of the upper abdomen.
   5. Consider insertion of a nasogastric tube and aspiration of gastric content.
   6. Continue general anesthesia and cricoid pressure.
   7. Go to steps A5–7 (above) at completion of surgery.

C. If ventilation is inadequate (clinically or SpO_2 < 90% on 100% O_2),
   1. Administer 100% O_2 and maintain cricoid pressure.
   2. Obtain anesthetic help and equipment for cricothyrotomy.
   3. Insert oropharyngeal airway and try triple-airway maneuver.
   4. If still inadequate, insert LMA.

   5.1. If ventilation remains inadequate and, depending on time elapsed and level of oxygenation,
   - reinsert LMA after releasing cricoid pressure transiently (reapply cricoid when satisfactorily positioned) or
   - insert nasopharyngeal airway or
   - go to steps 5.2 or 5.3 (below).

   5.2. If spontaneous ventilation is resuming and the patient awakening, turn her to the left-lateral, head-down position, oxygenate and reassess.

   5.3. If ventilation remains inadequate and the woman is paralyzed, leave supine with pelvic tilt and establish transtracheal ventilation via percutaneous cricothyrotomy.

   6. If unsuccessful, perform surgical cricothyrotomy or tracheostomy.
   7. If successful during steps C2–5, make decision regarding urgency of surgery and go to A or B (above).

LMA, laryngeal mask airway.

lem in those with a difficult airway (132,142), although cricoid pressure significantly reduces the chance of successful insertion and ventilation (132,142,144). Since the first description of its successful use after failed obstetric intubation and difficult ventilation (145), many reports attest to its value. It is not always the answer, however (146), and, as LESP is reduced compared to spontaneously breathing face-mask anesthesia, the latter is preferable when ventilation proves satisfactory initially (147). When LMA insertion fails, a choice must be made between trying a nasopharyngeal airway, with the risk of epistaxis (which may be catastrophic) (148), and transient release of cricoid pressure in the supine tilted position while attempting to reposition the LMA. This should be followed by reapplication of cricoid pressure if successful. If the LMA is successfully positioned, blind intubation via the LMA is possible (149,150), even during spontaneous ventilation with cricoid pressure applied (151,152). This is not recommended, however, since aids such as the gum elastic bougie or Cook airway exchange catheter are unreliable, and since all blind techniques have high failure rates (132,143,153), risking regurgitation with channeling of gastric fluid through the LMA. If intubation is considered essential, fiberoptic endoscopic-guided intubation may be the safest and most effective approach (132,154).

Fortunately, continued inability to ventilate is rare (up to 2 per 10,000) (123). Continued failure to oxygenate and ventilate necessitates transtracheal ventilation, though few anesthetists have personal experience (98). This may be very difficult, since anatomic landmarks are often impalpable in obese women, and the risk of serious complications in an emergency or in inexperienced hands is high (155,156). Techniques are well reviewed (122, 124,157,158). Left-tilt should be maintained and transtracheal ventilation achieved [preferably using percutaneous cricothyrotomy, via either a commercial kit or a large-bore (at least 14 gauge) IV cannula, appropriate connector, and means of high-pressure oxygen delivery, such as an oxygen flush valve on the anesthetic machine or a Sanders injector] (157). Surgical cricothyrotomy or tracheotomy commonly fail or cause bleeding and airway obstruction (18,158); they should be considered a last resort.

During the first stages of the drill, the anesthetist and obstetrician/surgeon must determine whether the operation must proceed or can be postponed or deferred. The safest course of action is the latter. Unfortunately, surgical delay may sometimes result in adverse outcome. This is most frequently potential fetal demise at an urgent Cesarean section. The preferred option is to allow the woman to wake and to institute subarachnoid and/or epidural anesthesia (depending on time constraints and expertise) or, if central neuraxis block is contraindicated, to perform awake intubation under local anesthesia, followed by GA. *Since maternal well-being is paramount, the decision to continue GA should be made only if the anesthetist is confident that cricoid pressure is effective and sustainable, and control of the maternal airway and ventilation are completely reliable.* Local infiltration anesthesia or transtracheal ventilation with IV anesthesia should not be undertaken unless staff are experienced with these techniques. Mask anesthesia can be deepened using volatile inhalational anesthetics [traditionally halothane (Fluothane), due to its lack of pungency] and nitrous oxide, assuming pulse oximetry indicates normal arterial hemoglobin oxygen saturation. Cricoid pressure must be maintained and surgery expedited. External pressure over the epigastrium is best avoided during delivery. Regurgitation is unlikely at a depth of surgical anesthesia, especially with spontaneous ventilation. Continuation under neuromuscular block should be considered in only exceptional circumstances (159).

As discussed earlier, the possibility of upper airway trauma, edema, and subsequent postextubation obstruction must also be considered after failed intubation. In those who have been subsequently intubated by other means, an option is to continue ventilation postoperatively, although this should rarely be necessary.

REFERENCES

1. Brocke-Utne JG, Downing JW, Seedat F. Laryngeal edema associated with pre-eclamptic toxemia. *Anaesthesia* 1977;32:556.
2. Brimacombe J. Acute pharyngolaryngeal edema and pre-eclamptic toxemia. *Anaesth Intensive Care* 1992;20:97.
3. Rocke DA, Scones GP. Rapidly progressive laryngeal edema associated with pregnancy-aggravated hypertension. *Anaesthesia* 1992;47:141.
4. Salt PJ, Nutbourne PA, Park GR, Glazebrook CW. Laryngeal edema after Caesarean section. *Anaesthesia* 1983;38:693.
5. Hein HAT. Cardiorespiratory arrest with laryngeal edema in pregnancy-induced hypertension. *Can J Anaesth* 1984;31:210.
6. Fayek SS, Isaac PA, Shah J. Awake fibreoptic intubation in a 38-week pregnant patient with submandibular abscess. *Int J Obstet Anesth* 1994;3:103.
7. Mettam IM, Reddy TR, Evans FE. Life-threatening acute respiratory distress in late pregnancy. *Br J Anaesth* 1992;69:420.
8. Cohen SE. Physiological alterations of pregnancy. In: Ostheimer GW, ed. *Clinics in Anaesthesiology*. London: WB Saunders, 1986; 4(1):33.
9. Camann WR, Ostheimer GW. Physiological adaptations during pregnancy. *Int Anesthesiol Clin* 1990;28:2.
10. Archer GW, Marx GF. Arterial oxygen tension during apnoea in parturient women. *Br J Anaesth* 1974;46:358.
11. Vanner RG. Mechanisms of regurgitation and its prevention with cricoid pressure. *Int J Obstet Anesth* 1993;2:207.
12. Jones MJ, Mitchell WD, Hindocha N, James RH. The lower esophageal sphincter in the first trimester of pregnancy: comparison of supine with lithotomy positions. *Br J Anaesth* 1988;61:475.
13. Hey VMF, Cowley DJ, Ganguli PC, Skinner LD, Ostick DG, Sharp DS. Gastroesophageal reflux in late pregnancy. *Anaesthesia* 1977;2:372.
14. O'Sullivan G. Gastric emptying during pregnancy and the puerperium. *Int J Obstet Anesth* 1993;2:216.
15. Whitehead EM, Smith M, Dean Y, O'Sullivan G. An evaluation of gastric emptying times in pregnancy and the puerperium. *Anaesthesia* 1993;48:53.
16. Levy DM, Williams OA, Magides AD, Reilly CS. Gastric emptying is delayed at 8-12 weeks' gestation. *Br J Anaesth* 1994;74:237.
17. Macfie AG, Magides AD, Richmond MN, Reilly CS. Gastric emptying in pregnancy. *Br J Anaesth* 1991;67:54.
18. Sandhar BK, Elliott RH, Windram I, Rowbotham DJ. Peripartum changes in gastric emptying. *Anaesthesia* 1992;47:196.
19. O'Sullivan GM, Sutton AJ, Thompson SA, Carrie LE, Bullingham RE. Noninvasive measurement of gastric emptying in obstetric patients. *Anesth Analg* 1987;66:505.
20. Nimmo WS, Wilson J, Prescott LF. Narcotic analgesics and delayed gastric emptying during labour. *Lancet* 1975;1:890.
21. Wright PMC, Allen RW, Moore J, Donnelly JP. Gastric emptying during lumbar extradural analgesia in labour: effect of fentanyl supplementation. *Br J Anaesth* 1992;68:248.
22. Holdsworth JD. Relationship between stomach contents and analgesia in labour. *Br J Anaesth* 1978;50:1145.
23. Carp H, Jayaram A, Stoll M. Ultrasound examination of the stomach contents of parturients. *Anesth Analg* 1992;74:683.
24. Vanner RG, Goodman NW. Gastroesophageal reflux in pregnancy at term and after delivery. *Anaesthesia* 1989;44:808.
25. Gin T, Cho AMW, Lew JKL, et al. Gastric emptying in the postpartum period. *Anaesth Intensive Care* 1991;19:521.
26. MacLennan FM. Maternal mortality from Mendelson's syndrome: an explanation? *Lancet* 1986;1:587.
27. Bogod DG. The postpartum stomach—when is it safe? *Anaesthesia* 1994;49:1.
28. Cormack RS, Lehane J. Difficult tracheal intubation in obstetrics. *Anaesthesia* 1984;39:1105.
29. Samsoon GLT, Young JRB. Difficult tracheal intubation: a retrospective study. *Anaesthesia* 1987;42:487.
30. Mallampati SR, Gatt SP, Gugino LD, et al. A clinical sign to predict difficult tracheal intubation: a prospective study. *Can J Anaesth* 1985;32:429.
31. Fahy L, Horton WA, Charters P. Factor analysis in patients with a history of failed tracheal intubation during pregnancy. *Br J Anaesth* 1990;65:813.
32. Endler GC, Mariona FG, Sokol RJ et al. Anesthesia-related maternal mortality in Michigan, 1972 to 1984. *Am J Obstet Gynecol* 1988;159:187.
33. Farcon EL, Kim MH, Marx GF. Changing Mallampati score during labour. *Can J Anaesth* 1994;41:50.
34. Yeo SW, Chong JL, Thomas E. Difficult intubation: a prospective study. *Singapore Med J* 1992;33:362.
35. Savva D. Prediction of difficult tracheal intubation. *Br J Anaesth* 1994;73:149.
36. Rocke DA, Murray WB, Rout CC, Gouws E. Relative risk analysis of factors associated with difficult intubation in obstetric anesthesia. *Anesthesiology* 1992;77:67.
37. Frerk CM. Predicting difficult intubation. *Anaesthesia* 1991;46:1005.
38. Rose DK, Cohen MM. The airway: problems and predictions in 18,500 patients. *Can J Anaesth* 1994;41:372.
39. Mendelson CL. The aspiration of stomach content into the lungs during obstetric anesthesia. Am J Obstet Gynecol 1946;52:191.
40. Stephens ID. ICU admissions from an obstetrical hospital. *Can J Anaesth* 1991;38:677.
41. Ong B, Cohen MM, Cumming M, Palahnuik RJ. Obstetric anesthesia at Winnepeg Women's Hospital 1975-83: anesthetic techniques and complications. *Can J Anaesth* 1987;34:294.
42. Kallar SK, Everett LL. Potential risks and preventative measures for pulmonary aspiration: new concepts in preoperative fasting guidelines. *Anesth Analg* 1993;77:171.
43. Glassenberg R. General anesthesia and maternal mortality. *Semin Perinatol* 1991;15:386.

44. Department of Health. *Report on Confidential Enquiries into Maternal Deaths in England and Wales 1973-75, 1976-78, 1979-81, 1982-84, 1985-87, 1988-90*. London: HMSO.
45. Hawkins J, Koonin L, Palmer S, Gibbs C, Lawson H, Atrash H. Anesthesia-related maternal deaths in the United States: a twelve year review 1979-1990. [Abstr] *Anesthesiology* 1993;79:A982 .
46. Peskett WGH. The anesthetic contribution to maternal mortality in New Zealand. *Int J Obstet Anesth* 1991;1:179.
47. Scott DB. Endotracheal intubation: friend or foe. *Br Med J* 1986;292: 157.
48. Sachs B, Oriol N, Ostheimer G et al. Anesthetic-related maternal mortality, 1954 to 1985. *J Clin Anesth* 1989;1:333.
49. Gonzalez ER, Kallar SK. Reducing the risk of aspiration pneumonitis. *Ann Pharmacotherapy* 1989;23:203.
50. Greenhalgh CA, McLean JL. A survey of acid aspiration chemoprophylaxis in academic departments of obstetric anesthesia in the United States and Canada. [Abstr] *Anesthesiology* 1993;79:A1005.
51. Helbo-Hansen HS, Bang U. Current Danish practice for aspiration prophylaxis in obstetric anesthesia: a survey. *Int J Obstet Anesth* 1993;2:233.
52. Greiff JMC, Tordoff SG, Griffiths R, May AE. Acid aspiration prophylaxis in 202 obstetric units in the UK. *Int J Obstet Anesth* 1994;3: 137.
53. Morgan M. Getting there. [Editorial] *Anaesthesia* 1991;46:709.
54. Thomas TA. Maternal mortality. [Editorial] *Int J Obstet Anesth* 1994; 3:125.
55. Elkington KW. At the water's edge: where obstetrics and anesthesia meet. *Obstet Gynecol* 1991;77:304.
56. Lewis M, Crawford JS. Can one risk fasting the obstetric patient for less than 4 hours? *Br J Anaesth* 1987;59:312.
57. Lam KK, So HY, Gin T. Gastric pH and volume after oral fluids in the postpartum patient. *Can J Anaesth* 1993;40:218.
58. Michael S, Reilly CS, Caunt JA. Policies for oral intake during labour. A survey of maternity units in England and Wales. *Anaesthesia* 1991;46:1071.
59. Teabeaut JR II. Aspiration of gastric contents. An experimental study. *Am J Pathol* 1952;28:51.
60. James CF, Modell JH, Gibbs CP, Kuck EJ, Ruiz BC. Pulmonary aspiration—effects of volume and pH in the rat. *Anesth Analg* 1984;63: 665.
61. Piper DW, Fenton BH. pH stability and activity curves of pepsin with special reference to their clinical importance. *Gut* 1965;6:506.
62. Schwartz DJ, Wynne JW, Gibbs CP, Hood CI, Kuck EJ. The pulmonary consequences of aspiration of gastric contents at pH values greater than 2.5. *Am Rev Respir Dis* 1980;121:119.
63. Taylor G. Acid pulmonary aspiration syndrome after antacids. A case report. *Br J Anaesth* 1975;47:615.
64. Raidoo DM, Rocke DA, Brock-Utne JG, Marszelak A, Engelbrecht HE. Critical volume for pulmonary acid aspiration: reappraisal in a primate model. *Br J Anaesth* 1990;65:248.
65. May AE. The confidential enquiry into maternal deaths 1988-1990. [Editorial] *Br J Anaesth* 1994;73:129.
66. Brocke-Utne JG, Rout C, Moodley J, Mayat N. Does preoperative gastric emptying decrease the risk of acid aspiration in obstetrical anesthesia? [Abstr] *Anesth Analg* 1989;68:S39.
67. Murphy DF, Nally B, Gardiner J, Unwin A. Effect of metoclopramide on gastric emptying before elective and emergency Caesarean section. *Br J Anaesth* 1984;56:1113.
68. McNeill MJ, Ho ET, Kenny GNC. Effect of iv metoclopramide on gastric emptying after opioid premedication. *Br J Anaesth* 1990;64: 450.
69. Rowbotham DJ, Bamber PA, Nimmo WS. Comparison of the effect of cisapride and metoclopramide on morphine-induced delay in gastric emptying. *Br J Clin Pharmacol* 1988;26:741.
70. Popat MT, Dyar OJ, Blogg CE. Comparison of the effects of oral nizatidine and ranitidine on gastric volume and pH in patients undergoing gynaecological laparoscopy. *Anaesthesia* 1991;46:816.
71. Ewart MC, Yau G, Gin T, Kotur CF, Oh TE. A comparison of the effects of omeprazole and ranitidine on gastric acid secretion in women undergoing elective Caesarean section. *Anaesthesia* 1990;45: 527.
72. Bill KM, Flynn RJ, Moore J. Prolonged suppression of gastric acid secretion in the obstetric patient. [Abstract] *Can J Anaesth* 1989;36: S53.
73. Rocke DA, Rout CC, Gouws E. Intravenous administration of the proton pump inhibitor omeprazole reduces the risk of acid aspiration at emergency Cesarean section. *Anesth Analg* 1994;78:1093.
74. Yau G, Kan AF, Gin T, Oh TE. A comparison of omeprazole and ranitidine for prophylaxis against aspiration pneumonitis in emergency Caesarean section. *Anaesthesia* 1992;47:101.
75. Gibbs CP, Spohr L, Schmidt D. The effectiveness of sodium citrate as an antacid. *Anesthesiology* 1982;57:44.
76. Dewan DM, Floyd HM, Thistlewood JM, Bogard TD, Spielman FJ. Sodium citrate pretreatment in elective Cesarean section patients. *Anesth Analg* 1985;64:34.
77. Knight PR, Rutter T, Tait AR, Coleman E,Johnson K. Pathogenesis of gastric particulate lung injury: a comparison and interaction with acidic pneumonitis. *Anesth Analg* 1993;77:754.
78. Gibbs CP, Schwartz DJ, Wynne JW, Hood CI, Kuck EJ. Antacid pulmonary aspiration in the dog. *Anesthesiology* 1979;51:380.
79. Rout CC, Rocke DA, Gouws E. Intravenous ranitidine reduces the risk of acid aspiration of gastric contents at emergency Cesarean section. *Anesth Analg* 1993;76:156.
80. O'Sullivan G, Sear JW, Bullingham RES, Carrie LES. The effect of magnesium trisilicate mixture, metoclopramide and ranitidine on gastric pH, volume and serum gastrin. *Anaesthesia* 1985;40:246.
81. Gillett GB, Watson JD, Langford RM. Ranitidine and single-dose antacid therapy as prophylaxis against acid aspiration syndrome in obstetric practice. *Anaesthesia* 1984;39:638.
82. Thompson EM, Loughran PG, McAuley DM, Wilson CM, Moore J. Combined treatment with ranitidine and saline antacids prior to obstetric anesthesia. *Anaesthesia* 1984;39:1086.
83. Lykens MG, Bowton DL. Aspiration and acute lung injury. *Int J Obstet Anesth* 1993;2:236.
84. White PF. Intubation, aspiration prophylaxis in mid-trimester abortions? [Letter] *Anesthesiology* 1984;61:223.
85. Vanner RG. Gastroesophageal reflux and regurgitation during general anesthesia for termination of pregnancy. *Int J Obstet Anesth* 1992;1: 123.
86. Mankowitz E, Khan MFR, Downing JW, Brock-Utne JG, Holloway AM. Inhalation of gastric contents. *Br J Anaesth* 1981;53:778.
87. Crosby ET, Halpern SH. Supplemental maternal oxygen therapy during Caesarean section under epidural anesthesia: a comparison of nasal prongs and facemask. *Can J Anaesth* 1992;39:313.
88. Norris MC, Kirkland MR, Torjman MC, Goldberg ME. Denitrogenation in pregnancy. *Can J Anaesth* 1989;36:523.
89. Russell GN, Smith CL, Snowden SL, Bryson THL. Pre-oxygenation and the parturient patient. *Anaesthesia* 1987;42:346.
90. Norris MC, Dewan DM. Preoxygenation for Cesarean section: a comparison of two techniques. *Anesthesiology* 1985;62:827.
91. Gambec AM, Hertzka RE, Fisher DM. Preoxygenation techniques: Comparison of three minutes and four breaths. *Anesth Analg* 1987;66: 468.
92. Myers RE, Stange L, Joelsson I, Huzell B, Wussow C. Effects upon the fetus of oxygen administration to the mother. *Acta Obstet Gynecol Scand* 1977;56:195.
93. Longo LD, Power GG. Placental oxygen transfer: a systems approach. *Rev Perin Med* 1976;1:1.
94. Marx GF, Mateo CV. Effects of different oxygen concentrations during general anesthesia for elective Caesarean section. *Can Anaesth Soc J* 1971;18:587.
95. Baraka AS, Hanna MT, Jabbour SI et al. Preoxygenation of pregnant women and nonpregnant women in the head-up versus supine position. *Anesth Analg* 1992;75:757.
96. Howells TH, Chamney AR, Wraight WJ, Simons RS. The application of cricoid pressure. *Anaesthesia* 1983;38:457.
97. Lawes EG, Duncan PW, Bland B, Gemmel L, Downing JW. The cricoid yoke—a device for providing consistent and reproducible cricoid pressure. *Br J Anaesth* 1986;58:925.
98. Glosten B. Obstetric anesthesia risk: a review of recent literature. *Int J Obstet Anesth* 1994;3:7.
99. Bonney G, Lyons G. Failed intubation drill: a review of its use in obstetric practice. [Abstr] *Int J Obstet Anesth* 1994;3:108.
100. Crowley DS, Giesecke AH. Bimanual cricoid pressure. *Anaesthesia* 1990;45:588.
101. Crook TM, McCrirrick A. A survey of airway management during induction of general anesthesia in obstetrics. *Int J Obstet Anesth* 1994;3:143.

102. Ralph SJ, Wareham CA. Rupture of the esophagus during cricoid pressure. *Anaesthesia* 1991;46:40.
103. Whittington RM, Robinson JS. Thompson JM. Fatal aspiration (Mendelson's) syndrome despite antacids and cricoid pressure. *Lancet* 1979;2:228.
104. Vanner RG. Tolerance of cricoid pressure by conscious volunteers. *Int J Obstet Anesth* 1992;1:195.
105. Carter B, Van Decar T, Herman N, Knape K. Cricoid pressure: teaching the recommended range. [Abstr] *Int J Obstet Anesth* 1994;3:107.
106. Holdcroft A, Morgan M. Intravenous induction agents for Caesarean section. [Editorial] *Anaesthesia* 1989;44:719.
107. Blackburn CL, Morgan M. Comparison of the speed of onset of fazadinium, pancuronium, tubocurarine and suxamethonium. *Br J Anaesth* 1978;50:361.
108. Baraka A, Wakid N, Noueihed R, Karam K, Bolotova N. Pseudocholinesterase activity and atracurium versus suxamethonium block. [Abstr] *Br J Anaesth* 1986;58:S91.
109. Carmie JC, Street MK, Kumar B. Emergency intubation of the trachea facilitated by suxamethonium. Observations in obstetric and general surgical patients. *Br J Anaesth* 1986;58:498.
110. Crawford JS. Suxamethonium muscle pains and pregnancy. *Br J Anaesth* 1971;43:677.
111. Thind GS, Bryson THL. Single dose suxamethonium and muscle pain in pregnancy. *Br J Anaesth* 1983;55:743.
112. Baraka A, Jabbour S, Tabboush Z, Sibai A, Bijjani A, Karam K. Onset of vecuronium neuromuscular block is more rapid in patients undergoing Caesarean section. *Can J Anaesth* 1992;39:135.
113. Hawkins JL, Johnson D, Kubicek MA, Skjonsky BS, Morrow DH, Joyce TH III. Vecuronium for rapid-sequence intubation for Cesarean section. *Anesth Analg* 1990;71:185.
114. Baraka A, Noueihid R, Sinno H, Wakid N, Agoston S. Succinylcholine vecuronium (ORG NC45) sequence for Cesarean section. *Anesth Analg* 1983;62:909.
115. Abouleish E, Abboud T, Lechevalier T, Zhu J, Chalian A, Alford K. Rocuronium (Org 9426) for Caesarean section. *Br J Anaesth* 1994;73:336.
116. Williams KN, Carli F, Cormack RS. Unexpected, difficult laryngoscopy: a prospective survey in routine general surgery. *Br J Anaesth* 1991;66:38.
117. Lyons G. Failed intubation. *Anaesthesia* 1985;40:759.
118. Hood DD, Dewan DM. Anesthetic and obstetric outcome in morbidly obese parturients. *Anesthesiology* 1993;79:1210.
119. Graham SG, Luxon MC. The requirement for intensive care support for the pregnant population. *Anaesthesia* 1989;44:581.
120. Chadwick HS, Posner K, Caplan RA, Ward RJ, Cheney FW. A comparison of obstetric and nonobstetric anesthesia malpractice claims. *Anesthesiology* 1991;74:242.
121. American Society of Anesthesiologists Task Force report. Practical Guidelines for Management of the Difficult Airway. *Anesthesiology* 1994;78:597.
122. Fear DW. Failed intubation in the parturient. [Editorial] *Can J Anaesth* 1989;36:614.
123. Tunstall ME. Failed intubation in the parturient. [Editorial] *Can J Anaesth* 1989;36:611.
124. Benumof JL. Difficult laryngoscopy: obtaining the best view. [Editorial] *Can J Anaesth* 1994;41:361.
125. Davies JM, Weeks S, Crone LA, Pavlin E. Difficult intubation in the parturient. *Can J Anaesth* 1989;36:668.
126. Benumof JL. Management of the difficult adult airway. With special emphasis on awake tracheal intubation. *Anesthesiology* 1991;75:1087.
127. Mokriski BK, Malinow AM, Gray WC, McGuinn WJ. Topical nasopharyngeal anesthesia with vasoconstriction in preeclampsia-eclampsia. *Can J Anaesth* 1988;35:641.
128. Rosenberg DB, Gross JB. Awake, blind nasotracheal intubation for Cesarean section in a patient with autoimmune thrombocytopenic purpura and iatrogenic Cushing's syndrome. *Anesth Analg* 1993;77:853.
129. Ovassapian A, Krejcie TC, Yelich SJ, Dykes MHM. Awake fiberoptic intubation in the patient at high risk of aspiration. *Br J Anaesth* 1989;62:13.
130. Tunstall ME. Failed intubation drill. *Anaesthesia* 1976;31:850.
131. Tunstall ME, Sheikh A. Failed intubation protocol: oxygenation without aspiration. *Clin Anaesth* 1986;4:171.
132. Brimacombe J, Berry A. The laryngeal mask airway for obstetric anesthesia and neonatal resuscitation. *Int J Obstet Anesth* 1994;3:211.
133. Rosen M. Difficult and failed intubation in obstetrics. In: Latto IP, Rosen M, eds. *Difficulties in Tracheal Intubation*. London: Bailliere Tindall, 1984:152.
134. Wilson ME, Spiegelhalter D, Robertson JA, Lesser P. Predicting difficult intubation. *Br J Anaesth* 1988;61:211.
135. LaLande P, Knill RL. B.U.R.P. is more effective than backward pressure on the thyroid cartilage in managing difficult laryngoscopy. *Can J Anaesth* 1994;41:A65.
136. Tunstall ME, Geddes C. "Failed intubation" in obstetric anesthesia. An indication for the use of the "esophageal gastric tube airway." *Br J Anaesth* 1984;56:659.
137. Baraka A, Salem R. The combitube esophageal-tracheal double lumen airway for difficult intubation. [Letter] *Can J Anaesth* 1993;40:1222.
138. Akhtar TM. esophageal vent—laryngeal mask to prevent aspiration of gastric content. *Br J Anaesth* 1994;72:52.
139. Boys JE. Failed intubation in obstetric anesthesia. A case report. *Br J Anaesth* 1983;55:187.
140. Chung DC. Failed intubation: a different perspective. *Can J Anaesth* 1990;37:486.
141. Cheam EWS. The use of tracheal tubes as esophageal obturators.[Letter] *Anaesthesia* 1994;49:734.
142. Brain AIJ. Three cases of difficult intubation overcome by the laryngeal mask airway. *Anaesthesia* 1985;40:353.
143. Asai T, Barclay K, Power I, Vaughan RS. Cricoid pressure impedes placement of the laryngeal mask airway and subsequent tracheal intubation through the mask. *Br J Anaesth* 1994;72:47–51.
144. McClune S, Regan M, Moore J. Laryngeal mask airway for Caesarean section. *Anaesthesia* 1990;45:227.
145. Christian AS. Failed obstetric intubation. [Letter] *Anaesthesia* 1990;45:995.
146. Rabey PG, Murphy PJ, Langton JA, Barker B, Rowbotham DJ. Effect of the laryngeal mask airway on lower esophageal sphincter pressure in patients during general anesthesia. *Br J Anaesth* 1992;69:346.
147. Ansermino M, Blogg CE. Failed tracheal intubation at Caesarean section and the laryngeal mask. *Br J Anaesth* 1992;69:465.
148. Crowhurst JA. Failed intubation management at Caesarean section. *Anaesth Intensive Care* 1991;19:305.
149. Heath JL, Allagain J. Intubation through the laryngeal mask: a technique for unexpected difficult intubation. *Anaesthesia* 1991;46:545.
150. Frerk CM. Intubation through the laryngeal mask. *Anaesthesia* 1991;46:985.
151. Swayne P, Greenslade GL. Emergency intubation through the laryngeal mask airway. *Anaesthesia* 1994;49:696.
152. Hasham FM, Andrews PJD, Juneja MM, Ackerman WE. The laryngeal mask airway facilitates intubation at Cesarean section. A case report of difficult intubation. *Int J Obstet Anesth* 1993;2:181.
153. Brimacombe J, Berry A. Failed obstetric intubation: use of the laryngeal mask as an airway intubator? [Letter] *Int J Obstet Anesth* 1994;3:120.
154. Hasham F, Kumar CM, Lawler PGP. The use of the laryngeal mask airway to assist fibreoptic orotracheal intubation. [Letter] *Anaesthesia* 1991;46:891.
155. Smith RB, Babinski M, Klain M, Pfaeffle H. Percutaneous transtracheal ventilation. *J Am Coll Emerg Phys* 1976;5:765.
156. Neff CC, Pfister RC, Van Sonnenberg E. Percutaneous transtracheal ventilation: experimental and practical aspects. *J Trauma* 1983;23:84.
157. Yealy DM, Stewart RD. Translaryngeal cannula ventilation: continuing misconceptions. *Anesthesiology* 1987;67:445.
158. King TA, Adams AP. Failed tracheal intubation. *Br J Anaesth* 1990;65:400.
159. Duffy B. To paralyse a failed intubation or not? [Letter] *Anaesth Intensive Care* 1991;19:135.

Airway Management, edited by
L.H. Hanowell, M.D. and R.J. Waldron, M.D.,
Lippincott-Raven Publishers, Philadelphia © 1996.

CHAPTER 21

Airway Management of the Patient with Cervical Spinal Injury and Disease

Vance E. Shearer, Adolph H. Giesecke, Jr., and Mark T. Murphy

HISTORICAL PERSPECTIVE

The potentially devastating results of cervical spinal injury have been recognized since antiquity. The Edwin Smith papyrus (written circa 1600 BC) describes the effects of dislocation of the cervical vertebrae: "... there is paralysis of the arms, legs and sphincters with bad prognosis" (1). Homer's eighth Iliad describes instant death from a wound at the junction of the skull and the spine (1). Galen (129–200 AD), with his physiologic experiments on animals, described the various neurologic deficits that occurred when the spinal cord was severed (1). Hippocrates (460–370 BC), in his treatise on fractures, dislocations, and wounds of the head, recognized that "... rest and immobilization are of capital importance" (1).

Bohlman (2), analyzing care of spine-injured patients presenting to Baltimore hospitals between 1950 and 1972, found that clinically important fractures were missed in one-third of these patients. Failure to immobilize the spine resulted in an incidence of secondary neurologic injury of 10% to 25%. During the 1970s, Cales and Trunkey (3) found that up to 30% of trauma-related deaths could be prevented if appropriate systems for trauma care were developed (4–8). An important advance in the management of the traumatized patient was the institution of advanced trauma life support (ATLS) by the American

V.E. Shearer, A.H. Giesecke, Jr., and M.T. Murphy: Department of Anesthesiology, University of Texas, Southwestern Medical School, Dallas, Texas 75235-9068.

College of Surgeons Committee on Trauma. The ATLS protocol gives first priority to airway maintenance with cervical spinal control (9). As a result of the improvement in both prehospital and hospital care delivered to trauma patients over the last 20 years, the New York University-Bellevue Medical Center reported a fourfold increase in the percentage of trauma patients admitted with preserved neurologic function below the level of cord injury, as compared with the percentage 20 years earlier (10).

However, delay in the diagnosis of clinically significant fractures still occurs in 10% of spine-injured patients (11). These delays result from failure to perform radiographic investigation or the misinterpretation of x-ray films. Neurologic sequelae of these undiagnosed injuries are similar to those of 20 years ago. In the series of 274 patients reported by Reid et al. (12), cervical spinal injury was missed in 14%, with a resulting secondary neurologic injury rate 7.5 times greater than the rate in those patients whose injuries were appropriately diagnosed and treated on admission. Woodring and Lee (13), studying the limitations of routine cervical radiography for evaluation of acute cervical trauma, found that 5% of asymptomatic patients had cervical spinal injuries detected by computed tomography (CT) (13).

Currently, there is no best technique in managing the airway of the patient with suspected/known cervical spinal injuries. This chapter reviews the various techniques of airway management and evaluates their advantages and disadvantages. The clinician must evaluate the patient's specific injuries and, taking into account his or her own airway-management skills, determine the best method of airway control.

FUNCTIONAL ANATOMY OF THE CERVICAL SPINE

Before considering airway management in the patient with an abnormal cervical spine, a review of the anatomy of the normal cervical spine is in order (Fig. 1). There are seven cervical vertebrae. The spinous processes of C-2 through C-6 are unique in that they are bifid (Fig. 2). Since C-1 (the atlas) and C-2 (the axis) are anatomically and functionally different from C-3 through C-7, they are discussed separately.

Upper Cervical Spine (C-1 and C-2)

The atlas, named after the Titan of classical mythology, supports the head (occiput) (Fig. 3). It is the only vertebra without a vertebral body (normally the weight-bearing portion); instead, it consists of an anterior and posterior arch. It also has a pair of lateral masses (instead of articular processes) formed at the junction of the anterior and posterior arches. These lateral masses are the site of the superior and inferior articular surfaces, which

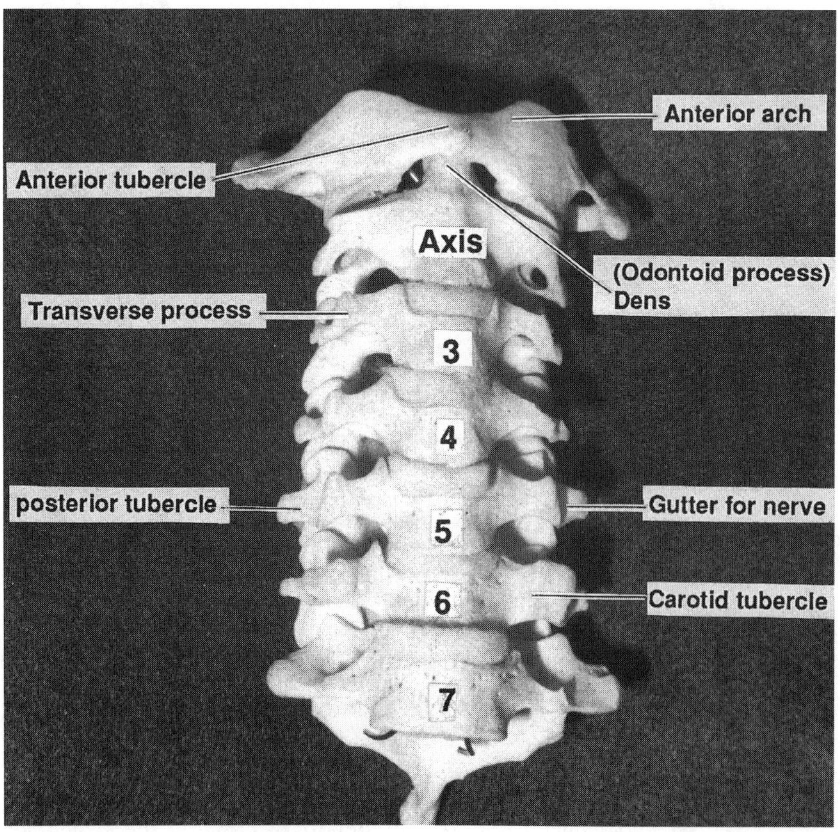

FIG. 1. Anterior-posterior view of the cervical spine.

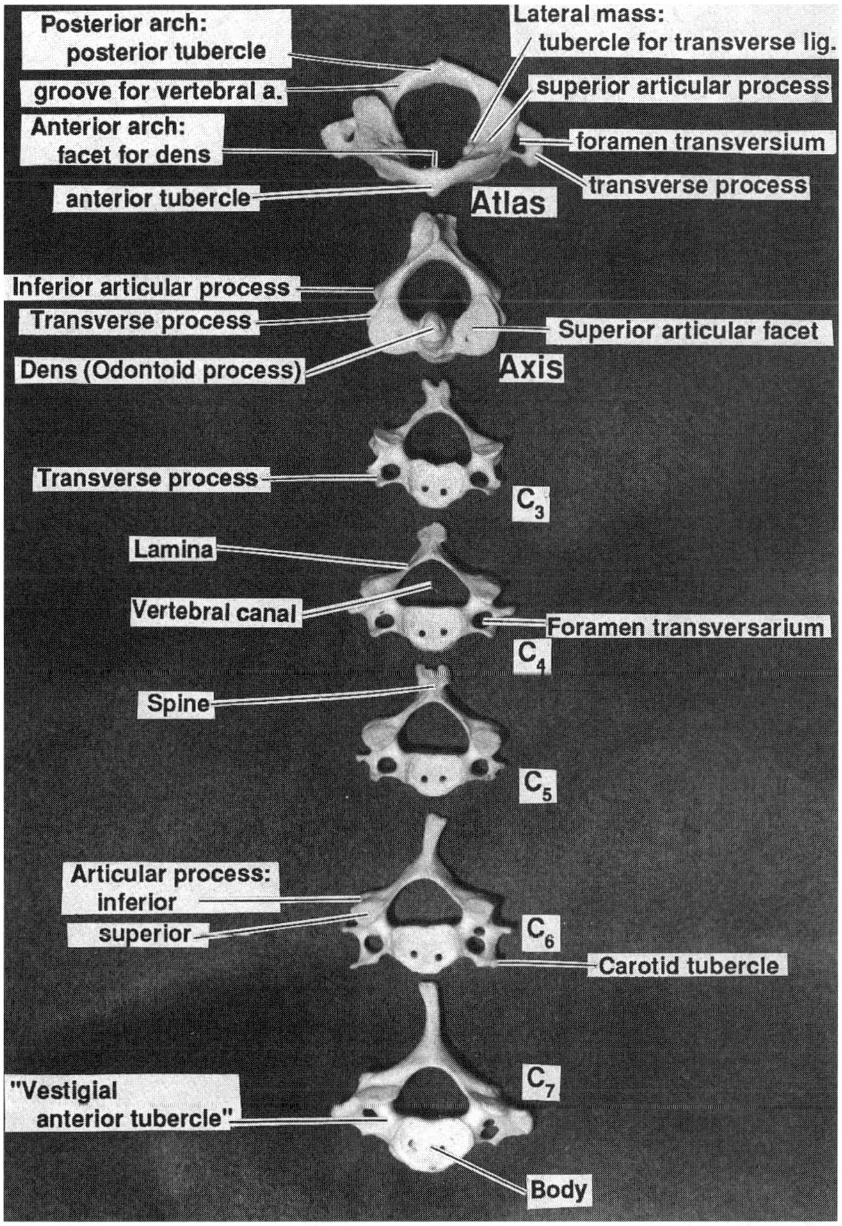

FIG. 2. Anatomic structures of the cervical spine.

articulate with occipital condyles above and the superior facet joints of the axis (C-2) below. Projecting medially from the two lateral masses are bony tubercles, to which is attached the transverse ligament (Fig. 3). When the atlas and axis are articulated, the upward projection of the axis, the dens, lies behind the anterior arch of the atlas and is retained in this position by the transverse ligament (Fig. 3). Projecting laterally from the lateral masses of C-1 are the transverse processes. Each transverse process from C-1 through C-6 has a foramen through which the vertebral artery passes. The vertebral vein also passes through these foramina, and that of C-7 as well.

The axis (C-2) is the pivot on which the atlas, and therefore the head, rotates (Fig. 4). The body of the axis gives rise to the dens (odontoid process), which projects vertically through the atlas and attaches to the anterior margins of the foramen magnum by the alar and apical ligaments (Fig. 5). This attachment forms the occipito-atlanto-axial complex. The laminae of the axis are thicker than those of any other cervical vertebra and provide attachment to the ligamenta flava. They fuse posteriorly with the large and powerful spinous processes, to which the muscles that extend, retract, and rotate the head attach.

Lower Cervical Spine (C-3 to C-7)

The lower five cervical vertebrae are anatomically more typical of the remaining vertebrae, except for the presence of the foramen transversarium (Fig. 2). C-7 has

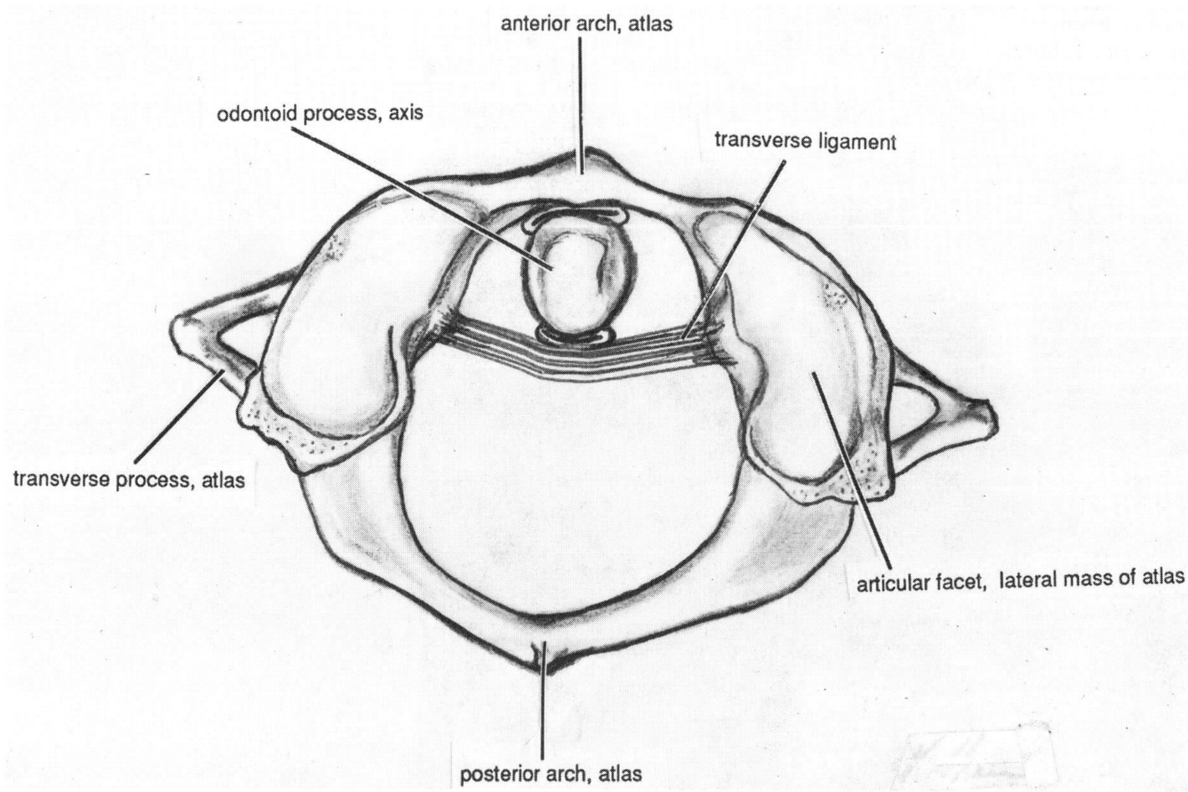

FIG. 3. Articulation of the odontoid process of the axis with the atlas.

a single, long spinous process that is sometimes visible under the skin at the base of the neck (vertebra prominens). The ligamentum nuchae is attached to the spinous process of C-7.

Ligaments and Articulations

The atlanto-occipital joint is a synovial joint that allows flexion and extension, but no rotation or lateral bending of the head on the atlas. The atlas and axis articulate at three sites to allow rotation of the atlas on the axis and a small amount of flexion and extension. Synovial cavities exist between the anterior arch of the atlas and the dens, and between the dens and the transverse ligament to allow rotation (Fig. 3). The dens is also held in place by the cruciform ligament complex, which consists of fibers that attach the body of the axis to the occiput (Fig. 5). Alar ligaments attach the dens to the occiput laterally and restrict rotation. The ligamentous attachments of the atlas to the occiput are the anterior and posterior atlanto-occipital membranes, which are the continuations of the anterior longitudinal ligament and the ligamentum flavum, respectively. The superior continuation of the posterior longitudinal ligament is the tectorial membrane.

The articulations of the lower five cervical vertebrae are the vertebral bodies and the superior and inferior pedicles, which articulate horizontally to form the facet joints (Fig. 2). These osseous articulations are synovial joints and are separated by synovial capsules.

The cervical spine is stabilized anteriorly by the anterior and posterior longitudinal ligaments, which extend the length of the cervical spine. Narrow intertransverse ligaments are located between the transverse processes but add little strength to the spine.

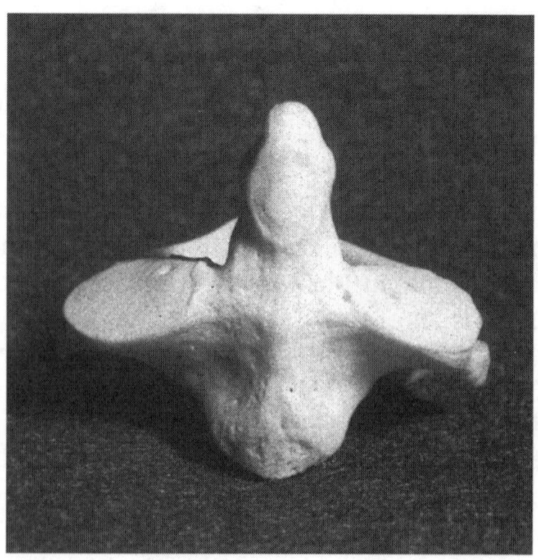

FIG. 4. Anterior-posterior view of the axis.

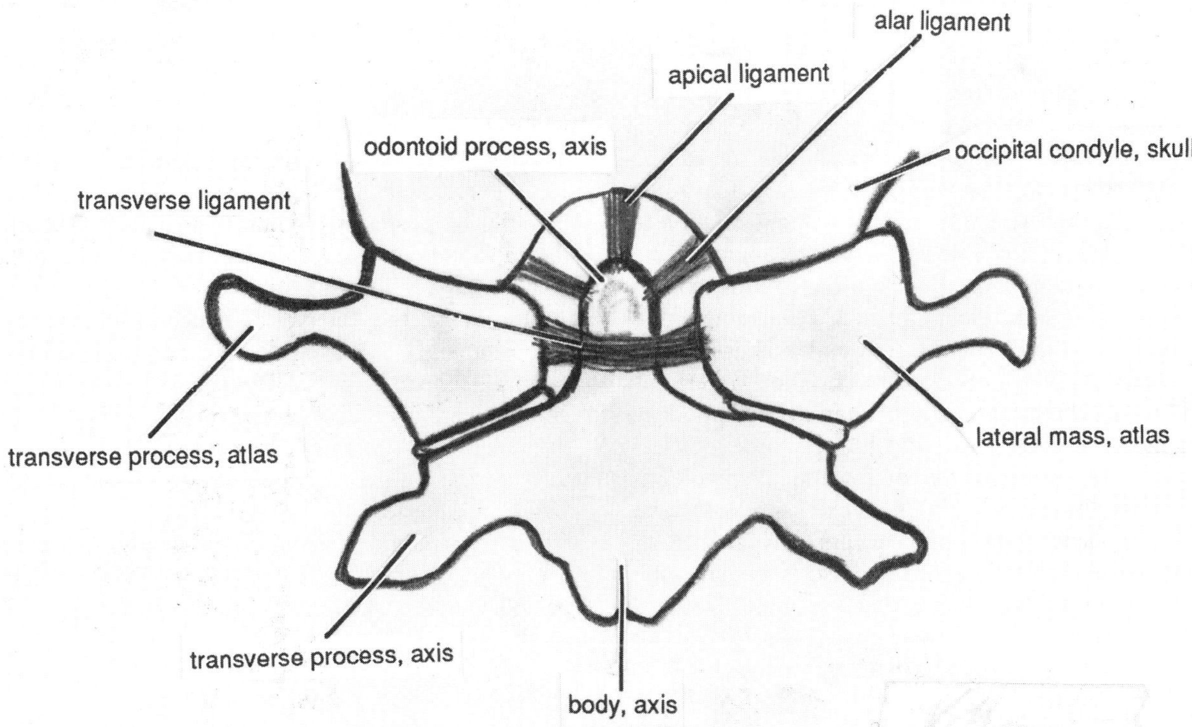

FIG. 5. Coronal view of the occipito-atlanto-axial complex.

The anterior longitudinal ligament joins adjacent vertebral bodies anteriorly and anterolaterally and travels along the anterior surface of the vertebral bodies. It terminates superiorly over the anterior arch of the atlas, forming the anterior atlanto-occipital ligament, which inserts on the base of the skull. The posterior longitudinal ligament courses upwards along the dorsal surface of the vertebral bodies and fans out over the body of the axis and the odontoid process to terminate as a tectorial membrane, which inserts at the base of the occiput. The anterior longitudinal ligament limits extension, and the posterior longitudinal ligament (with the other posterior column ligaments) tends to limit flexion.

The spine is also stabilized posteriorly by the supraspinous and interspinous ligaments and the ligamenta flava. The supraspinous ligament courses between the tips of the spinous processes and imparts a significant degree of structural integrity to the cervical spine. The weaker interspinous ligaments connect one spinous process to the next along the length of the processes. The ligamenta flava, which connect adjacent laminae, consist of paired elastic ligaments.

The Pediatric Cervical Spine

The pediatric cervical spine differs from that of adults in that it is cartilaginous and exhibits ongoing epiphyseal development and progressive vertebral ossification. The tip of the dens is not ossified at birth and is attached to the body of C-2 by a cartilaginous band. By the age of 6 years, ossification of the tip begins, and there is subsequent fusion of the dens to the body of C-2. Complete ossification of C-3 through C-7 does not occur until 3 to 6 years of age. Although children's ligaments are similar to those of adults, the elastic properties of these ligaments do not develop until about 8 years of age. This can result in abnormal mobility between vertebral bodies with minor trauma. Furthermore, ossification of the facets does not occur until 7 to 10 years of age; therefore, significant stability is not present until that time.

Kinematics of the Cervical Spine

The normal range of motion of the occipito-atlanto-axial complex in flexion and extension is about 23.4° (14). Flexion within this complex is limited by the contact between the odontoid process and the anterior border of the foramen magnum, the tectorial membrane, and the posterior elements (15). Extension is limited by the contact of the occiput, the posterior arch of the atlas, and the arch of the axis (15). A narrow atlanto-occipital gap and, to a lesser extent, a short interspace between the posterior arches of the atlas and axis have been associated with difficult intubations caused by restricted extension (16–18).

Up to 50% of the total axial rotation of the neck is achieved at the atlantoaxial complex. This degree of rotation has been associated with the development of vertebrobasilar ischemia resulting from kinking of the vertebral arteries. No lateral bending (movement) occurs at the C-1 and C-2 complex. Lateral displacement of the C-1 and C-2 complex greater than 4 mm is abnormal. Anteroposterior translation greater than 1 mm is abnormal at the occipito-atlanto-axial complex. Movement in the vertical, horizontal, and lateral directions without rotation is called "translation." Because of the various angles of the facet joints, a motion in one direction can simultaneously cause a motion in a different direction. For example, the axial rotation at the C-1 and C-2 complex is associated with as much as 2 mm of vertical translation. Overrotation can result in the rupture of the alar and occipitodentate ligaments.

The range of motion of the lower cervical spine contributes an additional 66° of flexion/extension (14). The largest component of this motion occurs between the C-5 and C-7 vertebrae. Although the cause is unclear, the range of motion of the lower cervical spine in the adult decreases as much as 25% between the ages of 20 and 80. Most of this decrease occurs at the C-5 through C-7 segments (19).

Stability and Instability of the Cervical Spine

Stability is defined as the ability to maintain normal anatomic relationships between vertebrae under conditions of normal physiologic loading (20). Conversely, instability occurs when normal physiologic loads can cause displacement of the vertebral elements, thereby jeopardizing the spinal cord, nerve roots, and/or vasculature (21).

The stability of the occipito-atlanto-axial complex is secured by the transverse, alar, and apical ligaments and the superior terminations of the anterior and posterior longitudinal ligaments (21). The vertebral canal is largest at the occipito-atlanto-axial complex. At C-1, this canal is divided into thirds. One-third of the space at C-1 is odontoid, one-third spinal cord, and the other third empty space (22). Although no more than 3 mm of anterior-posterior translocation between the dens and the anterior arch of the atlas normally occurs, an isolated rupture of the transverse ligament with intact alar and apical ligaments may allow 5 mm of movement. As much as 10 mm of displacement can occur if all these ligaments are disrupted (21). The size of the normal vertebral canal at C-1 is approximately 20 mm, and cord compression is not seen when this distance is greater than 18 mm. However, cord compression can occur with a decrease to less than 14 mm (23). The previously mentioned one-third empty space in the vertebral canal allows for some margin of safety at the level of C-1.

The lower cervical spine consists of an anterior and a posterior column. The anterior column is supported by structures anterior to the posterior longitudinal ligament; likewise, the posterior column is supported by those elements posterior to the posterior longitudinal ligament. Those structures supporting the anterior column are the anterior longitudinal ligament, the intervertebral disk, and the posterior longitudinal ligament, as well as the facet joints with the capsular and intertransverse ligaments. The posterior column is primarily supported by the supraspinous and interspinous ligaments and the ligamenta flava (20,24).

Studies on the cadaveric model of the spine, with extension and flexion under physiologic loads, found the cervical spine to be unstable when all the elements of one column were disrupted. Furthermore, if only one element of the motion segments of one column was intact and all the segments of the other column were intact, either posterior or anterior, the cervical spine remained stable under physiologic loads (24). Clinically, this condition cannot be assumed, and therefore the cervical spine must be considered unstable until proved otherwise.

EPIDEMIOLOGY OF CERVICAL SPINAL INJURIES

Considering the long-term disability entailed and the demands made on both patient and governmental resources, cervical spinal cord injury poses a major public health problem. Cervical spinal injuries occur in about 1.5% to 3% of all major trauma patients who arrive at the hospital alive (25–33). The victims of fatal blunt trauma have a 16% to 25% incidence of cervical spinal injury (34,35). In 1981, approximately 6000 automobile passengers died in the United States of cervical spinal injury (36). The wearing of shoulder-lap-belt restraint systems has been effective in reducing fatal neck injuries (37). It is hoped that these injuries will decrease further with the institution of air bags as a standard feature on all automobiles, especially for those who do not wear the three-point belts.

The majority of spinal cord injuries result from motor vehicle accidents and account for about 50% of the spinal injuries seen throughout the United States (36,38). In California, the incidence of spinal cord injuries was estimated at 53 per million population per year, occurring mostly in males 15 to 35 years of age and those greater than 65 years of age (39,40). Although much focus has been placed on football as a cause of spinal cord injury, water sports (diving, surfing, and waterskiing) and skiing accounted for more than 80% of the athletically related spinal cord injuries seen in California (38,41). Younger children are less likely to suffer a cervical spinal injury, as a result of their decreased body weight and cartilaginous cervical spine (42–44). Children tend to have higher-level cervical spinal injuries, with those under 2 years of age suffering C-1 or C-2 injuries almost exclusively, owing to their more horizontal facet joints and lax ligaments (45).

SPECIFIC INJURIES AND MECHANISMS

Atlanto-occipital Dislocations

Atlanto-occipital dislocation is an extremely rare injury. In 1980, Pang and Wilberger (46) found only 13 case reports in the world literature, with only 6 of these patients reported as surviving after admission to the hospital. Although survivors with this injury are rare, it is the most common cervical spinal injury in fatal motor vehicle accidents (35,47,48). Death appears to be caused by transection of the medulla oblongata or of the spinomedullary junction (2,48,49).

The mechanism of injury appears to be a combination of hyperextension of the head, with an associated distraction force on the cranium. Frequently, there are abrasions on the chin, cheeks, or forehead, suggesting that there has been a hyperextension force sufficient to tear the transverse ligament, the tectorial and cruciform membranes, and the alar ligaments. With atlanto-occipital dislocation, the atlas itself remains in position, held by the anterior and posterior occipital atlantal membranes and the anterior and posterior longitudinal ligaments. This results in the slippage of the occiput backward on the atlas. Along with the subsequent damage to the medulla, compression of the vertebral arteries between the condyles and the laminae of C-1 may also occur. The radiologic diagnosis of atlanto-occipital dislocation may not be readily visible on plain lateral cervical films and therefore easily missed. The diagnosis can be suggested by the demonstration of retropharyngeal swelling on the lateral cervical spinal film. The distance between the anterior edge of the foramen magnum and the tip of the posterior arch of the atlas should be equal to the distance between the anterior arch of the atlas and the posterior edge of the foramen magnum. If this ratio is greater than 1, then the head is forward relative to the spine (50). Atlanto-occipital dislocation is a treacherously unstable injury. Even the slightest amount of traction on the patient's cervical spine can result in cardiorespiratory arrest (51).

Although airway management is discussed later in this chapter, special mention should be made of this injury. If possible, these patients should be kept awake in order to assess their cardiorespiratory and neurologic status continuously, and they should be immobilized as soon as possible. Since respiration may be severely impaired, they may need an emergency airway. Any motion of the cervical spine during intubation attempts may be extremely dangerous. Therefore, a surgically placed airway in an awake patient with minimal motion of the neck is probably the intubation technique of choice with this injury.

Injuries to the C-1 and C-2 Complex

Among traffic accident fatalities associated with severe cervical spinal cord injury, 80% involve the articulations between the occiput, C-1, and C-2. Conversely, serious neurologic injury is less common in survivors of injury to the upper cervical spine than in survivors of injury to the lower cervical spine. Since the spinal cord occupies only one-third of the vertebral canal at the C-1 and C-2 level, survivors with these lesions rarely have neurologic sequelae (52,53).

Fracture of the Atlas

Fractures of the atlas (Jefferson fracture, 1920) can be either stable or unstable. Those fractures with an intact transverse ligament are stable, whereas those fractures associated with rupture of this ligament are unstable. If posterior movement of the dens is greater than 3 mm behind the anterior ring of the atlas, significant injury to the transverse ligament is probable (21).

Jefferson described bilateral fractures of the posterior arch of the atlas as a result of a direct vertical blow to the head causing compression of the atlas. As a result of this compression, the lateral masses are displaced outward. Since the bursting fragments are displaced outward, with resulting widening of the spinal canal, the cervicomedullary junction may remain unharmed. Patients present with occipital or neck pain and signs of nuchal rigidity with limitation of motion (54). The patient may support the forehead in the hands when looking downward and support the head posteriorly when looking upward. Dysphagia and thick speech occasionally may be associated with a rotary dislocation. In cases of fracture of the anterior arch, palpation of the pharynx may detect a protuberance. CT is useful in demonstrating the Jefferson fracture.

Transaxial Cervicomedullary Injury

Transaxial cervicomedullary injury involves a deadly direct blow to the vertex without the fracture of the skull or cervical spine. After rebounding from this blow, the brain stem and cervical spinal cord are herniated caudally through the foramen magnum to the level of the C-2 segment, resulting in immediate cardiorespiratory arrest and death. A fatal football accident of this type was caught on motion pictures and the mechanism for this injury was duplicated in monkeys (54–56).

Odontoid Fractures

The odontoid process is almost completely interarticular, and because of its close relationship with the atlas, it is susceptible to injury with any injury of the atlas. Although the exact mechanism for odontoid fracture is not known, it may result from high-velocity blows to the face or the side or back of the head. Lateral loading combined with other forces may be responsible for this injury. Anterior displacement from flexion forces of the transverse ligament occur in about 80% of these fractures, whereas in 20%, extension forces the anterior ring on the odontoid, with posterior displacement (57). Odontoid fractures comprise about 75% of cervical spinal injuries in children and about 10% to 15% in adults (58). Clinically, these fractures produce severe high cervical pain and muscle spasm. Pain may also radiate to the back of the head. The diagnosis of odontoid fracture can be made by anterior-posterior plain films or lateral tomograms. This injury can be confused with os odontoideum, which is the congenital nonunion of the dens with the axis.

There are three types of odontoid fractures. Type I fractures involve only the tip of the odontoid (Fig. 6). These fractures usually occur from disruption of the apical or alar ligaments. Since the transverse ligament is intact, the cervical spine remains stable, and since the blood supply is not disturbed, these injuries have a good prognosis (59–61).

Type II fractures occur at the base of the dens at the site of its union with the vertebral body (Fig. 6). The blood supply is disrupted, and except in children, nonunion of this injury is common. Type II fractures are the most common odontoid fracture, and this injury can result in displacement of the odontoid.

Type III fractures occur to the body of the axis and heal well, since this fracture occurs through cancellous bone (Fig. 6). Displacement associated with this fracture can occur (62).

Fractures of the odontoid process may result in atlantoaxial dislocation. Atlantoaxial dislocation can also occur from congenital deformities of the bones and ligaments,

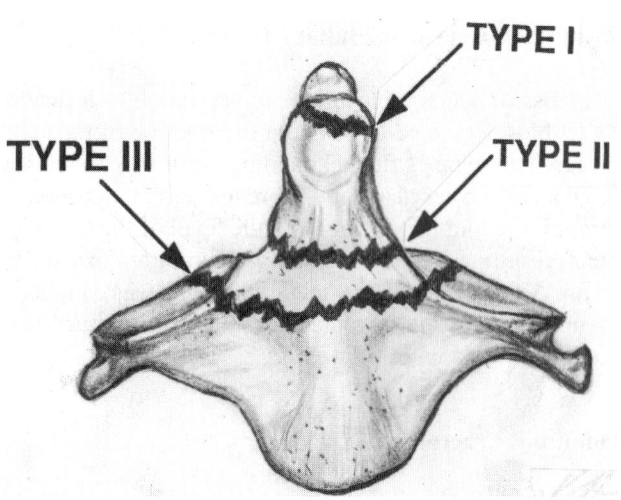

FIG. 6. Classification of anatomic fractures of the odontoid process.

as in os odontoideum, and with ligamentous injuries not associated with bony fracture. Tears of the transverse and alar ligaments as well as avulsion of the tectorial and cruciform membranes can occur with severe hyperextension or flexion. Anterior atlantoaxial dislocations are more common with this injury. These patients present with neck soreness and stiffness, with pain later radiating to the shoulders. This injury can be diagnosed by cautious extension/flexion, during which the anterior ring of the atlas dislocates either forward or backward. These injuries require surgical repair, as the soft tissue ligaments do not heal spontaneously.

Bell (63) described the "brachial cruciate paralysis syndrome." This syndrome, which mimics central cervical cord syndrome, results from the dens pressing into the base of the medulla, causing pressure on the pyramidal tracks in the midline. This occurs with atlantoaxial dislocation and results in paralysis of the upper extremities. With proper traction and positioning, this neurologic picture usually reverts to normal.

Traumatic Spondylolisthesis of the Axis ("Hangman's Fracture")

In 1913, Wood-Jones (64) described this fracture, which results from judicial hanging performed by the platform-drop technique. This injury occurs with the avulsion of the laminar arches of C-2 and some dislocation of the vertebral body of C-2 on C-3 (Fig. 7). In a proper judicial hanging, the knot is placed in the submental position and the platform-drop technique is used; the weight of the body pulls downward. The clivus of the skull and the C-1 and C-2 vertebral bodies move as a unit, causing avulsion of the laminar arches. The resulting mechanism of hyperextension with sudden violent distraction causes complete transection of the cord and vertebral arteries, destroying the cervicomedullary junction and resulting in immediate death (65). Today, the majority of patients with this lesion are injured in either motor vehicle or diving accidents (65,66). Schneider et al. (66) reported eight cases of hangman's fracture that occurred as a result of motor vehicle accidents. Two of the patients in their series did not lose consciousness and described themselves as hanging on the steering wheel or dashboard of the vehicle. Both of these patients had abrasions on their chins and faces (66). The mechanism of injury in these cases was severe hyperextension. However, unlike what occurs in a judicial hanging, the weight of the body in such cases is supported without a further drop, so the avulsed arches decompress the cervicomedullary junction and neurologic deficit may not occur. Neurologic injury is probably uncommon because of the large diameter of the vertebral canal at this level. Although a neurologic injury is relatively uncommon in survivors, this injury is the second-most-common lesion

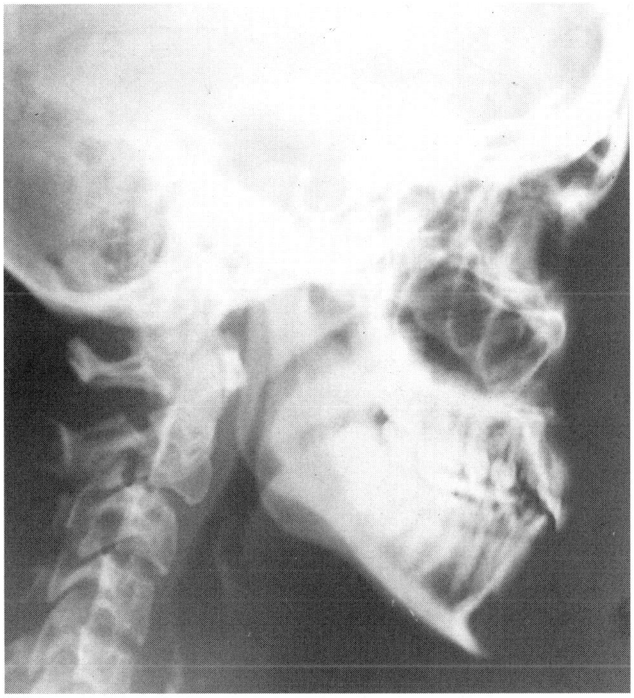

FIG. 7. Extension and distraction causing a fracture of the posterior elements of C-2 with subluxation of C-2 on C-3 ("hangman's fracture").

in victims of fatal motor vehicle accidents (46,47,67). Head trauma and mandibular fractures occur in approximately 70% of these patients, and other upper cervical spinal lesions are common (65).

The diagnosis of this injury is easily made on lateral or oblique plain films and can be classified into three types (Fig. 7). Type I fractures are without angulation and have less than 3 mm of displacement. Type II fractures are bipedicular fractures with significant angulation and translation. Type III fractures are characterized by severe angulation and displacement with unilateral or bilateral facet dislocations. This type of fracture results in the separation of the skull and the first two cervical vertebrae from the remainder of the cervical spine and is extremely unstable (68).

Lower Cervical Fractures and Dislocations

The various fractures and dislocations of the lower cervical spine depend on the mechanism of injury. Most of these injuries are the result of indirect forces originating in the head or the trunk that subject the cervical spine to forces of flexion, rotation, extension, and vertical compression.

Hyperflexion can cause a strain injury that results from partial tearing of the posterior ligamentous structures. Radiographic evaluation of these patients frequently demonstrates a normal spine; however, flexion views may demonstrate separation of the interspinous ligaments. The primary consequence of this injury is the syndrome of chronic neck ache, and involvement of the spinal cord and nerve roots is rare.

Unilateral facet dislocation occurs with the combination of forward flexion and rotation. There is tearing of the interspinous ligaments and the facet capsule on the involved side, resulting in forward displacement over the inferior facet at the level of the dislocation. The most common vertebral levels of facet dislocation are as follows: C-5 on C-6, followed by C-6 on C-7, and then C-4 on C-5. Unilateral facet dislocation frequently results in cervical nerve root entrapment and the potential for spinal cord injury at the level of subluxation.

Bilateral facet dislocation occurs when the flexion forces are greater than those contributed by rotation (Fig. 8). This injury involves disruption of the interspinous ligaments as well as both facet capsules, with the potential for disruption of the posterior and anterior longitudinal ligaments. Greater than 50% subluxation between the vertebral bodies is frequently seen. The spinal canal may be compromised by bilateral facet dislocation, often resulting in severe spinal cord injury.

A wedge compression fracture occurs with the combination of hyperflexion and a compressive force applied to the anterior portion of the vertebral body. This injury

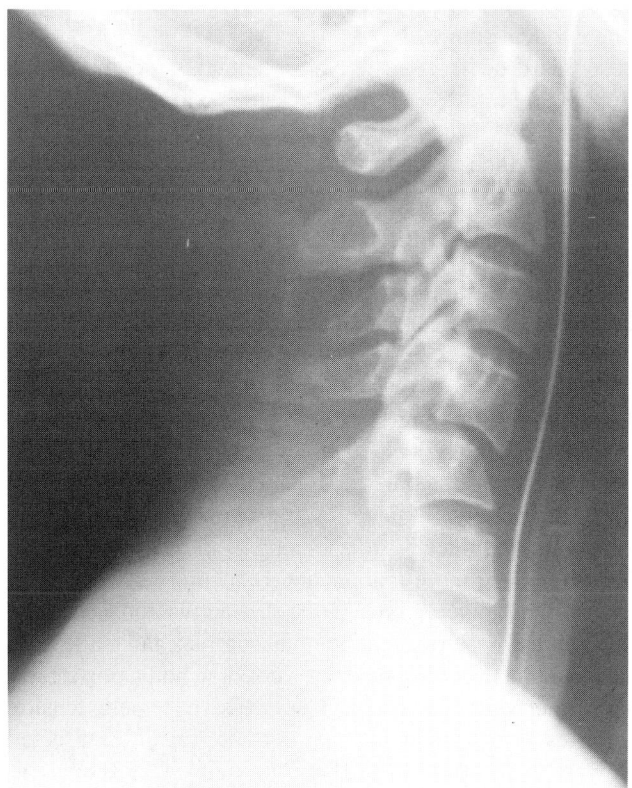

FIG. 8. Hyperflexion injury with bilateral facet dislocation of C-4 on C-5.

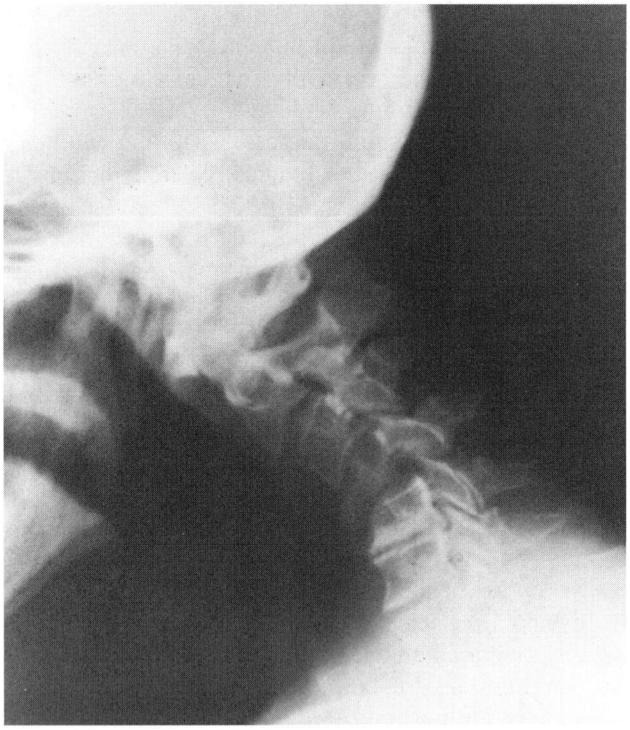

FIG. 9. Severe flexion deformity with fracture of the body of C-4.

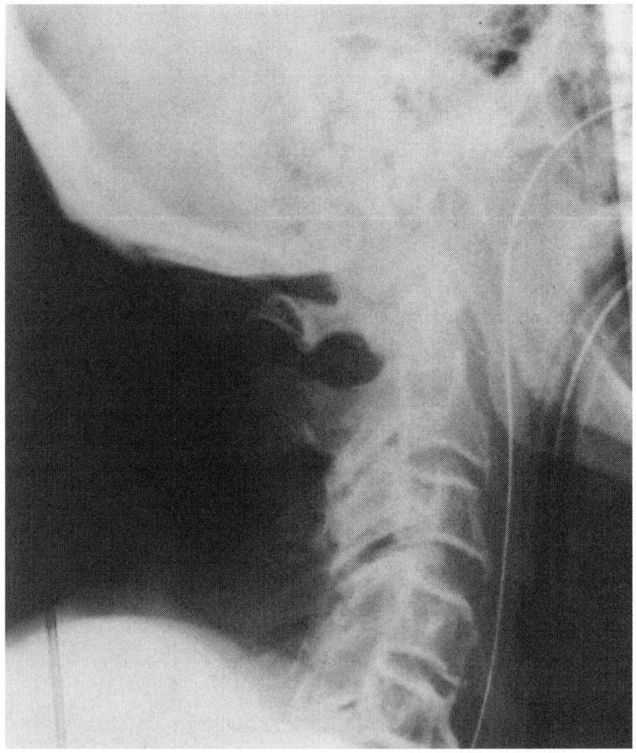

FIG. 10. Hyperextension injury with widening of the C3-4 intervertebral disk space.

causes disruption of the posterior ligamentous structures, with separation of the spinous processes and instability of the cervical spine.

A teardrop fracture occurs when major compressive forces are applied with the neck in flexion. This mechanism results in a comminuted fracture of the vertebral body in which the anterior-inferior vertebral fragment is triangular (Fig. 9). The posterior fragments of the vertebral body are commonly displaced into the spinal canal, causing major spinal cord damage.

Hyperextension injuries probably account for the majority of cervical spinal injuries (69,70). Hyperextension injuries may be divided into two subgroups, distractive and compressive (69). With distractive hyperextension injuries, the forces are directed away from the trunk, placing the anterior elements of the cervical spine under tension. Either the anterior ligamentous complex fails or the vertebral body fractures transversely. This may be seen radiographically by widening of the disk space (Fig. 10); however, these injuries are frequently missed on initial radiographic exams. If the distractive force is more severe, the posterior ligamentous complex fails, allowing displacement of the superior vertebral body posteriorly into the vertebral canal. Compressive hyperextension injuries occur when the major force vector is directed toward the trunk while the head is extended, causing compression of the posterior elements. The resulting injury, depending on the degree of force, can vary from unilateral vertebral arch fracture (with or without displacement), to bilateral laminar fracture without other tissue failure, to bilateral vertebral arch fracture with full vertebral body displacement anteriorly.

Common Spinal Cord Trauma Syndromes

The extent and pattern of spinal cord injury depend on the amount of force and the mechanism of injury applied to the spinal cord. The initial injury may be complicated by secondary ischemia or hemorrhage, which adversely affects the ultimate outcome.

Transverse myelopathy is the most severe consequence of spinal cord trauma. With this injury, all neurologic function below the level of the lesion is lost. This injury occurs as a result of anatomic disruption of the cord, physiologic disruption as a result of compression or ischemia, or a combination of both.

Anterior cervical cord syndrome results from injury to the anterior two-thirds of the spinal cord, with involvement of the corticospinal tracks and the anterolateral spinothalamic systems. This injury involves loss of all voluntary motor activity as well as temperature and pain sensation below the level of the lesion. Proprioception, which is a posterior column function, remains intact. Unlike what occurs in the central cord syndrome, the degree of motor deficit in both the upper and lower extremities is generally the same.

The central cord syndrome results from a lesion within the centrum of the cervical spinal cord, with preservation of a rim of tissue at the periphery. This may occur from a hemorrhagic contusion, mechanical disruption, ischemia, or a combination of these mechanisms. With this syndrome, the upper extremities are disproportionately weak compared with the lower extremities, and sensory loss is minimal. The central cord syndrome is frequently associated with degenerative disease of the cervical spine, for example, cervical spondylosis, a congenitally narrow spinal canal, or a midline posterior herniated nucleus pulposis.

The patient with Brown-Séquard syndrome presents with hemisection of the spinal cord. Clinically, there is ipsilateral motor paralysis starting just below the level of injury and contralateral sensory and temperature loss from two to three segments below the lesion. This lesion usually results from penetrating rather than blunt trauma; however, a *contrecoup* injury, vascular compromise, or foreign bodies in the spinal canal may also produce this injury.

Penetrating Injuries to the Cervical Spine

Although penetrating injuries to the neck and the cervical spine can occur with industrial and motor vehicle accidents, they are most likely to occur with stab and gunshot wounds. With the ever-increasing urban violence and gang warfare on the city streets, as well as the ready availability of weapons, penetrating trauma to the neck is becoming increasingly common. The authors recently found a 1% incidence of cervical spinal injury with penetrating neck trauma (71). Penetrating trauma to the neck is also frequently associated with injuries to other major structures, namely, airway and vascular structures, which further complicates the airway management of these patients.

Diseases and Anomalies of the Cervical Spine

Although much discussion focuses on trauma to the cervical spine and the subsequent airway management of these patients, congenital and inflammatory disease processes may also affect the cervical spine and greatly influence airway management. Those practitioners who routinely manage the airway must be familiar with these conditions in order avert a disastrous outcome.

The inflammatory diseases include rheumatoid arthritis, enteropathic arthritis, Reiter's syndrome, Still's disease, psoriatic arthritis, and ankylosing spondylitis.

Rheumatoid arthritis is associated with osteoporosis, erosion of bone, synovial overgrowth, and destruction of ligaments (72). Atlantoaxial subluxation is the most common radiographic finding in rheumatoid arthritis, occurring in 25% of patients (73). Although subluxation may occur in any of four plains, the incidence of anterior subluxation is about 80% (72). It is more commonly seen in male patients with long-standing disease, and in patients with subcutaneous nodules and seropositive disease (72). This lesion involves an attenuation or disruption of the transverse ligament that results in anterior movement of the atlas on the axis. Atlantoaxial subluxation is best seen on the lateral cervical spinal x-ray, which demonstrates an increased atlas-dens interval (73). Those patients with alar and apical ligament involvement may have an atlas-dens interval of greater than 10 mm (22). From 10% to 33% of the patients with atlantoaxial subluxation develop signs of cord compression (72,75,76). Another condition that commonly occurs in conjunction with anterior subluxation is vertical subluxation of the odontoid process through the foramen magnum into the posterior fossa; this may occur in 4% to 35% of patients with rheumatoid arthritis (72,76).

Although less common, with a 6% to 7% incidence, posterior subluxation typically results in cord compression (72). Another condition found in 20% to 40% of patients with rheumatoid arthritis is erosion of the odontoid process, making anterior-posterior subluxation and cord compression possible (72).

Arthritic involvement of the temporomandibular and cricoarytenoid joints may further add difficulty to airway management. Prior to elective intubation of patients with rheumatoid arthritis, the cervical spine should be carefully evaluated. If physical examination reveals limited motion, lateral cervical spinal films should be attained in the neutral position and with flexion/extension views. The lower cervical spine should also be reviewed for the presence of subaxial subluxation. Subaxial subluxation may occur in about 7% to 29% of patients with rheumatoid arthritis (72).

Keenan et al. (77) reported airway deviation in patients with polyarticular arthritis affecting the cervical spine. They described the larynx as displaced caudally, deviated to the left, rotated to the right, and angulated anteriorly. Therefore anterior-posterior films should also be examined for laryngeal deviation.

Rheumatoid arthritis is characterized by osteoporosis and erosion of bone. Ankylosing spondylitis, another inflammatory arthropathy, is characterized by infiltration of ligaments and joint capsules by granulation tissue that progressively undergoes fibrosis, calcification, and ankylosis (78). These processes eventually result in complete ankylosis of the cervical spine, and cervical fracture may result from even minor extension injuries (79,80). These fractures typically occur between C-5 and C-7 and extend through the ossified disk spaces, with resultant transection of the spinal column. Epidural hemorrhages are also common complications with these fractures (2). Since even minor extension can cause injuries in these patients, they should be immobilized in flexion. Like the rheumatoid arthritis patients, these patients may also have temporomandibular joint involvement, making endotracheal intubation extremely difficult.

TABLE 1. *Syndromes associated with odontoid hypoplasia*

Congenital scoliosis
Disproportionate dwarfism
Klippel-Feil syndrome
Morquio syndrome
Neurofibromatosis
Osteogenesis imperfecta
Trisomy 21 (Down syndrome)

Similar to the inflammatory arthropathies, congenital anomalies may also affect the cervical spine and subsequent airway management. Just as rheumatoid arthritis is associated with atlantoaxial subluxation, so are Down syndrome, odontoid anomalies, and muccopolysaccharidoses. Congenital anomalies may involve hypoplasia or failed fusion of bony structures, laxity of ligamentous structures, or excess ossification. General hypoplasia of the odontoid process is associated with several congenital anomalies (Table 1) and can result in anterior subluxation of the atlas on the axis during hyperextension.

The anomaly of os odontoideum occurs as a primitive articulation between the odontoid process and the axis, leaving a gap between the free ossicle and the axis (51). This ossicle is free to move in all directions, which results in considerable instability of the cervical spine.

Patients with trisomy 21 (Down syndrome) exhibit excessive laxity of their joints, and the transverse ligament is no exception. The incidence of atlantoaxial instability in children with Down syndrome is estimated at 14% to 24% (81–83). These patients are at risk for subluxation of the atlas anteriorly on the axis, with resultant cord compression. Other conditions found with Down syndrome are cervical spondylosis, spina bifida of the atlas, os odontoideum, vertebral occipitalization, and Klippel-Feil syndrome (84). Klippel-Feil syndrome is associated with ankylosis of the cervical spine and fusion of several cervical vertebrae (85).

For an elective intubation, all patients with congenital anomalies associated with cervical spinal involvement should have lateral cervical spinal x-rays obtained in the neutral, flexed, and extended positions. Evidence of atlantoaxial subluxation, as well as cervical spondylosis, should be sought. Prior planning and preparation for a difficult intubation will greatly decrease both morbidity and mortality. Elective intubation (either blindly or with fiberoptic observation) is best conducted in the awake patient, after topical anesthesia.

INITIAL MANAGEMENT OF THE TRAUMA PATIENT

All trauma patients must be managed according to ATLS protocol as prescribed by the American College of Surgeons Committee on Trauma (9). The first priority during the primary survey is airway maintenance with cervical spinal control. Cervical spinal immobilization should be initiated in all trauma patients who are unconscious or who have multisystem injuries or penetrating neck injury. Those patients with a high likelihood of cervical spinal trauma are best stabilized with a hard (Philadelphia) collar, sandbags, and taping of the head and body to a rigid backboard (86–88). Hard collars alone may allow up to 73% of normal flexion and extension (88,89). Awake, alert, and sober patients with no other major distracting injuries, no complaints of neck pain, and no tenderness or neurologic deficit probably do not have a cervical spinal injury (90–93,25,28). However, before ruling out a cervical spinal injury by the above criteria, one must remember that most trauma patients either are intoxicated with alcohol or drugs, have multiple injuries, or both. Therefore, adherence to these criteria is essential.

Shock in the trauma patient has many causes. Although hypovolemia from hemorrhage is the most common cause, cardiogenic shock and neurogenic shock are often seen, sometimes in combination. Spinal injuries above T-7 cause hypotension and areflexia, and those above T-5 also produce bradycardia because of the loss of sympathetic innervation. These patients may also have significant respiratory compromise, depending on the level of injury. Hypovolemia and/or hypoxia may complicate any spinal cord injury. Therefore, shock and hypoxia should be rapidly treated. It is essential to remember to correct hypovolemia and restore the volume status before considering administration of vasopressors. Vasopressors administered before the restoration of volume may add ischemic insult to an already injured spinal cord. Central venous pressure monitoring is recommended in managing this complex problem. The correction of hypoxia and airway management are discussed later in this chapter.

RADIOLOGIC EXAMINATION

Three standard plain radiographic views of the cervical spine are the cross-table lateral, anterior-posterior, and open-mouth (odontoid) views. When interpreting cervical spinal radiographs, one must remember the "ABCs"—alignment, bones, and cartilage—and soft tissue spaces.

Because of the many various overlying structures and shadows, cervical spinal x-ray films can be difficult to interpret, and subtle findings can be easily missed. The recent quote, "A man needs to know his limitations," is good advice for those practitioners who interpret cervical spinal x-ray films. Failure to recognize a cervical fracture or evidence of cervical instability may result in subsequent severe neurologic sequelae.

The first view to obtain is the cross-table lateral (CTL) (Fig. 11). C-1 through the upper levels of T-1 must be depicted on these films because 7% to 20% of all cervi-

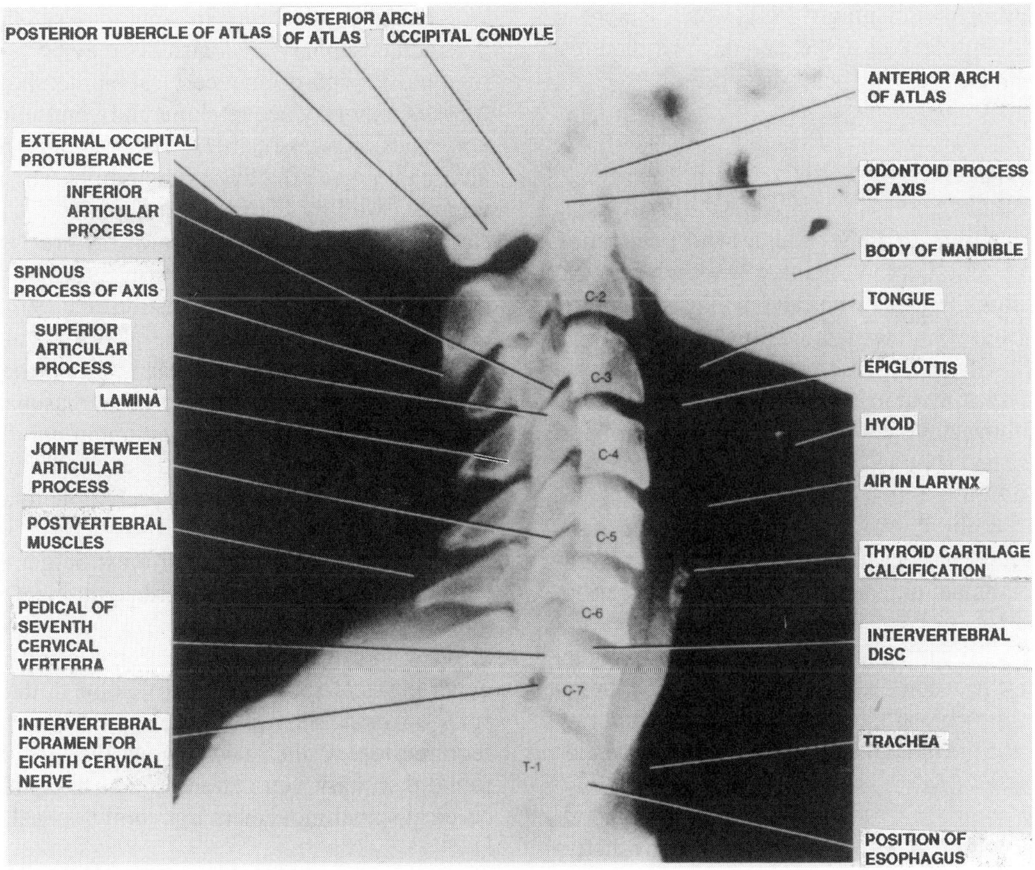

FIG. 21-11. Adequate lateral cervical spinal x-ray.

cal spinal injuries occur at C-7 or at the junction of C-7 and T-1 (94–97). When reviewing the CTL, one should address the normal lordotic curve of the cervical spine, the anterior and posterior borders of the vertebral bodies, the junctions between the laminae and the spinous processes, and the tips of the spinous processes. These should all form smooth curves. Lateral films should also be assessed for the normal alignment of the occipito-atlanto-axial complex. At each vertebral level, abnormalities of the bony structure of the vertebral bodies, intervertebral disk spaces, articular facet joints, spinous processes, and interspinous distances should be evaluated. The anterior prevertebral soft tissue should be measured at the inferior aspect of C-3. A measurement greater than 5 mm may indicate a hematoma secondary to cervical spinal injury. The sensitivity of the CTL alone, however, is only 74% to 82% (32,95,98,99).

The anterior-posterior view is assessed for the vertical alignment of the spinous and articular processes and any abnormalities of the joint and disk spaces. For example, rotation of a spinous process may indicate a unilateral facet dislocation. The sensitivity of radiography for detecting cervical spinal fractures may be increased to 92% with the addition of the anterior-posterior and odontoid views (32,95–97).

The third view, the open-mouth or odontoid view, assesses the integrity of the atlanto-occipital and atlanto-axial joints as well as the odontoid process. The gap between the lateral masses of C-1 and the dens should be equal, and the lateral masses should not extend beyond the body of C-2. Deviation indicates a fracture of the vertebral arch of C-1 (Jefferson fracture).

Oblique views may be added to visualize the intervertebral foramen and the vertebral arches. Since the standard cross-table lateral, anterior-posterior, and odontoid views offer only 92% sensitivity, further studies may be indicated in symptomatic patients.

Extension/flexion views may detect ligamentous injuries. Extension/flexion views should be done only under the direct supervision of a physician and not when the patient is unconscious.

Some authors recommend the liberal use of CT to rule out cervical spinal injury (13). CT is useful when plain radiographs are suggestive of injury or equivocal, or when clinical symptoms persist. CT is also useful for the evaluation of the unconscious patient, and it offers the advantage of evaluating the spinal canal. CT has limited value for examining odontoid and anterior atlantal fractures, since they are parallel to the plane of the CT scan.

Magnetic resonance imaging (MRI), which is able to detail the bone, muscle, soft tissue, and neural structures, is helpful in making more difficult diagnoses.

AIRWAY MANAGEMENT PRINCIPLES

The first priority in treating patients with penetrating or multiple trauma is airway maintenance with cervical spinal stabilization. Patients who can talk have an airway; however, depending on the injuries, this airway may be only tenuous, as some of these patients can quickly decompensate. Therefore, it is important to evaluate the airway and breathing continually. The practitioner should search for signs and symptoms of upper and lower airway obstruction: dyspnea, hoarseness, stridor, dysphonia, subcutaneous emphysema, and hemoptysis. The neck should be carefully inspected for deformity, edema, crepitation, tracheal deviation, and jugular venous distention. The practitioner should auscultate the chest for heart and breath sounds and the neck for bruits and stridor that may not be otherwise heard in a noisy emergency room. Some of these signs may be subtle, but their recognition may avert a disaster if the patient subsequently requires endotracheal intubation.

The airway should be kept clear of mucous, blood, vomitus, and foreign bodies. Cervical radiographs should be reviewed for the presence of cervical spinal injury as well as tracheal deviation and soft tissue air. Chest radiographs are reviewed for hemothorax, pneumothorax, widening of the mediastinum, tracheal deviation, enlarged cardiac silhouette and aortic knob, rib fractures, and pulmonary contusions. Many of these conditions occur concurrently with cervical spinal injury.

Although many trauma patients are intoxicated with alcohol or drugs, a trauma patient who is agitated or obtunded should first be assumed to have hypoxia or hypercarbia until proved otherwise. Patients who are obviously obstructed, apneic, or cyanotic require immediate intervention. Most such patients require endotracheal intubation. Basic maneuvers to open an airway, such as carefully applied chin lift and bag-valve-mask ventilation, may be sufficient. The neck should not be hyperextended when the chin-lift maneuver is performed. ATLS protocol recommends the chin-lift maneuver as the method of choice (9). Aprahamian et al. (100) surgically created complete ligamentous instability of C-5 and C-6 in a fresh cadaver. They found that any maneuver that created extension of the head on the neck produced anterior subluxation and widening of the disk space at that level. The chin-lift and jaw-thrust maneuvers created an increase in disk space greater than 5 mm, which was more than the change created by oral tracheal intubation (3 to 4 mm). When these maneuvers were repeated with the aid of Philadelphia and soft collars, these devices were found to have no consistent effect and produced a worsening of instability in some cases. The oropharyngeal and nasopharyngeal airways may be associated with less movement of the cervical spine; however, these devices may produce retching and vomiting in the semiconscious or awake patient. The nasopharyngeal airway, although not as effective as the oropharyngeal airway, is tolerated well by the responsive patient. ATLS protocol states that if a cribriform plate fracture is suspected, a nasopharyngeal airway may be inserted and used to facilitate the passage of a nasogastric tube (9). The chin-lift and jaw-thrust maneuvers are also difficult to perform with a hard Philadelphia collar in place; therefore, a nasopharyngeal airway appears to be a reasonable choice to relieve airway obstruction. The important objective is to establish a patent airway, and the careful application of any of these techniques is far preferable to an obstructed airway.

Bag-valve-mask ventilation must be gently applied to help avoid inflation and overdistention of the stomach with air. Using a fresh cadaver model, Hauswald et al. (101) found that mask ventilation caused flexion in the upper cervical spine and retroflexion in the midcervical spine, which seemed to be secondary to the force required to seal the mask against the face. They further found that mask ventilation produced significantly more cervical spinal movement than oral tracheal intubation.

Aspiration Prophylaxis

All acutely traumatized patients should be considered to have a full stomach (102). Gastric emptying is delayed as a result of pain, fear, anxiety, intoxication, shock, and loss of consciousness (103–105). Furthermore, many of these patients may have eaten or drunk immediately prior to their injury. The time interval between the last intake and the painful injury is more important in predicting a full stomach than the interval between the last intake and the intubation (106). As many as 24 to 48 hours may be required for the stomach to empty in a severely traumatized patient.

Factors that increase the risk of aspiration pneumonitis are gastric volume greater than 0.4 mL/kg, increased acidity (pH < 2.5), and presence of particulate matter (107). Patients with head injuries and those requiring bag-valve-mask ventilation are prone to vomiting or regurgitation and are at increased risk for aspirating these contents into the lungs. Rapid intubation of the trachea with either a cuffed endotracheal tube in patients over 8 years of age or a tracheostomy tube is the best method to prevent aspiration. One method of decreasing the risk for aspiration is the placement of a nasogastric tube. Although the nasogastric tube cannot evacuate the stomach completely, it can empty the gas along with some fluid, thereby reducing intragastric pressure. Placement of a nasogastric tube is contraindicated in patients with potential cribriform plate fractures (108). Placement of the nasogastric tube is associated with retching and coughing, which can elevate the intracranial pressure in head-injured patients and intra-ocular pressure with open-globe injuries. Retching and coughing may also cause movement of unstable cervical spinal injuries.

Although complications may be associated with the placement of the nasogastric tube, and complete evacuation of gastric contents cannot be ensured, most severely traumatized patients benefit from careful placement of this tube. Some feel that the gastric tube may act as a wick by defeating the competence of the lower esophageal sphincter and also render cricoid pressure ineffective (109). However, a more recent study demonstrated that the nasogastric tube did not decrease the effectiveness of cricoid pressure (110).

Properly applied cricoid pressure is a well-accepted standard for effectively preventing regurgitation of gastric contents in the unconscious patient during endotracheal intubation. Cricoid pressure and the prevalent use of muscle relaxants have contributed to the low incidence (8/10,000) of regurgitation in emergency anesthetics (111). However, the use of cricoid pressure in patients with unstable cervical spinal injuries is controversial, since the potential for subluxation exists at the site of instability, especially injuries of C-5 and C-6 (112,113). Properly applied cricoid pressure compresses the esophagus between the vertebral body of C-6 and the cricoid ring with a force of 44 newtons or about 10 lb. This amount of force may cause further subluxation and spinal cord injury (100). However, others have reported the use of orotracheal intubation after rapid-sequence induction with cricoid pressure and manual in-line axial stabilization (MIAS), and no evidence of new neurologic injury appeared with this technique (33). Since cricoesophageal compression is effective in preventing regurgitation and aspiration pneumonitis, we support the use of this technique in trauma patients with potential cervical spinal injury. For those patients with known unstable injuries of the lower cervical spine, especially of C-5 and C-6, the risk for spinal cord injury with cricoid pressure may be greater than the risk for regurgitation if an otherwise straightforward orotracheal intubation is anticipated.

Controversies About Endotracheal Intubation

No consensus exists as to the best technique for tracheal intubation of the patient with a cervical spinal injury. Different authors recommend awake tracheal intubation (100,113–117), direct laryngoscopy with cricoid pressure and head/neck stabilization (MIAS) (31,33,118, 119), cricothyroidotomy (120,121), or a fiberoptic technique (oral or nasal) (122–124). ATLS protocol offers an algorithm for airway management in the unconscious blunt trauma patient (9). This algorithm gives preference to nasotracheal intubation. However, algorithms are rigid and dogmatic and do not account for the individual skills of the practitioner or the varying clinical presentations of the patient. Crosby and Lui (125), in their recently published review of adult airway management with cervical spinal injuries, suggest that the method of intubation is not as important as recognizing the possibility of a cervical spinal injury and taking appropriate care. Hastings and Marks (126), in another recent review, recommended that those working with trauma patients use their professional judgment to establish a management plan for cervical spinal injuries. They advocated a case-specific strategy for airway management incorporating the airway management skills and expertise of the practitioner. We agree with the authors of both these reviews and feel that airway management should be administered with great care and managed on a case-by-case basis according to the practitioner's skills. These airways should be managed only by experienced practitioners; this patient population is not suitable for novices who need to practice their airway-management skills.

When the various intubation techniques are being considered, the anatomic aspects and mechanism of injury must be recalled. In review, the anterior column stabilizes the spine in extension and the posterior column stabilizes the spine in flexion. Therefore, hyperextension tends to injure the anterior elements and hyperflexion, the posterior elements. Both columns may be injured when extreme compressive or rotational forces are added to the mechanism. For example, if only the anterior column has been injured as a result of hyperextension, the cervical spine tends to be more stable in flexion, and therefore a small amount of flexion may be possible. However, when both columns are disrupted, no movement is permitted.

TECHNIQUES OF AIRWAY MANAGEMENT

Nasotracheal Intubation

Awake nasotracheal intubation following topical anesthesia is a well-accepted technique for the patient with cervical spinal injury or disease. This technique has been strongly advocated by many clinicians. Awake nasotracheal and orotracheal intubations are especially useful for securing an airway in patients with anatomic anomalies or diseases (e.g., rheumatoid arthritis) that make direct laryngoscopy difficult or impossible.

Some anatomic predictors of a difficult intubation are a receding mandible, small mouth, macroglossia, a short muscular neck, protruding maxillary incisors, and limited mobility of the mandible or neck. The degree of visibility of the posterior intra-oral structures with the tongue maximally protruded is also helpful in predicting the difficulty of intubation (127,128). For example, if the soft palate, fauces, uvula, and tonsilar pillars are readily seen, then intubation will probably be easy. Conversely, if nothing in the posterior pharynx can be seen, intubation may be very difficult. These methods of evaluation have only limited value in the trauma patient, especially in the patient wearing a rigid cervical collar.

Nasotracheal intubation avoids excessive extension of the occipito-atlanto-axial complex and the flexion of the lower cervical spine that is required to view the glottis with direct laryngoscopy. However, Aprahamian et al. (100) found that blind nasotracheal intubation produced more than 5 mm of posterior subluxation when the neck was stabilized anteriorly by hand pressure. This was reduced to 2 mm by omitting the stabilization. Furthermore, flexion/extension of the neck, which should be avoided in the unstable spine, is often necessary to achieve successful blind nasal intubation of the trachea.

Awake intubations have not been shown to worsen neurologic injury in acute cervical trauma patients (129, 130). When Holley and Jordan (131) retrospectively reviewed the airway management of 113 patients with unstable injuries who required intubation for surgical fixation, they found no new neurologic changes after either nasal or oral intubation. In another retrospective report, Meschino et al. (130) found a similar neurologic outcome between cervical spine-injured patients after awake tracheal intubation and those patients who were not intubated (130). Although some authors have reported a better than 90% success rate for blind nasal intubation in the emergency room (113,132), Dronen et al. (133) reported the success rate of blind nasal technique to be 65% vs. 100% for oral intubation by direct laryngoscopy. They found that multiple attempts at nasal intubation were not unusual and produced a complication rate of 86%. The most frequent complication was epistaxis (69%); however, vomiting occurred in 17% of these patients, with a 10% aspiration rate. Although Dronen et al. were studying cases of poisoning, a 10% incidence of aspiration is excessive and would be poorly tolerated in severely traumatized patients. Death resulting from hypoxic cardiac arrest after a failed, traumatic blind nasotracheal intubation has been reported (134). We also reported a death as a result of a failed attempt at blind nasal intubation in a patient with a gunshot wound to the neck in our retrospective study of airway management for patients with penetrating neck trauma (71). A rapidly expanding hematoma that resulted from the intubation attempt obliterated the airway, and the patient expired before a surgical airway could be established. This death occurred in one of the four patients in the blind nasal group. Having seen this same sequence of events occur in others, we concluded that for the patient with penetrating neck injury, blind attempts at intubation should be avoided unless there is no other way to establish the airway.

Although the unconscious patient who is spontaneously breathing can be intubated using the blind nasal technique, many of these patients have intact reflexes and are likely to cough, retch, and vomit. Since these patients cannot protect their airway, they are prone to aspiration. Awake blind nasal techniques also require a cooperative patient, and time is required to prepare the airway properly for this technique. Although coughing can be controlled with translaryngeal anesthesia, some believe that this anesthesia may increase the risk for aspiration (135). However, Ovassapian et al. (136) found no evidence of aspiration after laryngeal anesthesia for fiberoptic intubation in 105 patients. In the severely traumatized patient, blood and secretions may also interfere with the ability to properly anesthetize the airway.

Epistaxis is a common complication of blind nasotracheal intubation, and this bleeding increases the difficulty of subsequent direct laryngoscopy if it becomes necessary. Epistaxis may make a fiberoptic technique impossible. Coughing, vomiting, and the hypertensive response to intubation may all increase intracranial pressure and intra-ocular pressure in patients with head injuries and open-globe injuries, respectively, and blind nasal intubation should be avoided in these patients. Blind intubation techniques may also cause airway obstruction in patients with laryngeal injuries and are contraindicated in the presence of basilar skull fractures. Movement of the cervical spine has not been adequately studied in living patients. Unconscious and semiconscious patients may respond to intubation with excessive movement. Therefore, the authors have reservations about use of the blind nasotracheal technique for emergency intubation in patients with a cervical spinal injury.

For those patients who are awake, alert, and cooperative without co-existing head, airway, and eye injuries, awake nasotracheal intubation in the well-anesthetized airway is a reasonable technique. Treating the nasal passages with phenylephrine or oxymetazoline helps to reduce epistaxis. Placing a suction catheter through a warmed 6.5- to 7-mm-inner-diameter endotracheal tube and then through the nasal passages, using the suction catheter as a leader, helps to prevent submucosal tunneling (137). The use of a whistle (e.g., Beck airway air flow monitor; Great Plains Ballistic Co., Lubbock, Texas) or measurement of end-tidal carbon dioxide is helpful in identifying the proximity to the airway. Since the cervical spine-injured patient is to be maintained in the neutral position and since extension, flexion, and manipulation of the neck are to be avoided, successful intubation is more difficult. If the endotracheal tube does not easily pass into the larynx, inflation of the tube cuff may direct the advancing tip of the endotracheal tube toward the larynx. If an increase in breath sounds is heard, then the cuff is deflated and the tube can be gently passed into the larynx on inspiration (138). The light wand has been recommended by some as an aid to blind oral or nasal tracheal intubation (139–141) (Fig. 12). The light wand is a flexible stylet with a light bulb at the distal end, which serves to illuminate the trachea, allowing placement of

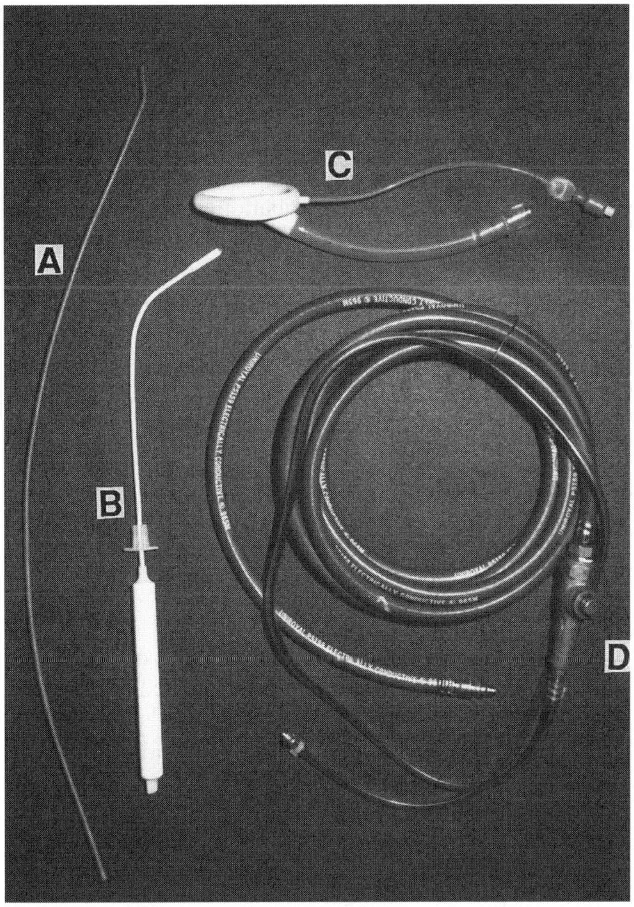

FIG. 12. Suggested intubating equipment: gum elastic bougie *(A)*, light wand *(B)*, laryngeal mask airway *(C)*, and Sanders jet ventilator *(D)*.

the endotracheal tube. This device has only a limited success rate (63% to 88%) (141). Manipulation of either the jaw or the larynx is required in some cases for successful intubation. Confirmation of proper intubation with this technique is best detected by end-tidal capnography. Outside the operating room, where capnography is not generally available, a self-inflating bulb is useful in detecting esophageal intubations, thus avoiding inflation of the stomach when auscultating breath sounds (142). A compressed, self-inflating bulb attached to the adapter of an endotracheal tube will not reinflate with an esophageal intubation but will rapidly reinflate with endotracheal intubation (Fig. 13). If a patient can talk with an endotracheal tube cuff inflated, the tube is in the esophagus.

Fiberoptic Bronchoscopy

Fiberoptic-aided oral or nasotracheal intubation has gained wide popularity for overcoming difficult intubations. The use of fiberoptic intubation with cervical spinal pathology has been well established and documented (123,143–145). We found fiberoptic intubation useful for airway management in patients with penetrating neck trauma; all eight patients in our reported series were safely intubated with this technique (71). It provides adequate laryngeal visualization without neck manipulation, as well as confirmation of intubation. Messeter and Pettersson (122) compared the fiberoptic technique with standard laryngoscopy in 41 patients with advanced rheumatoid arthritis presenting for cervical fusion. No patient in either group developed neurologic changes as a result of intubation. The use of the bronchoscope resulted in a reduction in the number of intubations rated as difficult when compared with direct laryngoscopy. This technique has an almost 100% success rate for elective intubations by skilled clinicians (124). However, it may not always be appropriate in acute situations. It requires time and may be impossible in the presence of excessive secretions, blood, and vomit (145,146). These factors not only interfere with visibility but also prevent adequate local anesthesia, which is essential in the awake patient to prevent bucking or coughing. Although fiberoptic intubation is technically easier in the sitting position, this is not possible in the severely traumatized cervical spine-injured patient.

With skilled hands and proper patient selection, fiberoptic bronchoscopy is probably the technique of choice for elective intubation of patients with cervical spinal pathology. Orotracheal fiberoptic intubation is more difficult, but the oral route avoids the complications of nasal intubations—nasal trauma and sinusitis. The oral route also allows placement of a larger-diameter endotracheal tube, which makes respiratory care and weaning from the ventilator easier. However, many practitioners are not proficient in the use of the fiberoptic bronchoscope, and many severely injured patients are not good candidates for this technique; therefore, other techniques must be considered.

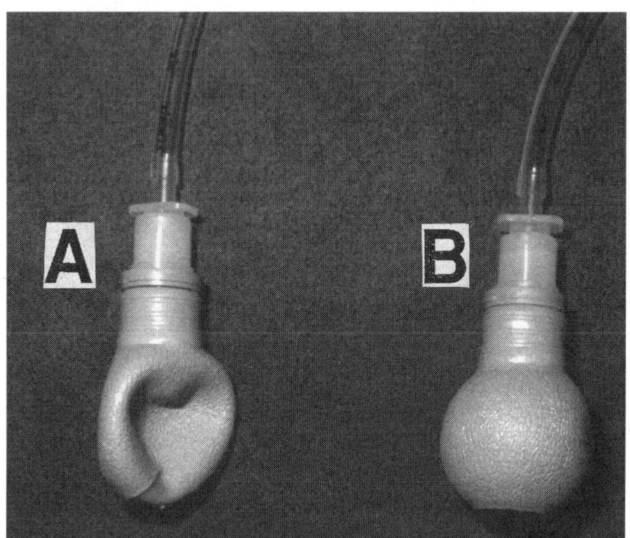

FIG. 13. Self-inflating bulb depicts an esophageal intubation *(A)*. Bulb rapidly inflates with a tracheal intubation *(B)*.

Direct Laryngoscopy

Direct laryngoscopy with cricoid pressure and MIAS is the fastest and surest method of intubating the trachea. However, some authors believe that the degree of atlanto-occipital extension necessary to align the airway and view the larynx may injure an unstable spine (113,116, 117). Fitzgerald et al. (147) studied cervical supine motion, comparing blind oral intubation using the Augustine guide (Augustine Medical Inc., Eden Prairie, Minnesota) vs. direct laryngoscopy. They found that direct laryngoscopy resulted in a mean 46° extension of the occiput–C-3 unit, vs. a 29° extension with the Augustine guide (147). However, MIAS was not used in this study. Horton et al. (148) also found significant atlantoaxial extension with direct laryngoscopy but minimal movement in the lower cervical spine in anesthetized volunteers. Therefore, patients with unstable upper cervical spinal injuries may be more vulnerable to neurologic damage from the atlanto-occipital extension necessary to visualize the glottis during direct laryngoscopy, whereas the majority of cervical spinal injuries (C-3 to C-7) may be less vulnerable to further injury, since they are less affected by extension (148).

The addition of the Hoffman prism, as on the Belscope, seems to produce less cervical spinal motion, especially extension. However, Gajraj et al. (149) found no difference in motion of the cervical spine between direct laryngoscopy with the Macintosh 3 blade and indirect laryngoscopy with the Belscope. Two patients in this study could not be intubated with the Belscope because of the technical difficulties with indirect visualization of the glottis.

Another device that requires an indirect technique is the Bullard laryngoscope. This laryngoscope has an anatomically shaped blade with a fiberoptic light and visual path. It has been used successfully in both adult and pediatric patients with unstable cervical spinal injury (150,151). However, since intubation requires placement of an endotracheal tube under indirect vision, the insertion of the endotracheal tube may be difficult. Threading the tracheal tube over a guide wire may improve the success of intubation (152). Both the Bullard laryngoscope and the Belscope require practice and proficiency, and these devices are not immediately available at many institutions.

Clinically, sudden worsening of neurologic deficits has occurred with traction (153,154). Many authors refer to the use of manual in-line traction to stabilize the cervical spine during direct laryngoscopy. Since application of excessive traction may result in neurologic injury, *the term "traction" should be eliminated* from descriptions of cervical spinal stabilization for intubation. The proper maneuver should be *manual in-line axial stabilization.* The concept of this maneuver is to stabilize the head in the neutral position, using just the force required to prevent movement of the head and neck during intubation attempts. Some movement of the cervical spine, especially extension of the occipito-atlanto-axial complex, is unavoidable with direct laryngoscopy. MIAS should allow only that motion necessary to view the glottis, and if this motion is deemed excessive (for example, with an anterior airway), then the intubation attempt should be aborted and other means to secure the airway should be implemented.

Manual in-line stabilization reduces cervical supine movement during orotracheal intubation by about 60% (112). Nolan and Wilson (155) evaluated the gum elastic bougie as an intubation aid and found that about 45% of patients had at least one grade of decreased visibility of the larynx when the intubating position of the head and neck were changed from the sniffing to the neutral position. When movement of the head and neck was restricted by stabilization and cricoid pressure applied, the glottis was not seen in 22% of patients in the neutral position. In this study of 157 intubations, they found that patients managed with the bougie could be intubated in a mean time of 26 seconds. There were five failures in the group managed without the bougie; all of these subjects were, subsequently, successfully intubated with the aid of the gum elastic bougie. However, this study did not compare cervical spinal motion with x-ray studies. We strongly recommend the routine use of the gum elastic bougie as an aid to intubation of the cervical spine-injured patient (Fig. 12).

During direct laryngoscopy with or without the gum elastic bougie (or a similar device), the larynx often has to be intubated blindly. With any technique that involves blind intubation of the trachea, it is important not to apply excessive pressure when ventilating through the endotracheal tube until proper endotracheal intubation can be confirmed. Whenever possible, it is best to auscultate the epigastrium for air in the stomach prior to auscultating the chest for breath sounds. This technique allows detection of an esophageal intubation earlier, thereby decreasing the amount of air insufflated into the stomach. Cricoid pressure should not be removed until proper confirmation of endotracheal intubation. When the esophagus is inadvertently intubated, it is best to leave the endotracheal tube in the esophagus in order to vent vomitus away from the airway. The presence of an endotracheal tube in the esophagus generally does not hamper further intubation attempts, and it also indicates to the intubator where not to place the endotracheal tube. As described in published reports, some degree of cervical spinal motion is inevitable with direct laryngoscopy. However, this motion does not appear clinically to affect neurologic outcome (30,33,118,131,156,157). This low incidence of neurologic injury probably results from the relatively large canal of the upper cervical spine. Since one-third of the canal at C-1 is occupied by the dens, one-third by the spinal cord, and one-third by empty space, there appears to be some margin of safety.

No large studies compare intubation techniques and neurologic outcome specifically in patients with unstable cervical spinal injuries. In a small series, Rhee et al. (156) found no adverse effect of direct laryngoscopy in seven patients with C-1 or C-2 injuries. Grande et al. (33) found orotracheal intubation was successful in more than 3000 trauma patients at the Maryland Institute for Emergency Medical Services; however, only 30 of these patients were proved subsequently to have a cervical spinal injury, and none developed a decrease in neurologic function as a result of intubation. They further emphasized the importance of oxygenation and ventilation with cricoid pressure before intubation.

Conscious patients and hemodynamically stable patients who are semiconscious, have a closed head injury, or have sustained an open-globe injury should receive an anesthetic and a muscle relaxant prior to direct laryngoscopy. Cricoid pressure and manual in-line stabilization should be used during these intubations. Etomidate 0.2 to 0.3 mg/kg followed by succinylcholine 2 mg/kg or rocuronium 0.6 mg/kg or vecuronium 0.2 mg/kg will allow intubation of the trachea within 60 to 90 seconds. (Higher doses of rocuronium may yield more prompt onset of intubation in the patient with a full stomach; this is currently under further investigation.) Succinylcholine can be safely administered within the first 24 to 48 hours following injury, after which time its use can cause significant hyperkalemia in those patients at risk (158). Before the administration of succinylcholine, we do not preblock with a nondepolarizing agent, since observation of the termination of fasciculations allows the intubator access to the airway at the earliest possible time. Adequate relaxation is vital in order to prevent coughing and bucking on the endotracheal tube.

The use of high-dose nondepolarizing muscle relaxants has been criticized for the prolonged period of paralysis after their administration and the inability to perform neurologic examinations subsequently. For example, the duration of neuromuscular block produced by vecuronium (0.28 mg/kg) that precedes 25% recovery (twitch height) is approximately 90 minutes. This objection is usually academic, since many of these patients undergo diagnostic studies and/or surgery within that time period. We do not recommend pancuronium, since large doses result in significant tachycardia and interfere with the ability to use tachycardia as a sign of hemodynamic instability. For those hemodynamically stable patients with closed head injuries or a history of cardiovascular disease, we recommend careful intravenous administration of an opioid (fentanyl 3 to 5 μg/kg or alfentanil 20 μg/kg) in addition to etomidate to blunt the hypertensive response to intubation. For those conscious patients who are unstable and do not have major vascular or intracranial injuries, we recommend ketamine 1 to 2 mg/kg as the induction agent of choice. When neuromuscular relaxation is required for intubation, hemodynamically unstable unconscious patients require only succinylcholine 2 mg/kg (or another drug regimen providing prompt neuromuscular relaxation if succinylcholine is contraindicated or undesirable).

To prevent hypoxia and hypercarbia, prolonged attempts at intubation should be avoided. We recommend that intubators hold their breath during the intubation attempt so as to determine the patient's need for oxygen and ventilation. Pulse oximetry should be employed in all areas where intubations are performed. However, the pulse oximeter has some limitation in the hemodynamically unstable trauma patient with vasoconstriction secondary to hypovolemia or hypothermia. If the time to complete the intubation is deemed too long, the patient should be ventilated and oxygenated by careful and gentle bag-valve-mask ventilation with cricoid pressure. This technique has been reported to be safe for acute trauma patients with full stomachs (33).

If bag-valve-mask ventilation is difficult or impossible, a laryngeal mask airway (LMA) (Fig. 12) can be quickly and atraumatically inserted and may provide a conduit for ventilation until other intubation techniques can be pursued (159). The LMA has achieved wide acceptance for ventilating patients under anesthesia during elective surgery, and its successful use has been reported with unstable spinal injury (160,161). An airway algorithm proposed by Benumof (162) suggests using the LMA in the "can't intubate, can't ventilate" scenario prior to attempting transtracheal ventilation. We have found the LMA extremely valuable in establishing ventilation in the "cannot intubate, cannot ventilate" scenario in our surgical patients. The successful use of the LMA in emergency patients after failed intubation and bag-valve-mask ventilation at Parkland Hospital has averted several emergency surgical airways. Although aspiration of gastric contents is still possible, a properly placed LMA may minimize the amount of air insufflated into the stomach and therefore decrease the risk for regurgitation. The LMA is generally contraindicated in the conscious and semiconscious patient and in patients with upper airway pathology. (It may, however, be used to assist ventilation or intubation in the patient who cannot be mask ventilated or intubated by standard methods. See Chapter 13.) Although the LMA can usually be placed into the hypopharynx quickly and without difficulty, practice and proficiency with this device are required before its use. An airway emergency is not the appropriate time to use the LMA for the first time. A No. 6 (internal diameter) endotracheal tube can be passed through the laryngeal mask and blindly inserted into the trachea (163) (see Chapter 13 for a discussion of this technique). Since there is cervical spinal motion associated with mask ventilation, the LMA may be superior to bag-valve-mask ventilation; however, further investigation will be required in the emergent and severely injured patient to confirm the safety of this device (101).

Penetrating Neck Trauma

We have found that direct laryngoscopy has a 98% success rate when intubating patients with penetrating neck trauma (71). Two patients required an emergency surgical airway after failed intubation by direct laryngoscopy; one patient received an emergency tracheostomy, and the other received a cricothyroidotomy with a 14-gauge cannula and jet ventilation. However, only one patient in this series of 107 patients had a cervical spinal injury, which was a complete transection of the cord at C-5. He was intubated by direct laryngoscopy without further neurologic complication. Although most patients with penetrating trauma to the cervical spinal cord have devastating and irreversible neurologic deficit, one must protect and immobilize the cervical spine to prevent extension of injury. Patients with penetrating cervical spinal trauma may also have co-existing airway and vascular injuries, which greatly complicate airway management. Since one patient in our series died as a result of a failed blind nasotracheal intubation attempt, we recommend that patients with penetrating neck trauma be intubated either by direct laryngoscopy, fiberoptic bronchoscopy, or a surgical airway, depending on the patient's hemodynamic stability and injuries. For example, those patients with penetrating trauma to the larynx should receive an emergency surgical airway (9,71,164).

Surgical Airway Techniques

There are four methods to establish a surgical airway. The first two methods require a surgical incision: cricothyroidotomy and tracheostomy. The second two methods are somewhat less invasive and require a percutaneous puncture of the cricothyroid membrane. One method is performed by carefully puncturing the cricothyroid membrane with a 12- to 14-gauge needle or catheter and administering oxygen by a high-pressure source. This method is frequently referred to as "transtracheal jet ventilation." The last method is retrograde intubation, which involves the blind insertion of a tracheal tube into the trachea over a guide wire or catheter passed in retrograde fashion into the oral or nasal pharynx through the cricothyroid membrane.

When an immediate airway is needed and direct laryngoscopy has failed or is impossible because of airway trauma, a cricothyroidotomy is immediately indicated (9). A surgical cricothyroidotomy is well described in the ATLS course (9). ATLS protocol does not recommend a cricothyroidotomy in children under 12 years of age because the cricoid ring is the narrowest part of the airway in these individuals, and complications of tracheal stenosis may later occur. The ATLS manual states that surgical cricothyroidotomy is easily performed by making a skin incision extending through the cricoid membrane. This is more easily said than done. We have observed many bloody disasters in attempts to perform cricothyroidotomy for establishing emergency airways. The use of this technique in the emergency room has been associated with an immediate complication rate of 32% (120). The inexperience of residents was cited as the cause of these complications. We often find that in the haste to establish a surgical airway, inexperienced practitioners fail to identify properly the cricothyroid membrane and/or fail to stabilize the site of incision with their hand or other instrument and lose their surgical track. The cricothyroid membrane is the shallowest portion of the anterior neck and usually provides a site of easy access to the airway with minimal trauma. We offer some suggestions for performing a cricothyroidotomy; be calm and deliberate, take the time to identify the cricothyroid membrane properly, stabilize the site of incision with the thumb and index finger of the nonoperative hand, and do not remove the nonoperative hand until the airway is either instrumented or intubated.

The next surgical technique is tracheostomy. Except in patients under 12 years of age, a tracheostomy is not indicated for establishing an emergency airway unless there is co-existing injury to the larynx. For those patients with large penetrating wounds to the airway, it is often necessary to intubate the trachea through these wounds. There are no studies of cervical spinal motion with either cricothyroidotomy or tracheostomy. It is important to take care not to manipulate the neck excessively and avoid neck extension in patients with potential cervical spinal injury. The inability to extend the neck in these patients may also increase the degree of difficulty in performing a surgical airway.

Transtracheal Ventilation

Transtracheal jet ventilation can circumvent the need for a surgical cricothyroidotomy and can provide an effective mode of oxygenation and ventilation until the trachea can be formally intubated (165). This technique does not protect against aspiration and may not allow adequate hyperventilation for patients with increased intracranial pressure. Another disadvantage of this technique is that the equipment (i.e., a Sanders jet ventilator) (Fig. 12) must be readily at hand to provide ventilation after placement of a 12- to 14-gauge cannula through the cricothyroid membrane. Smith et al. (166) found a 29% complication rate with emergency transtracheal jet ventilation. Tension pneumothorax, pneumomediastinum, subcutaneous emphysema and/or abdominal distention may result with this technique. Transtracheal jet ventilation is preferred over surgical cricothyroidotomy in patients under 12 years of age.

Retrograde Intubation

Retrograde intubation has been used successfully in trauma patients. Barriot and Riou (167) studied 19 patients who were intubated with the retrograde technique. Twelve patients had severe maxillofacial trauma, and 7 patients had cervical spinal injury. Conventional oral or nasal intubation techniques failed in 13 of these patients. All 19 patients in their series were intubated with the retrograde technique on the first attempt in less than 5 minutes. They found that despite the restrictions on head and neck movement, cricoid membrane puncture was accomplished without difficulty.

One problem encountered with the retrograde technique is that the endotracheal tube can hang up on the epiglottis. This problem can be overcome by threading the guide wire through the suction port of a fiberoptic bronchoscope. Alternatively, a firm tube such as a Salem sump tube can be passed over the guide wire. Either method lends support and helps guide the endotracheal tube past the epiglottis. The effectiveness of this technique may also be improved by passing the guide wire through the Murphy eye of the endotracheal tube (168). There are commercially available kits (Cook Retrograde Intubation Set, Bloomington, Indiana) to perform retrograde intubations. Our first-time use of this kit resulted in a successful intubation on the first attempt in less than 1 minute. This technique has great potential for managing patients with difficult airways, specifically patients with an injured cervical spine. With proper patient selection and adequate anesthesia of the airway, this technique can be easily performed in the awake patient. The unconscious or anesthetized patient can also be intermittently ventilated during this procedure. Although we favor this technique and believe that retrograde intubation provides a reasonable approach to intubate the trachea, further studies with larger patient populations are indicated.

Another method of intubating the trachea, which has had limited use to date, is blind oral intubation with the Augustine guide. The Augustine guide consists of an intubation guide that is placed orally into the vallecula and a stylet with a flexible hollow shaft that acts both to find the glottic opening and to facilitate the introduction of the endotracheal tube. When the stylet is placed correctly into the trachea, the aspiration of 30 mL of air is possible without resistance, whereas the plunger of the syringe recoils after aspiration (because of the soft muscular walls) when it is placed in the esophagus. Fitzgerald et al. (147) studied the excursions of the cervical spine, comparing the Augustine guide vs. direct laryngoscopy. They found that the median time necessary for intubation with the Augustine guide was 41 seconds, as compared with 21 seconds with direct laryngoscopy. The success rate for direct laryngoscopy was 100%. The success rate for the Augustine guide on the first attempt was 75%, with an overall 100% success rate by the second attempt. Using the Augustine guide, cervical spinal extension of the occiput–C-3 unit was significantly less (20 vs. 46) than when direct laryngoscopy was used. These data were collected with the patient's head in the neutral position, but the investigators did not apply MIAS in their methods. Although this technique has merit in minimizing cervical spinal movement, further study is justified in the severely traumatized patient (see Chapter 15, Figs. 27–31).

MANAGEMENT PLANS

Immediate Airway Intervention

The severely traumatized patient frequently needs immediate airway intervention because of hemodynamic instability, hypoxia, airway obstruction, or elevated intracranial pressure. We believe that direct laryngoscopy is probably the method of choice for immediate airway control of trauma patients with actual or potential cervical spinal injuries. Direct laryngoscopy is the quickest and surest method of establishing an airway in these patients. With the use of MIAS and cricoid pressure, studies to date have not shown worsened neurologic outcome with this technique.

For patients who cannot be intubated or ventilated, or who have upper airway pathology (for example, a laryngeal fracture or massive maxillofacial trauma), we believe that immediate cricothyroidotomy in the hands of a skilled practitioner is the technique of choice. Transtracheal jet ventilation can be an alternative in pediatric patients, in patients without increased intracranial pressure, or in those who are not *in extremis*.

Urgent Airway Management

When urgent airway intervention is necessary, either for emergency surgery or respiratory failure, direct laryngoscopy with cricoid pressure and manual in-line stabilization is preferable. Retrograde intubation is also a reasonable alternative if a difficult intubation is anticipated. For those rare patients with atlanto-occipital dislocation or patients with extensive maxillofacial trauma or airway trauma, a cricothyroidotomy or tracheostomy would be the technique of choice. Awake techniques may be used if time permits, but multiple attempts should be avoided.

Elective Intubation for Cervical Spinal Surgery

Stable trauma patients who require intubation primarily for surgical repair of their injuries are probably best intubated by awake fiberoptic bronchoscopy. Although no data indicate its superiority over direct laryngoscopy, the neurologic status of the awake patient can be continuously assessed, and the awake patient can position himself or herself for surgery when appropriate. If fiberoptic bronchoscopy has failed (insufficient patient cooperation, secretions or blood in the airway, edema, lack of practitioner skill), then other methods of intubation must be considered. For patients with a difficult airway and upper cervical spinal injuries in whom fiberoptic intubation has failed, the retrograde intubation technique should be considered. If this technique fails, an elective cricothyroidotomy is also a reasonable choice, especially if the patient is immobilized in tongs or a halo. Since limited outcome studies have shown no worsening in the neurologic outcome with intubation by direct laryngoscopy and manual in-line axial stabilization, this technique may also be chosen if an easy intubation is anticipated. Blind intubation through an LMA would also be a reasonable alternative.

SUMMARY

This chapter has reviewed the anatomy of the cervical spine along with its supporting ligamentous structures. The epidemiology and mechanisms of cervical spinal injury have been presented. We have discussed the patterns of injury with both upper and lower cervical spinal injury. Basic airway management of the multiply traumatized patient has been presented. The advantages and disadvantages, as well as the results of outcome studies, of various airway techniques have been discussed. Until large studies of airway management for patients with unstable cervical spines are published, there is no best method to manage the airway of such patients. This chapter has offered some suggestions that are supported by the literature and influenced by the authors' experience and bias. However, practitioners should manage their patients with cervical spinal injury to the best of their individual skills. The most important beneficial factors in managing these severely traumatized patients are the recognition of the potential for cervical spinal injury, spinal immobilization, and appropriate care. In the words of Hippocrates, "I will use treatment to help the sick according to my ability and judgment, but never with a view to injury and wrongdoing" (1).

REFERENCES

1. Garrison FH. *History of Medicine*, 4th ed. Philadelphia: WB Saunders; 1929: 86,98,115.
2. Bohlman HH. Acute fractures and dislocations of the cervical spine. *J Bone Joint Surg* 1979;61:1119–1142.
3. Cales RH, Trunkey DD. Preventable trauma deaths: a review of trauma care systems development. *JAMA* 1985;254:1059–1063.
4. Boyd DR. Comprehensive regional trauma and emergency medical service delivery systems: goal of the 1980s. *Crit Care Q* 1982;5:1
5. Gertner HR, Baker SP, Rutherford RB, Spitz WU. Evaluation of the management of vehicular fatalities secondary to abdominal injury. *J Trauma* 1972;12:425–431.
6. Foley RW, Harris LS, Pilcher DB. Abdominal injuries in automobile accidents: review of care of fatally injured patients. *J Trauma* 1977; 17:611–615.
7. Faist E, Bauer AE, Dittmer H, Heberer G. Multiple organ system failure in polytrauma patients. *J Trauma* 1983;23:775–787.
8. Trunkey DD. Trauma. *Sci Am* 1983;249:28–35.
9. American College of Surgeons Committee on Trauma. *Advance Trauma Life Support Course*. Chicago: American College of Surgeons; 1989.
10. Young W, Ransohoff J. Injuries to the cervical cord. In: The Cervical Spine Research Society, ed. *The Cervical Spine*, 2nd ed. Philadelphia: JB Lippincott; 1989:464–495.
11. Rosen P, Wolfe RE. Therapeutic legends of emergency medicine. *J Emerg Med* 1989;7:387–389.
12. Reid DC, Henderson R, Saboe L, Miller JD. Etiology and clinical course of missed spine fractures. *J Trauma* 1987;27:980–986.
13. Woodring JH, Lee C. Limitations of cervical radiography in the evaluation of acute trauma. *J Trauma* 1993;34:32–39.
14. Jofe MH, White AA, Panjab MM. Kinematics. In: The Cervical Spine Research Society, ed. *The Cervical Spine*. Philadelphia: JB Lippincott; 1983:23–35.
15. Ragozzino MW, Deluca SA. Upper cervical spine trauma. *Am Fam Physician* 1985;32:113–119.
16. White A, Kander PL. Anatomical factors in difficult direct laryngoscopy. *Br J Anaesth* 1975;47:468–473.
17. Zuck D. Difficult tracheal intubation. *Anaesthesia* 1985;40:1016–1077.
18. Nichol HC, Zuck D. Difficult laryngoscopy—the anterior larynx and the atlanto-occipital gap. *Br J Anaesth* 1983;55:141–144.
19. Hayashi H, Okada K, Harrada M, Tada K, Veno R. Etiologic factors of myelopathy. A radiographic evaluation of the aging changes in the cervical spine. *Clin Orthop* 1987;214:200–209.
20. White AA, Southwick WO, Panjabi MM. Clinical instability in the lower cervical spine. *Spine* 1976;1:15–27.
21. Johnson RM, Wolf JW Jr. Physiology and biomechanics, stability. In: The Cervical Spine Research Society, ed. *The Cervical Spine*. Philadelphia: JB Lippincott; 1983:35–53.
22. Steel HH. Anatomical and mechanical considerations of the atlanto-axial articulations. *J Bone Joint Surg* 1968;50:1481–1490.
23. Hensineer RN. Congenital anomalies of the atlantoaxial joint. In: The Cervical Spine Research Society, ed. *The Cervical Spine*. Philadelphia: JB Lippincott; 1983:155–160.
24. White AA, Johnson RM, Panjabi MM, Southwick WO. Biomechanical analysis of clinical stability in the cervical spine. *Clin Orthop* 1975;109:85–95.
25. Bachulis B, Long W, Hynes G, Johnson M. Clinical indications of cervical spine radiographs in the traumatized patient. *Am J Surg* 1987;153:473–477.
26. Bryson B, Mulkey M, Murnford B, Schwedhelm M, Warren K. Cervical spine injury: incidence and diagnosis. *J Trauma* 1986;26:669.
27. Cadoux C, White J, Hedberg M. High-yield roentgenographic criteria for cervical spine injures. *Ann Emerg Med* 1987;16:738–742.
28. Bayless P, Ray VG. Incidence of cervical spine injuries in association with blunt head trauma. *Am J Emerg Med* 1989;7:139–142.
29. Kreipke DL, Gillespie KR, McCarthy MC, Mail JT, Lappas JC, Broadie TA. Reliability of indications for cervical spine films in trauma patients. *J Trauma* 1989;29:1438–1439.
30. Talucci RC, Shaikh KA, Schwab CN. Rapid sequence induction with oral endotracheal intubation in the multiply injured patient. *Am Surg* 1988;54:185–187.
31. Ross SE, Schwab CN, David ET, Delong WG, Born CT. Clearing the cervical spine. Initial radiographic evaluation. *J Trauma* 1987;27: 1055–1060.
32. O'Malley KF, Ross SE. The incidence of injury to the cervical spine in patients with craniocerebral injury. *J Trauma* 1989;28:1476–1478.
33. Grande CM, Barton RB, Stene JK. Appropriate techniques for airway management of emergency patients with suspected spinal cord injury. *Anesth Analg* 1988;67:714–715.
34. Alker GJ, Oh YS, Leslie EL. Postmortem radiology of head and neck injuries in fatal traffic accidents. *Radiology* 1975;114:611–617.
35. Bucholz RW, Burkhead WZ, Graham W. Occult cervical spine injuries in fatal traffic accidents. *J Trauma* 1979;19:768–771.

36. Huekle DF, O'Day J, Mendelsohn RA. Cervical injuries suffered in automobile crashes. *J Neurosurg* 1981;54:316.
37. Watson N. Road traffic accidents, spinal injuries and seat belts. *Paraplegia* 1983;21:63.
38. Heiden JS, Weiss MH. Cervical spine injuries with and without neurological deficit: part I. *Contemp Neurosurg* 1980;2:1–6.
39. Kraus JF. A comparison of recent studies on the extent of the head and spinal cord injury problem in the United States. *J Neurosurg* 1980;53:S35.
40. Kraus JF, Franti CE, Riggins RS. Incidence of traumatic spinal cord lesions. *J Chron Dis* 1975;28:471.
41. Heiden JS, Weiss MH, Rosenberg AW, Apuzzo MLJ, Kurze T. Management of cervical spinal cord trauma in Southern California. *J Neurosurg* 1975;43:732–736.
42. Rachesky I, Boyce T, Duncan B, Bjelland J, Sibley B. Clinical prediction of cervical spine injuries in children. *Am J Dis Child* 1987; 141:199–201.
43. Lally K, Senal M, Hardin W, Haftel D. Kaehler M, Mahour G. Utility of the cervical spine radiograph in pediatric trauma. *Am J Surg* 1989;158:540–542.
44. Roshkow JE, Haller J, Hotson G, Sclafni S, Mezzacappa PM, Rachlin S. Imaging evaluation of children after fall from a height: review of 45 cases. *Radiology* 1990;175:359–363.
45. Fesmire F, Luten R. The pediatric cervical spine: developmental anatomy and clinical aspects. *J Emerg Med* 1989;7:133–142.
46. Pang D, Wilberger JE Jr. Traumatic atlanto-occipital dislocation with survival: case report and review. *Neurosurgery* 1980;7:503–508.
47. Alker GJ, Oh YS, Leslie EV. High cervical spine and craniocervical junction injuries in fatal traffic accidents: a radiologic study. *Orthop Clin North Am* 1978;9:1003–1010.
48. Dorr LD, Harvey JP Jr. Traumatic lesions in fatal acute spinal column injuries. *Clin Orthop* 1981;157:178–190.
49. Evarts C. Traumatic occipito-atlantal dislocation: report of a case with survival. *J Bone Joint Surg* 1970;52:1653–1660.
50. Powers B, Miller MD, Kramer RS. Traumatic anterior atlanto-occipital dislocation. *Neurosurgery* 1979;4:12–17.
51. Gabrielsen TO, Maxwell JA. Traumatic atlanto-occipital dislocation, with case report of patient who survived. *Am J Roentgenol Radium Ther Nucl Med* 1966;97:624–629.
52. Ersmark H, Lowenhielm P. Factors influencing the outcome of cervical spine injuries. *J Trauma* 1988;28:407–410.
53. Levine AM, Edwards CC. Treatment of injuries in the C1-C2 complex. *Orthop Clin North Am* 1986;17:31–34.
54. Fielding JW, Hawkins RJ. Atlanto-axial rotary fixation. *J Bone Joint Surg* 1979;59:37–44.
55. Schneider RC, Crosby EC. Craniocerebral, cervicomedullary, and spinal injuries. In: Schneider RC, Kahn EA, Crosby EL, Taren JA, eds. *Correlative Neurosurgery*, 3rd ed. Springfield, Illinois: Charles C. Thomas; 1982:1175–1300.
56. Gosch HH, Gooding E, Schneider RC. Distortion and displacement of the brain in experimental head injuries. *Surg Forum* 1969;20:425–426.
57. Mouradian WH, Fietti, Cochran GV. Fractures of the odontoid: a laboratory and clinical study of mechanisms. *Orthop Clin North Am* 1978;9:985–1001.
58. Sherk HH. Fractures of the atlas and odontoid process. *Orthop Clin North Am* 1978;9:973–984.
59. Anderson LD, D'Alonzo RT. Fractures of the odontoid process of the axis. *J Bone Joint Surg* 1974;56:1663–1674.
60. Ryan MD, Taylor TK. Odontoid fractures: a rational approach to treatment. *J Bone Joint Surg* 1982;64:416–421.
61. Schatzker J, Rorabeck CH, Waddell JP. Fractures of the dens (odontoid process). An analysis of thirty-seven cases. *J Bone Joint Surg* 1971;53:392–405.
62. Hanssen RD, Cabenela ME. Fractures of the dens in adult patients. *J Trauma* 1987;27:928–934.
63. Bell HS. Paralysis of both arms from injury of the upper portion of the pyramidal decussation: cruciate paralysis. *J Neurosurg* 1970;33: 376–380.
64. Wood-Jones F. The ideal lesion produced by judicial hanging. *Lancet* 1913;1:53.
65. Francis WR, Fielding JW, Hawkins RJ. Traumatic spondylolisthesis of the axis. *J Bone Joint Surg Br* 1981;63:313–318.
66. Schneider RL, Livingston RE, Cave AJE. Hangman's fracture of the cervical spine. *J Neurosurg* 1965;22:141.
67. Bucholz RW, Burkhead WZ. The pathologic anatomy of fatal atlanto-occipital dislocations. *J Bone Joint Surg* 1979;61:248–250.
68. Levine AM, Edwards CC. The management of traumatic spondylolisthesis of the axis. *J Bone Joint Surg* 1985;67:217–226.
69. Allen BL, Ferguson RL, Lehman TR. A mechanistic classification of closed, indirect fractures and dislocations of the lower cervical spine. *Spine* 1982;7:1–27.
70. Gehweiler JA Jr, Clark WM, Schaaf RE, Powers B, Miller MD. Cervical spine trauma: the common combined conditions. *Radiology* 1979;130:77–86.
71. Shearer VE, Giesecke AH. Airway management for patients with penetrating neck trauma: a retrospective study. *Anesth Analg* 1993; 77:1135–1138.
72. Komusi T, Munro T, Harth M. Radiologic review: the rheumatoid cervical spine. *Semin Arthritis Rheum* 1985;14:187–195.
73. Grantham SA. Rheumatoid arthritis and other noninfectious inflammatory diseases. Atlantoaxial instability. In: The Cervical Spine Research Society, ed. *The Cervical Spine*. Philadelphia: JB Lippincott; 1983:356–362.
74. Weissman BN, Aliabadi P, Weinfeld MS, Thomas WH, Sosman JL. Prognostic features of atlantoaxial subluxation in rheumatoid arthritis patients. *Radiology* 1982;114:745–751.
75. Mathews JA. Atlantoaxial subluxation in rheumatoid arthritis. *Ann Rheum Dis* 1969;28:260–266.
76. Harris ED. Rheumatoid arthritis, the clinical spectrum. In: Kelley WN, Harris ED, Reddy S, Sledge LB, eds. *Textbook of Rheumatology*, 2nd ed. Philadelphia: WB Saunders; 1985:927–930.
77. Keenan MA, Stiles CM, Kaufman RL. Acquired laryngeal deviation associated with cervical spine disease in erosive polyarticular arthritis. *Anesthesiology* 1983;58:441–449.
78. Calin A. The spondyloarthropathies. *Scientific American Medicine. Rheumatology*. New York; Scientific American; 1985.
79. Sinclair JR, Mason RA. Ankylosing spondylitis. The case for awake intubation. *Anaesthesia* 1984;39:3–11.
80. Broom MJ, Raycroft JF. Complications of fractures of the cervical spine in ankylosing spondylitis. *Spine* 1988;13:763–766.
81. Dyck P. Os odontoideum in children: neurological manifestations and surgical management. *Neurosurgery* 1978;2:93–99.
82. Pueschel SM, Scola FH. Atlantoaxial instability in individuals with Down's syndrome: epidemiologic, radiographic and clinical studies. *Pediatrics* 1987;80:555–560.
83. Moore RA, McNicholas KW, Warren SP. Atlantoaxial subluxation with symptomatic spinal cord compression in a child with Down's syndrome. *Anesth Analg* 1987;66:89–90.
84. Poznanski AK. Congenital anomalies of the cervical spine. In: Bailey RW, ed. *The Cervical Spine*. Philadelphia: Lea and Febiger; 1974;47–90.
85. Pizzutillo PD. Klippel-Feil syndrome. In: The Cervical Spine Research Society, ed. *The Cervical Spine*. Philadelphia: JB Lippincott; 1983:174–187.
86. Cline JR, Scheidel E, Bigsby EF. A comparison of the methods of cervical immobilization used in patient extraction and transport. *J Trauma* 1985;25:649–653.
87. Soderstrom CA, Brumback P. Early care of the patient with cervical spine injury. *Orthop Clin North Am* 1988;17:3.
88. Podolsky S, Baraff LJ, Simon RR, Hoffman JR, Larmon B, Ablon W. Efficacy of cervical spine immobilization methods. *J Trauma* 1983; 23:461–465.
89. McCabe JB, Nolan DJ. Comparison of the effectiveness of different cervical immobilization collars. *Ann Emerg Med* 1986;15:93–96.
90. Fisher RP. Cervical radiographic evaluation of alert patients following blunt trauma. *Ann Emerg Med* 1984;13:905–907.
91. Roberge RJ, Wears RC, Kelley M, Evans TC, et al. Selective application of cervical spine radiography in alert victims of blunt trauma: a prospective study. *J Trauma* 1988;28:784–788.
92. Neifeld G, Keene J, Hevesy G, Leckin J, Provst A, Thisted R. Cervical injury in head trauma. *J Emerg Med* 1988;6:203–207.
93. Ringenberg BJ, Fisher AK, Urdaneta LF, Midthum MA. Rational ordering of cervical spine radiographs following trauma. *Ann Emerg Med* 1988;17:792–796.
94. Gisbert V, Hollerman J, Ney A. Incidence and diagnosis of C7-T1 fractures and subluxations in multiple-trauma patients: evaluation of the advanced trauma life support guidelines. *Surgery* 1989;106:702–709.

95. Streitwieser D, Knopp R, Wales L, Williams J, Tonnemacher K. Accuracy of standard radiographic views in detecting cervical spine fractures. *Ann Emerg Med* 1983;12:538–542.
96. Miller MD, Gehweiler JA, Martinez S, Charlton OP, Daffner RH. Significant new observations on cervical spine trauma. *AJR Am J Roentgenol* 1978;130:659–663.
97. Nichols CG, Young DH, Schiller WR. Evaluation of cervicothoracic junction injury. *Ann Emerg Med* 1987;16:640–642.
98. Schaffer MD, Doris PE. Limitation of the cross table lateral view in detecting cervical spine injuries. A retrospective analysis. *Ann Emerg Med* 1981;10:508–513.
99. Blahd WH, Iserson KU, Bjelland JC. Efficacy of the post-traumatic cross table lateral view of the cervical spine. *J Emerg Med* 1985;2: 243–249.
100. Aprahamian C, Thompson BM, Finger WA, Darin JC. Experimental cervical spine injury model: evaluation of airway management and splinting techniques. *Ann Emerg Med* 1988;17:25–29.
101. Hauswald M, Sklar DP, Tandberg D, Garcia JF. Cervical spine movement during airway management: cinefluoroscopic appraisal in human cadavers. *Am J Emerg Med* 1991;9:535–538.
102. Howard JM. Gastric and salivary secretion following injury: the systemic response to injury. *Ann Surg* 1955;141:342–346.
103. Simpson KH, Stakes AF. Effects of anxiety on gastric emptying in preoperative patients. *Br J Anaesth* 1987;59:540.
104. Todd JG, Nimmo WS. Effect of premedication on drug absorption and gastric emptying. *Br J Anaesth* 1983;55:1189.
105. Zaricznyj B, Rockwood CA Jr, O'Danaghue DH, Ridings GR. Relationship between trauma to the extremities and stomach motility. *J Trauma* 1977;17:920–930.
106. Giesecke AH, Hodgson RMH, Phulchand PR. Anesthesia for severely injured patients. *Orthop Clin North Am* 1970;1:21–48.
107. Bynum LJ, Pierce AK. Pulmonary aspiration of gastric contents. *Am Rev Respir Dis* 1976;114:1129–1136.
108. Seebacher J, Nozik D, Matthew P. Inadvertent intracranial introduction of a nasogastric tube, a complication of severe maxillofacial trauma. *Anesthesiology* 1975;42:100–102.
109. Satiani B, Bonner JT, Stone HH. Factors influencing intraoperative gastric regurgitation. *Arch Surg* 1978;113:721–723.
110. Salem MR, Joseph NJ, Heyman HJ, Belani B, Paulissian R, Ferrara TP. Cricoid compression is effective in obliterating the esophageal lumen in the presence of a nasogastric tube. *Anesthesiology* 1985;63: 443–446.
111. Olsson GL, Hallen B, Hambraeus-Jonzon K. Aspiration during anesthesia: a computer-aided study of 185,338 anesthetics. *Acta Anaesthesiol Scand* 1986;30:84.
112. Majernick TG, Bieniek R, Houston JB, Hughes HG. Cervical spine movement during orotracheal intubation. *Ann Emerg Med* 1986;15: 417–420.
113. Danzel AF, Thomas DM. Nasotracheal intubation in the emergency department. *Crit Care Med* 1980;8:677–682.
114. Giuffrida JG, Bizzari DV, Latteri FS. Prevention of major airway complications during anesthesia by intubation of the conscious patient. *Anesth Analg* 1960;39:201–211.
115. Gold MI, Buechel DR. A method of blind nasal intubation for the conscious patient. *Anesth Analg* 1960;39:257–263.
116. Bivins HG, Ford S, Bezakinovic Z, Price NM, Williams JL. The effect of axial traction during orotracheal intubation of the trauma victim with an unstable cervical spine. *Ann Emerg Med* 1988;17:25–29.
117. Walls R. Orotracheal intubation and potential cervical spine injury. *Ann Emerg Med* 1987;16:373.
118. Doolan S, O'Brien J. Safe intubation and potential cervical spine injury. *Ann Emerg Med* 1987;16:373.
119. Shearer VG, Giesecke AH. Anesthetic considerations in cervicothoracic trauma. *Semin Anesth* 1994;13:110–148.
120. McGill J, Clinton J, Ruiz E. Cricothyroidotomy in the emergency department. *Ann Emerg Med* 1982;11:361–364.
121. Kress D, Balasubramaniam S. Cricothyroidotomy. *Ann Emerg Med* 1982;11:199–201.
122. Messeter KH, Pettersson KI. Endotracheal intubation with the fibre-optic bronchoscope. *Anaesthesia* 1980;35:294–298.
123. Rogers SN, Benumof JL. New and easy techniques for fiberoptic-aided tracheal intubation. *Anesthesiology* 1983;59:569–572.
124. Ovassapian A, Dykes M. The role of fiberoptic endoscopy in airway management. *Semin Anesth* 1987;6:93–104.
125. Crosby E, Lui A. The adult cervical spine: implications for airway management. *Can J Anaesth* 1990;37:77–93.
126. Hastings RH, Marks JM. Airway management for trauma patients with potential cervical spine injuries. *Anesth Analg* 1991;73:471–482.
127. Samson G, Young J. Difficult tracheal intubation: a retrospective study. *Anaesthesia* 1987;42:487.
128. Mallampati SR, Gatt SP, Gugino LD. A clinical sign to predict difficult tracheal intubation: a prospective study. *Can Anaesth Soc J* 1985; 32:429.
129. Kapp JR. Endotracheal intubation in patients with fractures of the cervical spine. *J Neurosurg* 1975;42:731–732.
130. Meschino A, Devitt JH, Schwartz ML, Koch JR. The safety of awake tracheal intubation in cervical spine injury. *Can J Anaesth* 1988;35: 531–532.
131. Holley J, Jorden R. Airway management in patients with unstable cervical spine fractures. *Ann Emerg Med* 1989;18:1237–1239.
132. Tintinalli JE, Claffey J. Complications of nasotracheal intubation. *Ann Emerg Med* 1981;10:142–144.
133. Dronen SC, Merician KS, Hodges JR, Hoekstra JW, Borron SW. A comparison of blind nasotracheal and succinylcholine-assisted intubation in the poisoned patient. *Ann Emerg Med* 1987;16:650–652.
134. Layman PR. An alternative to blind nasal intubation. *Anaesthesia* 1983;38:165.
135. Claeys DW, Lockhart CH, Hinke JE. The effects of translaryngeal block and Innovar on glottic competence. *Anesthesiology* 1973;38: 485–486.
136. Ovassapian A, Krejcie T, Yelich S, Dykes M. Awake fiberoptic intubation in the patient at high risk of aspiration. *Br J Anaesth* 1989;62: 13–16.
137. Brodman G, Duncalf D. Avoiding the trauma of nasotracheal intubation. *Anesth Analg* 1981;60:618.
138. Gorback MS. Inflation of the endotracheal tube cuff as an aid to blind nasal endotracheal intubation. *Anesth Analg* 19871;66:913.
139. Fox Dg, Caspro T, Rastrelli AJ. Comparison of intubation techniques in the awake patient: the Flexiline surgical light (lightwand) versus blind nasal approach. *Anesthesiology* 1987;66:69–71.
140. Verdile VP, Chiang JL, Dedger R, Steward RO, Kaplan R, Paris PM. Nasotracheal intubation using a flexible lighted stylet. *Ann Emerg Med* 1990;506–518.
141. Ellis DG, Stewart RD, Kaplan RM, Jokymec A, Freeman JA, Bleyaert D. Success rates of blind orotracheal intubation using a transillumination technique with a lighted stylet. *Ann Emerg Med* 1988; 15:138–142.
142. Salem MR, Wafai Y, Joseph NJ, Baraka A, Czinn A. Efficacy of the self-inflating bulb in detecting esophageal intubation. *Anesthesiology* 1994;80:42–48.
143. Mulder DS, Wallace DH, Woolhouse FM. The use of the fiberoptic bronchoscope to facilitate endotracheal intubation following head and neck trauma. *J Trauma* 1975;15:638-640.
144. Wang JF, Reves JG, Gutierrez FA. Awake fibreoptic laryngoscopic tracheal intubation for anterior cervical spinal fusion in patients with cervical cord trauma. *Int Surg* 1979;64:69–71.
145. Delaney KA, Hessler R. Emergency flexible fibreoptic nasotracheal intubation: a report of 60 cases. *Ann Emerg Med* 1988;17:919–926.
146. Mlinek EJ, Clinton JE, Plummer D, Ruiz E. Fibreoptic intubation in the emergency department. *Ann Emerg Med* 1990;19:359–362.
147. Fitzgerald RD, Kraft P, Skrbensky G, Pernerstarfer T, Steiner E, Kapral S, Weinstabl C. Excursions of the cervical spine during tracheal intubation: blind oral intubation compared with direct laryngoscopy. *Anaesthesia* 1994;49:111–115.
148. Horton WA, Fahy L, Charters P. Disposition of cervical vertebrae, atlanto-axial joint, hyoid and mandible during X-ray laryngoscopy. *Br J Anaesth* 1989;63:435–438.
149. Gajraj N, Chason DP, Shearer VE. Cervical spine movement during orotracheal intubation: comparison of the Belscope and Macintosh blades. *Anaesthesia* 1994:49:732–744.
150. Saunders PR, Giesecke AH. Clinical assessment of the adult Bullard laryngoscope. *Can J Anaesth* 1989;36:5118–5119.
151. Berland LM, Casselbrant M. The Bullard laryngoscope: a new indirect oral laryngoscope (pediatric version). *Anesth Analg* 1990;70: 105–108.
152. Dyson A, Harris J, Bhatia K. Rapidity and accuracy of tracheal intubation in a mannequin: comparison of the fibreoptic with the Bullard laryngoscope. *Br J Anaesth* 1990;65:268–270.

153. Fried L. Cervical spinal cord injury during skeletal traction. *JAMA* 1974;229:181–183.
154. Kauffman NH, Harris JH, Spencer JA, Kopanisky DR. Danger of traction during radiography for cervical trauma. *JAMA* 1982;247:2369.
155. Nolan JP, Wilson ME. Orotracheal intubation in patients with potential cervical spine injuries: an indication for the gum elastic bougie. *Anaesthesia* 1993;48:630–633.
156. Rhee KJ, Green W, Holcroft SW, Mangili JA. Oral intubation in the multiply injured patient: the risk of exacerbating spinal cord damage. *Ann Emerg Med* 1990;19:511–514.
157. Stellin GP, Barkers,S, Murdock KM, Waxman K. Oral-tracheal intubation in trauma patients with cervical fractures. *Crit Care Med* 1989; 17:534.
158. Gronert GA, Theye RA. Pathophysiology of hyperkalemia induced by succinylcholine. *Anesthesiology* 1975;43:89–99.
159. Pennant JH, Pace NA, Gajraj N. Role of the laryngeal mask airway in the immobile cervical spine. *J Clin Anesth* 1993;5:226–230.
160. Calder I, Ordman AJ, Jackowski A, Crockared HA. The brain laryngeal mask airway. An alternative to emergency tracheal intubation. *Anaesthesia* 1990;45:137–139.
161. Logan A. Use of the laryngeal mask in a patient with an unstable fracture of the cervical spine. *Anesth Analg* 1991;46:987.
162. Benumof JL. Management of the difficult adult airway, with special emphasis on awake tracheal intubation. *Anesthesiology* 1991;75: 1087–1110.
163. Heath ML, Allagain J. Intubation through the laryngeal mask: a technique for unexpected difficult intubation. *Anaesthesia* 1992;46:545–548.
164. Trone JH, Schaefer SD, Carder HM. Blunt and penetrating laryngeal trauma: a 13-year review. *Otolaryngol Head Neck Surg* 1980;88:257–261.
165. Zornow, M, Thomas T, Scheller M. The efficacy of three different methods of transtracheal ventilation. *Can J Anaesth* 1989;36:624–628.
166. Smith RB, Schaer WB, Pfaeffle J. Percutaneous transtracheal ventilation for anesthesia and resuscitation: a review and report of complications. *Can Anaesth Soc J* 1975;22:607–612.
167. Barriot P, Riou B. Retrograde technique for tracheal intubation in trauma patients. *Crit Care Med* 1988;16:712–713.
168. Bourke D, Levesque PR. Modification of retrograde guide for endotracheal intubation. *Anesth Analg* 1974;53:1013–1014.

Airway Management, edited by
L.H. Hanowell, M.D. and R.J. Waldron, M.D.,
Lippincott-Raven Publishers, Philadelphia © 1996.

CHAPTER 22

Airway Management of Head-Injured Patients

Peter G. Moore

INTRODUCTION

Epidemiology of Head Injuries

Head injuries constitute a significant medical and socioeconomic problem in both developed and underdeveloped countries (1–5). Although death rates have improved over the last 20 years because of improved trauma care systems (6,7) and safety legislation (e.g., helmet laws) (8–10), the death rate remains unacceptably high. The latest figures show that head injury prevails as the most common cause of death following trauma in the United States (48.5% of all trauma deaths)(11,12). This translates to an overall annual mortality of 15 deaths per 100,000 population (11). Motor vehicle trauma accounts for about 66% of all trauma deaths caused by head injury (12). Hospital admissions for head injury in the United States are approximately 200 to 300/100,000 admissions. Although most patients have minor head injuries (13) and require basic observation for 24 to 48 hours, about one-third of head injuries are classified as moderate (about 20%) (14) to severe (10%), with an overall mortality rate of 14.5% (12). In addition, a victim of severe head injury usually sustains associated injuries involving the face, neck, cervical spine, chest, abdomen, and skeleton (15–18). Therefore, triage must be performed as soon as possible and must precisely define priorities in care so that effective management strategies can be instituted.

P. G. Moore: Department of Anesthesiology, University of California, Davis Medical Center, Sacramento, California 95817.

Goals for Management of Head Injuries: Role of Airway Management

The modern management of the head-injured patient focuses on 1) prompt resuscitation, 2) early diagnosis and management of space-occupying lesions, and 3) supportive care to minimize secondary effects resulting from hypoxia, hypercarbia, and hypotension that contribute to extension of the area of injury (13,19). These objectives require close attention to airway management to ensure adequate resuscitation and cardiopulmonary stability.

PATHOPHYSIOLOGY OF HEAD INJURIES

The logical management of the head-injured patient is based on a good understanding of the nature, pathophysiology, and effects of head trauma.

Pathology of Head Injuries

The damage of head injuries results from direct forces applied to the head—blunt trauma subjacent to the site of the injury (*coup* injuries), rapid deceleration forces on the opposite side of the brain (*contrecoup* injuries), penetrating injuries (primarily gunshot wounds), hypoxic/ischemic injuries, and secondary damage from cerebral edema leading to intracranial hypertension and the intracranial herniation of brain tissues.

Coup injuries are caused by direct or focal impact to the head, which can lead to localized bleeding and hematoma formation or direct tissue injury coincident with the site of impact (Table 1). *Contrecoup* injuries occur at sites anatomically opposed to the site of impact. They are caused by the rapid movement of relatively compliant brain and meningeal tissue being subjected to rapid deceleration forces while held within the constraining limits of the skull. The inertia of the relatively malleable brain causes it to be pushed against the side of the skull that has been struck (*coup*) and to be pulled away from the skull on the contralateral side. That is, owing to the relatively spherical nature of the brain, a swirling motion is imparted to it, and the brain may then suffer injury during impact against rough bony and dural prominences. Mortality from *contrecoup* injuries approached 55% in one study; combined *coup-contrecoup* injuries represent considerably greater force applied to the brain, and their mortality rate may approach 80% (20).

Intracranial hematomas can be defined in terms of their anatomic site. This classification is useful, as it allows distinctions to be made in terms of the mechanism of injury, patient presentation, and prognostic outlook. For example, extradural injuries often involve a concomitant skull fracture and are relatively localized. The prognosis may be relatively favorable, as underlying brain contusions may be relatively minimal provided they can be evacuated in a timely manner. However, significant neurologic injury can result from the space-occupying nature of the lesion, which leads to displacement and shift of intracranial contents and herniation. Therefore, prompt diagnosis, control of bleeding, and evacuation of the hematoma confer a favorable outcome for cases of extradural hematoma. The evolution of extradural hematomas is reflected in their clinical course, during which injury is accompanied by a brief loss of consciousness, followed by an improvement in level of consciousness (lucid period), followed in turn by progressive deterioration ("talk and deteriorate"), resulting in the death of the patient if definitive surgery is not performed. When promptly treated, a patient with an extradural hematoma should recover with minimal neurologic deficit. However, the talk-and-deteriorate clinical pattern is also seen with other intracranial hematomas (21). For example, in one study (21), approximately 25% of all severely head-injured patients talked at some time prior to deterioration into coma. Of those 25% who talked and deteriorated, 42% were subsequently shown to have intracerebral contusion/hematoma, 22% an extradural hematoma, 17% a subdural hematoma, and 19% no focal mass lesion. While prompt evacuation of an extradural hematoma may result in favorable outcome, the outlook for subdural and intracerebral hematomas may be less promising.

TABLE 1. *Pathology of head injury*

Skull injuries
Vault fracture
Linear
Depressed
Basilar fracture
Focal injuries
Epidural hematoma
Subdural hematoma
Contusion
Intracerebral hematoma
Diffuse brain injuries
Mild concussion
Classic cerebral concussion
Prolonged coma
Mild DAI
Moderate DAI
Severe DAI
Cerebral edema
Hypoxic encephalopathy

DAI, diffuse axonal injury.

Acute subdural hematoma implies significant, violent injury that results in concomitant injury to underlying brain tissue. An acute subdural hematoma can also progressively expand and requires urgent surgical evacuation. In general, the more rapid the onset, the less favorable the outcome, regardless of the speed of diagnosis, as rapid onset implies more extensive hemorrhage and brain damage (22). Patients with acute subdural hematoma require intensive supportive care following surgery in order to restrict the formation of cerebral edema in marginally damaged brain tissue.

Traumatic subarachnoid hemorrhage is less common but indicates severe injury to deep structures (23) or venous sinuses that may be difficult to reverse. In surviving patients, secondary hydrocephalus may ensue and require permanent ventricular drainage to avoid cerebral compression.

Intracerebral hematomas may be diffuse or focal and are often multiple. Intracerebral hematomas and contusions are associated with adjoining tissue injury and edema formation. Isolated or superficial hematomas can be potentially evacuated, but in many cases the injury is not amenable to surgical intervention. The focus of treatment is to control intracranial edema and limit secondary effects.

Direct concussive forces can produce diffuse axonal injury (DAI), which if severe causes irreversible brain damage (23). In its milder forms, DAI is reversible provided edema formation is prevented. The disease pattern of mild DAI is characterized by a brief period of unconsciousness at the time of injury, with initial recovery and variable loss of memory and orientation to person, time, and place. This presentation may mimic to some degree the early course of a patient with an extradural hematoma (21). However, exact diagnosis must be achieved, as extradural hematoma requires immediate surgery, whereas DAI is managed conservatively. Mild DAI usually resolves over the ensuing weeks or months, with full neurologic recovery expected. In more severe instances of DAI, there is a variable potential for recovery that can be optimized provided secondary brain injury is avoided.

The progressive nature of head injury emphasizes the importance of early resuscitation to reduce the degree of secondary damage, precise diagnosis of pathology with definitive surgery as indicated, and continued management to control intracranial pressure-volume relations (13). Additionally, it must be remembered that airway management and management of concomitant exsanguinating injuries take priority during resuscitation.

Intracranial Pressure-Volume Relationships

Intracranial pressure (ICP) in a resting supine subject is normally less than 10 mm Hg. The intracranial contents consist of the brain, interstitial fluid, cerebrospinal fluid (CSF), and cerebral blood (Table 2). For the most part, the contents are relatively incompressible yet are contained within a rigid space, thereby placing rigid limits on expansion or swelling. This point is illustrated by examination of the pressure-volume relationship in the skull (Fig. 1). Therefore, when bleeding or edema occurs in response to trauma, there is only a modest capacity for reduction in the CSF or intracranial blood spaces to accommodate the expanding brain tissue. This initial accommodation, when intracranial compliance is relatively high, minimizes the effects of volume expansion. As this compensation is exhausted, compliance is profoundly reduced, so that any further increases in volume precipitate marked increases in ICP. Consequently, cerebral perfusion pressure is reduced, thus precipitating ischemic injury, further edema formation, and extension of injury. In turn, ICP is further compromised and, if held unchecked, results in herniation of brain contents and

TABLE 2. *Intracranial contents*

Blood
Cerebrospinal fluid
Interstitial fluid
Cells
Neurons
Constitutive cells

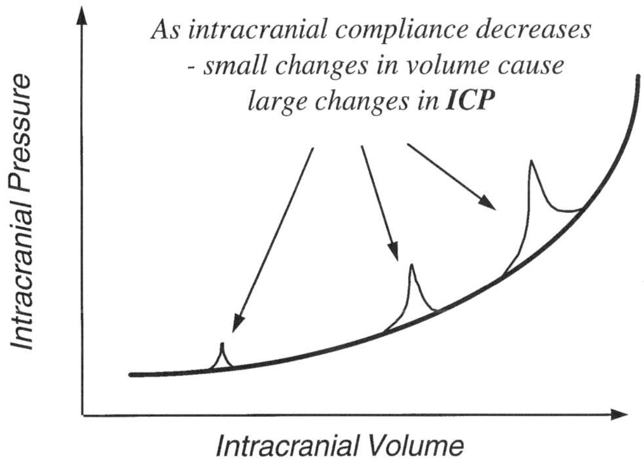

FIG. 1. Schematic diagram of the intracranial pressure-volume relationship.

brain death. This mechanism accounts for the secondary damage that accompanies brain injury and may be responsible for determining outcome and recovery.

Secondary Brain Injuries

Clinicians have the potential to influence outcome by minimizing the degree of secondary damage that often follows head injury; however, little can be done to reverse the cell death that occurs with the initial traumatic event. Indeed, it can be argued that neurologic outcome may be largely influenced by the degree of secondary brain injury that follows the primary injury (24,25).

Cellular and interstitial edema formation contribute significantly to the secondary damage that follows brain injury. The edema may be both vasogenic (caused by microcirculatory mechanisms) or cytotoxic (caused by cellular injury). Disruption of the integrity of the capillary membrane following injury leads to a breakdown in the blood-brain barrier and the extravasation of fluid, electrolytes, and protein into the brain. In the head-injured patient, metabolic disturbances within cells are primarily caused by hypoxia or ischemia, with consequent intracellular edema, cell swelling, and death (26).

The adequacy of oxygen supply to the brain largely depends on the maintenance of an adequate cerebral blood flow. In normal brain, blood flow is relatively constant over a wide range of perfusion pressures as a result of autoregulation (Fig. 2). Cerebral blood flow bears a relatively direct linear relationship to the arterial pressure of carbon dioxide ($PaCO_2$) over the normal physiologic range (Fig. 2). However, the oxygen tension (PaO_2) becomes important under conditions of hypoxia (Fig. 2).

In injured brain (Fig. 3), there may be areas of irreversible damage where there is negligible blood flow and marginal areas that have lost their autoregulatory capacity

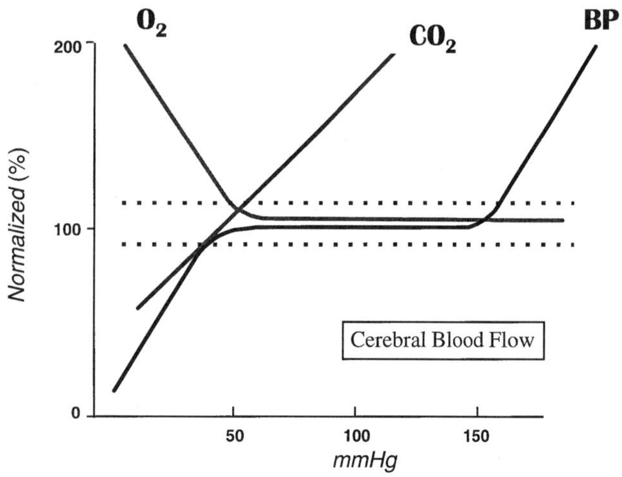

FIG. 2. Physiologic determinants of cerebral blood flow.

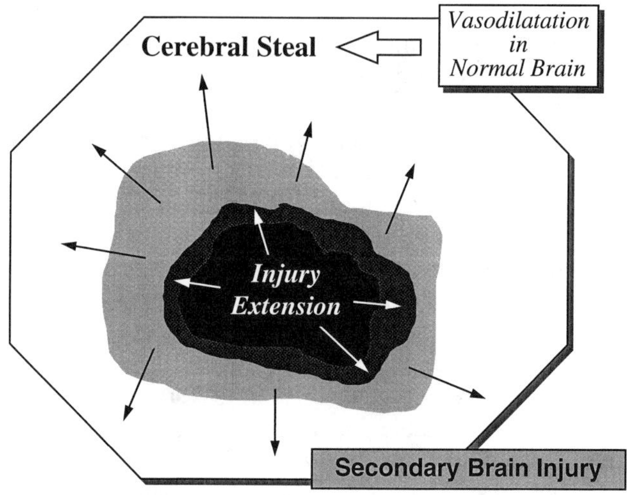

FIG. 4. Secondary extension of injury occurs through intracerebral steal. Vasodilation of normal brain regions reduces perfusion pressure to marginal areas, causing steal and impaired oxygenation.

(perfusion pressure-dependent). These marginal areas are potentially recoverable provided that their oxygen demands are satisfied. They are also potentially subject to the phenomenon of cerebral steal, whereby any vasodilation in the normal cerebral microvasculature can reduce local perfusion pressure to these marginal areas. This can result in a relative reduction in blood flow to the marginal area (i.e., "steal") that precipitates ischemic injury, edema formation, and extension of irreversible injury (Fig. 4). Cerebral steal can be initiated by hypoxia- or hypercarbia-induced cerebral vasodilation or by anesthetic agents with vasodilator properties.

Secondary damage can be minimized by controlling ICP (27,28). This can be accomplished by avoiding precipitating factors such as hypotension, hypoxia, hypercarbia, venous distention, and airway obstruction (Fig. 5). Direct therapeutic measures such as hyperventilation (to produce hypocarbia and cerebral vasoconstriction), CSF drainage, osmotic agents, alkalinizing buffers, and barbiturate coma therapy can successfully reduce edema in the short term (Table 3).

Cerebral Perfusion Pressure

Cerebral perfusion pressure (CPP) under normal conditions is defined as the mean arterial pressure (MAP) minus the jugular venous pressure. However, in damaged

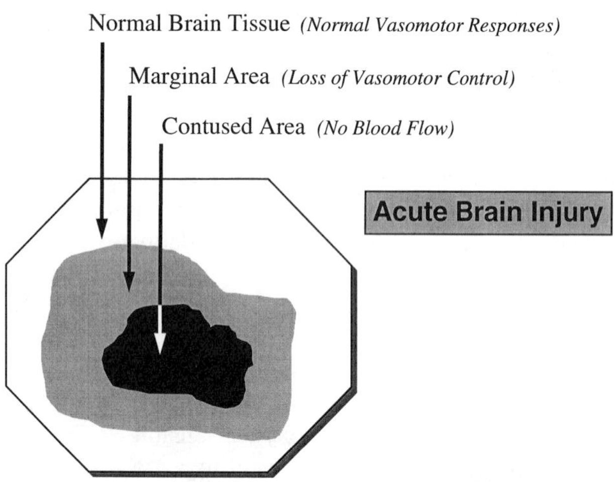

FIG. 3. Injured brain consists of areas of irreversible injury (no blood flow) and marginal areas with compromised autoregulatory capacity (i.e., perfusion-pressure-dependent zone).

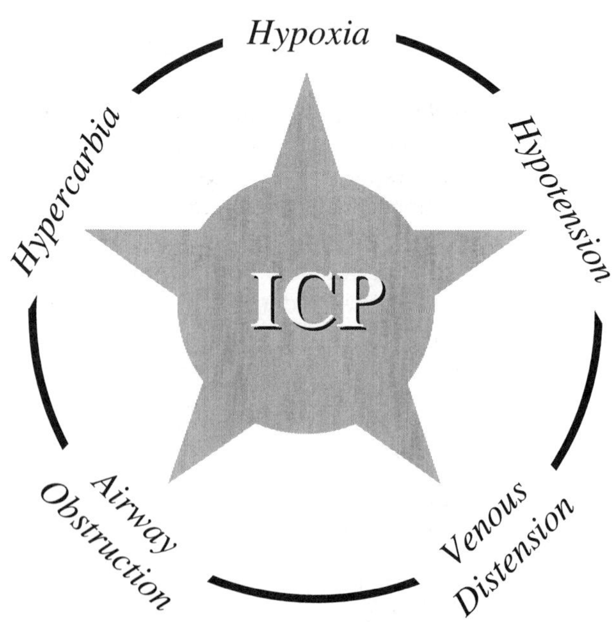

FIG. 5. Intracranial pressure is increased by hypotension, hypoxia, hypercarbia, venous distention, and airway obstruction in head-injured patients.

TABLE 3. *Management of intracranial hypertension*

Evacuate intracranial mass lesions
Reduce CSF volume
CSF drainage
Reduction of CSF formation
Furosemide
Acetazolamide
Reduce cerebral blood volume
Maintenance of blood pressure
Head-up position
Avoidance of high central venous pressures
Avoidance of high peak ventilatory pressures
Avoidance of coughing and straining
Hyperventilation
Cerebral vasoconstriction
Reduce cerebral edema with
Osmotic diuretics
Corticosteroids
Surgical decompression

CSF, cerebrospinal fluid.

TABLE 4. *Glasgow coma score*

	Points[a]
Eye opening	
spontaneous	4
to speech	3
to pain	2
nil	1
Best motor response	
obeys commands	6
localizes to pain	5
withdraws to pain	4
abnormal flexion	3
extensor response	2
nil	1
Verbal response	
oriented	5
confused	4
inappropriate words	3
incomprehensible sounds	2
nil	1

[a]Maximal possible score, 15; minimum possible score, 3.

brain ICP may exceed venous pressure. Concomitantly, CPP would be equal to the MAP-ICP difference. Therefore, systemic hypotension (decline in MAP) or intracranial hypertension (rise in ICP) reduces CPP and compromises blood flow to marginal areas. Increases in ICP can also be produced by coughing, straining, or stertorous breathing, which increase venous pressures and reduce CPP. Intracerebral venous distention increases ICP directly by increasing the intracerebral blood volume and indirectly by reducing CPP to evoke ischemia, as outlined above.

MANAGEMENT OF HEAD INJURIES

Outcome following head injuries can be favorably influenced by effective prehospital care and resuscitation, rapid diagnosis and triage, and active efforts to control ICP and minimize secondary pathophysiologic insults. Effective airway management is a key intervention in these efforts to minimize the extent of injury. As previously mentioned, these efforts are directed at avoiding hypotension, hypoxia, hypocarbia, venous distention, and airway obstruction (Fig. 5).

Emergent Care

The initial management of the trauma patient involves rapid assessment of airway patency, ventilatory efforts, adequacy of the circulation, and extent of the injuries. In assessing the extent of head injuries, the Glasgow coma score (GCS) provides rapid determination of the severity of head injury and predictive value of outcome and directs further triage of the patient (Table 4, Fig. 6). Airway management must be achieved in the severely injured patient with a GCS less than 8 before further investigative measures are undertaken in order to avoid deterioration in uncontrolled circumstances, e.g., while in the CT scanner.

Airway Management

Airway management involves assessment of patency and intervention to avoid airway obstruction, hypoxia, and hypercarbia, as these factors have significant deleterious effects on ICP.

In the suboptimal conditions of the prehospital environment, advanced airway intervention should be under taken only to relieve airway obstruction, to protect the airway in an unconscious, unresponsive patient, or to facilitate ventilation in a nonbreathing patient. In many instances, basic airway management involving clearance of blood, foreign material, and vomitus and the use of oropharyngeal or nasopharyngeal devices with oxygen supplied by face mask will suffice. There is reason for caution because of the high association of cervical spinal injuries with head injuries and the difficulty of preventing neck movement in the prehospital setting (18).

In the emergent field situation, intubation can be accomplished by direct laryngoscopy and oral endotracheal intubation when cervical injury is unlikely. In the struggling patient or the patient with increased muscle tone or spasm, the neuromuscular-blocking drug succinylcholine (1 mg/kg IV) can facilitate intubation. However, there must be a reasonable expectation of success on the part of the caregiver that ventilation by face mask can be achieved because succinylcholine abolishes respiratory efforts. When endotracheal intubation is required, axial fixation of the neck should be practiced. Direct lar-

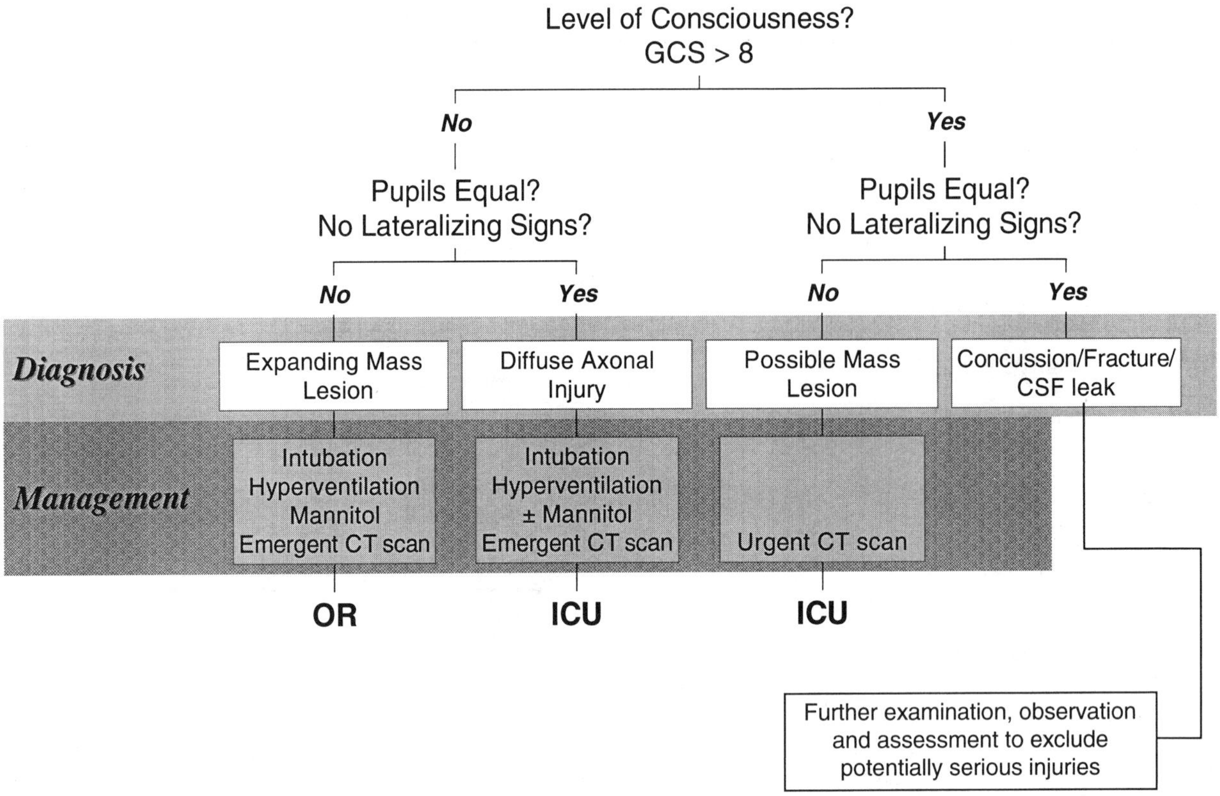

FIG. 6. Triage algorithm for the management of head injury using Glasgow coma score of 8 as the primary decision trigger.

yngoscopy may also be dangerous, as mandibular retraction may cause neck movement. Blind nasal intubation may also be dangerous, particularly in patients with concomitant facial injuries or CSF rhinorrhea, as injury to the cribriform plate can occur.

Performing percutaneous cricothyroidotomy (29) or using a laryngeal mask airway, provided the procedure is skillfully performed, may provide the best safety margin in the severely head-injured patient in the field. Emergency intubation may be necessary as the priority intervention in the field, prior to transport to hospital, to protect or provide a patent airway. Blind nasal intubation is appropriate when there is no significant injury to the base of the skull. Cricothyroidotomy may be useful when there is significant faciomaxillary injury. The caregiver must be conscious of the high incidence of concomitant injury to the cervical spine. All airway intubation techniques should be carried out with axial traction and/or with a cervical collar applied to the patient.

The emergency room provides a more controlled environment for airway management, and here more definitive procedures can be performed. The prehospital airway should be evaluated and alternatives provided if this is inadequate. Elective intubation can be accomplished if the patient requires transport to diagnostic imaging. In patients scheduled for surgery, elective endotracheal

TABLE 5. *Indications for endotracheal intubation in head injury*

Emergent
Obstruction
Associated injuries
Impaired consciousness
Ventilation
Correct hypoventilation
Reverse hypoxemia
Protection
Elective
Impaired protective reflexes
Prevention of pulmonary complications
Protection from aspiration
Tracheobronchial secretions
Access for ventilation
Concomitant use of muscle relaxant, sedative, or hypnotic drugs
Deliberate hyperventilation
For anesthetic management during surgery

intubation is best accomplished in the operating room as part of the anesthetic induction.

Indications for Endotracheal Intubation

The severely head-injured patient must have a rapid and comprehensive triage to determine patency of the airway, effectiveness of ventilation, hemodynamic status, level of consciousness, and neurologic status. Also, there must be a prompt assessment of concomitant injuries to the face, neck, chest, abdomen, and skeleton. Endotracheal intubation is indicated as an emergency measure (see previous section) or electively for airway protection or as a method of affording appropriate oxygenation and ventilation (Table 5). Elective endotracheal intubation is a planned procedure. Therefore, prophylactic measures should be applied to minimize any potential increases in ICP associated with intubation.

Precautions to Minimize Increases in Intracranial Pressure

Elective intubation is a planned process involving adequate preparation to avoid increases in ICP and precautionary measures to limit the risk for inhalation of vomitus (Table 6). Procedures to prevent and limit increases in ICP are essential, as endotracheal intubation can be associated with precipitous increases in ICP. **Instrumentation, coughing, straining, or the elevated venous pressure that accompanies increased intrathoracic pressure during controlled positive-pressure ventilation** *all* potentially increase ICP.

Increases in ICP can be minimized by various means—in particular, adequate oxygenation, voluntary hyperventilation to avoid hypercarbia, and muscle relaxation to prevent coughing and straining (Table 7). The conscious patient should be adequately anesthetized to avoid sympathoexcitation (release of catecholamines). For similar reasons, ketamine should be avoided. Thiopental sodium is particularly useful, as it reduces ICP and cerebral metabolic demands. Although anesthesia may be unnecessary in unconscious patients, thiopental sodium can be used in unconscious patients for its beneficial effects on ICP.

TABLE 6. *Elective intubation*

Preparation
Maintain axial traction
Pre-oxygenate
Encourage hyperventilation
Lidocaine (1.5 mg/kg IV)
Mannitol?
Defasciculating dose of nondepolarizing blocker
Rapid-sequence technique
Cricoid pressure
Thiopental
Succinylcholine (2 mg/kg)[a]

[a]If contraindicated, use a suitable non-depolarizing neuromuscular blocking agent (see Chapter 11).

TABLE 7. *Preventative measures to minimize increases in ICP during intubation*

Maintain normal oxygen levels
Encourage hyperventilation
Avoid respiratory depressants
Avoid coughing, straining, or vomiting
Prophylactic medication
Lidocaine (1–2 mg/kg IV)
Alfentanil (low dose)
Choose induction anesthetic that reduces ICP
Thiopental sodium (5 mg/kg)
Use maximal dose of neuromuscular blocker

ICP, intracranial pressure.

In addition to the above-mentioned, various techniques are useful in reducing the stimulus of intubation. These include the use of lidocaine (1.5 mg/kg IV). The intravenous administration of a low dose of synthetic narcotic may be helpful prior to airway instrumentation; however, higher doses of synthetic narcotic may reduce cerebral perfusion pressure (30). Infusion of mannitol (0.5 mg/kg IV) can also be used to reduce ICP, although it acts more slowly and may not provide useful protection for intubation (31).

Apnea time during instrumentation should be minimized, and the shift to positive-pressure ventilation should be undertaken initially with small tidal volumes (5 to 7 mL/kg ideal body weight) and low peak inspiratory pressures. Deliberate hyperventilation should be employed to minimize any increases in ICP associated with intubation and to provide long-term regulation of ICP.

Resuscitation Fluids

Hypovolemic hypotension is counterproductive to control of ICP (32). Therefore, once hemorrhage is controlled, the circulating blood volume should be restored. In the head-injured patient, excessive administration of water must be avoided, as this adversely affects cerebral edema formation, whereas a sodium load appears to be salutary (33). Recent studies suggest that the use of hypertonic saline-dextran solutions are beneficial in patients with severe head injury (34).

Continuing Airway Management

Patients with GCS of less than 8 or concomitant injuries causing respiratory failure require prolonged ventilation. Following the initial resuscitative and stabilization period, this is best managed by tracheostomy so as to avoid damage to the larynx, prevent oral and antral (sinus) infections, and facilitate subsequent weaning and nursing care. Because the risk for silent aspiration and nosocomial pneumonia is high in unconscious patients, percutaneous feeding gastrostomy is also performed to facilitate enteral nutrition (35). Those patients whose neurologic status is expected to improve promptly can be ventilated without resort to tracheostomy. They can be fed through an enteral feeding tube that is passed into the duodenum via the oral or nasal route with the aid of gastroscopy or fluoroscopy. In this way, patients requiring short-term ventilatory support pending neurologic recovery can subsequently be extubated after meeting ventilatory weaning criteria. They can resume regular feedings on recovery of protective airway reflexes and sufficient swallowing function.

The use of positive end expiratory pressure (PEEP) should be minimized in head-injured patients, as increases in intrathoracic pressure may result in venous distention and therefore increased ICP. However, in patients with concomitant respiratory failure, hypoxemia must be avoided. Careful titration of PEEP, measures to optimize oxygen supply/demand (pressure-support ventilation), and administration of muscle relaxants (when indicated) can be employed without significant deterioration in ICP (36).

Prolonged hyperventilation is usually performed as a means to minimize cerebral edema formation. Although prolonged hyperventilation produces systemic respiratory alkalosis, progressive intracerebral and CSF acidosis intervene in response to the cerebral vasoconstriction. This phenomenon defeats the purpose of hyperventilation and is counterproductive to the goal of reducing cerebral edema (26). The use of tromethamine (THAM), a carbon dioxide-consuming buffer, can obviate the development of cerebral acidosis during prolonged hyperventilation and benefit the severely head-injured patient (37–39).

Secondary Airway Complications in Head-Injured Patients

Secondary airway complications are common in the head-injured patient, occurring in about a third of them (40). The factors that contribute to airway complications include the emergent circumstances surrounding airway intervention; the predisposition to oral, bronchial, and pulmonary infection (41,42); the prolonged duration of intubation; and neurologic deficits that affect airway and swallowing reflexes. These complications may be acute and self-limiting, such as postextubation stridor (common in the pediatric head-injured population) (43). Other, chronic complications may be mild, such as dysphonia, or more severe, such as vocal cord paralysis, tracheal stenosis, subglottic stenosis, glottic stenosis, and tracheomalacia (40,44,45). Because significant airway complications are common in severely head-injured patients who recover, it is recommended that all patients submitted to prolonged ventilatory care undergo direct endoscopic examination prior to planned decannulation of the airway and that decannulation be deferred in patients with positive findings until definitive correction can be performed (40).

SUMMARY: ROLE OF AIRWAY MANAGEMENT IN HEAD INJURIES

Airway management plays a key role in the care of the head-injured patient by correcting or preventing the factors that precipitate increases in intracranial pressure. The avoidance of hypoxia, hypercarbia, hypotension, venous distention, and airway obstruction is critical in minimizing secondary brain injury and improving outcome. Effective airway management is the major means of reversing or preventing these pathophysiologic insults.

REFERENCES

1. Champion HR, Copes WS, Sacco WJ, Lawnick MM, Keast SL, Bain LW, Flanagan ME, Frey CF. The major trauma outcome study: establishing national norms for trauma care. *J Trauma* 1990;30:1356–1365.
2. Daly KE, Thomas PR. Trauma deaths in the southwest Thames region. *Injury* 1992;23:393–396.
3. Lee ST, Lui TN, Chang CN, Wang DJ, Heimburger RF, Fai HD. Features of head injury in a developing country—Taiwan (1977–1987). *J Trauma* 1990;30:194–199.
4. Ratanalert S, Phuenpathom N. Management of head injury patients who talked and deteriorated. *Surg Neurol* 1990;34:27–29.
5. Tiret L, Hausherr E, Thicoipe M, Garros B, Maurette P, Castel JP, Hatton F. The epidemiology of head trauma in Aquitaine (France), 1986: a community-based study of hospital admissions and deaths. *Int J Epidemiol* 1990;19:133–140.
6. Gentleman D. Causes and effects of systemic complications among severely head injured patients transferred to a neurosurgical unit. *Int Surg* 1992;77:297–302.
7. Klauber MR, Marshall LF, Toole BM, Knowlton SL, Bowers SA. Cause of decline in head-injury mortality rate in San Diego County, California. *J Neurosurg* 1985;62:528–531.
8. Sosin DM, Sacks JJ, Holmgreen P. Head injury-associated deaths from motorcycle crashes. Relationship to helmet-use laws. *JAMA* 1990;264:2395–2399.
9. Fleming NS, Becker ER. The impact of the Texas 1989 motorcycle helmet law on total and head-related fatalities, severe injuries, and overall injuries. *Med Care* 1992;30:832–845.
10. McSwain NE Jr., Belles A. Motorcycle helmets—medical costs and the law. *J Trauma* 1990;30:1189–1197; discussion, 1197–1199.
11. Shackford SR, Mackersie RC, Holbrook TL, Davis JW, Hollingsworth-Fridlund P, Hoyt DB, Wolf PL. The epidemiology of traumatic death. A population-based analysis. *Arch Surg* 1993;128:571–575.
12. Gennarelli TA, Champion HR, Copes WS, Sacco WJ. Comparison of mortality, morbidity, and severity of 59,713 head injured patients with 114,447 patients with extracranial injuries. *J Trauma* 1994;37:962–968.
13. Jennett B. Diagnosis and management of head trauma. *J Neurotrauma* 1991;8(Suppl 1):S15-S19.
14. Colohan AR, Oyesiku NM. Moderate head injury: an overview. *J Neurotrauma* 1992;9(Suppl 1):S259–S264.
15. Hills MW, Deane SA. Head injury and facial injury: is there an increased risk of cervical spine injury? *J Trauma* 1993;34:549–553; discussion: 553–554.
16. Moore PG, James OF, Byth PL, Simpson IJ. Factors affecting outcome after chest injury. *Anaesth Intensive Care* 1985;13:362–369.
17. Bone LB, McNamara K, Shine B, Border J. Mortality in multiple

trauma patients with fractures. *J Trauma* 1994;37:262–264; discussion: 264–265.
18. Fox MA, Fabian TC, Croce MA, Mangiante EC, Carson JP, Kudsk KA. Anatomy of the accident scene: a prospective study of injury and mortality. *Am Surg* 1991;57:394–397.
19. Gentleman D, Jennett B. Audit of transfer of unconscious head-injured patients to a neurosurgical unit. *Lancet* 1990;335:330–334.
20. Jayakumar PN, Sastry Kolluri VR, Basavakumar DG, Subbakrishna DK, Arya BY, Das BS, Narayana Reddy GN. Prognosis in contrecoup intracranial haematomas—a clinical and radiological study of 63 patients. *Acta Neurochir (Wien)* 1991;108:30–33.
21. Lobato RD, Rivas JJ, Gomez PA, Castaneda M, Canizal JM, Sarabia R, Cabrera A, Munoz MJ. Head-injured patients who talk and deteriorate into coma. Analysis of 211 cases studied with computerized tomography. *J Neurosurg* 1991;75:256–261.
22. Kotwica Z, Brzezinski J. Acute subdural haematoma in adults: an analysis of outcome in comatose patients. *Acta Neurochir (Wien)* 1993;121:95–99.
23. Shigemori M, Tokutomi T, Kuramoto S, Moriyama T, Kikuchi N, Sasaguri Y. Diffuse axonal injury and early intracranial sequelae in severe head injury. *Neurol Med Chir* (Tokyo) 1991;31:390–395.
24. Sahuquillo J, Poca MA, Garnacho A, Robles A, Coello F, Godet C, Triginer C, Rubio E. Early ischaemia after severe head injury. Preliminary results in patients with diffuse brain injuries. *Acta Neurochir (Wien)* 1993;122:204–214.
25. Robertson CS, Contant CF, Gokaslan ZL, Narayan RK, Grossman RG. Cerebral blood flow, arteriovenous oxygen difference, and outcome in head injured patients. *J Neurol Neurosurg Psychiatry* 1992; 55:594–603.
26. Bouma GJ, Muizelaar JP, Choi SC, Newlon PG, Young HF. Cerebral circulation and metabolism after severe traumatic brain injury: the elusive role of ischemia. *J Neurosurg* 1991;75:685–693.
27. Chesnut RM, Marshall LF. Management of head injury. Treatment of abnormal intracranial pressure. *Neurosurg Clin N Am* 1991;2:267–284.
28. Miller JD. ICP monitoring—current status and future directions. *Acta Neurochir (Wien)* 1987;85:80–86.
29. DeLaurier GA, Hawkins ML, Treat RC, Mansberger ARJ. Acute airway management. Role of cricothyroidotomy. *Am Surg* 1990;56:12–15.
30. Hanowell LH, Thurston JD, Behrman KH, Disbrow EA. Alfentanil administered prior to endotracheal suctioning reduces cerebral perfusion pressure. *J Neurosurg Anesthesiol* 1993;5:31–35.
31. Feldman JA, Fish S. Resuscitation fluid for a patient with head injury and hypovolemic shock. *J Emerg Med* 1991;9:465–468.
32. Pietropaoli JA, Rogers FB, Shackford SR, Wald SL, Schmoker JD, Zhuang J. The deleterious effects of intraoperative hypotension on outcome in patients with severe head injuries. *J Trauma* 1992;33:403–407.
33. Ramming S, Shackford SR, Zhuang J, Schmoker JD. The relationship of fluid balance and sodium administration to cerebral edema formation and intracranial pressure in a porcine model of brain injury. *J Trauma* 1994;37:705–713.
34. Vassar MJ, Perry CA, Holcroft JW. Prehospital resuscitation of hypotensive trauma patients with 7.5% NaCl versus 7.5% NaCl with added dextran: a controlled trial. *J Trauma* 1993;34:622–632; discussion: 632–633.
35. D'Amelio LF, Hammond JS, Spain DA, Sutyak JP. Tracheostomy and percutaneous endoscopic gastrostomy in the management of the head-injured trauma patient. *Am Surg* 1994;60:180–185.
36. Miller RS, Nelson LD, DiRusso SM, Rutherford EJ, Safcsak K, Morris JA. High-level positive end-expiratory pressure management in trauma-associated adult respiratory distress syndrome. *J Trauma* 1992;33:284–290; discussion, 290–291.
37. Muizelaar JP, Marmarou A, Ward JD, Kontos HA, Choi SC, Becker DP, Gruemer H, Young HF. Adverse effects of prolonged hyperventilation in patients with severe head injury: a randomized clinical trial. *J Neurosurg* 1991;75:731–739.
38. Marmarou A, Holdaway R, Ward JD, Yoshida K, Choi SC, Muizelaar JP, Young HF. Traumatic brain tissue acidosis: experimental and clinical studies. *Acta Neurochir Suppl (Wien)* 1993;57:160–164.
39. Wolf AL, Levi L, Marmarou A, Ward JD, Muizelaar PJ, Choi S, Young H, Rigamonti D, Robinson WL. Effect of THAM upon outcome in severe head injury: a randomized prospective clinical trial. *J Neurosurg* 1993;78:54–59.
40. Nowak P, Cohn AM, Guidice MA. Airway complications in patients with closed-head injuries. *Am J Otolaryngol* 1987;8:91–96.
41. Pickworth KK, Falcone RE, Hoogeboom JE, Santanello SA. Occurrence of nosocomial pneumonia in mechanically ventilated trauma patients: a comparison of sucralfate and ranitidine. *Crit Care Med* 1993;21:1856–1862.
42. Hsieh AH, Bishop MJ, Kubilis PS, Newell DW, Pierson DJ. Pneumonia following closed head injury. *Am Rev Respir Dis* 1992;146: 290–294.
43. Kemper KJ, Benson MS, Bishop MJ. Predictors of postextubation stridor in pediatric trauma patients. *Crit Care Med* 1991;19:352–355.
44. Woo P. Acquired laryngomalacia: epiglottis prolapse as a cause of airway obstruction. *Ann Otol Rhinol Laryngol* 1992;101:314–320.
45. Woo P, Kelly G, Kirshner P. Airway complications in the head injured. *Laryngoscope* 1989;99:725–731.

Airway Management, edited by
L.H. Hanowell, M.D. and R.J. Waldron, M.D.,
Lippincott-Raven Publishers, Philadelphia © 1996.

CHAPTER 23

Blunt Trauma to the Major Airways

Richard J. Waldron and Leland H. Hanowell

INTRODUCTION

Blunt trauma to the major airways (larynx, trachea, and major bronchi) is unusual. Blunt laryngeal trauma occurs in about 1:43,000 emergency room admissions (1). The incidence of blunt tracheobronchial trauma is in the order of 3% to 7% of patients presenting with blunt chest trauma (2,3,4). However, acute blunt trauma to the major airways (BTMA) presents an incomparable challenge to physicians specialized in the management of airways. The management of the emergency difficult airway is covered in protocols and algorithms as suggested by the American Society of Anesthesiologists (5), Advanced Trauma and Life Support (ATLS) (6), and the Early Management of Severe Trauma (EMST) (7). This chapter will focus on a small portion of these protocols. We will review the epidemiology, biomechanics, pathology, and presentation of acute BTMA, and suggest management protocols. The problems associated with use of percutaneous cricothyrotomy, cricothyroid puncture, and transtracheal jet ventilation (TTJV) in such cases will also be highlighted.

R.J. Waldron: Department of Anaesthetic Services, Royal Hobart Hospital, and University of Tasmania, Hobart, Tasmania, Australia 7001.

L.H. Hanowell: Department of Anesthesiology, University of California, Davis School of Medicine and Medical Center, Sacramento, California 95817.

Bronchoscopy in some form (rigid or flexible) is a technique that may be one of the cornerstones of successful early intervention and treatment (7,8,9). It cannot be too highly recommended that all practicing anesthesiologists become familiar with the use of flexible fiberoptic bronchoscopy (FFB).

HISTORY

As early as 1848, Webb (10) reported a case of a man run over by a cart who subsequently died as a result of a ruptured liver. At autopsy, a ruptured left main bronchus was found. In 1912, Schönberg (11) published 16 case reports of major bronchial tears. Ruptures of the trachea and bronchi were believed to carry a 100% mortality rate at this time. However, in 1927, Krinitzki (12) described rupture of the right main stem bronchus and right lung atelectasis in a 30-year-old woman, the result of injuries sustained 20 years previously.

Surgical repair of a total rupture of the bronchi was first described in 1914 (13) for a 2-year-old girl run over by a wine cart, suffering a tension pneumothorax due to left main bronchus rupture. Despite thoracotomy and repair,

This chapter is reprinted from: Waldron RJ, Hanowell LH, Grande CM. Blunt airway trauma. *Seminars in Anesthesia.* Philadelphia: WB Saunders, 1994:13;129–135, with permission.

the girl died 4 days later. In 1931, Nissen (14) described successful treatment by pneumonectomy of an injury to a main stem bronchus that was complicated by stricture formation and purulent bronchiectasis. Griffith (15) in 1949 described the first successful delayed repair of total rupture of a bronchial lesion (2 months after the injury); in 1957, Beskin described the first successful primary repair of complete tracheal transection. As we are concentrating on the management of the acute presentation of BTMA, there will be no further discussion of surgical treatment.

EPIDEMIOLOGY, MECHANISMS, BIOMECHANICS, AND PATHOLOGY

Epidemiology

There are many logistic difficulties in accurately establishing the exact incidence of acute blunt trauma to the larynx and tracheobronchial tree (16). One significant study was reported in 1972 by Bertelsen and Howitz (3). Their report was divided into two parts, the major portion being a necropsy report of 1178 patients dying after trauma between 1961 and 1966. There were 33 (2.8%) cases with lesions to the trachea and bronchi. Motor vehicle accidents (MVAs) accounted for 28 (85%) of the 33, death being instantaneous in 27 (82%). Multiple fatal injuries were found in 24 patients. Of the six patients alive on admission to hospital, five died within 45–120 minutes. Of these five, three had total unilateral rupture of one main stem bronchus, and one patient had total rupture of the distal trachea.

Ecker et al. (4) at the same time reviewed 105 injuries to the trachea and bronchi (30 due to blunt trauma and 75 penetrating) in Dallas County over the 10-year-period of 1958 to 1967. Data from the Medical Examiner's Office was included in the study. The male:female ratio was 5.5:1 in total, with an average age of 31 years (average age of 46 years for all chest trauma patients). Seventy-one patients were dead on arrival (DOA), compared to thirty-four alive on arrival. Ecker et al. (4) found the cervical trachea to be the most common site of injury in patients who survived, while the distal trachea and bronchi were more frequent in the DOA group. The DOA group also had a higher incidence of associated injuries (138), including spinal fractures and injuries to the heart, aorta, and liver.

The incidence of tracheobronchial injuries relative to other injuries associated with blunt chest trauma is summarized in Table 1. Note that the frequency is comparable to that of aortic dissection. There is also a high incidence of associated injuries (Table 2). When there is associated trauma to the major thoracic vessels, the mortality rate increases dramatically (17).

TABLE 1. *Thoracic injuries resulting from crush injury of chests*

	Incidence (n=86)
Flail chest/multiple rib fractures	59%
Hemothorax	34%
Pneumothorax	32%
Documented pulmonary injury	32%
Injuries of heart or pericardium	15%
Fracture of sternum	15%
Rupture of diaphragm	14%
Bronchial rupture	7%
Rupture of aorta or major vessel	5%

From Besson and Seagesser, ref. 2.

TABLE 2. *Associated injuries*

Recurrent laryngeal nerve
Cervical spine
Esophagus
Major thoracic vessels
Head injuries

Mechanism of Injury

The mechanisms of injury can be conveniently divided into two categories, according to the anatomic site of injury, i.e., the cervical portion of the trachea and the intrathoracic portion of the tracheobronchial tree (18).

With the cervical portion, the mechanism of injury is generally a direct blow, typically young children striking the handlebars of bicycles (19), steering wheel injuries in MVAs (20), or wires/cables across the neck. This is the same mechanism as for blunt laryngeal trauma and presents with the same symptoms and signs, i.e., dyspnea, voice change, cervical subcutaneous crepitus, hemoptysis. There are numerous case reports describing the anesthetic management of such cases (9,21,22). With such mechanisms, it is advisable to be suspicious of both cervical spine and esophageal injuries.

The majority of lesions occur with the intrathoracic portion of the major airways. Up to 80% of lesions occur within 2.5 cm (1 in) (Fig. 1) of the carina (16). Generally, these are high kinetic-energy (acceleration/deceleration) injuries. The patients are frequently young, male, unrestrained front seat drivers/passengers striking the steering wheel or the dashboard of a car. Other frequent causes are industrial accidents and sporting injuries.

Another, more important, mechanism for the practicing anesthesiologist is rupture of the posterior wall of the trachea or bronchus associated with insertion of endotracheal/endobronchial tubes, overinflation of cuffed endotracheal tubes (ETTs), or the use of so-called tube-changers. One series reported 5 cases of tracheobronchial injury out of 2700 endobronchial intubations with double-lumen ETTs (Carlens type) (23).

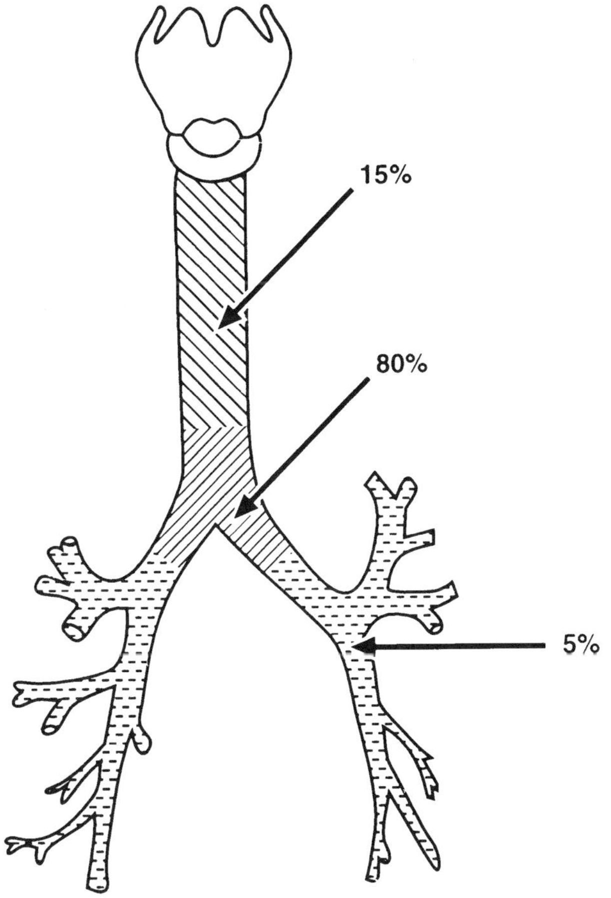

FIG. 1. Sites of frequency of injuries to the major airways. Note that 80% occur within 1 in (2.5 cm) of the carina.

Biomechanics and Pathology

The pathogenesis of tracheobronchial tear/rupture is due to three mechanisms that may occur either alone or in concert (Fig. 2) (16,24,25).

1. A decrease in the anteroposterior diameter of the thorax occurs, widening the transverse diameter. The lungs remain in contact with the chest wall and, thus, are pulled apart, creating traction at the carina. If this force exceeds the elasticity of the tracheobronchial tree, rupture occurs.
2. When the trachea and major bronchi are crushed between the sternum and vertebral column with a closed glottis, the sudden increase in intrabronchial pressure produced is greatest in the larger bronchi, and rupture may occur. Schönberg first postulated in 1912 that there may be reflex closure of the glottis associated with closed chest trauma (23). This, associated with thoracic compression, causes an increase in intraluminal pressure, which Schönberg argued would be greatest in the larger airways. This theory is supported by experimental work involving the impacting of 25-kg weights onto the anterior chest walls of anesthetized, intubated dogs. There was a fivefold increase in the incidence of bronchial rupture when the ETT was clamped at the time of impact (2).
3. Rapid deceleration may result in shearing forces at the areas of relative fixation, namely, the carina and cricoid cartilage.

The pathology of resulting injuries may range from simple partial tears of the airway to complete airway transections, with dislocation of the two ends of the airway (Fig. 3). In complete transections, the distal trachea may retract into the mediastinum, behind the manubrium (26). The rupture itself may be complex as well, i.e., transverse and longitudinal lesions. Symbas et al. (27) reviewed the pathology findings in 189 cases, observing transverse rupture in 74% of patients. Longitudinal and complex lesions occurred in 18% and 8% of patients, respectively. Proximal injuries have a generally better outcome than do the more distal injuries.

PRESENTATION AND DIAGNOSIS

Clinical Presentation

As with many forms of blunt injuries, the diagnosis of BTMA may not be immediately apparent (26,28). The

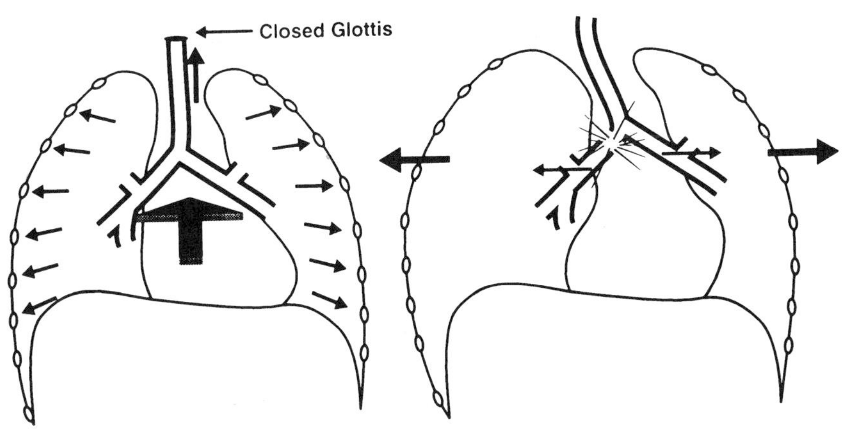

FIG. 2. Biomechanics of blunt trauma to the major airways *(intrathoracic portion)*. Note that a closed glottis at the time of impact increases the frequency of injury (by up to 5 times).

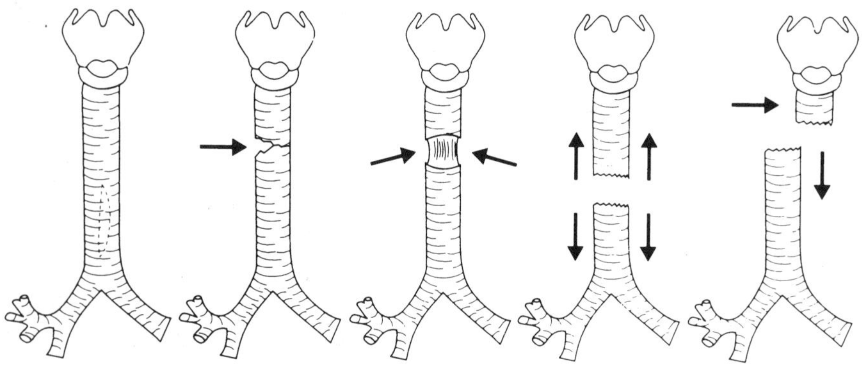

FIG. 3. Variations in the pathology of blunt trauma. Note that longitudinal and complex injuries *(not shown)* may occur.

clinician must have a high index of suspicion (similar to abdominal and cervical spine injuries). Blunt trauma to the major airways is a life-threatening condition, both immediately (up to 75% mortality at the scene) and when the diagnosis is delayed. The mortality rate is still 30% to 60% (29) when patients are diagnosed on arrival to the hospital, and 15% will die within the first hour.

The underlying principle is to secure the airway below the level of the lesion to allow ventilation to the gas-exchanging portion of the respiratory system. This is the same principle as in neoplastic or inflammatory conditions of the major airways. Note that the patient may be already optimizing the airway when initially assessed. It is also important to note that presentation may be paradoxical, i.e., symptoms and signs may not correlate well with the degree of injury. Typically, patients who arrive in emergency rooms may be initially stable and then suddenly deteriorate (2,30).

Diagnosis

Important clues to the diagnosis are summarized in Table 3. The history of MVA involving an unrestrained front seat passenger/driver in association with subcutaneous cervical emphysema suggests airway injury, particularly if there is no rib fracture. Subcutaneous emphysema/crepitus may be extensive. Voice changes indicate either structural damage to the larynx or involvement of the recurrent laryngeal nerve. Any patient with persisting pneumothorax despite chest tubes and suction, worsening subcutaneous emphysema, or persistent atelectasis should be considered a potential victim of BTMA (31).

TABLE 3. *Diagnosis*

Symptoms[a]
History of direct blow, MVA, crush injury
Dyspnea
Signs[a]
Voice change, hemoptysis, subcutaneous emphysema/crepitus, tachypnea
Radiology
Chest x-ray: subcutaneous emphysema, pneumomediastinum, pneumothorax, pneumopericardium
CT scan

[a]Symptoms and signs often bear no relation to the degree of injury

MVA, motor vehicle accident; CT, computed tomography.

Radiology may be useful in the stable patient. On chest x-ray, appearances of cervical or extensive subcutaneous emphysema of the chest wall, pneumomediastinum, pneumothorax, and/or pneumopericardium—particularly in the absence of rib fractures—should be investigated. Computerized tomography (CT) will diagnose this condition. However, CT may not be advisable in the compromised patient.

The most reliable form of diagnosis and management is direct visualization of the injury. This can be best achieved by bronchoscopy (FFB or rigid) or surgical exposure (tracheotomy, sternotomy, thoracotomy).

The decision on which method to use will rely on a combination of factors, i.e., recognition of the severity of the injury, level of the injury, available equipment, and the level of expertise of the treating physician(s). A multidisciplinary (team) approach will also expedite treatment of these trauma victims. Solely diagnostic direct and indirect laryngoscopy are of secondary importance in the management of these patients, as the priority is to secure the airway.

ANESTHETIC MANAGEMENT

Considerations

In the situation of blunt major airway trauma, the usual principles of emergency anesthesia airway control may not apply (Table 4). These patients have increased airway resistance, so they are prone to hypercarbia and, thus, sensitive to respiratory depressant medication such

TABLE 4. *Precautions in the patient with blunt major airway trauma*

Sensitive to respiratory depressant drugs
Unable to apply cricoid pressure
Muscle relaxation contraindicated (until the airway is properly secured)
IPPV relatively contraindicated (increases pneumothorax/surgical emphysema)
"Blind" intubation may not secure the airway/create false passages

IPPV, intermittent positive pressure ventilation.

as opiates and benzodiazepines. Similarly, muscle relaxants are relatively contraindicated (19,20,32,33) as many patients will be optimizing their airway with their own neck musculature, i.e., the "sniffing" position (20). Maintenance of spontaneous ventilation in this way avoids the need for positive pressure ventilation (PPV) in patients who are at significant risk of tension pneumothorax (19,21). Spontaneous ventilation also may be preferable to PPV in patients with chest tubes already *in situ*, to avoid losing significant ventilation through these tubes. Cricoid pressure may be inadvertently applied at the point of disruption to the airway, causing obstruction. Even if a "modified" rapid sequence induction/intubation is performed and a good view of the laryngeal structures and inlet is obtained, securing the airway in this situation is not guaranteed. The ETT may not traverse the lesion or a false passage may be created (19,20,34,35).

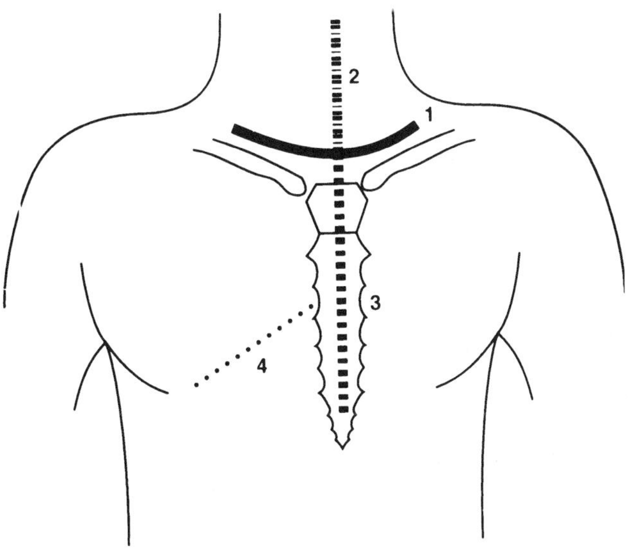

FIG. 4. Surgical incisions for control of the airway. Note a low transverse cervical incision *(1)* to allow access behind the manubrium. It may be necessary to extend incisions *1* and *2* to include a sternotomy *(3)*. Occasionally, a right posterolateral thoracotomy *(4)* may be required.

Tracheotomy

Early awake tracheotomy is the method of choice, we believe, for securing the airway (1,7,29,36–38). This allows definitive diagnosis and immediate treatment, avoids manipulations of the cervical spine, and lessens concerns regarding aspiration. The usual tracheotomy incision is made along the skin crease midway between the laryngeal prominence and the top of the manubrium. Some physicians recommend a low transverse neck incision (Fig. 4) so that access behind the manubrium is possible (18,20,39). The surgeon should be prepared to extend this incision downward over the sternum. An alternative would be a longitudinal neck incision. Other alternatives include right posterolateral thoracotomy (40) (for access to lesions at the carina).

Such procedures require a level of proficiency, equipment, and personnel with suitable experience. During these resuscitative measures, patients are often hypoxic (or becoming hypoxic), frequently becoming uncooperative. The normal surface anatomy is distorted, due to the trauma (as well as from the surgical emphysema), resulting in bleeding and poor identification of structures.

Bronchoscopy

An alternative to awake tracheotomy is bronchoscopy (41). Rigid (27) or FFB (42) should be performed by suitably trained physicians. Relative contraindications to performing FFB include lack of patient cooperation (combative behavior), excessive bleeding, and inexperience with the FFB. With rigid bronchoscopy, it must be remembered that the technique of insertion requires manipulation of the head and cervical spine, potentially hazardous in these patients. Before beginning any form of bronchoscopy, infiltration of local anesthetic is recommended in anticipation of emergent tracheotomy, should there be loss of the airway during this procedure (21).

Other Procedures

In some situations, neither of these two approaches may be feasible. The first is the multiply injured, severely shocked patient. The second is the pediatric patient. With the former, it may be that a "modified" rapid sequence intubation is the only feasible option (e.g., in the field or emergency room). Our suggestions here would be to use a small ETT (either microlaryngoscopy tubes or size 6.0/7.0 conventional ETTs). Bilateral chest tubes should be in place (or 14-gauge cannulae). Only two attempts at intubation should be performed. If unsuccessful, consider leaving the ETT in position as a guide for surgical tracheotomy. There are also case reports of successful blind oral intubation (43), blind nasal intubation (35), passage of a rigid bronchoscope (9,44), and cardiopulmonary bypass (the risks of heparinization in the multiply injured patient must be considered) (27).

In stable, pediatric patients, awake procedures are desirable but not practical all the time. In these situations, successful inhalational induction has been described (19, 33,45,46). A surgeon prepared for either tracheotomy or rigid bronchoscopy should be present during induction of anesthesia.

Cricothyrotomy, Cricothyroid Puncture, and Transtracheal Jet Ventilation

Although a "fail-safe" plan in managing patients with difficult airways and failed intubations includes percutaneous cricothyrotomy (47,48) and TTJV, BTMA is a situation where such procedures may be relatively contraindicated. There are a number of reasons for this.

Most of these "emergency airway" devices rely on normal surface anatomy, which may be distorted in trauma patients. There may be gross swelling of the neck, due either to vascular damage or to surgical emphysema, making palpation of the cricothyroid membrane difficult (18,35). Unilateral tension pneumothorax or vascular damage (paratracheal hematoma) may displace the trachea, so that location of the trachea may be difficult. Surgical emphysema may allow suction of air into the syringes used for location of the trachea (18). Transtracheal jet ventilation in such situations may easily further increase surgical emphysema, making tracheotomy more difficult.

Because the level of trauma has not been evaluated, successful insertion may be above the level of the lesion so that access to the gas-exchanging portion of the airway has not been achieved. There may be increased damage to the affected airway, as well as bleeding into it, further compromising the patient.

SUMMARY

BTMA is an infrequent cause of a difficult airway. It is thought to occur in approximately 3% to 5% of blunt chest trauma victims. Patients are typically young, unrestrained front seat drivers/passengers involved in MVAs. Although it is usually seen in association with other injuries, BTMA also may be the only serious injury (2). The keys to successful diagnosis and treatment are high index of suspicion (49), maintaining an alert, self-ventilating patient for as long as possible, and visualization of the lesion, either by surgical exploration or by bronchoscopy. A suggested management plan is shown in Fig. 5.

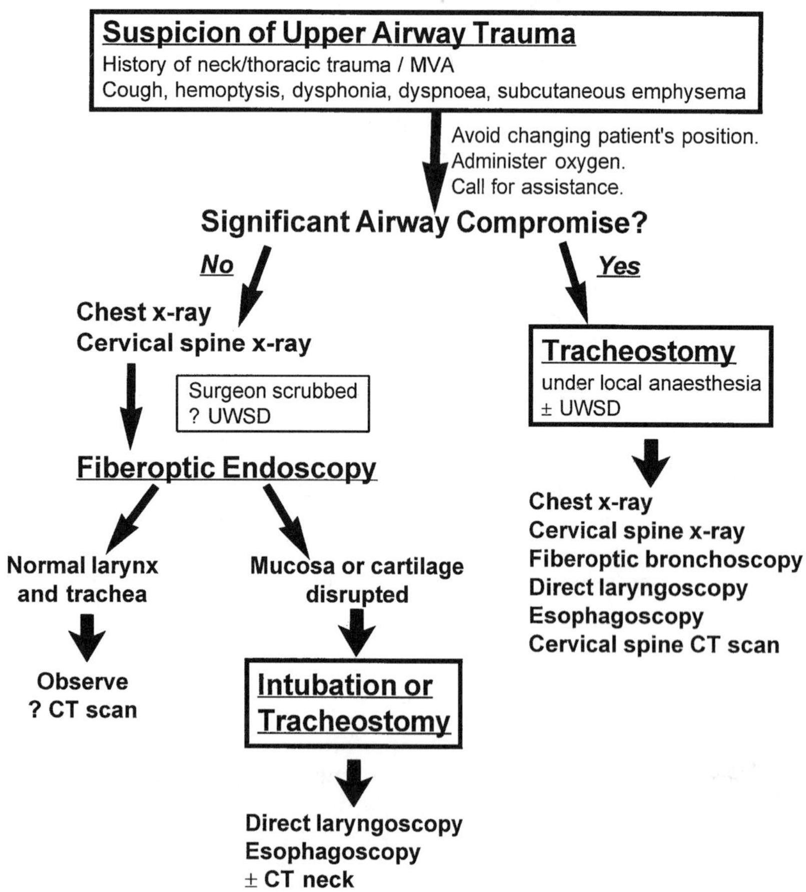

FIG. 5. Algorithm for the management of blunt airway trauma. UWSD, underwater sealed drain (chest tube).

REFERENCES

1. Schaefer SD. The treatment of acute laryngeal injuries. *Arch Otolaryngol Head Neck Surg* 1991;117:35–39.
2. Besson A, Seagesser F. A colour atlas of chest trauma and associated injuries. *Wolfe Medical Publications* 1983;2:10–80.
3. Bertelsen S, Howitz P. Injuries of the trachea and bronchi. *Thorax* 1972;27:188–194.
4. Ecker RR, Libertini RV, Rea WJ, Sugg WL, Webb WR. Injuries of the trachea and bronchi. *Ann Thorac Surg* 1971;11:289–298.
5. Benumof JL. Management of the difficult airway. *Anesth* 1991;75: 1087–1110.
6. Thoracic Trauma. In: *Advanced Trauma Life Support Course for Physicians*, 5th ed. 1993.
7. Reece GP, Shatney CH. Blunt injuries of the cervical trachea: review of 51 patients. *South Med J* 1988;81:1542–1548.
8. Hood RM, Sloan HE. Injuries of the trachea and major bronchi. *J Thorac Cardiovasc Surg* 1959;38:458–480.
9. Baumgartner F, Sheppard B, de Virgilio C, Esrig B, Harrier D, Nelson RJ, Robertson JM. Tracheal and main bronchial disruptions after blunt chest trauma: presentation and management. *Ann Thorac Surg* 1990;50:569–574.
10. Webb A. *Pathologica Indica or the Anatomy of Indian Diseases*, 2nd ed. Calcutta: Thacker 1848:147.
11. Schönberg S. Bronchialrupturen bei Thorax–kompression Klin. *Wocheschr Berlin* 49;2218 1912.
12. Krinitzki SI. Zur Kasuistik einer vollstandigen. Zerreibung des rechten Luftrohrenastes. *Virchows Arch Pathol Anat* 1928;266:815–819.
13. Vierheilig J. Die sukutane Bronchuszerreibung. *Beitr Klin Chir* 1914; 93:201 221.
14. Nissen R. Exstirpation eines ganzen Lungenflügels. *Zentralbl Chir* 1931;58:3003.
15. Griffith JL. Fracture of the bronchus. *Thorax* 1949:4;105–109.
16. Kirsh MM, Orringer MB, Behrandt DM, Sloan H. Management of tracheobronchial disruption secondary to nonpenetrating trauma. *Ann Thorac Surg* 1976;22:93–101.
17. Kelly JP, Webb WR, Moulder PV, Everson C, Burch BH, Lindsay FS. Management of airway trauma: tracheobronchial injuries. *Ann Thorac Surg* 1985;40:551–555.
18. Waldron RJ, Young RJ. Traumatic tracheal transection. *Anaesth Intensive Care* 1993;20:103–105.
19. Donchin Y, Vered IY. Blunt trauma to the trachea. *Br J Anaesth* 1976;48:1113–1114.
20. Capan LM , Miller S, Turndorf H. Management of neck injuries. In: *Trauma: Anesthesia and Intensive Care*. Philadelphia: J.B. Lippincott Company, 1991;430–438.
21. Flood LM, Astley B. Anesthetic management of acute laryngeal trauma. *Br J Anaesth* 1982;54:1339–1342.
22. Goodie G, Paton P. Anesthetic management of blunt airway trauma—three cases. *Anaesth Intensive Care* 1991;19:271– 274.
23. Roxburgh JC. Rupture of the tracheobronchial tree. *Thorax* 1987;42: 681–688.
24. de la Rocha AG, Kayler D. Traumatic rupture of the tracheobronchial tree. *Can J Surg* 1985;28:68–71.
25. Grover FL, Ellestad C, Arom KV, Root D, Cruz, Trinkle JK. Diagnosis and management of major tracheobronchial injuries. *Ann Thorac Surg* 1979;28:384–391.
26. Pate JW. Tracheobronchial and esophageal injuries. *Surg Clin North Am* 1989;69:111–123.
27. Symbas PN, Justicz AG, Ricketts RR. Rupture of the airways from blunt trauma: treatment of complex injuries. *Ann Thorac Surg* 1992; 54:177–183.
28. Sirker D, Clark MM. Rupture of the cervical trachea following a road traffic accident. *Br J Anaesth* 1973;45:909–911.
29. Travis SPL, Layer GT. Traumatic transection of the thoracic trachea. *Ann Royal Coll Surg Engl* 1983;65:240–241.
30. Edwards WH, Morris JA, DeLozier JB, Adkins RB. Airway injuries: the first priority in trauma. *Am Surg* 1987;53:192–197.
31. Flynn AE, Thomas AN, Schecter WP. Acute tracheobronchial injury. *J Trauma* 1989;29:1326–30.
32. Atkinson RS, Rushman GB, Lee JA.In: *A Synopsis of Anaesthesia*, 10th ed. London: Butterworth-Heinemann, 1987;475–476.
33. Murrin KR. Intubation procedure and causes of difficult intubation. In: Latto IP, Rosen M, eds. *Difficulties in Tracheal Intubation*. London: Bailliere Tindall, 1985.
34. Donlon JV. Anesthesia and eye, ear, nose, and throat surgery. In: Miller RD, ed. *Anaesthesia*, 3rd ed. Edinburgh: Churchill Livingstone, 1990.
35. Dash HH, Grode GR. Blunt trauma to the cervical portion of the trachea: a case report. *Br J Anaesth* 1983;55:1271–1272.
36. Camnitz PS, Shepherd SM, Henderson RA. Acute blunt laryngeal and tracheal trauma. *Am J Emerg Med* 1987;5:157–162.
37. Reece GP, Shatney CH. Blunt injuries of the cervical trachea: review of 51 patients. *South Med J* 1988;81:1542–1548
38. Urschel HC, Razzuk MA. Management of acute traumatic injuries of tracheobronchial tree. *Surg Gynecol Obstet* 1973;136:113–117.
39. Lawhorne TW, Jeyasingaham K, Kieffer RF. Transection of the trachea secondary to blunt trauma. *Br J Surg* 1978;65:176–178.
40. Lazar HL, Thomaston B, King TC. Complete transection of the intrathoracic trachea due to blunt trauma. *Ann Thorac Surg* 1984;37: 505–507.
41. Ramzy AI, Rodriguez A, Turney SZ. Management of major tracheobronchial ruptures in patients with multiple system trauma. *J Trauma* 1988;28:1353–1357.
42. Hara KS, Prakash UB. Fibre-optic bronchoscopy in the evaluation of acute chest and upper airway trauma. *Chest* 1989;96:627–30.
43. Olson RO, Johnsons JT. Diagnosis and management of intrathoracic tracheal rupture. *J Trauma* 1971;11:789–792.
44. McCleave DJ, Fenwick DG, MacDonald RR. Management of tracheal rupture involving both bronchi. *Anaesth and Intensive Care* 1975;3:53–57.
45. Brown TCK, Fisk GC. *Anaesthesia for Children*. Oxford: Blackwell, 1979;317– 318.
46. Seed RF. Traumatic injury to the larynx and trachea. *Anaesthesia* 1971;26:55–65.
47. Weaver T. Diagnostic and management strategies for chest trauma. In: Kerr D, Thirlwell J, eds. *Australas Anaesthesia* 1992;59–60.
48. Griggs WM, Myburgh JA, Worthley LIG. Urgent airway access—an indication for percutaneous tracheostomy. *Anaesth Intensive Care* 1991;19:586–587.
49. Mazzei Am, Mulder DG. Closed-chest injuries to the trachea and bronchus. *Arch Surg* 1970;100:677–680.

Airway Management, edited by
L.H. Hanowell, M.D. and R.J. Waldron, M.D.,
Lippincott-Raven Publishers, Philadelphia © 1996.

CHAPTER 24

Asthma, Anesthesia, and Airway Management

Thomas J. Gilman, Richard J. Waldron, and Anthony J. Bell

INTRODUCTION

Asthma is the most common cause of intrathoracic airway obstruction that significantly affects anesthesia (Table 1). Airway management of the asthmatic patient may require special considerations in choice of technique and/or drug selection. Asthma is a chronic disease characterized by acute exacerbations and a variable long-term prognosis. The disease is caused by bronchial inflammation and bronchospasm related to exposure to "trigger" factors that interact with the patient's immune system. The end result of these processes is reduced rates of air flow, air trapping, increased work of breathing, increased inspiratory pressures, and ventilation-perfusion mismatching. These conditions lead to hypoxia, hypercarbia, and respiratory acidosis. Asthmatic patients requiring surgery are cause for concern, as potential trigger factors are part of anesthesia and surgery (e.g., histamine-releasing drugs, surgical "stress," cold air, instrumentation of the airway).

T. J. Gilman: Department of Anesthesiology, University of California, Davis School of Medicine and Medical Center, Sacramento, California 95817.

R. J. Waldron: Department of Anaesthetic Services, Royal Hobart Hospital, and University of Tasmania, Hobart, Tasmania, Australia 7001.

A. J. Bell: Department of Critical Care Medicine, Royal Hobart Hospital, Hobart, Tasmania, Australia 7001.

This chapter reviews the epidemiology of asthma and new concepts about its pathophysiology, which relate to the current pharmacotherapy of asthmatic patients. The pre-anesthetic assessment, "optimization" of the asthmatic patient prior to elective surgery, intra-operative considerations, and treatment of acute bronchospasm are discussed (1,2,3). The discussion is also pertinent to airway management of asthmatic patients in settings outside the operating room.

CLINICAL FEATURES

Asthma affects 4% to 5% of the U.S. population and results in at least 5000 deaths per year. About 50% of asthmatic patients develop symptoms of the disease at less than 10 years of age, with another 30% developing symptoms before the age of 40. Males are affected two times more commonly than females.

Changing Concepts

Asthma has classically been defined as "a syndrome of increased responsiveness of the tracheobronchial tree to a variety of stimuli" (4). Recently, increasing recognition has been given to the inflammatory aspect of asthma (Table 2). Asthma can no longer be equated with bron-

TABLE 1. *Common obstructive airway diseases*

Disease	Etiology
Asthma	Allergic (IgE-mediated) Exercise-induced Aspirin-induced Infectious Occupational
Pulmonary emphysema	Environmental pollutants (e.g., smoking) Alpha$_1$-antitrypsin deficiency
Chronic bronchitis	Environmental pollutants (e.g., smoking) Infectious
Bronchiectasis	Infectious
Cystic fibrosis	Autosomal recessive inheritance
Kartagener's syndrome	Autosomal recessive inheritance
Tracheal stenosis	Iatrogenic

chospasm; instead, we know that this disease is the consequence of a combination of mucosal edema and inflammation, increased secretions, and bronchial smooth muscle contraction (5,6). These components of asthma are present in other disease states (e.g., cystic fibrosis), but the type of inflammatory response and induction of airway irritability are unique to asthma.

Morbidity and Mortality

Asthma affects more than 10 million Americans (7). Although fatalities caused by asthma are relatively rare and although the United States has one of the lowest asthma mortality rates in the developed world, there has been an increase in deaths related to asthma over the last 10 years in this country (1,8). Increases in asthma prevalence and rate of hospital admissions and deaths have been reported abroad (9,10). The reason for this increase in incidence and mortality associated with asthma is unclear.

There is evidence to suggest the increased morbidity and mortality may reflect reliance on inhaled beta$_2$-agonist therapy. This therapeutic regimen has the potential for masking the severity of asthma, either leading to the underutilization of anti-inflammatory agents or causing adverse cardiovascular effects and paradoxical bronchospasm. Morbidity and mortality may be further increased if there is inadequate assessment by patient and doctor of the severity of asthma exacerbations and inadequate hospital therapy.

TABLE 2. *1991 National Institute of Health definition of asthma*

1. **Airway obstruction** (or airway narrowing) that is reversible (but not completely so in some patients) either spontaneously or with treatment
2. **Airway inflammation** caused by immune mechanisms
3. **Airway hyperresponsiveness** to a variety of stimuli, including allergens, exercise, cold air, stress, instrumentation of the airway

A factor associated with increased risk for death is illness that is poorly defined in terms of diagnosis and severity; in many cases, objective parameters such as pulmonary function tests have not been performed, potential trigger factors have not been identified, and corticosteroids are underutilized. Death rates from asthma are three times higher in nonwhite patients from inner-city areas and may be related to less effective therapy. It is certain that more patients with asthma (with potentially more severe disease) are presenting for anesthetic and airway management (11,12).

Cellular Mechanisms

At present, asthma research is directed at identifying pathophysiologic mechanisms (13). As mentioned previously, asthma is a complex illness involving inflammatory and bronchospastic components. Pathologic evidence of inflammation has been found in virtually all asthmatic patients, including those with mild or asymptomatic disease. These findings include eosinophil and neutrophil infiltration of the airways with associated mast cell hyperplasia and degranulation (14). Epithelial damage is evidenced by sloughing, fluid exudation, thickening of the basement membrane, hypertrophy of smooth muscle, and hyperplasia of the goblet cells.

Mast cells release a variety of mediators; these include both directly bronchoconstrictive substances (histamine, leukotrienes, and prostaglandins) and locally acting factors that initiate the migration and activation of other inflammatory cells (eosinophils, neutrophils, basophils). The response to release of mast cell mediators is characterized by direct bronchoconstriction, enhanced vascular permeability, mucosal edema, and epithelial cell damage to the respiratory tract. Respiratory tract epithelial cells have recently been shown to play an important role in the pathogenesis of asthma. In addition to forming a physical barrier, epithelial cells produce endopeptidases responsible for the breakdown of bronchoconstrictive peptides; they also release epithelially derived relaxant factors, which are bronchodilators. The net effect of epithelial denudation in asthma is greater exposure of receptors to allergen, decreased breakdown of bronchoconstrictors, and decreased release of bronchodilating substances. With loss of integrity of the epithelial cells, the other inflammatory cells of the airway become involved with the release of local mediators. So, while mast cells play an important role in the acute bronchoconstrictor response to an allergen or other stimulus, secondary cellular infiltration is primarily responsible for initiating the subacute/chronic or second phase of the inflammatory response (15,16,17).

The mast cell activation of secondary-response cells (eosinophils, neutrophils, and T-cell lymphocytes) plays a key role in the chronic inflammatory response. The

TABLE 3. *Cells and factors involved in asthma*

Cell	Factors/mediators involved
Epithelial cells	Provide a physical barrier Produce a. Epithelial-derived relaxant factor (bronchodilator) b. Endopeptidases (break down bronchoconstrictors)
Mast Cells	Release a. Histamine b. Leukotrienes (chemotactic factors for eosinophils, neutrophils, basophils) c. Prostaglandins
Eosinophils	Associated with airway epithelial shedding
Helper T cells	Release lymphokines, particularly a. IL-1, IL-5, IL-6, IL-8, and tumor necrosis factor (involved in recruitment/activation) b. IL-3, IL-4, IL-5, and granulocyte-macrophage colony stimulating factor (affect inflammatory cell survival)

IL, interleukin.

number of activated eosinophils in the airway is associated with the severity of asthma. The cationic and major basic proteins of eosinophils damage airway epithelium and cause release of substance P and neurokinin A. These substances cause increased bronchospasm, increased vascular permeability, and mucous production. A subset of helper T cells (T_h2 cells) is activated and releases lymphokines, such as interleukin-5, which recruit and further activate eosinophils, thereby amplifying the immune response (18). These active cells (eosinophils and T lymphocytes), along with epithelial cells, macrophages, and fibroblasts, synthesize and release cytokines, which contribute to the chronic inflammatory state. Among the cytokines relevant to asthma are interleukin-1, interleukin-6, interleukin-8, and tumor necrosis factor, which are all involved in cell recruitment and activation; interleukin-3, interleukin-4, interleukin-5, and granulocyte-macrophage colony stimulating factor are important mediators of inflammatory cell survival (19) (Table 3).

This dual mechanism of asthma explains its poor response to specific antagonists of the primary inflammatory mediators, such as antihistamines. The initial inflammatory response, the secondary inflammatory response, and the persistence of the inflammatory feedback pathways emphasize the need to establish a therapy based on anti-inflammatory agents combined with bronchodilators. Therapy must be aimed at treating the chronic inflammatory process (20).

PRE-ANESTHETIC ASSESSMENT

Anesthesia care providers need to recognize the asthmatic patient who is at increased risk for perioperative bronchospasm, objectively assess pulmonary function, and understand which pre-anesthetic interventions are effective in minimizing risk. They should be familiar with the management of acute asthma attacks intra-operatively and with the postoperative care of the patient with severe asthma. The presence of asthma affects the risk for pulmonary complications both intra-operatively and postoperatively.

Evaluating the "At-Risk" Asthmatic Patient

Patients with any form of obstructive lung disease are at an increased risk for postoperative pulmonary complications (21). Studies have shown up to a 24% incidence of significant complications and a postoperative mortality approaching 5% (22). Most of these studies included patients with obstructive pulmonary diseases (other than asthma), such as tobacco smokers with chronic bronchitis and irreversible obstructive lung disease. Recent data show that patients with relatively severe asthma who are well controlled before undergoing surgery have minimal pulmonary complications and no mortality, and exhibit no significant excess risk compared with nonasthmatics (23).

The foundation of the preoperative assessment is the history. The patient is asked about current and past severity of symptoms. A history of emergency department visits, hospital admissions, and intubations for respiratory failure provides an assessment of the severity of disease and, more importantly, the rapidity with which the patient can develop severe bronchospasm. A review of the patient's pharmacologic regimen, especially past and current oral systemic corticosteroid use, identifies patients with relatively severe disease and those at risk for adrenal suppression (24).

Other co-existing factors that may increase the risk for pulmonary complications include a history of smoking, morbid obesity, and upper abdominal or thoracic surgical site (25,26) (Table 4).

Investigations

Spirometry is a simple, reproducible, and objective technique for assessing the asthma patient and provides a convenient means of determining the response to therapy

TABLE 4. *Conditions that increase risk for perioperative complications*

Thoracic/upper abdominal surgery
Age > 70 years
Morbid obesity
Smoking
Pre-existing pulmonary disease

From Gravenstein N, ed. *Manual of Complications During Anesthesia.* Philadelphia: JB Lippincott; 1991:304.

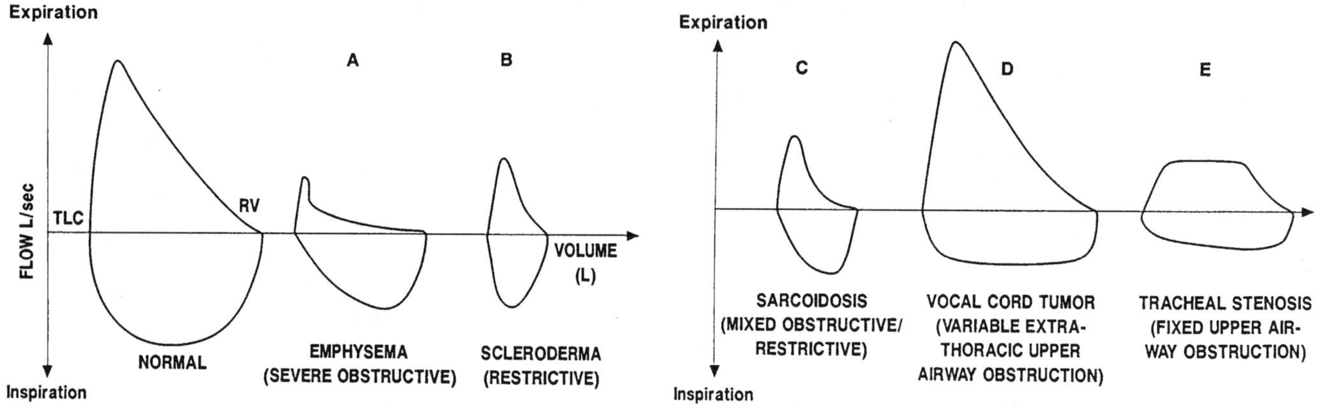

FIG. 1. Flow-volume loops showing the typical shapes in obstructive lung disease (**A**), restrictive disease (**B**), mixed obstructive and restrictive pattern (**C**), variable airway obstruction (**D**), and fixed airway obstruction (**E**). (From Siefkin AD. Perioperative care of the asthmatic. In: Hanowell LH, Junod FL, eds. *Pulmonary Care of the Surgical Patient.* Mt. Kisco, New York: Futura; 1994, with permission.)

(27). Spirometry is affected by patient effort, and variability is thus greater than for most clinical tests. The spirogram is expressed as a plot of expired volume as a function of time, or as a flow-volume loop with flow in liters per second as a function of volume. Figure 1 demonstrates characteristic flow-volume loops for various abnormalities of lung mechanics. The patient is asked to perform a maximal exhalation. The results are also affected by fatigue, neuromuscular function, and level of patient cooperation. Spirometry is essential in the assessment of asthma.

Useful values obtained through spirometry include the forced vital capacity (FVC), which is the maximum volume of air that can be exhaled after a maximal inhalation, and the forced expiratory volume in 1 second (FEV_1), which is the volume that can be exhaled during the first second of maximal exhalation. Normally, at least 80% of the FVC can be expired in the first second. When these values are expressed as a ratio (FEV_1/FVC), one can differentiate between a decreased FEV_1 caused by airway obstruction ($FEV_1/FVC < 80\%$) and a reduced FEV_1 in restrictive pulmonary disease, in which the FEV_1/FVC ratio is usually high ($> 80\%$) and FVC low. The forced expiratory flow over the middle half of the FVC ($FEF_{25-75\%}$) is less effort-dependent and more sensitive for small-airway obstruction. This value may be abnormal in early airway obstruction caused by smoking or in asymptomatic asthma after bronchodilator therapy, when the FEV_1/FVC ratio is normal (28).

Peak expiratory flow rate (PEFR) is the maximum rate of gas exhalation and is measured in liters per second. It can be measured using a hand-held device at the bedside or by the patient at home. PEFR is useful in documenting trends in airway resistance and response to treatment.

The graphic plots obtained from simple spirometry (flow-volume loops) demonstrate characteristic shapes depending on the pattern of airway disease, i.e., obstructive, restrictive, or mechanical upper airway obstruction.

Pulmonary function tests are frequently performed before and immediately following treatment with bronchodilators. Improvements of 15% to 20% in FEV_1 or of 25% to 30% in $FEF_{25-75\%}$ indicate a significant reversal of airway obstruction with therapy (29,30).

Arterial blood gas analysis is of limited value in the routine evaluation of asthma patients preoperatively, although studies have shown these patients are often mildly hypoxemic even at their baseline. This may reflect ventilation-perfusion mismatch caused by obstruction and mucous plugging as well as decreased oxygen diffusion secondary to airway inflammation (31). In the hospitalized patient with severe symptoms, serial blood gas analysis becomes one of the cornerstones of management. In these patients, hypercarbia implies a loss of the capacity to compensate fully for the increase in airway resistance by increasing ventilation, and represents impending respiratory failure (32).

The chest x-ray is not helpful in assessing the severity or guiding the management of asthma. However, it is useful in the evaluation of associated complications, such as pneumothorax, pneumonia, or atelectasis, or in ruling out aspiration of a foreign body in the differential diagnosis of wheezing (33).

Pre-anesthetic "Optimization"

Ideally, pre-anesthetic preparation of the asthma patient should begin at least 1 week before scheduled surgery (7) (Table 5). Elective operations should be delayed until optimization—the elimination of wheezing, treatment of infections, cessation of smoking, and maximization of pulmonary status—can be achieved. The patient

TABLE 5. *Pre-anesthetic assessment of the asthmatic patient*

History	Look for specific triggers (allergens, exercise, stress) Frequency of wheezing/attacks Current medications (take theophylline levels if appropriate) Number of hospital admissions/intubations Overweight, site of surgery
PEFR	Normally 400–600 L/min Review patient's log book (if available)
Pulmonary function tests	Improvement of 15–20% in FEV_1 and/or $FEF_{25-75\%}$ indicates suboptimal treatment
Chest X-ray	Limited value in the optimally managed asthmatic patient Excludes pneumothorax, inhaled foreign bodies, infection in the patient with acute exacerbation
ABG	Limited value in the optimally managed asthmatic patient May indicate the asthmatic patient is utilizing hypoxic drive

PEFR, peak expiratory flow rate; FEV_1, forced expiratory volume in 1 second; $FEF_{25-75\%}$, forced expiratory flow over middle half of FVC; ABG, arterial blood gases.

should be asked about adverse reactions to drugs, including allergic reactions to inhaled steroids, cromolyn sodium, ipratropium bromide, aspirin-like drugs and beta blockers. Intensive therapy is indicated to ensure that the secondary (subacute/chronic) inflammatory response is resolved before surgery.

Intensification of asthma therapy is indicated prior to surgery in anticipation of the increased airway irritation associated with perioperative events.

Drug Therapy

Beta-adrenergic Agonists

As inhaled agents, beta agonists are the most effective bronchodilators in clinical practice. The agents of choice are the selective $beta_2$-adrenergic agents. These agents relax bronchial smooth muscle and block mast cell $beta_2$ receptors. Their clinical effect occurs within minutes. Oral $beta_2$ agonists such as terbutaline and albuterol usually produce more tachycardia and tremor, and they are rarely more effective than the inhaled preparations. They may, however, be useful in children who are unable to use the metered-dose inhaler.

The $beta_2$ agents have traditionally formed the foundation of therapy and can be used prophylactically in asymptomatic patients in preparation for surgery. In those with severe symptoms, doses of $beta_2$ agonists can be repeated until there is relief of symptoms or side effects become intolerable (34,35). Although rapidly effective in the acute situation, the secondary inflammatory response and response to allergens is not inhibited.

Theophylline and Aminophylline

The response to theophylline is not as reliable as the response to $beta_2$ agonists and is complicated by a narrow therapeutic index. Common side effects of theophylline include nausea, anorexia, headache, insomnia, and, at toxic levels, seizures. Plasma theophylline levels are affected by processes that alter liver function and also by cigarette smoking, and laboratory monitoring of blood levels is required. The mechanism of action of theophylline is unclear. Postulated mechanisms of action include inhibition of phosphodiesterase and/or prostaglandins, stimulation of endogenous catecholamine release or beta-receptor agonist, and adenosine-receptor antagonism. Experimental data suggest that theophylline may also possess significant immune modulator effects (36).

Steroids

Inhaled corticosteroids are underutilized in the routine management of asthma (19,37). Based on improved understanding of the pathophysiology of asthma, these agents should be used in any patient experiencing daily asthma symptoms in order to reduce inflammation and decrease airway hyperreactivity (19). No adverse systemic effects of inhaled steroids, such as adrenal suppression, have been shown at doses of less than 800 μg/day of beclomethasone (38).

Patients who have no history of steroid use and who have been treated with bronchodilators alone may benefit from moderate doses of inhaled steroids given for 5 to 7 days before surgery. In patients who routinely use inhaled corticosteroids or who have required systemic steroids in the past, some authors recommend prednisone, 30 to 40 mg orally, each morning for 5 days before surgery (23,27). Bronchial hyperreactivity has been shown to correlate well with the degree of airway inflammation (39–43). In addition to reducing inflammation, inhaled and systemic glucocorticoids may have an important role in decreasing airway mucous secretions and in potentiating the bronchodilator effect of $beta_2$ agonists (6,44–46). This effect must be weighed against side effects, including delayed wound healing and an increased rate of gastrointestinal bleeding and infection.

Asthma patients who are taking inhaled steroids in doses greater than 800 μg/day of beclomethasone or its equivalent, and those who have required systemic steroids in the last 9 months, are regarded as being at risk for an Addisonian crisis in the perioperative period (24,27). In addition to the interventions listed above, these patients should receive 'stress' doses of corticosteroids, e.g., hydrocortisone 100 mg, prior to surgery and every 8 hours until the pulmonary status is stable (23).

The use of systemic steroids should be considered when the requirement for inhaled agents has increased significantly without adequate response. Intermittent courses of oral prednisone, methylprednisolone, or prednisolone in sufficient doses (30 to 80 mg/day of prednisone) should be prescribed, and pulmonary function monitored using spirometry or PEFR measurements. The dose is then tapered based on serial pulmonary function tests, and inhaled steroids are usually started during oral therapy (28).

Other Agents

Usual first-line drug therapy consists of the aerosolized agents, including beta agonists, anticholinergics, and corticosteroids (Table 6). Most patients also warrant a trial of inhaled cromolyn sodium, especially if there is a strong allergic component to their disease.

Second-line therapy is generally composed of oral agents, which are added when the response to inhaled drugs is inadequate. These include theophylline, sympathomimetics, and systemic corticosteroids.

Continuous systemic corticosteroids may be required for acute severe exacerbation that does not respond to other modes of treatment. Other agents include troleandomycin, a macrolide antibiotic that impairs the metabolism of methylprednisolone (47), and methotrexate, which also appears to have a steroid-sparing effect. These agents, though rarely required and not without potential adverse affects, are used to avoid or limit the side effects of chronic steroid therapy, including weight gain, skin thinning, glucose intolerance, gastrointestinal bleeding, hypertension, myopathy, hypokalemia, pathologic fractures, avascular necrosis, and cataracts. These adjunctive agents are usually discontinued perioperatively and then resumed in the postoperative period (28).

INTRA-OPERATIVE MANAGEMENT

The administration of an anesthetic to an asthmatic patient raises several interesting questions. Should the asthmatic patient be premedicated? Which anesthetic technique, regional vs. general, should be used? What is the risk for bronchospasm during induction? Which is better—topical or intravenous lidocaine? Which inhalational agent is preferred? What is the differential diagnosis and proper management of intra-operative wheezing? When is it time to extubate, and how should the patient be managed postoperatively?

Premedication

There are no controlled studies of specific premedications in asthma patients. In any patient with compromised pulmonary status, respiratory depressants should be avoided. Histamine$_1$ (H_1) antagonists possess sedative

TABLE 6. *Drug treatment of asthma*

Drug group	Drug name	Administration/dosage
Beta agonists[a]	Albuterol (Proventil, Ventolin)	Inhaler → titrate to effect (90 μg/dose) Jet nebulizer → 0.5 mL in 3 mL normal saline
	Metaproterenol (Alupent, Metaprel, MDI)	Inhaler → Titrate to effect (65 μg/dose) Jet nebulizer → 0.3 mL 5% solution in 3 mL normal saline
	Terbutaline (Brethaire)	Inhaler → 200 μg/dose SC → 0.25–0.5 mg q4h
	Epinephrine	SC/ETT → 0.2–0.5 mL of 1:1000 solution Children → 10 μg/kg
Anticholinergics	Atropine sulfate	Inhaler → 0.025–0.075 mg/kg Oral → 0.4–1.0 mg
	Glycopyrrolate	Inhaler/IM → 0.044 mg/kg
	Ipratropium	Inhaler → 18 μg/dose
Membrane stabilizers	Cromolyn	Used only in prophylaxis; of no use during acute attack
Methylxanthine derivatives	Aminophylline	IV bolus → 5–6 mg/kg IV infusion → 0.5–1.0 mg/kg/h
Steroids	Methylprednisolone	30–150 mg IV q6h
	Hydrocortisone	150–1000 mg IV q6h
Anesthetic agents	Ketamine	IV bolus → 0.75–1.0 mg/kg IV infusion → 0.15 mg/kg/h
	Volatiles (halothane, isoflurane)	Titrate according to blood pressure, PIP

[a]Many other inhaled selective beta$_2$ agonists are available.
MDI, metered dose inhaler; SC, subcutaneously; ETT, endotracheal tube; PIP, peak inspiratory pressure.

and drying properties and may be potentially helpful, while histamine$_2$ (H_2) antagonists should theoretically be avoided because of their role in the inhibitory feedback control of mediator release (33,48). Administration of some narcotics, particularly morphine, causes histamine release, although there is no evidence to suggest the levels achieved in the plasma cause significant bronchoconstriction.

Conduct of Anesthesia

The choice of regional anesthesia is not a guarantee against pulmonary complications or even against intraoperative bronchospasm (22,49). The use of regional techniques does, however, avoid the physiologic alterations of general anesthesia, such as reduced functional residual capacity, increased risk of atelectasis, ventilation-perfusion mismatching, and decreased pulmonary compliance (50). Tracheal intubation is known to be a potent stimulus of reflex bronchoconstriction (51,52). Given the above considerations, regional anesthesia, when feasible, is a logical choice. If a regional technique is chosen, the clinician must consider the potential complications. In particular, there is a high incidence of hemidiaphragmatic paresis with interscalene (up to 100%) and supraclavicular (28% to 80%) approaches to brachial plexus blockade (53). Patients for whom a regional technique is planned should receive the same preoperative preparation as those scheduled for general anesthesia.

Induction

There is no "best" anesthetic induction agent or anesthesia management plan. The approach must be individualized to the patient. The specific actions of the various agents and their interactions should be considered, particularly their potential to release histamine. Studies of the effect of thiobarbiturates on airway smooth muscle tone have found that human, rat, and dog bronchi all constrict when exposed to thiopental sodium (54). Subsequent studies have shown either an association or no association between thiopental (Pentothal) and bronchospasm (55,56). The goal during induction is to block reflex bronchospasm caused by tracheal intubation. Thiopental at doses commonly used for induction is known not to be a reliable blocker of this response. A reasonable approach may be to add an inhalational agent or give a second supplemental dose of thiopental to increase the depth of anesthesia just prior to intubation. Alternatively, a non-thiobarbituate agent may be selected for induction (33).

In asthmatic patients requiring rapid induction and tracheal intubation, emergency surgery, cardiopulmonary resuscitation, or mechanical ventilation for status asthmaticus, the use of inhalational anesthesia may not be practical. In such patients, induction with ketamine should be considered because of its bronchodilator properties (57). Ketamine has direct smooth muscle relaxant and vagal inhibitory effects, and it increases catecholamine secretion (34). In an animal model of hyperreactive airway disease, antigen-induced bronchospasm was prevented in Basenji greyhound dogs given ketamine. This protective effect was blocked when the animals were treated with beta antagonists, suggesting that it was the sympathomimetic effect of ketamine that was primarily responsible for the bronchodilator effect (58).

The use of local anesthetics to treat or prevent reflex bronchospasm has been the subject of many studies (59–61). Lidocaine has been shown to exert direct effects on airway smooth muscle, inhibit release of mediators such as histamine, and interrupt reflex arcs. At clinical concentrations, the mechanism of action appears to be limited to the interruption of airway reflex pathways. There has been no advantage demonstrated of inhaled vs. systemically administered lidocaine prior to airway instrumentation (58). A recent study concluded that inhaled 4% topical lidocaine and a 4% preservative-free lidocaine solution both induced bronchospasm in a significant proportion of asthmatic patients (62).

Halothane has traditionally been considered the inhalational agent of choice for preventing and reversing airway constriction (63,64). More recent studies in humans and animals demonstrate that isoflurane and enflurane at equivalent minimal alveolar concentrations are equally effective (65,66). Isoflurane and enflurane offer the advantage of not sensitizing the myocardium to catecholamines, which may be important in an asthmatic patient receiving beta-agonist agents (67). Although there is no evidence to indicate that one agent is superior to another in the treatment of bronchospasm or status asthmaticus, there are reports of patients failing to respond to one agent who subsequently have a good response to another.

Intra-operative Bronchospasm

When wheezing occurs intra-operatively, it is important to remember that it is a symptom and not a diagnosis (Table 7). Other possible life-threatening causes of wheezing should be considered. These include pulmonary edema, endobronchial placement of the endotracheal tube, mechanical obstruction of the tube, aspiration, pulmonary embolism, or tension pneumothorax. In addition, light anesthesia, secretions in the airway, and inadequate muscle relaxation may all cause audible wheezing and increased peak airway pressures (33,68).

When acute bronchospasm secondary to asthma is present, prompt therapy should be commenced. A suggested management plan is outlined in Table 8. Therapy should begin with inhaled Beta$_2$ agonists, and adequate depth of anesthesia should be ensured. An inhalational anesthetic agent (if not already being used) could be considered and oxygen concentration increased to avoid hypoxemia. Sub-

TABLE 7. *Conditions associated with wheezing under anesthesia*

1. Patient-related
   - Acute, e.g., croup, epiglottitis, bacterial tracheitis, aspiration (gastric contents/blood/particulate matter), pulmonary edema, pneumothorax
   - Chronic, e.g., asthma, cystic fibrosis, bronchiectasis, tracheal/bronchial stenosis or tumor, pulmonary edema
2. Anesthesia-related
   - Tracheal/carinal/bronchial stimulation
   - Equipment, e.g., kinked tracheal tube, overinflated cuff, prolonged intubation leading to tracheal edema/stenosis
   - Anaphylactic/anaphylactoid reactions caused by drugs, blood, latex
3. Surgery-related
   - Surgical stimulation/light anesthesia
   - Foreign bodies
   - Tracheal stenosis, tracheomalacia

TABLE 8. *Suggested management plan for intra-operative bronchospasm*

Confirm Bronchospasm	Exclude:
asculation	Anaphylaxis
increased airway pressure	ETT obstruction
coughing	Circuit obstruction
Primary Management	Aspiration
100 % oxygen	Light anesthesia/ surgical stimulation
assure adequate intravenous access	
expose patient to assess chest excursion	
check ETT, circuit, and oropharynx	
Asthma Confirmed	
deepen anesthesia (volatile anesthetic agent)	
cease surgical procedure (if possible)	
decrease respiratory rate and increase expiratory time	
Drug Therapy	
nebulized bronchodilator via side port in breathing circuit	
intravenous steroids	
If no improvement, consider:	
intravenous terbutaline	
intravenous aminophylline	
intravenous epinephrine	
intravenous ketamine	
keep patient intubated/discuss with intensivist	

ETT, endotracheal tube.

cutaneous or intravenous epinephrine may be given, although one must consider the risk for cardiac arrhythmias, especially when using halothane. Glucocorticoids should be added at doses equivalent to hydrocortisone 100 to 200 mg IV and continued every 6 to 8 hours postoperatively until the patient is stable. [In the U.S., methylprednisolone 1–2 mg/kg IV every 6 hours is conventional therapy.] The roles of anticholinergics and aminophylline in the acute setting are controversial. The use of aminophylline has been suggested to increase adverse drug interactions and may increase hypoxia through increased lung shunt fraction (69,70). The surgical procedure should be stopped if the respiratory compromise is severe and/or not responding to treatment.

If the intra-operative response is incomplete, the patient should remain intubated and mechanically ventilated. An intravenous bolus of ketamine followed by intravenous infusion can be administered. In severe acute asthma, limitation of air flow causes severe air trapping, hyperinflation of the lungs, barotrauma, cardiovascular collapse (caused by failure of venous return), and death. Clearly, during mechanical ventilation air cannot be continually pumped into the lungs when severe limitation of outflow is present. Controlled hypoventilation is characterized by high CO_2, but with control of peak inflation pressures it may be critical in life preservation (71). Since the major cause of mortality in the ventilated asthmatic patient is barotrauma and hemodynamic collapse, care must be taken to limit the peak airway pressures, preferably to 50 cm H_2O or less (72). [This may not always be possible.] A technique of mechanical ventilation with permissive hypercapnia, allowing the CO_2 to climb as high as 90 mm Hg, has been advocated (73). In refractory cases, partial femorofemoral bypass has been instituted in order to remove excess CO_2 (71).

The use of neuromuscular-blocking drugs in the operating room, to facilitate endotracheal intubation, and in the intensive care unit, to minimize peak airway pressures, is helpful in the asthmatic patient. However, these drugs can affect airway tone through two mechanisms. Some neuromuscular blockers cause histamine release, potentially precipitating bronchoconstriction. Because of their structural similarity to acetylcholine, these drugs may also interact with muscarinic receptors located in autonomic ganglia and on airway smooth muscle, resulting in airway constriction (34). Cholinesterase inhibitors (neostigmine, edrophonium), through their interference with acetylcholine metabolism at the muscarinic receptor, may also be detrimental (74). Given the few controlled studies addressing neuromuscular-blocking drugs and cholinesterase inhibitors in asthmatic patients, a logical approach might be to avoid those muscle relaxants known to cause histamine release, and to avoid cholinesterase inhibitors when possible in patients considered to be at risk for bronchospasm.

POSTOPERATIVE MANAGEMENT

Decisions about deep or awake extubation (extubation of the deeply anesthetized patient vs. extubation after nearly complete emergence from anesthesia) and about postoperative mechanical ventilation must be individualized. The belief of some authors that postoperative ventilation results in fewer pulmonary complications may be strongly influenced by the route and effectiveness of analgesia given (75). A prospective study of patients considered to be at high risk for pulmonary complications concluded that there were fewer postoperative complications in those patients who were given a 'light' general anesthetic combined with adequate epidural anesthesia and early extubation (76).

Postoperatively, asthmatic patients are more likely to become hypoxemic, even when asymptomatic (77). Supplemental oxygen and pulse oximetry are essential in the anesthesia recovery room (postanesthesia care unit). Ongoing or recurrent bronchospasm should be treated aggressively. The goal of postoperative analgesia is to allow adequate cough, tidal volumes, and early mobilization.

SUMMARY

Asthma is a common disease affecting well over 10 million patients in the United States. Despite dramatic advances in our understanding of the pathophysiology of asthma in recent years, the mortality rate of asthma is increasing. Our appreciation of the inflammatory nature of the disease has resulted in recommendations to alter our approach to the management of the asthmatic patient. This new approach is based on symptomatic therapy with beta agonists, the routine use of anti-inflammatory agents to reduce baseline inflammation and decrease the risk of bronchospasm, as well as the use of other bronchodilator agents to treat symptoms.

When a surgical procedure is planned for an asthmatic patient, the importance of assessment of the severity of the disease using objective and subjective criteria is stressed. Preoperative intensification of therapy is indicated. Data indicate that an asthmatic patient who has been well controlled pharmacologically may be anesthetized with minimal additional risk.

REFERENCES

1. Nicklas RA. Perspective on asthma mortality. *Ann Allergy* 1989;63: 578–584.
2. Strunk RC. Death due to asthma. New insights into sudden unexpected deaths, but the focus remains on prevention. *Am Rev Respir Dis* 1993;148:550–552.
3. Weiss KB, Wagener DK. Changing patterns of asthma mortality. Identifying target populations at high risk. *JAMA* 1990;264:1683–1687.
4. American Thoracic Society. Standards for the diagnosis and care of patients with chronic obstructive pulmonary disease (COPD) and asthma. *Am Rev Respir Dis* 1987;136:225-244.
5. Kaliner MA. How the current understanding of the pathophysiology of asthma influences our approach to therapy. *J Clin Immunol* 1993; 92:144–147.
6. US Department of Health and Human Services. Guidelines for the diagnosis and management of asthma: national asthma education program expert panel report. NIG-NHLBI 91:3042, 1991 (NIH publication no 91-3042).
7. Orfan N, Greenberger PA, Patterson R. Perioperative management of asthma and idiopathic anaphylaxis. *Ann Allergy* 1991;67:377–385.
8. Buist AS. Asthma mortality; trends and determinants. *Am Rev Respir Dis* 1987;136:1037–1039.
9. Sly RM. Increase in deaths from asthma. *Ann Allergy* 1984;53:20.
10. Jackson RT, Beaglehole R, et al. Mortality from asthma, a new epidemic in New Zealand. *BMJ* 1982;285:771–774.
11. Wilson JD, Sutherland DC, Thomas AC. Has the change to beta agonists combined with oral theophylline increased cases of fatal asthma? *Lancet* 1981;1:1235–1237.
12. Barger LW, Vollmer WM, Felt RW, et al. Further investigation into the recent increase in asthma deaths: a review of 41 asthma deaths in Oregon in 1982. *Ann Allergy* 1988;60:31–39.
13. Robin ED. Death from bronchial asthma. *Chest* 1988;93:614–618.
14. Busse W. Asthma in the 1990's. A new approach to therapy. *Postgrad Med* 1992;92:177–178, 183–186, 189–190.
15. Barnes PJ. New concepts in the pathogenesis of bronchial hyperresponsiveness and asthma. *J Allergy Clin Immunol* 1989;83:1013–1026.
16. McFadden ER Jr, Gilbert IA. Asthma. *N Engl J Med* 1992;327:1928–1937.
17. Lee TH, Lane SJ. The role of macrophages in the mechanisms of airway inflammation in asthma. *Am Rev Respir Dis* 1992;145:S27–30.
18. Hamid Q, Azzawi M, Ying S, et al. Expression of mRNA for interleukin-5 in mucosal bronchial biopsies from asthma. *J Clin Invest* 1991;87:1541–1546.
19. Barnes PJ. Anti-inflammatory therapy for asthma. *Annu Rev Med* 1993;44:229–242.
20. Rumbak MJ. New concepts in treatment of chronic persistent asthma. Using a stepwise protocol to control inflammation. *Postgrad Med* 1991;90:81–84, 89–90.
21. Wightman JAR. A prospective survey of the incidence of postoperative pulmonary complications. *Br J Surg* 1968;55:85–91.
22. Gold M, Helrich M. A study of the complications related to anesthesia in asthmatic patients. *Anesth Analg* 1963;42:283–293.
23. Pien L, Grammer L, Patterson R. Minimal complications in a surgical population with severe asthma receiving prophylactic corticosteroids. *J Allergy Clin Immunol* 1988;82:696–700.
24. Zora JA, Zimmerman D, et al. Hypothalamic-pituitary-adrenal axis suppression after short-term, high-dose glucocorticoid therapy in children with asthma. *J Allergy Clin Immunol* 1986;77:9–13.
25. Simonneau G, Vivien A, Sartene R, et al. Diaphragm dysfunction induced by upper abdominal surgery: role to postoperative pain. *Am Rev Respir Dis* 1983;128:899–903.
26. Garbaldi RA, Britt MR, Coleman ML, Reading JC, Pace ML. Risk factors for postoperative pneumonia. *Am J Med* 1981;70:677–680.
27. Seifkin AD. Using pulmonary function testing in the diagnosis and treatment of asthma. *Clin Rev Allergy* 1990;8:179–196.
28. Hanowell LH, Junod FL, eds. *Pulmonary Care of the Surgical Patient*. Mt. Kisco, New York: Futura; 1994.
29. Ries A. Response to bronchodilators. In: Clausen JL, ed. *Pulmonary Function Testing. Guidelines and Controversies*. Orlando: Grune & Stratton; 1984:215–221.
30. Shim C. Response to bronchodilators. *Clin Chest Med* 1989;10:155–164.
31. Nowak RM. Arterial blood gases and pulmonary function testing in acute bronchial asthma. *JAMA* 1983;249:2043–2046.
32. Tai E, Read J. Blood gas tensions in bronchial asthma. *Lancet* 1987; 1:644–646.
33. Hirshman CA. Perioperative management of the asthmatic patient. *Can J Anaesth* 1991;38(4 Pt 2):R26–28.
34. Hirshman CA, Bergman NA. Factors influencing intrapulmonary airway caliber during anesthesia. *Br J Anaesth* 1990;65:30–42.
35. Lee DKP, Ingbar DH. Aerosol delivery: what's best for your patient? *J Respir Dis* 1989;10:97–116.
36. Persson, CG. Xanthines as airway anti-inflammatory drugs. *J Allergy Clin Immunol* 1988;81:615–617.
37. Busse W. What role for inhaled steroids in chronic asthma? *Chest* 1993;104:1565–1571.
38. Geddes DM. Inhaled corticosteroids: benefits and risks. *Thorax* 1992; 47:404–407.
39. Bhagat RC, Grunsten MM. Effect of corticosteroids on bronchial responsiveness to methacholine in asthmatic children. *Am Rev Respir Dis* 1985;131:902–906.
40. Mattole S, Rosati G, Mormile F, Ciappi G. The immediate and short-

term effect of corticosteroids on cholinergic hyper-reactivity and pulmonary function in subjects with well-controlled asthma. *J Allergy Clin Immunol* 1985;76:214–222.
41. Ryan G, Ilatimer KM, Juniper EF, Roberts RS, Hargreave FE. Effect of beclomethasone dipropionate on bronchial responsiveness to histamine in controlled non-steroid-dependent asthma. *J Allergy Clin Immunol* 1985;75:25–30.
42. Dutoit JI, Salome CM, Woolcock AJ. Inhaled corticosteroids reduce the severity of bronchial hyperresponsiveness in asthma but oral theophylline does not. *Am Rev Respir Dis* 1987;136:1174–1178.
43. Costello JF, Clark TJH. Response of patients receiving high dose beclomethasone diproprionate. *Thorax* 1974;29:571–573.
44. Marom Z, Shelhamer J, Alling D, Kaliner M. The effect of corticosteroids on mucus glycoprotein secretion from human airways in vitro. *Am Rev Respir Dis* 1984;129:62–65.
45. Boggs DR, Athens JW, Cartwright GE, Wintrobe MM. The effect of adrenal glucocorticosteroids upon the cellular composition of inflammatory exudates. *Am J Pathol* 1964;44:763.
46. Shenfield GM, Hodson ME, Clark SW, Paterson JW. Interaction of corticosteroids and catecholamines in the treatment of asthma. *Thorax* 1975;30:430.
47. Wald J, Friedman B, Farr R. An improved protocol for the use of troleandomycin (TAO) in the treatment of steroid-requiring asthma. *J Allergy Clin Immunol* 1986;78:36–43.
48. Kingston HG, Hirshman CA. Perioperative management of the patient with asthma. *Anesth Analg* 1984;63:844–855.
49. Wang CY, Ong GS. Severe bronchospasm during epidural anesthesia. *Anaesthesia* 1993;48:514–515.
50. Benatar R. Anesthesia for the asthmatic. *S Afr Med J* 1981;409–411.
51. Aviado DA. Regulation of bronchomotor tone during anesthesia. *Anesthesiology* 1975;42:68–80.
52. Hirshman CA. Airway reactivity in humans. *Anesthesiology* 1983;58:170–177.
53. Urmey WF, Talts KH, Sharrock NE. One hundred percent incidence of hemidiaphragmatic paresis associated with interscalene brachial plexus anesthesia as diagnosed by ultrasonography. *Anesth Analg* 1991;72:498–503.
54. Adriane J, Rovenstein EA. The effect of anesthetic drugs upon bronchi and bronchioles of excised lung tissue. *Anesthesiology* 1943;4:253–262.
55. Shnider SM, Papper EM. Anesthesia for the asthmatic patient. *Anesthesiology* 1961;22:886–892.
56. Olsson HL. Bronchospasm during anesthesia: a computer-aided incidence study of 136,929 patients. *Acta Anaesthesiol Scand* 1987;31:244–252.
57. Corssen G, Gutierrez J, Reves JC, Huber FC Jr. Ketamine in the anesthetic management of asthmatic patients. *Anesth Analg* 1972;51:588–596.
58. Hirshman CA, Downes H, Farbood A, Bergman NA. Ketamine block of bronchospasm in experimental canine asthma. *Br J Anaesth* 1979;51:713–718.
59. Downes H, Loehning RW. Local anesthetic contracture and relaxation of airway smooth muscle. *Anesthesiology* 1977;47:430–436.
60. Weiss ER, Anderson WH, O'Brien KP. The effect of a local anesthetic, lidocaine, on guinea pig trachealis muscle in vitro. *Am Rev Respir Dis* 1975;112:393–400.
61. Downes H, Hirschman CA. Lidocaine aerosols do not prevent allergic bronchoconstriction. *Anesth Analg* 1981;60:28–31.
62. McAlpine LG, Thomson NC. Lidocaine-induced bronchoconstriction in asthmatic patients, relation to histamine airway responsiveness and effect of preservative. *Chest* 1989;96:1012–1015.
63. Gold MI, Helrich M. Pulmonary mechanics during general anesthesia. *Anesthesiology* 1970;32:422–428.
64. Korengs S, Takeda K, Ito Y. Differential effects of halothane on airway nerves and muscle. *Anesthesiology* 1984;60:309–318.
65. Heneghan CPH, Bergman NA, Jordan C, Lehane JR, Catley DM. Effect of isoflurane on bronchomotor tone in man. *Br J Anaesth* 1986;58:24–28.
66. Hirshman CA, Edelstein G, Peetz S, Wayne R, Downes H. Mechanism of action of inhalational anesthesia on airways. *Anesthesiology* 1986;56:107–111.
67. Jonston RR, Eger EI, Wilson C. A comparative interaction of epinephrine with enflurane, isoflurane, and halothane in man. *Anesth Analg* 1976;55:709–712.
68. Barbee WH. Bronchospasm in the operating room. *Anesthesiology* 1977;47:478.
69. Bowler SD, Mitchell CA, Armstrong JH, Scicchitano R. Nebulized fenoterol and IV aminophylline in acute severe asthma. *Eur J Respir Dis* 1987;70:280–283.
70. Siegel D, Sheppard D, Gelb A, Wienberg PS. Aminophylline increases the toxicity but not the efficacy of an inhaled beta adrenergic agonist in the treatment of acute exacerbations of asthma. *Am Rev Respir Dis* 1985;132:283–286.
71. Gattioni L, Kolobow T, Tomlinson R, et al. Low frequency positive pressure ventilation with extracorporeal carbon dioxide removal (LFPPV-ECCO_2R): an experimental study. *Anesth Analg* 1978;57:470.
72. Slinger PD. Perioperative respiratory assessment and management. *Can J Anaesth* 1992;30:R115–123.
73. Darioli R, Perret C. Mechanical controlled hypoventilation in status asthmaticus. *Am Rev Respir Dis* 1984;385–387.
74. Miller MM, Gish JF, Patterson R. Methacholine and physostigmine airway reactivity in asthmatic and non-asthmatic subjects. *J Allergy Clin Immunol* 1977;60:116–120.
75. Tarhan S, Moffitt EA, Sessler AD, Douglas WW, Taylor WF. Risk of anesthesia and surgery in patients with chronic bronchitis and chronic obstructive pulmonary disease. *Surgery* 1973;74:720–726.
76. Yeager MP, Glass DD, Neff Rk, Brink-Johnsen T. Epidural anesthesia and analgesia in high-risk surgical patients. *Anesthesiology* 1987;66:729–736.
77. Tyler IL, Tantisira B, Winter P, Montoyama EK. Continuous monitoring of arterial oxygen saturation with pulse oximetry during transfer to the recovery room. *Anesth Analg* 1985;64:1108–1112.

Airway Management, edited by
L.H. Hanowell, M.D. and R.J. Waldron, M.D.,
Lippincott-Raven Publishers, Philadelphia © 1996.

CHAPTER 25

Lasers and Shared Airways

Richard J. Waldron, Leland H. Hanowell and Roblee P. Allen

INTRODUCTION AND HISTORY

The challenges presented by pathology in or around a patient's airway have made successful treatment difficult. Resection of these lesions is one treatment option but often involves mutilating surgery (including tracheostomy and/or resection with or without primary anastomosis or grafts), which may be complicated by scarring and stenosis of the airway. Other problems include access to the lesion in the anesthetized patient, avoidance of pulmonary contamination, and the difficulties of controlling postoperative complications, particularly bleeding and edema. An anesthesiologist working in the field of airway surgery must be familiar with many techniques of airway control when "sharing" it with proceduralists. The introduction of lasers (Table 1) (Fig. 1) and endoscopic techniques has dramatically altered the surgical approach to many of these conditions, at the same time introducing new challenges to the anesthetist/anesthesiologist.

R.J. Waldron: Department of Anaesthetic Services, Royal Hobart Hospital, and University of Tasmania, Hobart, Tasmania, Australia 7001.
L.H. Hanowell: Department of Anesthesiology, University of California, Davis School of Medicine and Medical Center, Sacramento, California 95817.
R.P. Allen: Division of Pulmonary/Critical Care Medicine, Department of Internal Medicine, University of California, Davis School of Medicine and Medical Center, Sacramento, California 95817.

In this chapter, we will review the basic physics and hazards associated with the use of lasers in medicine. Lasers used in medicine produce nonionizing radiation, i.e., the effect on tissues is short-lived (1). The two most commonly used lasers in airway surgery are the carbon dioxide (CO_2) and the neodymium yttrium-aluminium-garnet (Nd:YAG) lasers. Hemostasis is a feature of laser surgery: The CO_2 laser coagulates vessels less than 0.5 mm in diameter, while the Nd:YAG lasers will coagulate vessels of larger diameter. We will examine their use in one of the more difficult areas of anesthetic and surgical care, the "shared" airway.

BASIC PHYSICS

Laser is an acronym derived from Light Amplification by Stimulated Emission of Radiation. Lasers are intense sources of electromagnetic radiation (light) in both the visible and invisible parts of the spectrum. Characteristics of laser "light"/radiation are:

1. *Monochromatic/coherent:* All photons have the same energy, wave length, and frequency. Ordinary light contains photons with a wide spectrum of wave lengths (Fig. 2).
2. *Collimation:* a focused beam that does not spread out. There is, therefore, very little loss of energy over distance. This also allows a beam of high energy to be concentrated in a small area and to remain so until impacting on its target. The end result is a monochro-

TABLE 1. *History of lasers in medicine*

1917	Einstein publishes paper outlining the quantum theory of radiation.
1960	Mainman and Javan performed the first simulated emission of laser light using ruby as activating material. Neodymium-in-glass laser discovered a year later.
1966	Yahr and Strully develop the CO_2 laser.
1970	Argon laser used in ophthalmic and dermatologic surgery.
1971	Jako uses CO_2 laser on dog. A micromanipulator is developed by Polanyi in 1974, enabling the CO_2 laser to be used with an operating microscope.
1975	Neodymium Yttrium-Aluminium-Garnet (Nd:YAG) laser introduced to medicine for the treatment of gastrointestinal hemorrhage.

matic, narrow, nondivergent, powerful beam, which is used to transfer energy to its target, usually in the form of heat.

Lasers are classified internationally according to maximum permissible exposure (MPE) (Table 2). Surgical lasers are used either in continuous working (CW) mode or in pulsed mode, the latter usually operating for a fraction of a second at higher power levels than the former. The radiant energy (joules) absorbed by tissues is a product of the power [watts (W)] multiplied by the duration. (2).

TABLE 2. *International classification of continuous working lasers*

Class 1	Powers do not exceed maximum permissible exposure for the eye
Class 2	Visible laser beams power only up to 1 mW Eye protected by blink-reflex time of 0.25 sec
Class 3a	Relaxation of class 2 to 5 mW for radiation, provided beam is expanded so that eye is still protected by blink reflex
Class 3b	Powers up to 0.5 W Direct viewing hazardous
Class 4	Powers over 0.5 W. Extremely hazardous

Generation of Laser Radiation

Absorption and Spontaneous Emission

According to the Bohr theorem, electrons of atoms/molecules are imagined as circling the nucleus in discrete

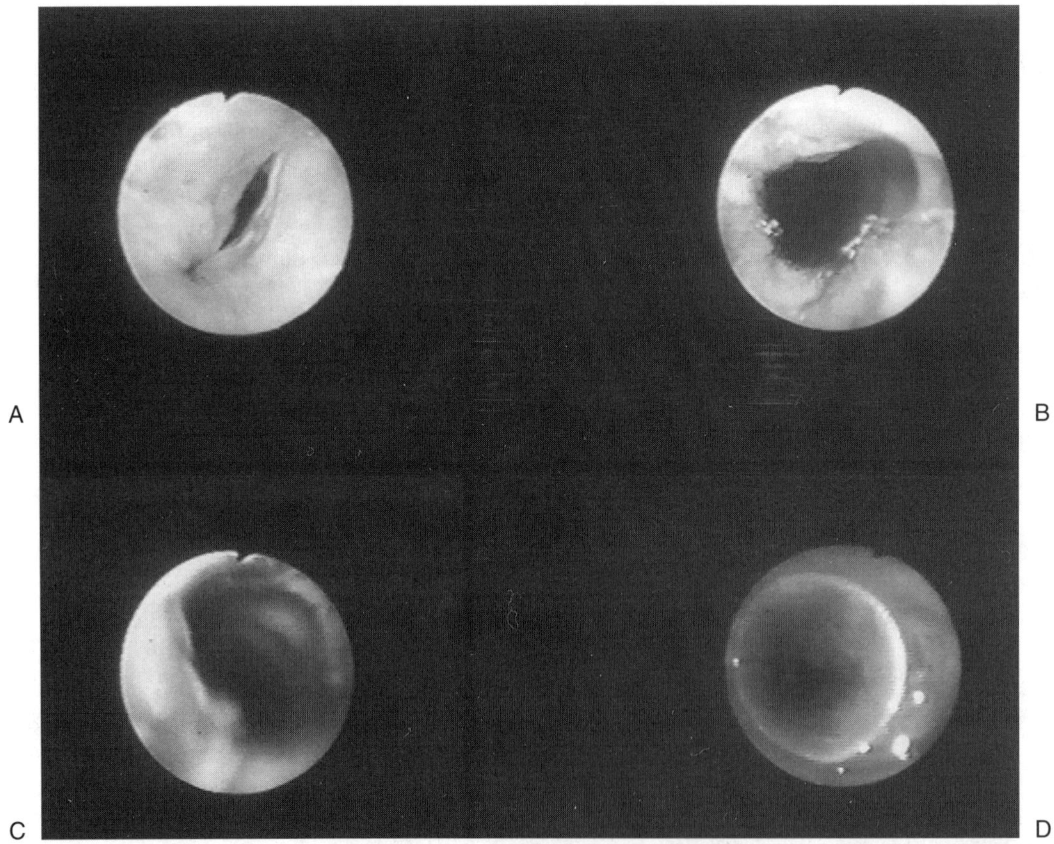

FIG. 1. Diagram demonstrates correction of a tracheal stenosis by laser therapy and placement of a tracheal stent. A near-complete stenosis of the trachea (**A**) was diagnosed in this patient, who had required prolonged intubation and was referred to our facility with stridor that persisted despite prior airway surgeries. The Nd:YAG laser was utilized to remove the stenosing tracheal scar with enlargement of the tracheal lumen (**B,C**). Subsequent to the laser resection of scar, a tracheal stent (**D**) was placed in the trachea through the rigid bronchoscope. Postoperatively, stridor was resolved.

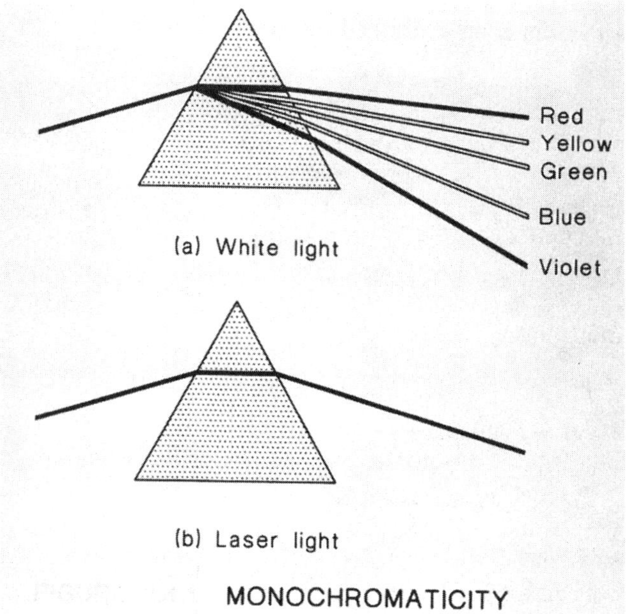

FIG. 2. Laser light, as compared with ordinary light, is all of the same wave length, as demonstrated by passing both forms of light through a prism. With permission from Standards Australia.

orbits, each having its own discrete energy level (Fig. 3). An atom or molecule tends to remain in its lowest possible energy (most stable) or "ground" state. Energy or photons can be absorbed by electrons, moving the electron to a different (higher energy level) orbit, thereby also promoting that atom/molecule to a higher energy level (excited state). Any atom/molecule in an excited state is regarded as unstable and tends to lose energy (i.e., emission) in the form of photons or discrete packages of light energy (the basis of the quantum theory of energy) as it attempts to return to its "ground" state. Atoms of a single element usually emit radiation at only one specific wave length and frequency.

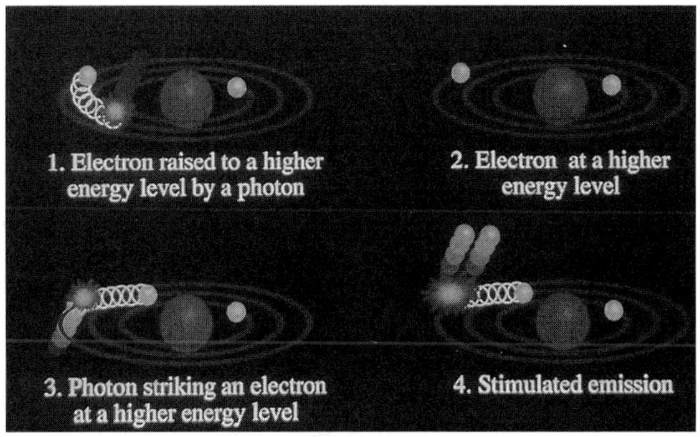

FIG. 3. The concepts of spontaneous absorption and emission, and stimulated emission. See text for details. (Courtesy of Mark Hassall, Laser Medics Pty, Ltd.)

Stimulated Emission

During stimulated emission, an atom/molecule in an excited state is exposed to radiation (photons) of energy levels exactly matching the energy difference (or wave length) between two orbits/shells. When this occurs, the excited atom/molecule can then emit the newly "absorbed" photon in addition to the one it releases as it attempts to return to its ground state (Fig. 3). Therefore, two photons are emitted, both having the same energy, frequency, and direction as does the stimulating radiation. Also, as there are now two photons released (one originally being used to stimulate the atom/molecule into a more excited state), the resulting beam is increased in intensity, or amplified (3).

Components of a Laser Device

Laser devices have three main components: a laser medium, an optical/resonating cavity or box, and a pumping source [or power supply (Fig. 4)].

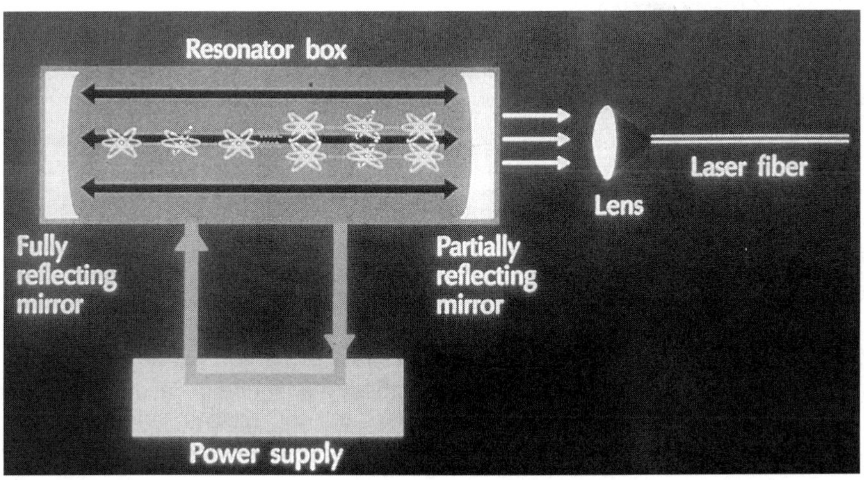

FIG. 4. Diagram of the main components of a laser: laser medium, resonating/optical cavity, and an energy pump/power supply. To allow a laser to work in pulsed mode, a device such as a Q switch *(not shown here)* is inserted in the resonator box, which generates pulses of less than one-millionth of a second. See text for details. (Courtesy of Mark Hassall, Laser Medics Pty, Ltd.)

Laser Medium

A laser medium is used to produce a laser beam. This medium can be solid, liquid, or gas (depending on the medium upon which they are based) and determines the wave length of the emitted laser radiation. For example, the ruby and Nd:YAG lasers use a solid cylindrical rod of material and are excited by a flash lamp coiled around the rod. The solid crystal may contain small ionic impurities (i.e., neodymium for the Nd:YAG, chromium in the ruby laser), known as a *dopant*. The liquid or dye lasers are excited either by a flash lamp or by another laser (i.e., argon-pumped dye laser). Gas lasers are usually excited by a high-voltage AC or DC electrical discharge. The main requirement is that the atoms or molecules of the medium can be excited to a higher energy level by the absorption of energy. Note that the quantity of energy emitted is a specific characteristic of the atom/molecule and may be less than the amount of energy absorbed.

Laser Tube/Optical Box or Cavity

The laser medium is confined in the optical (or resonator) cavity. Energy is pumped into the cavity, creating an increased state of raised energy levels in the molecules of the laser medium, followed by emission that occurs in all directions. The optical cavity is bounded by two mirrors, one at each end. One mirror reflects all photons back into the laser tube, which causes atoms/molecules to move to higher energy (unstable) states. The second mirror is only partially reflective and allows a small beam (along the "axis of propagation") to be emitted from the laser device. Immediately prior to this second mirror may be a device (e.g., a Q switch) that allows the generation of a "pulsed" beam.

Laser Wave Lengths

The wave length (or color) of laser radiation is a property of the laser medium (Fig. 5). Examples of typical lasers and wave lengths are given in Table 3. The Excimer laser has a short wave length, which gives it very good precision (very small spot size) for corneal shaping in ophthalmology. Lasers of longer wave lengths (e.g., the CO_2 laser) are not as precise. The Nd:YAG laser has many surgical applications as its shorter wave length allows it to be readily transmitted down optical fibers (as compared with the CO_2 laser).

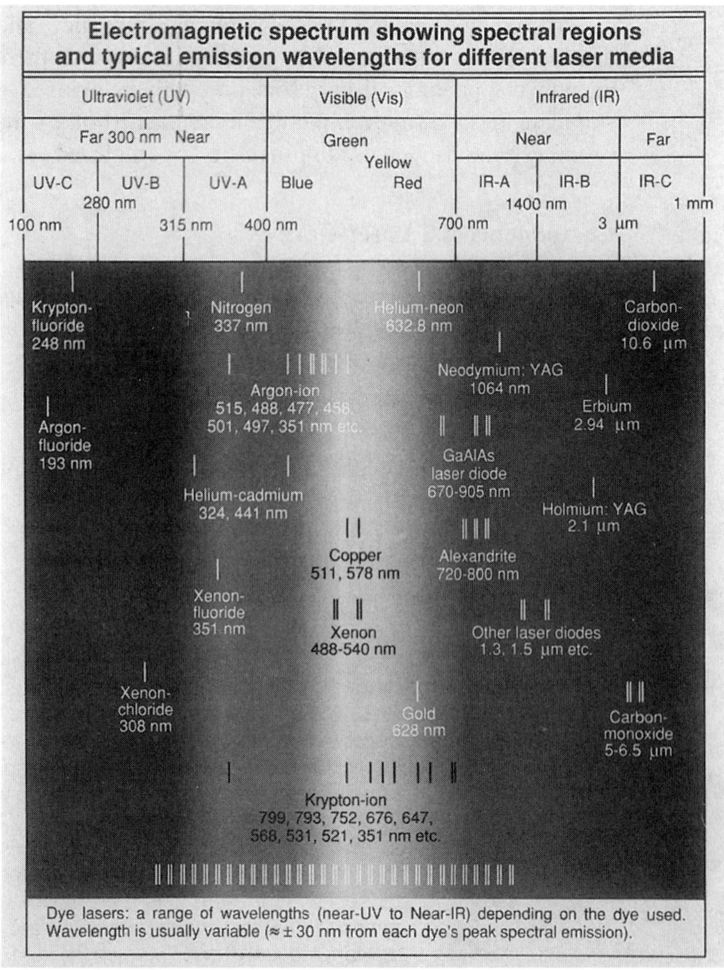

FIG. 5. Various wave lengths of lasers in medical use and their locations in the electromagnetic spectrum. Reprinted with permission for reprint from Standards Australia.

TABLE 3. *Wave lengths and medical uses of lasers (organized in increasing wave length)*

Laser	Medium	Wave length	Pumping	Typical energy	Medical uses
Excimer	Gas (ArF, XeCl)	125–350 nm (ultraviolet)	Electrical	0.5–50W	Ophthalmology, dermatology
Tunable dye	Rhodamine in liquid	360–670 nm (visible/ blue-red)	Argon-Krypton laser	<2 W	Ophthalmology, dermatology, oncology
Argon ion	Argon ion gas	488 (514) nm (blue)	Electrical discharge	3–20 W	Ophthalmology, dermatology, angioplasty, general surgery (photodynamic therapy)
KTP-YAG	Nd:YAG crystal	532 nm (green/yellow)	Krypton or xenon flashtube	5–15 W	Gynecology, general surgery
Helium neon	Helium-neon gas	632.8 nm (red)	Electrical discharge	1–30 mW	Aiming beams, pointers, acupuncture, x-ray alignment
Krypton	Krypton gas	647 nm (red)	Electrical discharge	1 W	Ophthalmology
Nd:YAG	Nd:YAG crystal	1060 nm (infrared)	Krypton or xenon flashtube	1–100 W	General surgery, endoscopy, angioplasty, ophthalmology, gynecology
CO_2	CO_2 in helium and nitrogen gas	10,600 nm (infrared)	Electrical discharge	1–80 W	General surgery, dermatology, gynecology, ENT

ArF, argon fluoride; XeCl, xenon chloride; KTP-YAG, potassium-titanyl-phosphate; Nd:YAG, neodymium yttrium-aluminium-garnet; ENT, ear, nose, and throat.

Other Characteristics

Modes of Operation

Most lasers used in medicine operate in one of two modes: CW or pulsed mode. With CW, the beam is in continuous operation. The beam may also be turned off for brief periods (e.g., 0.5 sec). This is often called *pulsed CW mode*. In pulsed mode, the beam operates for a very brief period. One example of this type of operation utilizes a device known as a Q-switch (not shown in Fig. 4), allowing a pulse of less than a millionth of a second duration to be generated.

Power

Power describes the overall strength of the beam, measured in W/cm^2. Focusing of a laser beam will result in a higher power density, e.g., an unfocused CO_2 laser beam approaches 1 cm^2 diameter, so that a 10 W laser has a power density of 10 W/cm^2. If the same laser beam is focused to a 1-mm^2 spot size, the same laser generates a power density of 1000 W/cm^2 (4). Continuous working mode lasers usually operate at <100 W, while pulsed lasers can produce powers of up to 10,000 W.

Laser Interactions with Biologic Tissue

Gamma radiation and x-rays travel greater distances through tissues than do lasers, causing ionization at a molecular level. When laser radiation strikes its target, it may undergo one or more of four processes (Fig. 6):

1. *Reflection* (also known as *backscatter*). For example, when laser radiation strikes a mirror or other shiny surface, it is reflected to another area with little loss of energy. When there is reflection from biologic tissue, it is more dispersed and associated with a loss of energy—this type of interaction is regarded as *backscatter*.
2. *Scatter* can occur when the beam strikes biologic tissue, resulting in dispersement of the beam and, thus, decreasing the power of the laser.
3. *Absorption*, where the energy (usually in the form of heat rather than ionization) is transferred to the tissue (Fig. 7). Tissue consistency, color, and water content will affect the amount of absorption. For example, the argon laser is highly absorbed by pigmented tissues; the CO_2 laser is highly absorbed by water.
4. *Transmission*, where no energy is lost during its passage through the tissue. The argon and Nd:YAG lasers are transmitted through clear fluids and structures.

The effect of a particular laser on human tissue depends on its wave length and power density. Generally, lasers with wave lengths >2500 nm (e.g., CO_2) will be absorbed by water in blood and tissues, whereas lasers with wave lengths <2500 nm (e.g., Nd:YAG, ruby, argon) are not absorbed by water, but by pigmented tissue. This explains why the cornea is injured with CO_2 lasers and why the Nd:YAG penetrates to the retina.

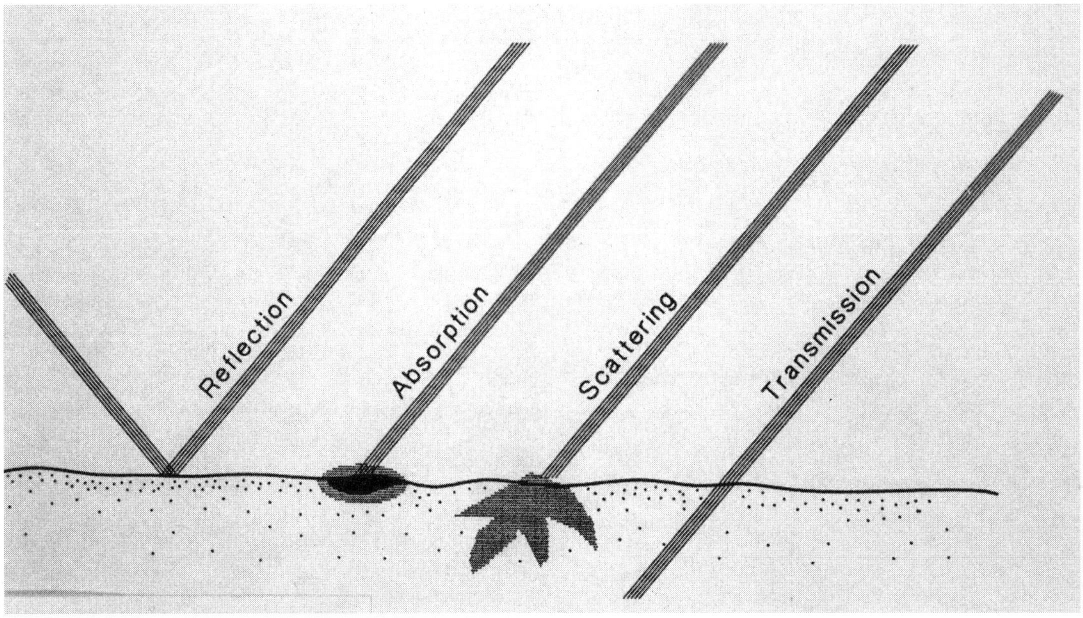

FIG. 6. The main interactions of lasers with biologic tissues. See text for details. Reprinted with permission for reprint from Standards Australia.

Lasers for Airway Surgery

There are many different lasers used in medicine, but the two most frequently used for airway lesions are the CO_2 and Nd:YAG lasers. Both have a rapid thermal drop, so that tissue surrounding the target area is relatively unaffected (although at 20 W, the Nd:YAG can produce thermal damage in tissue 10–15 mm away from the target) (5).

The CO_2 Laser

The CO_2 laser has been used to perform (or assist during) a wide variety of surgical procedures, including excision of skin lesions (e.g., telangiectasias, tattoos), splenectomies, mastectomies, tracheobronchial lesions, and even some vascular neurosurgical tumors. Ninety percent of the laser's energy is absorbed within 0.03 mm

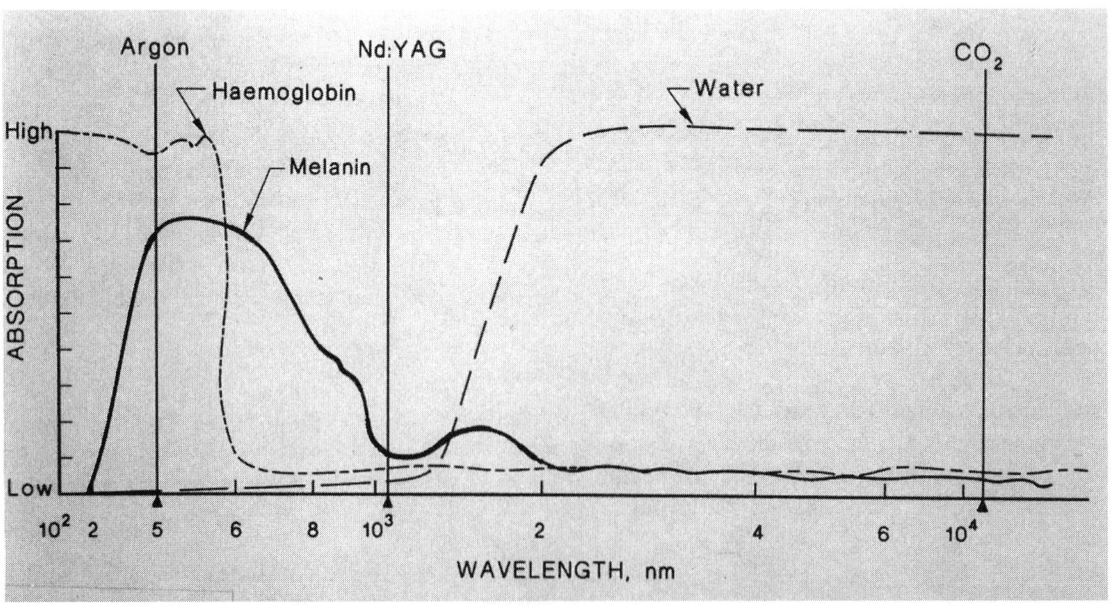

FIG. 7. Absorption characteristics and the relationships with various tissue types. Lasers with longer wave lengths (e.g., CO_2) generally have better absorption in water, whereas those with shorter wave lengths (e.g., Nd:YAG, Argon) are absorbed better in pigmented tissues. Reprinted with permission from Standards Australia.

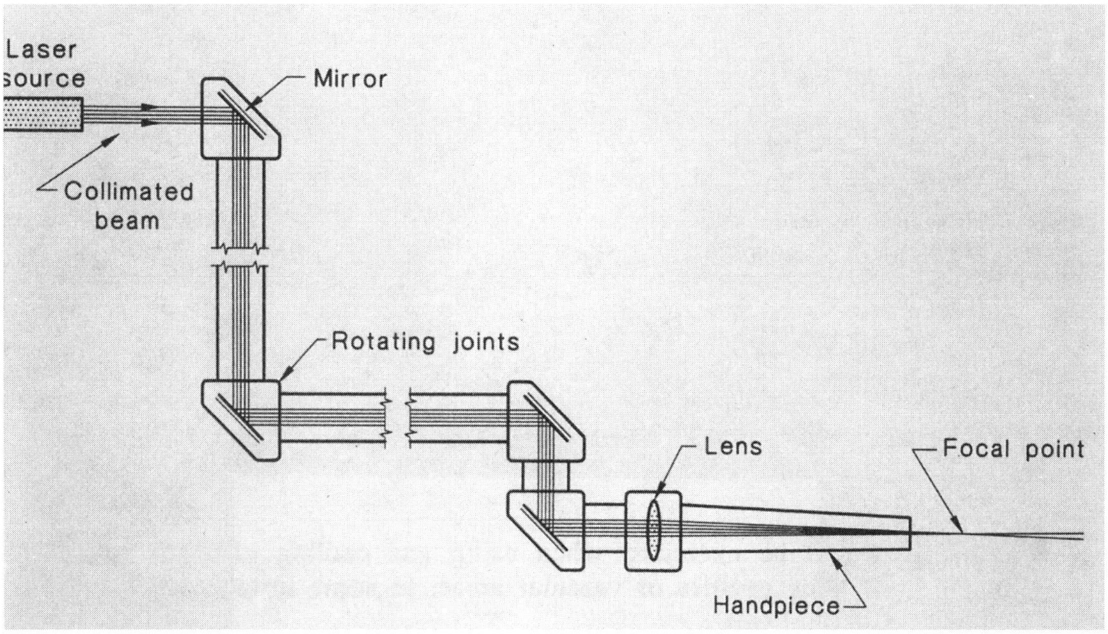

FIG. 8. An articulated arm delivery system via an operating microscope for a CO_2 laser. Reprinted with permission from Standards Australia.

of the surface [also known as the *extinction length* (EL)] onto which it is directed, making the CO_2 laser the most superficial of all medical lasers, with little reflection or scattering. Because the CO_2 laser is invisible, it is aimed by a relatively harmless (red) helium-neon laser as a marker. The operator must ensure that the two different laser beams are aligned before use.

The CO_2 laser is used in the treatment of laryngeal and tracheal pathology. It is less traumatic than are conventional surgery or diathermy and is a very precise form of surgical scalpel because of its shallow penetration (being strongly absorbed by water within cells) and because it produces only localized tissue damage, typically extending for less than 0.5 mm around the target. The field is also bloodless if the blood vessels in the target area are less than 0.5 mm in diameter. As a result, there is less postoperative edema as compared with other forms of surgery, e.g., electrocautery. The main practical limitation is that it cannot be transmitted through flexible optical fiber and requires an articulated arm with mirrors (Fig. 8). Thus, the target must be in direct line of sight.

Carbon dioxide laser radiation is readily absorbed by glass and plastic. Ordinary eyeglasses with side protectors are sufficient protection. Note, however, that contact lenses are not considered to provide adequate protection. If CO_2 laser radiation does strike the eye, injury is usually confined to the cornea, rather than extending to the retina.

The Neodymium Yttrium-Aluminium-Garnet (Nd:YAG) Laser

The Nd:YAG laser consists of a solid crystal of yttrium-aluminium-garnet, which is interspersed with the rare earth element, neodymium. It has greater penetration of tissues than does the CO_2 laser (EL of 60 mm in water and about 2 mm in soft tissue), one of the highest penetrations of all currently available medical lasers. It is transmitted by fiberoptic bundles (Fig. 9) that are surrounded by Teflon and silicon cladding; however, this results in loss of collimation by up to 12° when it exits the fiber bundle (6,7).

It is also invisible and is aimed using a helium-neon laser. It is not absorbed at the tissue interface and is scattered by water. The visible effect to the operator is minimal; damage to the tissues is concealed [has been likened to an iceberg (8)]. Tissue necrosis after use of this laser is slow, leading to delayed edema and possible orifice obstruction. In a new development, the Holmium YAG laser has a shallow penetration similar to the CO_2 laser but can be transmitted down optical fibers like the Nd:YAG laser.

HAZARDS OF LASER RADIATION IN THE OPERATING ROOM/THEATER

During the period January 1989 to June 1990, the American Food and Drug Administration (FDA) received 21 reports of injuries associated with the use of lasers (9). Of these, there were seven fatalities (33%). The hazards of lasers cannot be overemphasized.

Beam-Related

All staff involved with laser surgery should be familiar with the dangers and the safety measures required. The lasers currently in use do not cause ionization, are not

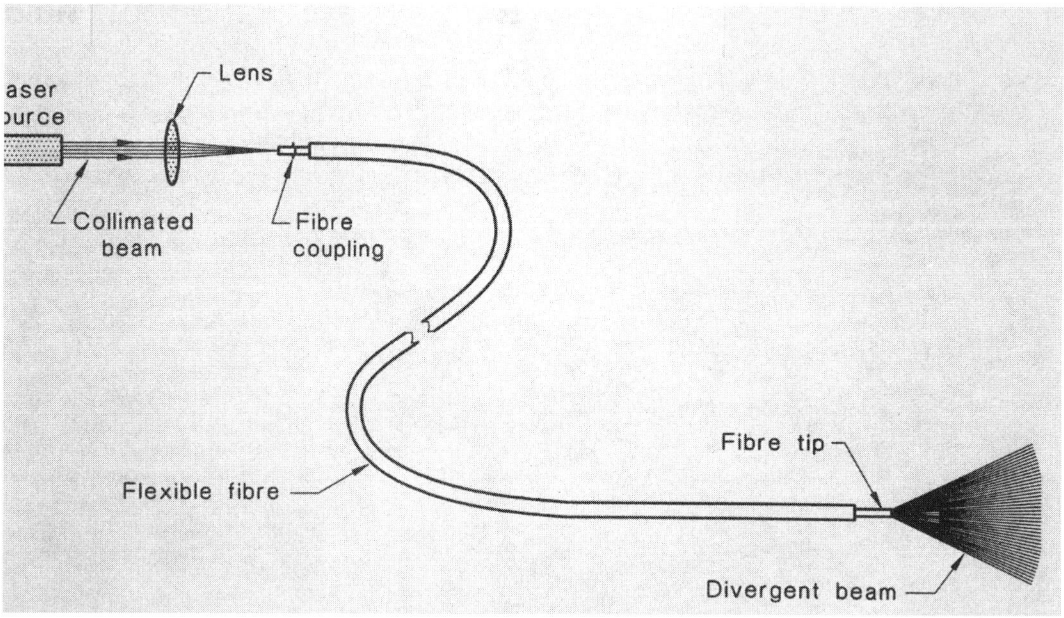

FIG. 9. A fiberoptic delivery system for Nd:YAG laser. Reprinted with permission from Standards Australia.

carcinogenic, and do not form a special hazard to pregnant women. However, they are intense sources of highly focused energy that do not lose significant amounts of energy over distance (hence the military interest in laser devices) or after reflection. The organs most at risk during a laser procedure (direct or reflected beam) are the eyes and the skin. Precautions for the use of lasers should include the following.

Operating Room/Theater Planning

Physicians, nurses, technicians, and administrators should all be involved in the setting up of a laser committee with the election of a Laser Safety Officer (LSO). The LSO is responsible for the implementation of the various standards [e.g., Australian and New Zealand Standards (AS/NZS) 4371:1994 (10)], credentialling of physicians and nursing staff for use of laser devices, and in-house education. When planning the layout of a laser operating room (OR), the setup of the entire OR, as well as positioning of the patient, must be considered. The setup should avoid having the laser beam directed toward any doors or windows. Consideration should be given to the permanent installation of blinds/shutters over windows for frequent use of lasers, particularly if they are not CO_2 lasers. The entrances to anesthetic and operating rooms should display approved laser warning signs (preferably at eye level with flashing lights), and traffic in and out of these locations should be minimized.

Similarly, the anesthetic machine (and anesthesiologist), breathing circuits, electrical equipment/patient monitors, and equipment with reflective surfaces should be kept out of "line of sight." Any equipment that may be subject to laser strike should be nonflammable and nonreflective. This includes surgical equipment such as drapes (paper or cloth), packs, scalpel blades, and retractors. The laser should never strike highly polished or mirrorlike surfaces; most instrumentation for use with lasers has a matte/dull finish.

Drapes are a problem. Cloth and paper drapes are combustible with sufficient exposure. They are useful in protecting the patient's skin from stray radiation, which can result in anything from mild erythema to full thickness burns. Special laser-resistant drapes are available; simply dampening the drapes has been successful (bear in mind that dampening may compromise the sterility of the operating field). A fire extinguisher (preferably CO_2) and a container of water or saline should be readily available.

Eye Protection

The visible lasers are the most dangerous because the radiation is focused by the lens (of the eye) onto the retina by a factor of up to 100,000 times. Thus, even low-power lasers can cause significant eye damage. All staff must wear appropriate safety glasses or goggles at all times during laser procedures. Ordinary glasses with no side pieces protect only against a frontal hit from a CO_2 laser; they are of no value with any other laser, nor can they protect from an incident beam from the side. Contact lenses are not appropriate protection, either. The patient also requires eye protection. This can be provided either by placing damp eye-pads/shields over the patient's eyes or by using the same protective eyewear used by OR staff.

TABLE 4. *Combustibility of endotracheal tubes using Nd:YAG laser*

Type of ETT	Time to smoke	Time to flame	Other comments
Rusch red rubber	2 sec (to penetration of ETT)	13 sec	ETT remained in one piece. Combustion ceased with interruption of oxygen.
Bivona "Fome-Cuf" laser tube	1 sec	12 sec ("blowtorch")	ETT remained in one piece. Flame terminated with cessation of oxygen.
Mallinckrodt Laser Flex®	6 sec	10 sec ("blowtorch")	Quick penetration by laser with rapid melting of steel. ETT in one piece/cessation of flame with interruption of oxygen.
Xomed "Laser-shield"	—	1 sec	ETT broke into several pieces in 12 sec.
Red rubber wrapped in 3M™ No. 425 aluminium tape or Venture copper foil	—	—	Unaffected after 1 min.

Table constructed from data from Sosis (ref. 41), using a LaserSonics (Santa Clara, California) model 1700 combined CO_2/Nd:YAG laser used in Nd:YAG mode. Laser output set to 50 W in continuous mode, beam diameter 0.68 mm. Endotracheal tubes placed on wet towels in room air with oxygen at 5 L/min flowing through them.

ETT, endotracheal tube; Nd:YAG, neodymium yttrium-aluminium-garnet.

Appropriate protective eyewear with side pieces should be labeled with the following:

1. The type of laser they are designed to protect against.
2. The wave length of the laser.
3. The degree of protection (optical density) provided.

Note that protective eyewear is not completely effective against a direct hit from a laser beam at close range; its main purpose is to protect the eyes from accidental reflections and scatter of the beam. All staff involved in laser surgery and anesthesia should have their eyes checked prior to their involvement with lasers.

Combustion

Lasers are capable of igniting most materials. Any combustibles in the surgical operating field are at risk, e.g., sponges, drapes, and towels. If such materials are at high risk of a laser strike, they should be either moistened with water or purchased as laser-resistant. A container of saline or water as well as a carbon dioxide fire extinguisher must be readily available. Hair spray, volatile skin preparations (alcohol, acetone) on patients, and high concentrations of volatile anesthetic agents [even the currently used agents (11)] should be avoided. Remember that during laser surgery of the bowel, methane, a combustible agent, should be evacuated (even though it is a gas that the laser beam will pass through, it will support combustion).

Endotracheal tubes (ETTs) as potential hazards for combustion are of greatest concern to the anesthetist/anesthesiologist. There is considerable literature debating which type of ETT [polyvinyl chloride (PVC) ETTs, PVC ETTs coated in a metallic tape, rubber ETTs, metallic ETTs (Table 4)] (12–14) and what gas mixture should be used during laser microsurgery of the upper airway (15–18). The important point, however, is that all ETTs can be ignited, irrespective of which mixture of anesthetic gases is used, although some are more supportive of fires than others.

Despite all precautions, it is still possible to be confronted by an airway fire. Understandably, there is no well-defined protocol for the management of this difficult situation, but the general recommendations are as follows (Table 5). The operator must indicate combustion as soon as possible. The laser should be turned off promptly. It is then imperative that delivery of all gases to the patient is ceased and the ETT is removed from the airway as quickly as possible. This is a difficult procedure for an anesthesiologist to perform as most anesthetic crisis management protocols call for 100% oxygen and maintenance of the airway. Oxygen and nitrous oxide both support combustion. The distal end of the ETT may still be burning, collapse, and/or separate from the rest of the ETT. Also, a burning PVC ETT produces hydrogen chloride (which can result in severe pneumonitis), and a burning red rubber ETT produces carbon monoxide. For this reason, the ETT should not be excessively secured in position at the start of the procedure. If the intubation was difficult, it may be prudent to use a tube changer prior to removing the burned ETT or to have a laryngeal mask

TABLE 5. *Management of airway fires*

1. Stop delivery of all gases to the patient.
2. Remove the endotracheal tube from the trachea as it may still be burning and no longer provide a patent airway.
3. Extinguish the fire.
4. Ventilate patient with 100% oxygen.
5. Laryngobronchoscopy to assess severity and extent of damage. Consider reintubation/tracheostomy, ventilation in intensive care, use of steroids and antibiotics.

airway (LMA) on hand. If the ETT, on removal, is still aflame, it should be doused immediately in a container of saline or water, as it is either in an oxygen-enriched environment or near materials that may ignite/support combustion (e.g., oxygen cylinders).

Once the fire is extinguished, the patient should then be ventilated with 100% oxygen via a face mask (or LMA, if appropriate). A laryngobronchoscopy should be performed to assess severity and extent of damage to the tracheobronchial tree as well as to remove any foreign bodies (pieces of ETT, metal foil, packs). Extensive burns should be managed with controlled ventilation via a new ETT or a tracheostomy. The use of antibiotics and steroids should be considered for the prevention of infection and scar/swelling minimization, respectively.

Non-Beam-Related

Patient Monitoring

Due to the protective eyewear and darkening of the OR to facilitate surgery, patient monitoring is compromised as are other tasks of the anesthetist/anesthesiologist (19). Most importantly, the vision of the anesthetist/anesthesiologist has been altered by restrictions in the field of vision and inability to use patient color as an indicator of well-being (20). Consequently, much more reliance must be placed on electrical monitoring (pulse oximetry, blood pressure, ECG, end-tidal CO_2). Care should be taken prior to commencement of surgery to ensure that these monitors and their probes are appropriately positioned so that reliable readings will be elicited during the operation. Note that these procedures may be quite long, with some endobronchial treatments taking up to 5.75 hours (21). Drug errors (i.e., misreading of medications, administration of the wrong drug) are more likely to occur with this type of OR environment.

Atmospheric Contamination

Vaporization of tissue, from either electrosurgery or laser radiation, produces fine particles with a mean size of 0.31 μ, a size that allows transport and deposition to alveoli (22). This has implications for contamination of staff and further contamination of patients. Cases have been reported of viable cells being collected from the laser plume (23,24), and human papilloma virus DNA has been retrieved from the plume of CO_2 laser (25). A smoke evacuation system (or scavenging system) and the use of high-filtration masks to filter particulate matter is recommended, particularly with use of the CO_2 laser, as it produces the most smoke. Currently, there have been no case reports of transmission of disease from patient to OR personnel as a result of laser surgery.

Embolism

Venous gas embolism can occur during endoscopic laser surgery, with reports of five fatalities in association with hysteroscopic surgery (26). Embolism has also occurred during Nd:YAG laser resection of tracheobronchial tumors (27,28). It appears that the coolant gas surrounding the laser may have been responsible for the deaths in association with the hysteroscopic surgery, and for this reason it is recommended that a liquid coolant be used wherever possible for these types of procedures (i.e., hysteroscopy, prostatectomy).

SHARED AIRWAYS

Although there are many different types of thoracic laser procedures (29–31), this chapter will concentrate on those involving the upper airway and respiratory system, as these procedures are perhaps the most difficult for the anesthetist/anesthesiologist to manage.

Preanesthetic Assessment

Patient Factors

In general, most patients presenting with airway pathology for laser surgery at our institutions have an American Society of Anesthesiologists (ASA) rating of 2 or greater (32). They are also usually elderly or very young. The elderly patient often has other concurrent disease (particularly hypertension and ischemic heart disease). The second group of patients, the pediatric patient, is complicated by differing airway anatomy and physiology (see relevant chapter). They usually present with conditions such as laryngomalacia (generally as a result of prolonged intubation or previous tracheotomy) or laryngeal papillomatosis (Fig. 10). Laryngeal papillomatosis is relatively rare, with an estimated 1500 new cases diagnosed each year (33). It is caused by the human papilloma virus and thought to be transmitted to the neonate from the birth canal. Periodic laser resection is often necessary to maintain an unobstructed airway, to treat recurrences, and to minimize risk of distal spread or carcinomatous transformation to squamous cell carcinoma (particularly human papilloma virus 16 or 18) (34).

Elderly patients require full workup for the cardiovascular system as well as careful evaluation of the respiratory system, particularly if the etiology of the lesion is tobacco-related. Features of ischemic disease should be sought in the preanesthetic workup, as laryngoscopic/bronchoscopic procedures may result in wide swings in blood pressure and heart rate. Similarly, preexisting complications of respiratory disease must be elicited. Tumors involving the airway may precipitate respiratory prob-

A 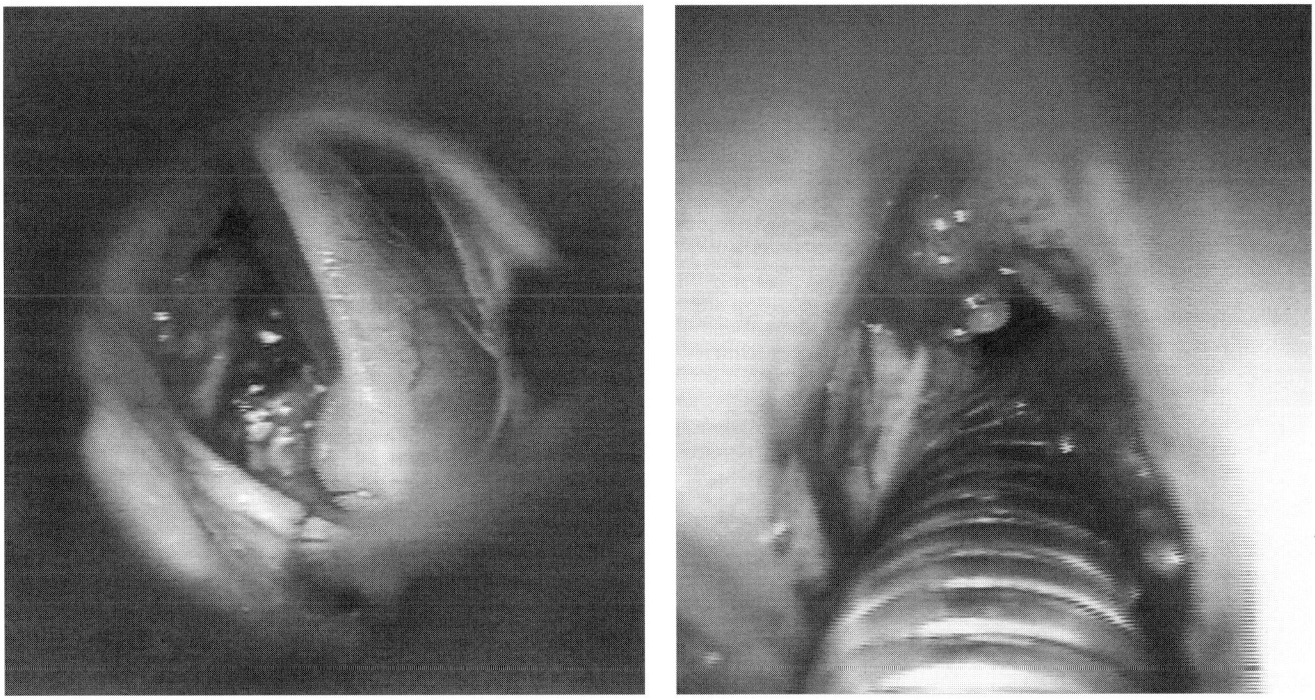 B

FIG. 10. Laser surgical techniques for laryngeal papillomatosis. **A:** Laryngeal papillomas distorted the vocal cords and nearly obliterated the trachea in this 5-year-old child. The carbon dioxide laser was utilized to remove the papillomas. **B:** Laryngoscopic view of the airway after resection of the majority of the papillomas. The metal endotracheal tube is here shown positioned between the cords; residual papillomas are noted anterior to the tube. These papillomas also were subsequently resected with the laser.

lems through hemorrhage, obstruction, infection, infiltration of lung parenchyma, and nonmetastatic manifestations, e.g., myasthenic syndrome that alters sensitivities to muscle relaxants.

Surgical Factors

There must be close communication and cooperation between operator and anesthesiologist to successfully manage laser surgeries of this area. The "shared airway" scenario is one where the operator and anesthesiologist/anesthetist are simultaneously requiring access to perform the operation and maintain adequate anesthesia. This is complicated by the fact that there is no agreement over the ideal method for the provision of safe and nonflammable anesthesia.

There are significant risks involved with surgery and anesthesia. Pneumothorax, pneumomediastinum, pneumopericardium (with tamponade) (35), fatal pulmonary hemorrhage, and esophageo(tracheo)bronchial fistulization have all been documented. Patients run the risk of significant hypoxia and hypercarbia during these procedures that can last up to 5 hours. This is complicated by the high frequency of cardiovascular disease in this patient population, the difficulty of monitoring end-tidal CO_2 with some rigid endoscope setups, and large swings in cardiovascular parameters during surgery. Many patients may present as difficult intubations, and appropriate consideration should be given to the technique of securing the airway prior to the use of the laser.

Anesthetic Factors

One of the major anesthetic goals with airway surgery is the quick return of the protective airway reflexes so as to be able to immediately assess the success of the procedure, any postoperative complications, and the likelihood of reintubation/postoperative ventilation. Long acting, sedative premedication is avoided in our institutions, and the use of short-acting anesthetic agents during the procedure assist in this aim. The anesthetic approach is also influenced by the preexisting medical condition of the patient and by other specific anesthetic problems, such as:

1. Difficult intubation
2. Monitoring of the patient, particularly with regard to changes in arterial blood gases (36), and assessing depth of anesthesia and effects on the cardiovascular system. Recall that the anesthetist will be wearing colored, protective eyewear in a darkened environment.

3. Level of the pathology in the patient's airway. For example, a lesion at the vocal cords may be unsuitable for jet ventilation. In an infant, an ETT may obscure the operator's field of vision.
4. Altered drug pharmacokinetics in elderly and pediatric patients. This can be complicated by nonmetastatic manifestations of lung cancers.
5. Preexisting tracheotomy or tracheotomy is part of the operative plan.

The following is a brief discussion of some of the techniques utilized in the "shared airway" scenario where a tracheostomy is not *in situ* prior to the induction of anesthesia.

Anesthetic Techniques

Local Anesthesia

Some procedures may require monitored anesthetic care only because the operator will use a flexible fiberoptic bronchoscope. In many situations, this can be performed under topical anesthesia. It is important to remember, however, that sedatives and local anesthetic agents do affect the sensitivity of the central chemoreceptors to CO_2. McCaughan et al. (36) noted that the changes in PaO_2 (decrease) and $PaCO_2$ (increase) were of the same magnitude in patients receiving general (29 cases) or local anesthesia (154 cases), although the pH change (a decrease) was greater for the general anesthesia group (mean drop of 0.073). George et al. (37) discuss the risk:benefit of local versus general anesthesia for endobronchial resections. Local anesthesia can be complicated by asphyxiation from hemorrhage or loss of airway, with a mortality as high as 2% in this study.

Advantages of a local anesthetic technique include:

1. Can avoid the "cannot-ventilate–cannot-intubate" scenario.
2. Avoids complications of general anesthesia, e.g., residual neuromuscular blockade, problems of oversedation postprocedure.
3. Patient can be used as a monitor of well-being (as well as other monitors).
4. Avoidance of ETT in airway, thus decreasing risk of airway fire.

General Anesthesia

General anesthesia can be maintained by either intravenous or inhalational agents. Maintenance of an adequate depth of anesthesia is important, particularly in regard to cardiovascular stability, patients with a bronchospastic component to their airway disease, and provision of good operating conditions for the operator. The most commonly used intravenous agent at our institutions is propofol, by either repeated bolus or infusion. It is ideal for use during jet ventilation and can be used if an ETT is in place or for sedation during local anesthetic techniques. In conjunction with other agents, it gives good control of blood pressure elevations and, with its rapid offset in action, allows good post procedure assessment of the patient.

The anesthetic vapors [halothane (Fluothane), enflurane (Ethrane), isoflurane (Forane), desflurane] are usually used via ETTs but can be used in conjunction with ventilating endoscopes. They are not combustible in the concentrations used to maintain satisfactory anesthesia (Table 6). It is also advisable to use the least concentration of oxygen consistent with adequate oxygenation of the patient because the higher the inspired oxygen concentration, the greater the risk that combustible material hit by the laser beam will ignite. Nitrous oxide should be avoided as it supports combustion. Room air, nitrogen, or helium are alternatives to reduce the inspired oxygen concentration. Helium is also useful in cases with critical airway obstructions.

General Anesthesia with Endotracheal Tubes

As mentioned previously, PVC, red rubber, and silicone ETTs can all be ignited by a laser beam in the presence of oxygen (see Table 4). Meyers (38) in 1981 conducted a series of tests using a CO_2 laser on PVC and red rubber ETTs in 50% and 100% oxygen and found that at 10 W, PVC ETTs produced flame when the duration of the beam was only 0.1 sec. *In vitro*, clear/transparent PVC ETTs will transmit a Nd:YAG laser, but not when contaminated by blood and/or mucus (39). PVC ETTs, as well as causing burns, also produce hazardous gases, whereas silicone ETTs tend to crumble and disintegrate when ignited. Red rubber ETTs are usually more resistant to ignition and do not disintegrate but produce carbon monoxide when ignited. All these ETTs can be wrapped with metallic tape (e.g., aluminium, copper) or metal-backed sponges from the cuff up. The tape must be applied evenly and smoothly to avoid separation/tears (in the metallic tape) (40) and rough edges. Tape reduces flexibility and increases the outer diameter of the ETTs. The cuff and distal tip of the ETT are generally not pro-

TABLE 6. *Lower limits of flammability of enflurane, isoflurane, and halothane in 20% oxygen in nitrous oxide and in 30% oxygen in nitrous oxide*

	Halothane (vol %)	Enflurane (vol %)	Isoflurane (vol %)
20% O_2 in N_2O	3.25	4.25	5.25
30% O_2 in N_2O	4.75	5.75	7.0

Reprinted with permission from *Brit J Anaesth,* ref. 11.

tected by the tape (to allow inflation of the cuff); some authors recommend the use of damp neurosurgical "cottonoids"/pledgets and filling the cuff with saline (or methylene blue) instead of air. Some will even tape the entire ETT (including the cuff and distal end) and use packing around the ETT to achieve a seal.

There have been many metal ETTs developed over the recent years, including ones by Norton and deVos, Hunton and Oswal, and the Laser-shield II (Xomed-Treace, US). We currently use a flexible, stainless steel ETT (the Laser-Flex®, Mallinckrodt Medical, Athione, Ireland) with a PVC Murphy eye tip and two cuffs filled with saline rather than air. Despite the advances in ETT tube design, these "laser-resistant" ETTs are still capable of ignition (41), particularly the PVC cuffs (same problem as ETTs with metal taping). In an effort to avoid the hazard of ETT combustion, withdrawal of a nasal red rubber ETT into the naso-oropharynx, out of range of the laser, has been advocated by some authors (42,43).

General Anesthesia with Rigid Endoscopes

Jet ventilation (high-frequency or otherwise) removes the requirement of an ETT for gaseous exchange during laser surgery of the airway, thus significantly decreasing the risk of airway fires. It can be performed either by supraglottic or infraglottic (44,45) approaches. Supraglottic approaches generally require the use of rigid endoscopes and a Venturi ventilation device such as a Sanders injector (Fig. 11) (46). Such devices are designed for use with a high-pressure gas source (such as a wall supply of oxygen at 310 kPa/50 psi) with an adjustable reducing valve, a manual toggle, and a metal injector (generally 12- to 14-gauge for adults, 16- to 18-gauge for pediatrics) that is securely attached to the endoscope. Although the Venturi principle entrains ambient gas, oxygen concentrations up to 86% at the distal end have been documented. The high-pressure gas source can include a blender to permit the addition of helium, nitrogen, or air. Jet ventilation should be commenced at low driving pressures and adjusted according to clinical criteria (chest wall movement, pulse oximetry, etc). The reducing valve is generally adjusted to 150–300 kPa for adults and used in short inspirations, entraining air. It must be remembered that it is a dynamic situation, i.e., the amount of driving pressure required will vary as the operator inserts/removes instruments, as bleeding occurs, and as material is removed from the airway.

When manual jet ventilation is used, intravenous anesthetic agents are recommended with complete neuromuscular blockade to maximize ease of ventilation (4,47). There are potential risks, particularly with barotrauma (pneumothorax, pneumomediastinum) as it is difficult to measure tracheal pressure. There are also risks with respect to the adequacy of ventilation as there is no means to measure end-tidal CO_2. Also there may be aspiration of resected material/blood, dehydration of respiratory epithelium, and residual neuromuscular blockade/reintubation (see below). This technique does, however, offer good surgical access, a relatively motionless surgical field (except for vocal cord surgery), and the minimization of flammable material in the airway. However, it is still possible for this approach to result in an airway fire and/or burns. Wegrzynowicz et al. (48) reported an airway fire using this technique, despite the use of a metal endoscope and appropriate patient protection. It appears that an errant beam ignited one of the surgeon's gloves, and some of the burning material was entrained by the oxygen-enriched jet ventilation.

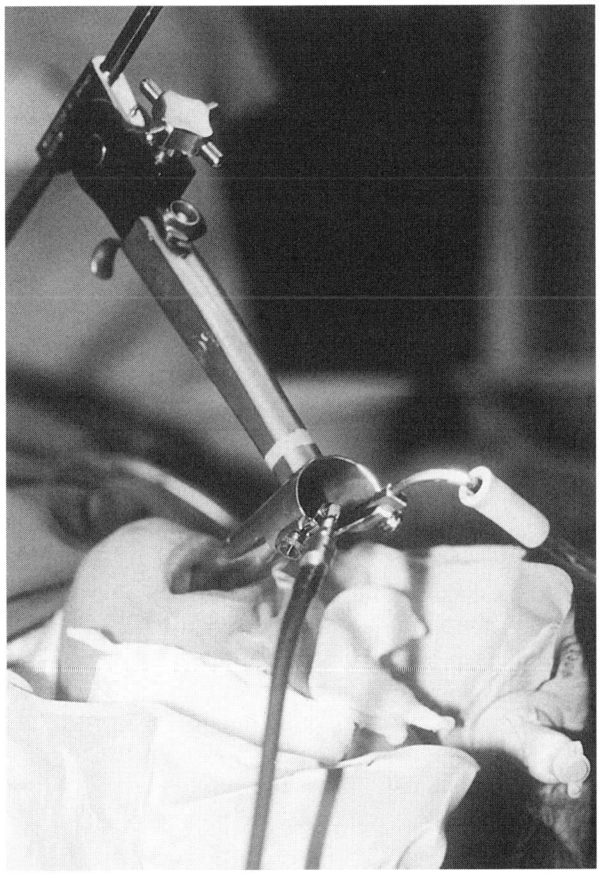

FIG. 11. Rigid bronchoscope with Sanders jet injector attached on the patient's left *(8 o'clock position)* and suction *(4 o'clock position)* in place. Note that the instruments have a shiny surface, which should be altered (either sandblasted or a matte finish) to minimize inadvertent reflection of laser beams. (Courtesy of Dr. T. Wong).

Lastly, there are bronchoscopes (e.g., Storz, Negus) that allow the breathing circuit from an anesthetic machine to be connected and to allow a patient to breathe spontaneously using volatile anesthetic agents. These are used particularly in pediatric airway surgery and have a standard 15-mm side port for the attachment either of a circle or Ayre's T-piece breathing circuit.

General Anesthesia with "Tubeless Anesthesia"/ Intermittent Apnea

Tubeless anesthesia and intermittent apnea, like the technique of jet ventilation, eliminate the need for an ETT in the laser surgical field (49,50). With jet ventilation, there is still the risk of barotrauma, particularly in the pediatric patient requiring airway surgery [e.g., laryngomalacia (51)] as well as movement of the vocal cords during inspiration. Tubeless anesthesia and/or intermittent apnea are techniques that avoid these problems and still allow a relatively unimpeded view of the operating field.

Intermittent apnea is perhaps used more for diagnostic airway procedures of short duration. It involves short, repeated periods where the anesthetic airway devices (usually a face mask) are removed to allow the operator access to the lesion. Lesions above the supraglottic region are usually selected. The patient must be fully monitored, particularly with a pulse oximeter. Anesthesia is induced in the normal manner; the patient can either be allowed to breathe spontaneously or be paralyzed with an airway maintained by a face mask or LMA. It is generally advisable to use as high a concentration of oxygen as is possible for this apneic technique, bearing in mind that this increases the risk of combustion with lasers.

With "tubeless anesthesia," the patient is allowed to breathe spontaneously (52). Oxygen, with or without anesthetic gases, may be delivered by a nasal cannula, nasopharyngeal airway, or a nasal ETT that is withdrawn out of the surgical field. Once again, care must be taken to ensure adequate depth of anesthesia (using inhalational or intravenous agents) with this technique to avoid laryngobronchospasm.

Recently, the LMA has been used for uvulopalato pharyngoplasty (53). It is an airway device that may find an expanding role in laser surgery in the airway for a number of reasons. It is useful in difficult intubations, does not cause the large swings in blood pressure and heart rate seen with conventional laryngoscopy and intubation, and allows good operator access to the subglottic region of the airway (with flexible fiberoptic Nd:YAG delivery systems).

Postprocedure

These patients are at high risk of postoperative complications, not surprisingly, predominantly of respiratory or cardiac origin. A 1991 study by Hanowell et al. (32) reviewed 73 patients requiring 87 treatments with Nd:YAG laser under general anesthesia (Table 7). There were complications in the postoperative management in 40 instances—almost 50%. The most frequent complication was a dysrhythmia (n = 14, or 16.1%), usually an ectopy (n = 6), followed by a tachyarrhythmia (SVT n = 4 and VT n = 1) and one case of complete heart block requiring pacemaker insertion. Hypotension requiring the administration of a vasopressor was required in almost 10% of cases. Variables predicting cardiovascular complications included increasing duration of general anesthesia and age. Reintubation was required in almost 10% of patients.

Of note, there was a 9.2% incidence of postoperative neuromuscular weakness (assessed clinically using nerve stimulators). Of these eight patients, six had squamous cell carcinomas and two had oat cell carcinomas. No patient had preoperative features of myasthenic syndrome (54), and there was no correlation between reintubation and the type of nondepolarizing neuromuscular blocker used nor the administration of antibiotics. This contrasts with the prospective study by Perrin et al. (55), in which there were no difficulties with residual muscle weakness in 124 consecutive laser procedures on 83 patients under general anesthesia without the use of muscle relaxants.

Another significant postprocedure problem is that of pulmonary edema (56–60). The mechanism of pulmonary edema following relief of airway obstruction is not entirely clear. Inspiratory effort against an airway obstruction generates an increased negative interstitial pressure that could promote edema formation, as explained by the Starling equation:

$$Q = K(Pc - Pt) - (c - t)$$

where Q is the rate of fluid flow across the capillary membrane; K is the filtration coefficient; Pc, Pt, c, and t represent the capillary hydrostatic, interstitial hydrostatic, capillary oncotic, and interstitial oncotic pressures, respectively (61).

If Pt becomes negative, movement of fluid out of capillaries and into the interstitium is facilitated. Stalcup and Mellins (62) measured mean pleural pressures up to –25.5 cm H_2O and peak inspiratory pressures of –38.8 cm H_2O in pediatric asthmatics. Capillary hydrostatic pressure can rise acutely during hypoxia, due to a shift of

TABLE 7. *Postoperative complications of patients requiring general anesthesia for Nd:YAG laser resection of endobronchial tumors*

Complication	No.[a]	Percent
Respiratory		
Reintubation	8	9.2
Neuromuscular		
Residual weakness	8	9.2
Cardiovascular		
Hypotension	8	9.2
Dysrhythmia	14	16.1
Ischemia	1	1.4
Infarction	1	1.4

From Hanowell et al. (32).
[a]n=87 procedures on a total of 73 patients.
Nd:YAG, neodymium yttrium-aluminium-garnet.

blood to the lung. Hypoxic pulmonary vasoconstriction in some segments of the lung can also shift blood flow in the lung. High intravascular pressures may injure capillary membranes, leading to increased membrane permeability. These factors may contribute to the development of this type of pulmonary edema.

SUMMARY

In their review of 1000 laser surgeries, Cavaliere et al. (63) noted the benefits of laser ablation of endobronchial tumors, including subsequent operability (initially precluded by airway obstruction), cure of benign lesions and carcinoid tumors, occasional long-term survival, and lifesaving acute intervention for critical airway stenosis. It is, therefore, clear that this modality of treatment is not a transient phenomenon.

A variety of new laser modalities are being investigated and incorporated into clinical management of airway disease. At present, many centers perform photodynamic therapy utilizing a tunable dye laser to treat obstructing airway lesions. This modality generally requires very short operating times and may be carried out with a fiberoptic bronchoscope in the majority of situations. In contrast to the Nd:YAG laser that thermally coagulates and vaporizes a tumor, the photodynamic therapy laser triggers a photochemical reaction that ultimately results in tumor cell death. The risks, therefore, of airway fire and acute airway hemorrhage are minimized during the acute treatment phase. However, 48–72 hours following treatment, a bronchoscopic debridement of the airway is generally required to remove necrotic tumor debris and exudative mucous plugs that develop secondary to the photodynamic reaction. The majority of these cases are still carried out utilizing fiberoptic techniques with conscious sedation and topical anesthesia. The risks, however, of hemorrhage, hypoxemia, and worsening airway compromise are taken into consideration during debriding procedures.

Anesthesiologists and anesthetists working in this difficult area must be in close communication with the operator. An understanding of the hazards presented by lasers, regular certification in laser safety, and frequent familiarization with drills for airway fire management are essential for the safe conduct of anesthesia.

REFERENCES

1. Padfield A, Stamp JM. Anesthesia for laser surgery. *Euro J Anaesth* 1992;9:353–366.
2. McKleskey CH. Anesthetic management of patients undergoing endoscopic laser surgery. *Anesth Clin North Am* 1989;7:611–629.
3. Davey A, Moyle JTB, Ward CS, eds. Lasers. In: *Ward's Anaesthetic Equipment*, 3rd ed. London: WB Saunders, 1992.
4. Van der Speck AFL, Spargo PM, Norton ML. The physics of lasers and implications for their use during airway surgery. *Br J Anaesth* 1988;60:709–729.
5. Boyce JR. Laser therapy for bronchoscopy. *Anesth Clin North Am* 1989;7:597–609.
6. Ball KA. The basics of laser technology. *Nurs Clin North Am* 1990; 25:619–634.
7. Sosis M. Anesthesia for laser surgery. *Intl Anesth Clin* 1990;28:119–131.
8. Keon TP. Anesthetic management during laser surgery. *Intl Anesth Clin* 1992;30:99–107.
9. Special report: laser safety. *Lasers Nursing* 1990;4:3–12.
10. Joint Standard AS/NZS 4173:1994. *Australian/New Zealand Standard: Guide to the Safe Use of Lasers in Health Care*. Standards Australia and Standards New Zealand, 1994.
11. Macdonald AG. A short history of fires and explosions caused by anesthetic agents. *Br J Anaesth* 1994;72:710–722.
12. Sosis M. Polyvinylchloride endotracheal tubes are hazardous for CO_2 laser surgery. *Anesthesiology* 1988;69:801.
13. Hunton J, Oswal VH. Anesthesia for carbon dioxide laser laryngeal surgery in infants. *Anaesthesia* 1988;43:394–396.
14. Kjeldsen L, Andersen APD, Hjorth A. Laser surgery in the airway. *Anesthesia* 1984;39:1146.
15. Cros AM. Lasers and the airway. In: Roberts JT, ed. *Clinical Management of the Airway*. Philadelphia: WB Saunders, 1992:355–367.
16. Hermens JM, Bennett MJ, Hirshman CA. Anesthesia for laser surgery. *Anesth Analg* 1983;62:218–229.
17. AlHaddad S, Brenner J. Helium and lower oxygen concentration do not prolong tracheal tube ignition time during potassium titanyl phosphate laser use. *Anesthesiology* 1994;80:936–938.
18. Pashayan AG, Gravenstein JS, Cassisi NJ, McLaughlin G. The helium protocol for laryngotracheal operations with CO_2 laser: a retrospective review of 523 cases. *Anesthesiology* 1988;68:801–804.
19. Boucek C, Freeman JA, Birchner NG, Tullock W. Impairment of anesthesia task performance by laser protection goggles. *Anesth Analg* 1993;77:1232–1237.
20. Vischoff D, Charest J. Propofol for pulsed dye laser treatments in paediatric outpatients. *Can J Anaesth* 1994;41:728–732.
21. Vanderschueren RG, Westermann CJ. Complications of endobronchial Neodymium-Yag (Nd:Yag) laser application. *Lung* 1990;168 Suppl:1089–1094.
22. Rampil IJ. Anesthetic considerations for laser surgery. *Anesth Analg* 1992;74:424–435.
23. Byrne PO, Sisson, PR, Oliver PD, Ingham HR. Carbon dioxide irradiation of bacterial targets in vitro. *J Hosp Infect* 1987;9:265–273.
24. Walker NPJ, Matthews J, Newson SWB. Possible hazards from irradiation with carbon dioxide laser. *Lasers Surg Med* 1986;6:84–86.
25. Kashima HK, Kessis T, Mounts P, Shah K. Polymerase chain reaction identification of human papilloma virus DNA on CO_2 laser plume from recurrent papillomatosis. *Otolaryngol Head Neck Surg* 1991; 104:191–195.
26. Baggish MS, Daniell JF. Catastrophic injury secondary to the use of coaxial gas-cooled fibers and artificial sapphire tips for intrauterine surgery: a report of 5 cases. *Lasers Surg Med* 1989;9:581–584.
27. Peachey T, Eason J, Moxham J, Jarvis D, Driver M. Systemic air embolism during laser bronchoscopy. *Anaesthesia* 1988;43:872–875.
28. Ross DJ, Mohsenifar Z, Potkin RT, Roston WL, Shapiro SM, Alexander JM. Pathogenesis of cerebral air embolism during neodymium-YAG laser photoresection. *Chest* 1988;94:660–662.
29. Barker SJ, Clarke C, Trivedi N, Hyatt J, Fynes M, Roessler P. Anesthesia for thoracoscopic laser ablation of bullous emphysema. *Anesthesiology* 1993;78:44–50.
30. Torre M, Grassi M, Nerli FP, Maioli M, Belloni PA. Nd-YAG laser pleurodesis via thoracoscopy. *Chest* 1994;106:338–341.
31. Fok M, Law SYK, Wong J. Neodymium:yttrium-aluminium-garnet laser for the treatment of tracheobronchial recurrences in esophageal carcinomas. *Ann Thorac Surg* 1994;58:1415–1418.
32. Hanowell LH, Martin WR, Savelle JE, Foppiano LE. Complications of general anesthesia for Nd:YAG laser resection of endobronchial tumors. *Chest* 1991;99:72–76.
33. Phelps WC, Alexander KA. Antiviral therapy for human Papillomaviruses: rationale and prospects. *Ann Intern Med* 1995;123:368–382.
34. Shah H, Garbe L, Nussbaum E, Dumon J, Chiodera PL, Cavaliere S. Benign tumors of the tracheobronchial tree. *Chest* 1995;107:1744–1751.
35. Vourc'h G, Le Gall R, Colchen. Pneumopericardium: an unusual

complication of endotracheal laser surgery. *Br J Anaesth* 1985;57: 451–452.
36. McCaughan JS, Barabash RD, Penn GM, Glavan BJ. Nd:YAG laser and photodynamic therapy for esophageal and endobronchial tumors under general and local anesthesia: effects on arterial blood gas levels. *Chest* 1990;98:1374–1378.
37. George PJ, Garrett CP, Nixon C, Hetzel MR, et al. Laser treatment for tracheobronchial tumours: local or general anesthesia? *Thorax* 1987; 42:656–660.
38. Meyers A. Complications of CO_2 laser surgery of the larynx. *Ann Otol* 1981;90:132–134.
39. Sosis M, Dillon F, Heller S. Hazards of a new specifically designed plastic endotracheal tube for use with the Nd-YAG laser. *Can J Anaesth* 1989;36:S91.
40. Hawkins DB, Joseph MM. Avoiding a wrapped endotracheal tube in laser laryngeal surgery: experiences with apneic anesthesia and metal Laser-Flex® endotracheal tubes. *Laryngoscope* 1990;100: 1283–1287.
41. Sosis M. What is the safest endotracheal tube for Nd-YAG laser surgery? A comparative study. *Anesth Analg* 1989;69:802–804.
42. Hatch DJ. Acute upper airway obstruction in children. In: Atkinson RS, Adams AP, eds. *Recent Advances in Anaesthesia and Analgesia*, vol 15. Edinburgh: Churchill Livingstone, 1985:133–153.
43. Hodges UM, Lloyd-Thomas A. Anesthesia for airway obstruction in the laryngo-onycho-cutaneous syndrome. *Anaesthesia* 1993;48:503–506.
44. Hunsaker DH. Anesthesia for microlaryngeal surgery: the case for subglottic jet ventilation. *Laryngoscope* 1994;104:1–30.
45. Schumacher P, Stotz G, Schneider M, Urwyler A. Laryngospasm during transtracheal high frequency jet ventilation. *Anesthesia* 1992;47: 855–856.
46. Lee ST. A ventilating laryngoscope for inhalation anesthesia and augmented ventilation during laryngoscopic procedures. *Br J Anaesth* 1972;44:874–878.
47. Conacher ID, Paes ML, Morritt GN. Anesthesia for carbon dioxide laser surgery on the trachea. *Br J Anaesth* 1985;57:448–450.
48. Wegrzynowicz ES, Niels NF, Pearson KS, Wachtel, Scamman FL. Airway fire during jet ventilation for laser excision of vocal cord papilloma. *Anesthesiology* 1992;76:468–469.
49 Wegrzynowicz ES, Niels NF, Pearson KS, Wachtel, Scamman FL. Airway fire during jet ventilation for laser excision of vocal cord papilloma. *Anesthesiology* 1992;76:468–469.
50. Aun CS, Houghton IT, So HY, Van Hasselt CA, Oh TE. Tubeless anesthesia for microlaryngeal surgery. *Anaesth Intensive Care* 1990; 18:497–503.
51. Baxter MRN. Congenital laryngomalacia. *Can J Anaesth* 1994;41: 332–339.
52. Williams SR, van Hasselt CA, Aun CS, Tong MC, Carruth JA. Tubeless anesthetic technique for optimal carbon dioxide laser surgery of the larynx. *Am J Otolaryngol* 1993;14:271–274.
53. Sher M, Brimacombe J, Laing D. Anesthesia for laser pharyngoplasty—a comparison of the tracheal tube with the reinforced laryngeal mask airway. *Anaesth Intensive Care* 1995;23:149–153.
54. Elmqvist D, Lambert EH. Detailed analysis of neuromuscular transmission in a patient with the myasthenic syndrome sometimes associated with bronchogenic carcinoma. *Mayo Clin Proc* 1968;43:689–709.
55. Perrin G, Colt HG, Martin C, Mak M, Dumon J, Gouin F. Safety of interventional rigid bronchoscopy using intravenous anesthesia and spontaneous assisted ventilation. *Chest* 1992;102:1526–1530.
56. Price SL, Hecker BR. Pulmonary edema following airway obstruction in a patient with Hodgkin's disease. *Br J Anaesth* 1987;59:518–21.
57. Lavertu P, Gervais AJ. Recurrent noncardiogenic pulmonary edema secondary to obstruction by hemiepiglottic remnant. *J Otolaryngol* 1988;17:229–232.
58. Scherer R, Dreyer P, Jorch G. Pulmonary edema due to partial upper airway obstruction in a child. *Intensive Care Med* 1988;14:661–662.
59. Galvis AG. Pulmonary edema complicating relief of upper airway obstruction. *Am J Emerg Med* 1987;5:294–297.
60. Kramer MR Melzer E, Sprung CL. Unilateral pulmonary edema after intubation of the right mainstem bronchus. *Crit Care Med* 1989;17: 472–474.
61. Starling EH. On the absorption of fluids from the connective tissue spaces. *J Physiol (Cambridge)* 1895–1896;XIX;19:312–326.
62. Stalcup SA, Mellins RB. Mechanical forces producing pulmonary edema in acute asthma. *N Engl J Med* 1977;297:592–596.
63. Cavaliere S, Foccoli P, Farina PL. Nd:YAG laser bronchoscopy. A five-year experience with 1,396 applications in 1000 patients. *Chest* 1988;94:15–21.

Airway Management, edited by
L.H. Hanowell, M.D. and R.J. Waldron, M.D.,
Lippincott-Raven Publishers, Philadelphia © 1996.

CHAPTER 26

Surgical Techniques in Airway Intervention

Richard S. Isaacs and Jonathan M. Sykes

INTRODUCTION

Tracheotomy has developed from an initial surgical intervention for the relief of airway obstruction into an elegant procedure that also has therapeutic utility in pulmonology. The first successful tracheotomy was recorded by Antonius Musa Brasavola in the fifteenth century, when he operated to relieve obstruction in a patient suffering from tracheal abscess (1). Since then, the evolution of tracheotomy has followed the necessity for intervention in a variety of diseases. For example, the surgical airway achieved prominence in the nineteenth century for the management of diphtheria and croup. It has also been incorporated into the management of patients with head and neck trauma, and of those with cancer of the upper aerodigestive tract.

In 1943, Galloway (2) recommended tracheotomy to assist in the treatment of respiratory paralysis secondary to poliomyelitis (2). This pulmonary application has expanded to assist in the management of those patients suffering from impending airway obstruction, depressed pulmonary function, aspiration, and unconsciousness. Tracheotomy is now used as an adjunct in neurologic and cardiothoracic surgery, where it offers great advantage in pulmonary toilet and respiratory control (3).

Airway management in the twentieth century has benefited from the very colorful evolution of surgical intervention. The transcervical airway has become a vital instrument in the armamentarium of the physician treating patients with airway distress. An understanding of the indications, techniques, and postoperative management of transtracheal intubation will allow the care provider to make full use of this important surgical airway intervention.

NOMENCLATURE

The terms *tracheotomy* and *tracheostomy* are used interchangeably in error. *Tracheotomy* is derived from the Greek words *tracheia arteria*, "rough artery" and *tome*, "to cut." *Tracheostomy*, on the other hand, is derived from the Greek suffix *stoma*, "to furnish with an opening or mouth." In 1923, Chevalier Jackson made the clinical

R. S. Isaacs: Department of Otolaryngology-Head and Neck Surgery, University of California, Davis Medical Center, Sacramento, California 95817; and Kaiser-Permanente, Northern California Region, Sacramento, California 95823.

J. M. Sykes: Department of Otolaryngology-Head and Neck Surgery, University of California, Davis School of Medicine and Medical Center, Sacramento, California 95817.

distinction between the terms *tracheotomy* and *tracheostomy* (4). *Tracheotomy* is "the operation of opening the trachea." Jackson performed tracheostomy only to treat airway obstruction where a more permanent opening was indicated. The tracheostomy was a procedure that exteriorized the trachea to the cervical skin until the opening had become epithelialized with epidermis to form a permanent stoma.

Therefore, the term *tracheostomy* should be reserved for those tracheotomy procedures in which a more permanent tracheal cutaneous fistula is desired.

CAUSES OF AIRWAY PROBLEMS

Assessment of Airway Compromise

Every patient with potential airway obstruction must be evaluated and managed in an expedient fashion. Upper airway obstruction must be differentiated from respiratory distress caused by pulmonary, cardiovascular, and neurologic disorders.

If the airway is stable, a careful medical history and thorough physical examination are essential for the effective management of airway obstruction. Historic points should address the nature and character of the onset of airway distress as well as the associated inciting factors. Important aspects of the physical examination include indirect laryngoscopy, digital examination of the oropharynx, and palpation of the neck. Chest auscultation and percussion may reveal important signs of lower airway compromise.

Depending on the severity of the upper airway obstruction, the signs and symptoms may vary from exertional dyspnea to severe stridor. Extreme airway obstruction may present as complete apnea. When stridor is present, the type of stridor may be suggestive of the location of the obstruction. Inspiratory stridor is typically indicative of partial supraglottic airway obstruction, while expiratory stridor may represent a lower airway lesion. Inspiratory and expiratory stridor suggest partial obstruction at the level of the glottis. When the obstruction is in the oropharyngeal or supraglottic region, a rattling type of noisy breathing is noted. This is most marked on inspiration, and relief may occur when the tongue or mandible are pulled forward. The following conditions should be considered in the differential diagnosis of airway obstruction.

Adults

Neoplasms

Neoplasms of the oral cavity, nasopharynx, oropharynx, hypopharynx, and larynx may give rise to airway obstruction. In the adult, the most common malignant neoplasm is squamous cell carcinoma. These tumors typically present with other signs and symptoms (e.g., local pain, dysphagia, and odynophagia) before they cause airway obstruction. Other malignant neoplasms that may cause airway obstruction include tumors of minor salivary gland origin and large tumors arising from the parapharyngeal space. Benign tumors from these origins may also cause obstruction. Lingual thyroid glands, hemangiomas, and vallecular cysts are a few examples of benign neoplasms that can cause obstruction. Although primary tracheal neoplasms are rare, tumors arising from the adjacent thyroid and esophagus may produce extrinsic masses that narrow the tracheal lumen. Typically, the airway obstruction in neoplasia occurs gradually, and some degree of respiratory compensation may be noted.

Trauma

The classic symptoms associated with blunt laryngeal trauma include hoarseness, laryngeal pain, dyspnea, and dysphagia. Alterations in the vocal cords, such as hematoma or edema, may produce hoarseness and pain. With progression of an injury, the hoarseness may worsen, and the patient may complain of more pain. At this point, the patient will usually have difficulty swallowing, due to the pain and to aerodigestive mechanical changes (i.e., edema, hypopharyngeal or esophageal laceration). Subcutaneous emphysema may be present. Dyspnea may worsen and progress to subsequent apnea. When significant laryngeal obstruction is present, emergent establishment of an alternative airway is indicated.

Another traumatic laryngeal injury that deserves special attention is that of laryngotracheal separation, or the so-called clothesline injury. This injury typically occurs when the victim is riding a motorcycle or snowmobile and the neck strikes a stationary object such as a wire fence or a tree branch. The force of impact is typically so great that the laryngeal cartilages become crushed, and the cricoid cartilage dissociates from the thyroid cartilage. Survivors of these injuries usually have a tenuous airway held together precariously by mucous membrane bridging the cartilages. This injury mandates urgent tracheotomy because intubation attempts may worsen the injury and produce false passages.

Operations on the upper aerodigestive tract may cause airway obstruction. The postoperative edema incurred following surgery of the oral cavity, oropharynx, and hypopharynx frequently necessitates close airway observation and even elective tracheotomy.

Postextubation Obstruction

Following prolonged intubation, the extubated patient may demonstrate signs and symptoms of upper airway obstruction. The presence of the endotracheal tube may produce upper aerodigestive tract edema, with resultant stridor and respiratory distress. The obstruction most commonly occurs at the level of the vocal cords or the subglottic region, and the obstruction is usually caused by the indwelling endotracheal tube. This is particularly true if the endotracheal cuff had been inflated to promote mechanical ventilation. Associated injuries include glottic, subglottic, and tracheal stenoses, as well as bilateral arytenoid fixation. When airway distress is imminent, reintubation should be avoided. A tracheotomy should be performed, followed by a diagnostic laryngoscopy. Once the cause of the airway distress is identified, subsequent treatment can be planned accordingly.

Infection and Inflammation

Severe tonsillar, peritonsillar, and retropharyngeal infection can present with airway obstruction. The adult form of epiglottitis is usually not as severe as the childhood form, although it can produce severe airway distress in the adult. Deep neck infections, in particular Ludwig's angina (severe infection in the floor of mouth, usually from dental origin), are known for their ability to produce upper airway obstruction.

Foreign Body

A foreign object may be aspirated into the larynx and trachea, with resultant partial or complete upper airway obstruction. A properly performed Heimlich maneuver may expel the foreign body from the airway. When only partial airway obstruction is present, the patient should be transferred to a local hospital for evaluation. Inspiratory and expiratory chest radiographs may identify the site of obstruction in preparation for endoscopic foreign body removal.

Neurogenic Disorders

The most common form of neurogenic airway obstruction in adults is bilateral vocal cord paralysis. This paralysis results in a paramedian vocal cord position and frequently produces a glottic opening of only 3 mm. This narrowed glottis can produce significant airway obstruction. In sedentary individuals, bilateral vocal cord paralysis may not produce significant airway symptoms. These larynges, however, are compromised and may become obstructed with minimal glottic edema of infection or trauma. The most common etiology of bilateral vocal cord paralysis in adults is iatrogenic (i.e., total thyroidectomy), although neoplasms of the mediastinum, thyroid, esophagus, and skull base can also produce this abnormality.

Laryngospasm

Acute laryngospasm can be precipitated by paroxysmal coughing, a laryngeal foreign body, or emergence from general anesthesia. Acute laryngospasm is usually self-limited. Occasionally, the stimulus of hypercarbia or hypoxia are necessary before laryngospasm resolves. Emergent airway intervention is rarely required.

Angioneurotic Edema

Allergic reactions may precipitate angioneurotic edema, particularly when the susceptible individual contacts the inciting allergen. The soft tissues of the lips, oral cavity, tongue, oropharynx, hypopharynx, and larynx become edematous, and airway obstruction ensues in the absence of prompt treatment. The treatment includes intravenous injection of epinephrine (0.5–1.0 cc repeated boluses of 1:10,000 dilution), intravenous injections of 25–50 mg of diphenhydramine hydrochloride (Benadryl™) with close airway observation, as well as the general treatment of allergic reactions. Intravenous steroids may be of benefit. Intubation or tracheotomy is performed in severe obstructive cases.

Children

Congenital Laryngeal Anomalies

Congenital laryngeal anomalies represent the most common causes of upper airway obstruction in children. Abnormalities of the nasal cavity, oral cavity, and pharynx may also contribute to airway obstruction. Although airway obstruction usually manifests at birth, some conditions do not present until the lesion has reached a critical size or associated inflammation contributes to further airway compromise.

Nasal Obstruction

Nasal obstruction may be responsible for respiratory distress in neonates. However, nasal obstruction rarely causes significant airway problems in older children or adults. The newborn is an obligate nasal breather until about 12 weeks of age. In neonates with bilateral nasal obstruction, asphyxiation may develop. The classic presentation of bilateral nasal obstruction is that of cyanosis and airway obstruction that absolves when the child cries and opens its mouth. This presentation may rarely be seen in cases of unilateral nasal obstruction. The nasal airway may be obstructed because of (1) bilateral choanal atresia; (2) nasal tumors and masses; (3) hypertrophied or inflamed adenoid tissue; and (4) inflammatory processes related to viral infections, drugs, and foreign bodies.

Oropharyngeal Obstruction

Oropharyngeal obstruction is generally related to congenital disorders of the tongue and its relation to the mandible. Obstruction may occur when the tongue is too large for the oral cavity, when the mandible is retrodisplaced, or when a disease process in the floor of the mouth displaces the tongue posteriorly. Characteristically, the obstruction is most marked when the patient is supine, and some relief is obtained when the patient is prone or the tongue is pulled forward.

Congenital disorders that may cause oropharyngeal obstruction include (1) the Pierre Robin sequence of micrognathia, glossoptosis, and cleft palate, (2) congenital macroglossia from Down syndrome or benign vascular tumors of the tongue (hemangioma), (3) tumors of the tongue and oropharynx (lingual thyroid or large thyroglossal duct cyst), and (4) congenital masses in the floor of the mouth or parapharyngeal space (ranula, salivary tumors, or cystic hygroma). Acquired causes of oropharyngeal obstruction include hypertrophic or inflamed tonsils and adenoids, and deep neck infections with abscesses of the peritonsillar, parapharyngeal, and retropharyngeal spaces.

Laryngeal Disorders

Laryngeal obstruction in children is caused most commonly by laryngomalacia (immature cartilaginous support of the supraglottic structures). The laryngeal disorders can be classified by location: supraglottic (large congenital cysts), glottic (bilateral vocal cord paralysis, glottic webs, and glottic stenoses), and subglottic (congenital and acquired stenoses and hemangiomas).

Tracheobronchial Obstruction

Tracheobronchial respiratory obstruction in children may be caused by congenital or acquired pulmonary abnormalities. These etiologies may be further divided as extrinsic (anomalous great vessels or tracheobronchogenic cysts) and intrinsic (foreign body, inspissated secretions, or tumors affecting the airway).

DECISION ANALYSIS IN AIRWAY MANAGEMENT

The airway decision process is a complex one and requires consideration of several factors to ensure the appropriate intervention for the individual patient. These factors include the relative risk–benefit analyses of tracheotomy versus alternative methods of intervention (algorithm).

AIRWAY DISTRESS ALGORITHM

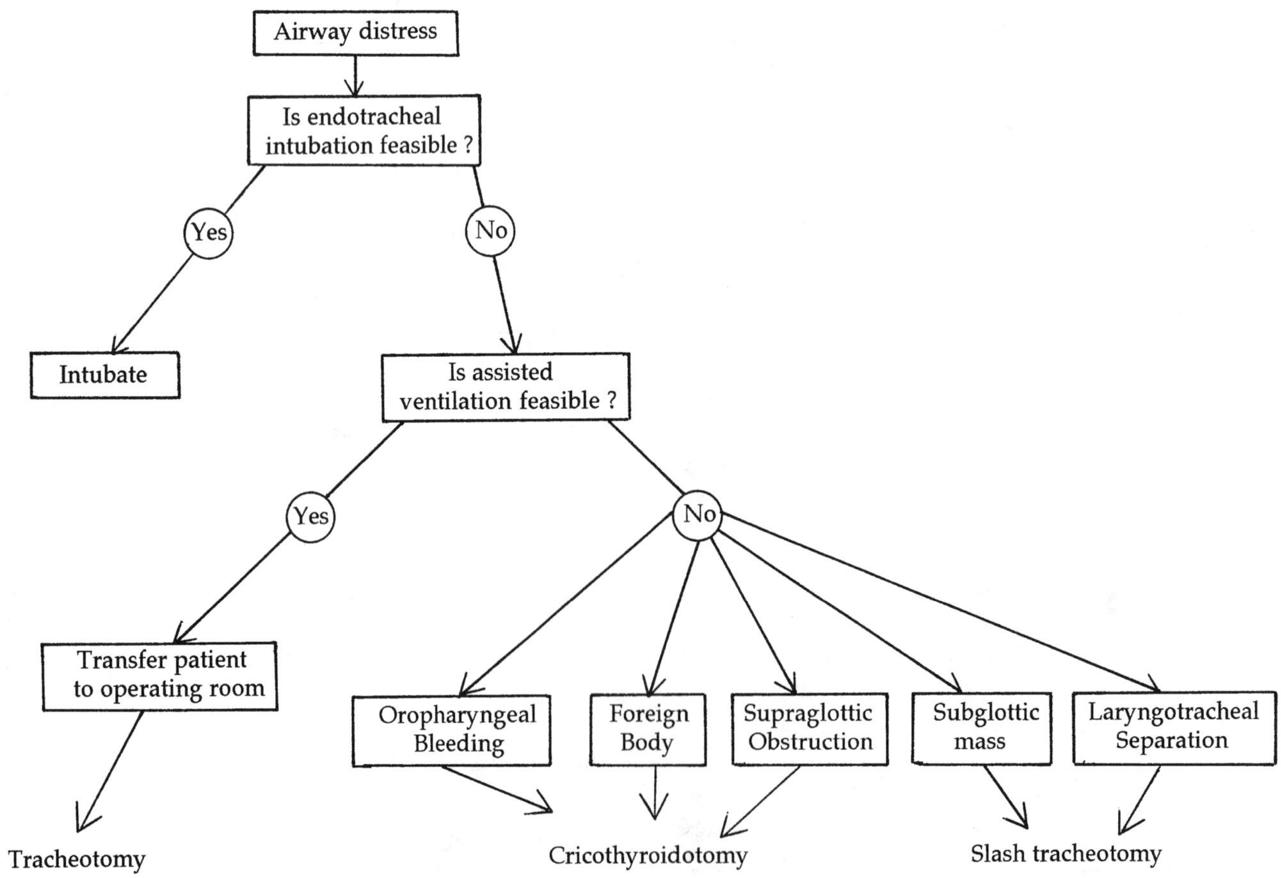

Preliminary Management

Patients in airway distress should be comforted as much as possible. They should be postured in a seated position and supported with supplemental oxygen. A face mask is usually well tolerated by adult patients, while children will typically tolerate oxygen provided by the mask held only near the face. The use of intravenous steroids remains debated. When the glottis has suffered injury, steroids may reduce the degree of laryngeal edema. However, expanding laryngeal hematomas and laryngeal fractures are largely unaffected by the use of steroids. Nevertheless, the potential benefits of steroids usually outweigh the risks and remain the authors' preference in many cases of airway distress.

Airway compromise should be managed expeditiously, preferably before an emergency ensues. Oroendotracheal intubation is the safest and the preferred method of emergent upper airway control. If endotracheal intubation is not feasible (i.e., in cases of nasopharyngeal or oropharyngeal obstruction), surgical intervention is required. Surgical management of the airway should be performed in a controlled setting, preferably in the operating room where all facilities will be available, including adequate lighting, specialized intubation equipment, and supplies for tracheotomy.

Indications for Tracheotomy

The primary objective of tracheotomy is to provide a secure airway. Current indications for tracheotomy are: (1) to relieve upper airway obstruction, (2) to provide a means for assisting mechanical ventilation, (3) to enable more efficient pulmonary hygiene, (4) for the elimination of pulmonary dead space, and (5) for the relief of obstructive sleep apnea.

Upper Airway Obstruction

Tracheotomy is emergently indicated when the cardinal signs of laryngeal obstruction are present and the placement of an endotracheal tube is not possible (Table 1). Anatomic obstruction to endotracheal intubation may result from foreign body, laryngeal trauma, laryngotracheal separation, maxillofacial trauma, or tumor.

Local anesthesia is usually necessary in cases in which endotracheal intubation is not feasible and can render the tracheotomy procedure entirely painless. Muscle relaxants should be avoided when an endotracheal tube cannot be placed. This will ensure maintenance of spontaneous respiration. Specialized anesthetic techniques are dependent on the age of the patient, the degree of respiratory obstruction, and the nature of the underlying disease.

TABLE 1. *Situation requiring emergency tracheotomy*

Musculoskeletal disorders
Ankylosis of the temporomandibular joint
Cervical arthritis
Trismus (inflammatory/neoplastic)
Infection
Ludwig's angina
Neoplasms
Obstructing oropharyngeal, laryngeal, and thyroid tumors
Trauma
Massive hemorrhage into tissues of the neck, pharynx, and tongue
Traumatic disruption of the trachea or larynx
Miscellaneous
Foreign body impacted into the larynx or upper trachea

Respiratory Support

Airway intervention may be indicated for prolonged respiratory support, particularly when a ventilator for positive pressure ventilation is needed. These patients usually have underlying pulmonary or neurogenic disease.

Pulmonary Hygiene

Frequently, patients with pneumonia, bronchiectasis, or other pulmonary inflammatory disorders will require airway intervention to provide access to suction the lower airway. The paralyzed or unconscious patient who is unable to clear normal secretions by an adequate cough mechanism is at risk for developing a life-threatening bronchorrhea. Similarly, the patient suffering central nervous system injury may develop a chronic aspiration that requires pulmonary toilet through an endotracheal tube or tracheotomy.

Elimination of Dead Space

The anatomic respiratory dead space includes those areas that are not available for gas exchange. The premiere area of gas exchange is at the alveoli and bronchioles. Minimal effective gas exchange takes place in the larger bronchi and upper aerodigestive tract. The oral and nasal cavities, the pharynx, and the larynx must be filled with inspired air. This dead space area represents approximately 150 ml. In the tachypneic pulmonary patient, a tracheotomy will usually help pulmonary function by reducing this nonuseful respiratory space.

Sleep Apnea

Patients suffering from sleep apnea represent a unique group that requires tracheotomy. These patients may have a normal upper airway while awake. During sleep, however, hypopharyngeal and upper airway collapse causes obstruction. Tracheotomy relieves the apneic symptoms and allows the otolaryngologist to identify and modify the upper airway, with hope for eventual tracheal decannulation.

Once the indication for tracheotomy has been reached, intervention should be carried out on an elective basis. This provides the best circumstances for both the surgeon and the patient. The procedure should be performed in a controlled setting, with adequate lighting, instrumentation, and assistance.

Indications for Cricothyroidotomy

Cricothyroidotomy is a technique that has been advocated as the most efficient and effective method of obtaining an emergency airway (Table 2). The procedure is quite simple to perform, and an emergent airway can be obtained in seconds. There are specific instances in trauma, foreign bodies, airway obstruction from neoplasms, and respiratory failure that dictate immediate entrance into the trachea. The insertion of an endotracheal tube may not be feasible simply because the appropriate skill and instrumentation are lacking, particularly outside of the hospital facility.

The safest and easiest point of tracheal entrance is the cricothyroid membrane. This section of the laryngotracheal complex is anatomically thin, relatively avascular, positioned above the thyroid isthmus, and is positioned below the level of the true vocal cords. The cricothyroid membrane lies just under the skin, making for a very rapid dissection to the level of the trachea. Cricothyroid entrance is accomplished with whatever instrument is available to cut the skin and the membrane. A scalpel, razor blade, pocket knife, scissors, hemostat, and large-bore needle have all been used successfully. Once the membrane is opened, a tube can be inserted into the subglottic trachea.

TABLE 2. *Cricothyroidotomy*

Indications
Emergent airway intervention when orotracheal intubation is not possible.
Advantages
Speed of tracheal entry (seconds)
Disadvantages
Bleeding (inferior laryngeal artery)
Pressure from the tube may induce necrosis of cricoid cartilage
Not effective for bypass of subglottic or tracheal obstructions
Allows for the insertion of only a small tracheotomy tube
Chondritis may result in stenosis; therefore, cricothyroidotomy should be converted to tracheotomy, electively within 24 hours.

TABLE 3. *Emergent tracheotomy "slash trach"*

Indications
Immediate tracheal entrance is imperative and cricothyroidotomy is not applicable (subglottic carcinoma, thyroid tumors)
Advantages
Can be performed by a single surgeon
Can be performed quickly
Disadvantages
Bleeding can be profuse
Hemostasis is achieved after the placement of the tracheal airway

When the patient's condition has stabilized, cricothyroidotomy should be converted to a tracheotomy at the third tracheal ring. In order to reduce the laryngeal complications associated with cricothyroidotomy, the elective tracheotomy should be performed within the first 24 hours (see section on complications of cricothyroidotomy).

Indications for Emergency Midline Tracheotomy

The emergency midline tracheotomy should be used in the rare emergent airway situation where the cricothyroidotomy is not applicable, for example, in cases of true subglottic obstruction (Table 3). Subglottic obstruction is usually caused by subglottic laryngeal carcinoma or large thyroid tumors. In some cases, the subglottic obstruction is identified during cricothyroidotomy, at which time the procedure is rapidly converted to the midline vertical "slash" tracheotomy.

Emergency midline tracheotomy should be considered a heroic, lifesaving measure when it is necessary. It is technically much more difficult, bloody, and dangerous when compared to elective tracheotomy or cricothyroidotomy.

TECHNIQUE

Figure 1 demonstrates the surface anatomy of the neck and the location of the transcervical airway interventions. The cricothyroid membrane has a relatively superficial location and is easily penetrated to establish an airway in an emergency situation. The trachea is located slightly deeper within the soft tissue of the anterior neck. The location of the trachea varies and, in some patients, can create significant technical difficulty when establishing a tracheal airway.

Elective Tracheotomy

Restoration of normal pulmonary ventilation with an oroendotracheal tube provides optimal operating condi-

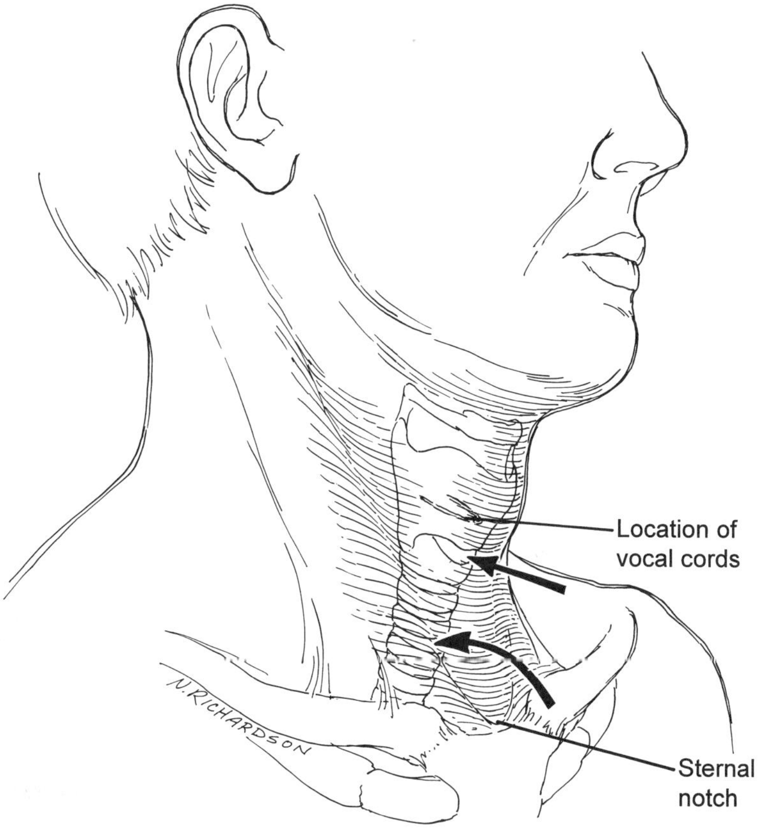

FIG. 1. Right anterior oblique view of the neck, showing the location of the laryngotracheal complex in relation to the anterior neck skin. Note the cricothyroid membrane *(straight arrow)*, where a cricothyroidotomy would be performed. The area for standard tracheotomy is indicated *(curved arrow)*. Of importance is the fact that the cricothyroid membrane is much closer to the skin than the tracheotomy site. This area also contains a marked decrease in superficial vasculature. The site for tracheotomy is much further from the skin and has more blood vessels in the region.

tions in elective tracheotomy. The placement of a tracheal tube or bronchoscope will maintain the airway and facilitate palpation of the trachea during dissection. This is very important in children, because their soft tracheal cartilages are difficult to palpate during the procedure.

The patient's neck is extended by the placement of a bolster under the shoulders. The incision site is infiltrated with local anesthesia (2% lidocaine with 1/100,000 epinephrine). The low anterior neck is infiltrated, then the injection is carried deeper through the underlying muscu-

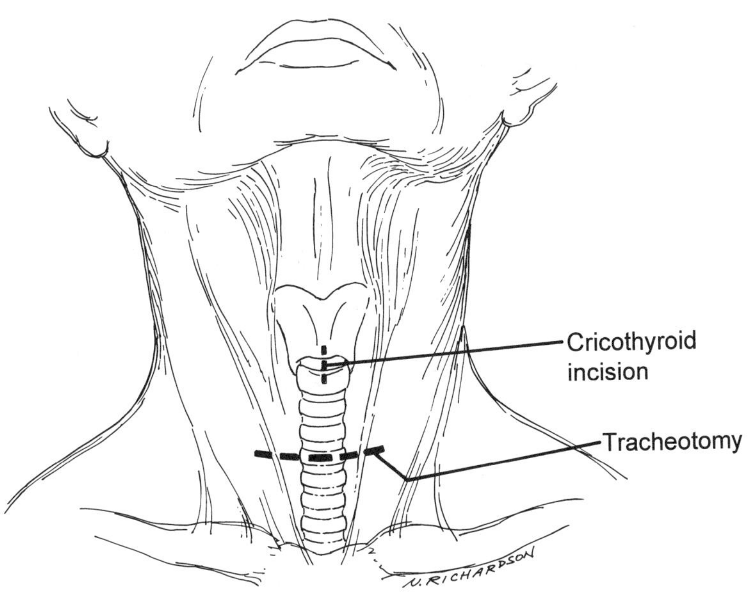

FIG. 2. Schematic diagram of the neck depicting the cricothyroidotomy and tracheotomy incisions. The cricothyroidotomy incision is usually made in a vertical orientation and the tracheotomy incision is made in the horizontal orientation along the relaxed skin tension lines approximately two fingers breadths above the sternal notch.

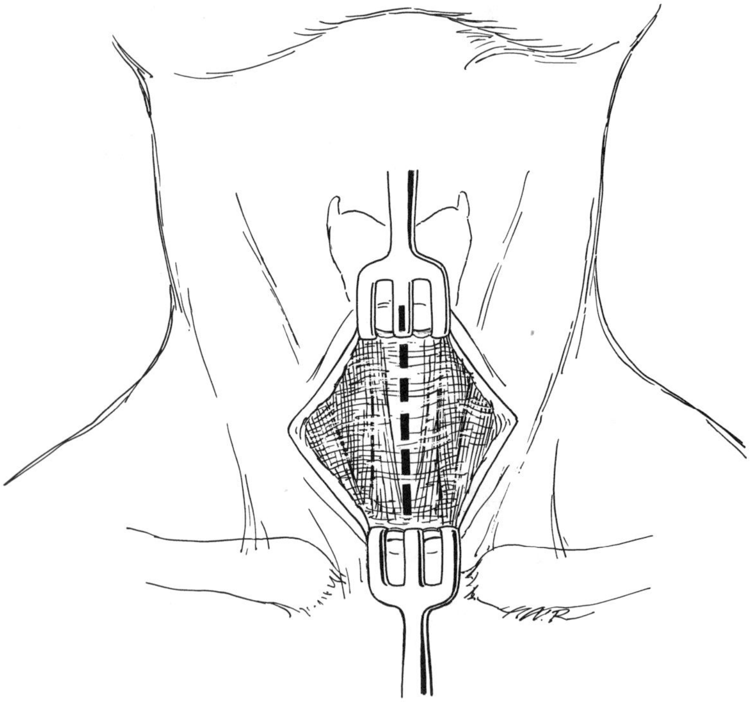

FIG. 3. Schematic diagram illustrating the investing layer of the deep cervical fascia, which is incised in a vertical fashion to expose the peritracheal fascia and trachea.

lar planes until the pretracheal fascia is infiltrated. The neck is then surgically prepared with a povidone-iodine scrub and paint, and the anterior neck is draped.

The laryngeal skeleton is palpated, and the space between the second and third tracheal cartilages is identified. A horizontal skin incision is made in a natural skin crease about 1–2 finger breadths above the sternal notch. Figure 2 shows the location of skin incisions in the anterior neck for tracheotomy and cricothyroidotomy. The skin and subcutaneous tissues are incised as the dissec-

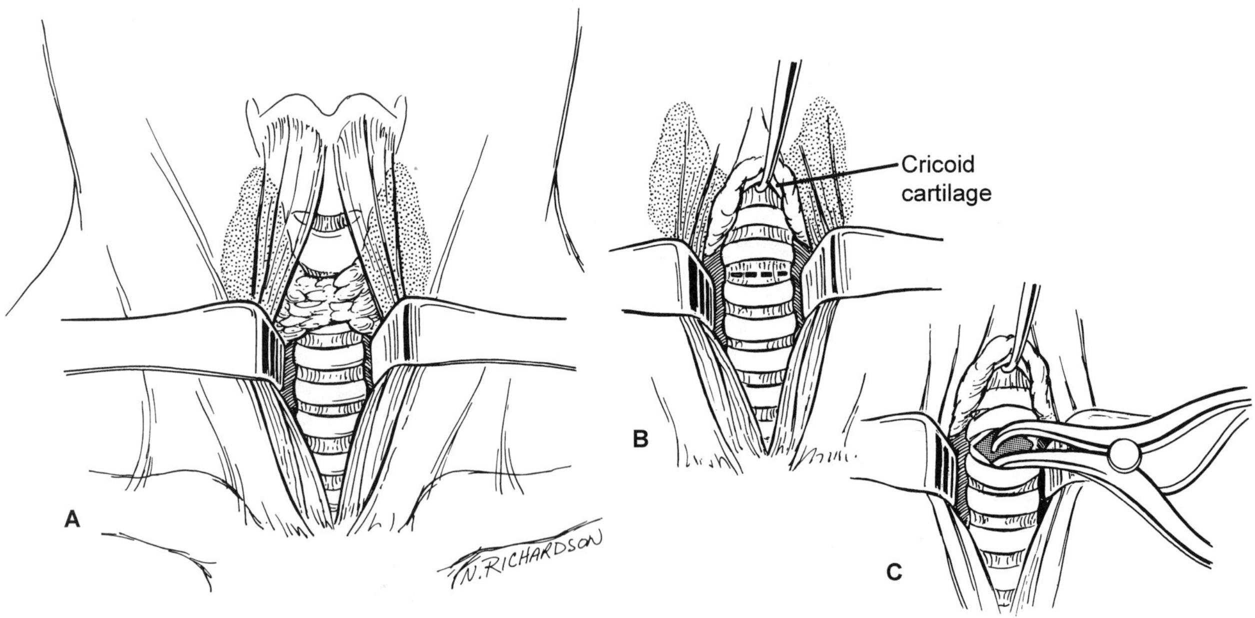

FIG. 4. A: Diagram illustrating lateral retraction of the sternohyoid and sternothyroid muscles to expose the trachea. **B:** A tracheal hook is inserted into the cricoid cartilage for elevation and immobilization of the trachea. A horizontal incision in the area between the second and third tracheal cartilages is illustrated *(dotted line)*. **C:** After horizontal incision in the intercartilaginous membrane, a tracheal dilator is inserted to maintain the open tracheotomy site. This facilitates the insertion of the tracheotomy tube.

tion continues to the investing layer of the deep cervical fascia. Here, the strap muscles and the midline raphe are identified (Fig. 3). Just superficial to the strap muscles, the anterior jugular veins can be identified in the investing fascia. It is usually not necessary to divide these vessels. A vertical midline incision is made that allows for lateral retraction of the sternohyoid and sternothyroid musculature (Fig. 4A). The thyroid isthmus is then identified at the second to fourth tracheal cartilages. The thyroid isthmus can be gently retracted cephalad or caudad, or the isthmus can be divided between two surgical clamps and tied with a suture ligature to expose the anterior tracheal wall (Fig. 4B).

A tracheal hook is inserted under the cricoid cartilage or under the first tracheal cartilage to elevate and immobilize the trachea. Before the tracheal incision is made, the endotracheal cuff is deflated, and the tip of the tube is withdrawn just to the level of the cricoid cartilage, in case there is a delay in the introduction of the tracheotomy tube. A small scalpel blade is used to make the tracheal opening. The Trousseau dilator maintains the opening during passage of the tube (Fig. 4C). The tracheal tube is inserted with the inner obturator in position. The distal end of the tube is initially directed posteriorly, and the tube is then gently pushed inferiorly, following the curve of the tube. The obturator is then removed, and the inner cannula is inserted and locked into position.

Ventilation commences through the tracheotomy tube. The tube is then secured with circumferential cloth trach ties. For added security, the tracheotomy tube flange can be sutured to the skin. A postoperative chest radiograph should be obtained to rule out pneumothorax and to determine proper tracheotomy tube positioning.

Incisions in the trachea can be varied and include the horizontal intercartilaginous, cartilaginous resection, cruciate, superiorly and inferiorly based tracheal flap inci-

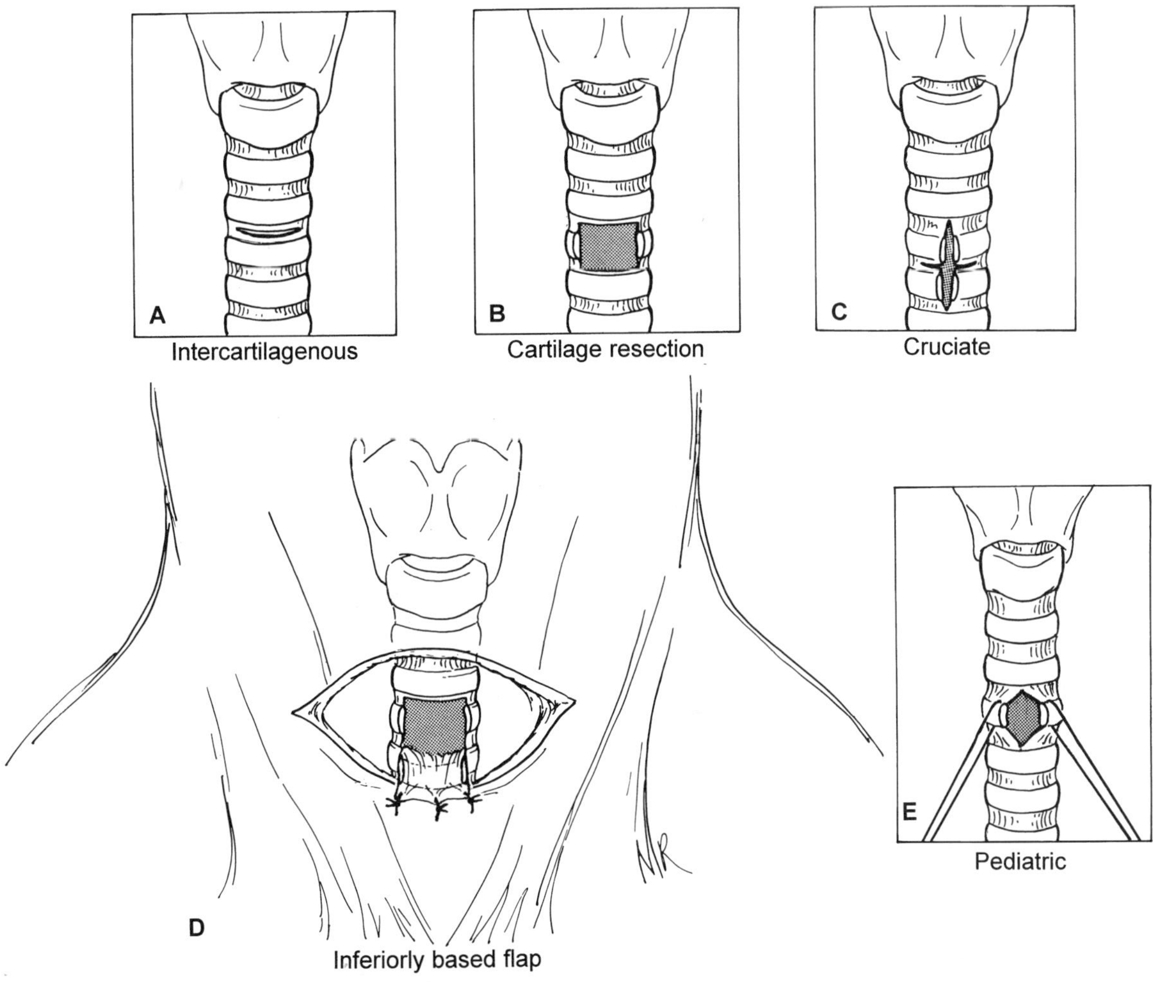

FIG. 5. Various incisions used to enter the trachea for insertion of the tracheotomy tube. **A:** Horizontal intercartilaginous incision. **B:** Cartilaginous resection with creation of an anterior tracheal window. **C:** Cruciate incision. **D:** Inferiorly based flap creating a semipermanent tracheostomy site. **E:** Vertical incision in the pediatric patient with the placement of left and right tracheal sutures, which are helpful in the case of accidental tracheotomy tube displacement.

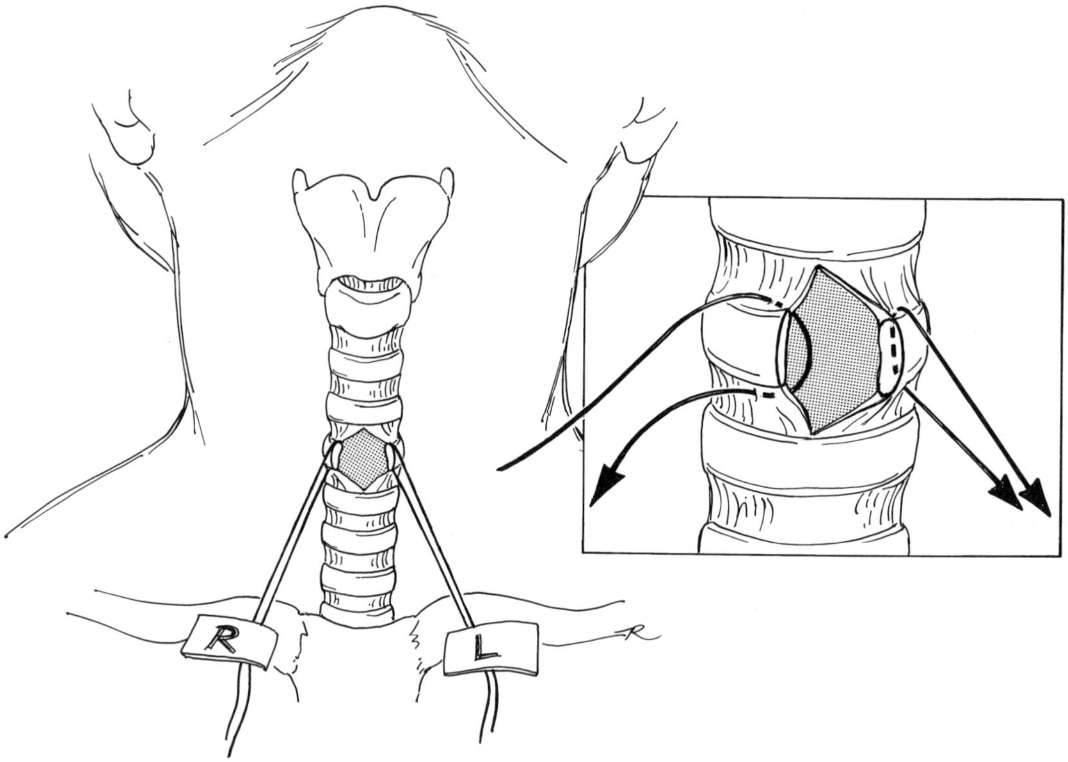

FIG. 6. Schematic diagram of the pediatric trachea showing the placement of right *(R)* and left *(L)* tracheal sutures for security and stabilization. The inset shows the placement of these sutures adjacent to the vertical tracheotomy incision.

sions, and the vertical cartilaginous incision (Fig. 5). In general, the incisions that disturb the anatomy of the trachea the least provide the best result. Destruction of the tracheal architecture can result in later tracheal stenosis following tracheal decannulation. In the patient requiring a long-term or more permanent tracheotomy, a tracheal flap pedicled on the trachea and sutured to the skin is desired.

The vertical cartilaginous incision is the preferred tracheal incision in children. The vertical cartilaginous tracheal incision, when performed in the child, should be performed through the third tracheal cartilage (Fig. 6). The placement of designated left and right tracheal sutures will assist in airway management in the event of accidental tracheotomy tube displacement.

Cricothyroidotomy

The technique of cricothyroidotomy is relatively simple. The neck is first hyperextended by the placement of a bolster or pillow under the shoulders. The laryngeal landmarks of the thyroid and cricoid cartilages are then palpated, and a vertical incision is made through the skin and underlying soft tissue at the superior aspect of the cricoid cartilage. The tough avascular cricothyroid membrane is then penetrated, and gas will exchange as the cricothyroid space is opened (Fig. 7A). The best instrument for cricothyroidotomy is a scalpel with a #11 blade; however, a pocket knife, scissors, or other available sharp object may be used in the field. Once the airway is entered, the blade is twisted to open the space that will allow the insertion of a standard tracheotomy tube (Fig. 7B). Any available tube can be inserted, including the barrel of a ballpoint pen, in an emergency.

Emergency Midline Tracheotomy

The patient is positioned as in elective tracheotomy, and the surface landmarks are rapidly palpated. A vertical incision is then made in the midline just below the cricoid cartilage and carried through the skin, subcutaneous tissue, and platysma in one stroke to about one finger breadth above the sternum. The trachea is immobilized with the surgeon's thumb and fingers of the left hand. The incision is then carried down to the level of the trachea. If possible, the thyroid isthmus is retracted. If the thyroid cannot be retracted, the isthmus is totally disregarded at this point. The trachea is split in the midline, and the left index finger is used to confirm the tracheal lumen. A tube is then inserted into the trachea, using the left index finger as a guide. Hemostasis is obtained after successful placement of the tracheotomy tube.

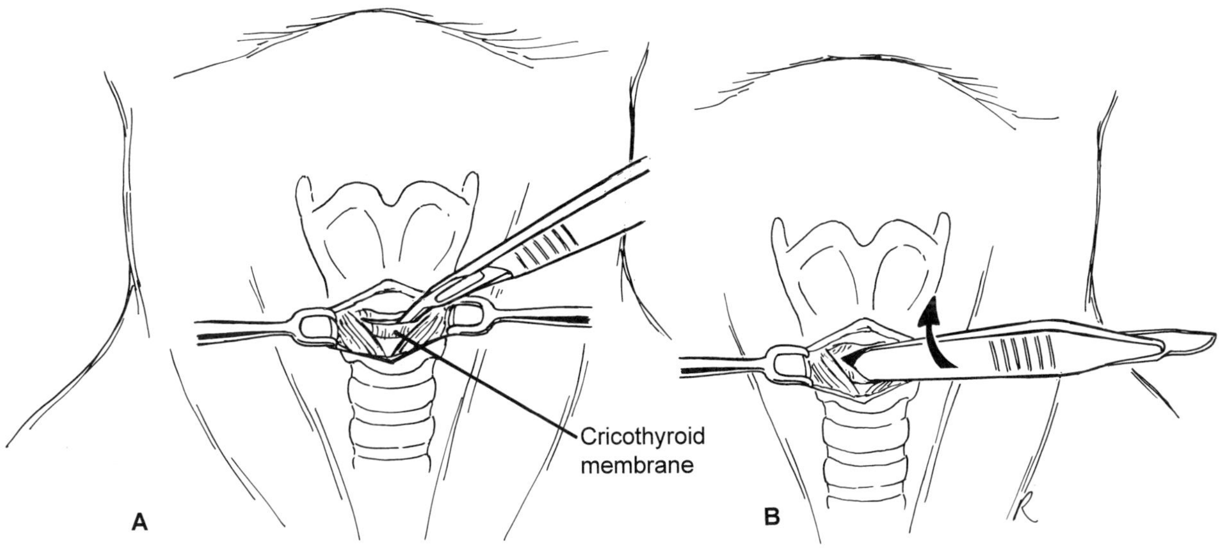

FIG. 7. A: Horizontal incision in the cricothyroid membrane during cricothyroidotomy. **B:** The handle of the knife blade is inserted into the cricothyroid incision and rotated 90° to allow insertion of standard tracheotomy tube.

Tracheotomy Tube Size Selection

The choice of a particular tracheotomy tube should be dependent on the indication for its use. For example, a patient requiring ventilatory support should be fitted with a tracheotomy tube having a low-pressure cuff. The low-pressure cuffs offer the broadest possible surface area, thereby reducing the chance of the development of a tube-related pressure ulcer. A cuffed tube is frequently utilized if aspiration is an anticipated problem. Although even the best of cuffed tubes do not completely prevent aspiration, their use can diminish the volume of aspirates.

TABLE 4. *Selection of tracheotomy tubes*

Age	French size	Internal diameter (mm)	Tracheotomy tube size
Infants and children			
Premature			00
Newborn	12	2.5	00–0
6 months	16	3.5	0–1
1 year	20	4.5	1–2
2 years	22	5.0	2
4 years	24	5.5	3
6 years	26	6.0	4
8 years	28	6.5	4
10 years	30	7.0	4
12 years	32	7.5	5
14 years	34	8.0	5
Adults			
Female	34–36	8.0–8.5	5
Male	36–40	8.5–9.5	6
Special cases			8–10

In the patient with an intact swallowing reflex, a fenestrated uncuffed trach tube is appropriate. This tube allows an unobstructed air flow through the glottis, which facilitates phonation when the tracheotomy tube is manually occluded with a finger. Some surgeons oppose the use of fenestrated tracheotomy tubes and state that these tubes may predispose to an increased incidence of tracheal granulation tissue.

Current manufacturers of tracheotomy tubes offer a wide variety of choices. Unfortunately, there is a lack of standardization of tube sizes. There is a system of tracheotomy tube sizes based on the outer diameter (OD) measurements in millimeters. Due to variability in the material used by the various tracheotomy tube producers, the correlation between OD dimension and size number is not consistent among manufacturers. Clinically, the inner diameter (ID) is used to determine the appropriate tracheotomy tube for a particular patient. Table 4 provides a general guideline to tube size selection, based on patient age. The following formula is useful in selecting the appropriate ID of the tracheotomy tube:

$$\text{Required inner diameter (mm)} = (\text{age in years})/4 + 4.5$$

For example, a child who is 4 years of age will require a tracheotomy tube with an inner diameter of 5.5 mm ($4/4 + 4.5 = 5.5$).

COMPLICATIONS

The complications associated with tracheotomy can be minimized by a thorough knowledge of the problems that result from surgical airway intervention. The complica-

TABLE 5. *Complications of tracheotomy*

Procedural
Subcutaneous emphysema, pneumomediastinum, pneumothorax
Hemorrhage
Tracheal/esophageal perforation
Postobstructive pulmonary edema
Early (immediate postoperative period)
Stoma infections
Tracheitis
Tracheotomy tube obstruction/dislodgement
Aspiration
Delayed
Tracheoinnominate artery fistula
Tracheoesophageal fistula
Tracheal granulations
Tracheal stenosis
Subglottic stenosis
Vocal cord dysfunction
Unattractive scar

tions are conveniently classified according to their time of presentation: (a) procedural, (b) early (immediately postoperative), and (c) delayed (Table 5).

Complications of Tracheotomy

Procedural Complications

Subcutaneous Emphysema, Pneumothorax, and Pneumomediastinum

The presence of air in the subcutaneous tissues is not an uncommon finding after tracheotomy. Subcutaneous emphysema can often extend diffusely over the face and chest. This frequently occurs by the surgical dissection during tracheotomy. It may also occur when the skin is closed tightly after the procedure, trapping coughed air into the subcutaneous space. Subcutaneous emphysema is not a serious problem and requires no treatment. However, it may also signify that air is present in the thoracic cavity.

Pneumomediastinum is caused by air dissecting through the fascial planes of the neck into the mediastinum. This complication usually resolves spontaneously. However, if mediastinal air is excessive, it may rupture into the pleural space and cause an either simple or tension pneumothorax.

Pneumothorax can result from the same factors that produce pneumomediastinum, although the etiology may also be injury to the cupulae of the pleura. Pneumothorax occurs more frequently in pediatric tracheotomies because the pleura of a child is higher in relation to the trachea than it is in the adult. Pneumothorax is detected on postoperative chest radiography and may require chest tube drainage for correction.

Hemorrhage

During tracheotomy, troublesome bleeding can originate from the anterior jugular venous system and the thyroid gland isthmus. Electrocautery is often not adequate for the control of bleeding from these sites. Large veins should be carefully identified and suture ligated when divided. Many patients requiring tracheotomy are hypotensive during the procedure, and the transected blood vessel may go unrecognized until the blood pressure is restored or the venous pressure is increased during coughing. This may produce bleeding in the early postoperative period. Bleeding of this type is best managed by exposing the open vessel and applying a suture ligature or electrocoagulation. If the vessel cannot be exposed, the bleeding can be controlled by packing gauze into the wound and around the tube. Delayed bleeding may occur postoperatively when the local vasoconstriction from the epinephrine is lost. This bleeding will also usually respond to gauze packing. Regardless of the cause, posttracheotomy bleeding must be attended to because the aspiration of small amounts of blood can produce serious pulmonary complications.

Tracheal/Esophageal Perforation

This unusual complication can lead to devastating consequences. The surgeon must be careful not to penetrate the posterior wall of the trachea and create a fistula between the trachea and the esophagus. The performance of a tracheotomy over a bronchoscope or endotracheal tube will help avoid this complication. In addition, the surgeon should inspect the posterior tracheal wall to ascertain lack of injury before inserting the tracheal cannula.

When a posterior tracheal wall injury and fistula has been created, it should be repaired at the time of occurrence. The trachea should be dissected from the esophagus, and each structure should be repaired separately. The placement of interposing soft tissue will facilitate wound healing and prevent the development of a delayed tracheoesophageal fistula. The patient should be maintained on nasogastric tube feedings until the area has completely healed.

Postobstructive Pulmonary Edema

The phenomenon of postobstructive pulmonary edema occurs more commonly in children, although it also occurs in adults. This condition results from the sudden relief of a long-standing obstruction. The bronchioles and alveoli are suddenly exposed to a diminished positive expiratory pressure that produces a hydrostatic pressure differential between the alveoli and the pulmonary capillaries. The result is pulmonary edema caused by an influx of interstitial fluid into the alveoli. This condition requires tracheal intubation with aggressive positive-end-expiratory-pressure support and intensive care monitoring.

Early Complications (Immediately Postoperative)

Stomal Infections

Even though tracheotomy may be performed under sterile conditions, it is a matter of only a few hours until the area is colonized by many species of microorganisms. The organisms are usually mixed and include *Pseudomonas, Escherichia coli,* as well as gram positive cocci. Colonizing bacteria are typically innocuous. When infection does occur, it usually responds well to local treatment. Rare cases of more serious infection have been reported in the literature, and these include mediastinal abscess (5) and necrotizing fasciitis (6).

Tracheitis

A dry tracheitis will result if humidity is not provided to the inspired air. Crusting and dehydration of the tracheal mucosa is managed by removing the larger crusts and applying antibiotic ointment to areas of secondary infection. Tracheitis can be avoided by adding humidification to the inspired air and by the instillation of sterile saline directly into the trachea (4–6 drops intermittently).

Tracheotomy Tube Obstruction/Dislodgement

Obstruction of the tracheotomy tube is usually due to the accumulation of crusts and is prevented by strict postoperative care (as discussed in the section on tracheotomy care). Essential to this care is adequate humidification of inspired air and frequent suctioning and cleaning of the inner cannula.

The tracheotomy tube may become dislodged if the cloth ties are inadequately secured or if the cloth ties loosen postoperatively. The tracheotomy tube flange may be sutured to the skin for enhanced security. A complete set of tracheotomy instruments should be readily available during the postoperative period in order to expose the trachea for reinsertion of the tube in the event of an accidental tracheotomy tube dislodgement.

Aspiration

Aspiration is a common problem that follows tracheotomy. Some patients experience difficulties with swallowing as the tracheotomy tube may limit laryngeal excursion. This creates an inadequate epiglottic closure with resultant aspiration. In addition, the subglottic trachea is exposed to rapid inspiratory flow rates and negative pressures that also promote aspiration. Swallowing dysfunction posttracheotomy will resolve gradually in the postoperative period. If a patient aspirates, the cuffed tube should remain inflated and the trachea suctioned frequently to remove secretions (7,8).

Delayed Complications

Tracheoinnominate Artery Fistula

Severe posttracheotomy bleeding can be caused by the erosion of a major vessel, usually the innominate artery. This erosion is commonly the result of trauma to the vessel—from surgery, infection, or repeated pressure from the cuff or tracheotomy tube. Predisposing factors include an inferiorly placed tracheotomy (below the third tracheal cartilage), an excessively curved tracheotomy tube, and infection. The classic presentation of tracheoinnominate artery fistula is a sentinel bleed several hours before a massive hemorrhage. A median sternotomy is required to achieve proximal arterial control in the chest. The vessel is then oversewn with nonabsorbable sutures. The hemorrhage typically occurs without warning and is fatal in the majority of cases.

Tracheoesophageal Fistula

Tracheoesophageal fistula can occur as the result of necrosis of the intervening wall between the posterior tracheal wall and the anterior wall of the esophagus. The etiology is pressure necrosis from the tracheotomy cuff or from the tip of a malpositioned tracheotomy tube. The necrosis may be compounded by the presence of an indwelling nasogastric tube.

The tracheoesophageal fistula should be corrected by open exploration. The esophagus and trachea should be repaired and an interposition muscle flap placed to provide vascularized support to the weakened areas.

Tracheal Granulations

Granulation tissue can cause delayed hemorrhage at the tracheostoma. This tissue develops in response to both the mechanical irritation from the indwelling tracheotomy tube and to chronic bacterial exposure. Granulomas usually form on the cephalad edge of the stoma. The initial tissue is soft and vascular, but as the granuloma matures, it may become fibrous and eventually become covered with epithelium. The soft vascular granulomas can produce nuisance bleeding, while the more mature granulomas can obstruct the tracheal lumen. Large granulomas can cause difficulties with decannulation.

Several approaches have been described to remove tracheal granulomas. The very soft tracheal granulomas are removed endoscopically using a #12 Frazier suction and a cup forceps. The granuloma can be removed through the stoma and the stalk divided and cauterized with electrocautery or silver nitrate. The more mature, harder granulomas can be delivered into the stoma and the base clamped and divided. Endoscopic removal can be facilitated by the use of the CO_2 laser, which effectively vaporizes the granuloma.

Tracheal Stenosis

The fundamental lesion in tracheal stenosis is mucosal ulceration, which leads to necrosis and dissolution of the underlying cartilage (9). The defect produces loss of the supportive tracheal and cricoid cartilages, with resultant airway stenosis.

The incidence of tracheal stenosis after tracheotomy can be reduced by maintaining minimal cuff inflation and a low pressure against the tracheal wall. The development of low-pressure cuffs in the 1970s has produced a dramatic reduction in the incidence of tracheal tube-related complications.

The treatment of tracheal stenosis is determined by its extent and location within the trachea. The air tracheogram and tracheal coronal computed tomography are the most useful diagnostic methods for determining the degree of stenosis (10,11). Once the stenosis is delimited, correction is performed by resection and end-to-end tracheal anastomosis (10), staged repair involving the advancement of adjacent skin with embedded cartilage grafts to reconstruct the anterior trachea (11), or placement of carefully designed costal cartilage grafts (12). In a small number of patients in whom less than one tracheal cartilage is stenotic, the stenoses may be corrected by the endoscopic application of the CO_2 laser (13).

Subglottic Stenosis

Stenosis of the subglottic region occurs from pressure injury to the subglottic mucosa, from chondritis of the cricoid or upper tracheal cartilages, or from direct injury to the cricoid cartilage. Subglottic stenosis may require endoscopic laser techniques or open surgical repair for correction (12).

Vocal Cord Dysfunction

The location of the recurrent laryngeal nerves in the tracheoesophageal groove usually protects them from harm during tracheotomy. Injury to the recurrent nerves is unusual but can occur if the midline orientation is lost during the operation, with resultant dissection lateral to the trachea. Injury to one recurrent laryngeal nerve produces a fixed vocal cord in the paramedian position, with associated hoarseness and temporary aspiration. Aspiration persists until the contralateral cord compensates for the gap between the cords. Section of both recurrent laryngeal nerves produces a bilateral vocal cord paralysis with midline cord position. The associated glottic obstruction in vocal cord paralysis may make tracheal decannulation impossible.

Unattractive Scar

In the authors' experience, the aesthetic result of a horizontal tracheotomy scar is superior to that of the vertical scar. The unattractive scar typically develops in cases of long-standing tracheotomy tube placement and in stomas that have been infected. An unsightly scar may require plastic surgical local flap techniques for repair.

Complications of Cricothyroidotomy

This procedure is useful for emergent airway intervention in adults. In children, this procedure is fraught with hazard and should be avoided. The cervical structures are smaller in preadolescent children, and the cricoid cartilage is prone to injury. Damage to the cricoid cartilage results in a very high incidence of both glottic and subglottic stenosis, which can be very difficult to repair.

The placement of a tracheotomy tube through the cricothyroid membrane creates an inflammatory response, with ultimate fibrosis and scarring. Because of the proximity to the delicate vocal cords and subglottic region, the scarring may produce troublesome glottic and subglottic stenoses that are very challenging to repair. A cricothyroidotomy should be utilized when alternative airway methods are not feasible. To avoid complications, a cricothyroidotomy should be converted to a tracheotomy within 24 hours.

Complications of Emergency Midline Tracheotomy

Bleeding can be profuse during the vertical slash procedure from injury both to the great vessels and to the thyroid isthmus. The procedure may also be associated with the complications discussed for elective tracheotomy.

TRACHEOTOMY CARE

The emphasis of posttracheotomy care is to maintain an adequate airway and to eliminate tracheal secretions. The hospital nursing staff must routinely examine the patency of the tracheotomy tube and the inner cannula. Coughing enables the patient to centralize tracheal secretions and bring them to the level of the tracheostoma, where suctioning is easily accomplished. Deep tracheal suctioning is frequently required in the postoperative period. Bloody, tenacious secretions can occlude the airway, and their aggressive cleansing is important for the maintenance of a patent airway. Using sterile technique, a flexible catheter is inserted carefully into the tracheotomy tube to the level of the carina. The suction is then applied, and the catheter is withdrawn slowly. The instillation of 5 cc of sterile saline will help loosen dried and thickened secretions.

The presence of ventilation through the tracheotomy site eliminates the physiologic functions of the upper aerodigestive tract. The tracheotomy patient must have these functions provided artificially. The most important function, humidification, is provided with humidified air through the tracheotomy collar. Humidification prevents tracheal dryness, discomfort, and the possibility of obstruction from crusting and mucous plug formation.

The inner cannula of the tracheotomy tube should be removed and cleaned every 3–4 hours. The cannula is easily cleaned with a soft brush. It may be necessary to soak the inner cannula in hydrogen peroxide to rid the tube of hardened crusts of mucous.

The tracheotomy tube should not be changed prior to the fifth postoperative day. This time period allows for the development of a cutaneous–mucosal tract, which allows for safe recannulation of the trachea. In the event that the tracheotomy tube requires replacement earlier than the fifth postoperative day, the appropriate operative conditions should be provided (lighting, instrumentation, and assistance).

Decannulation

Before decannulation can be considered, the disease process that required initial surgical intervention must no longer exist. The tube can be removed when the inciting obstruction has been corrected. Examination of the larynx with a mirror or by direct fiberoptic endoscopy will help determine vocal cord mobility and airway patency. Observation of the patient's ability to protect the airway from aspiration is also important.

A very practical approach to decannulation is to first test the patency of the airway by converting the tracheotomy tube to a smaller uncuffed tube. By manually occluding the tracheotomy tube and observing the patient's respiration through the nose and mouth, an accurate assessment of the airway can be made. If the patient has an adequate airway under the occluded circumstances, removal of the tube should be well tolerated. Tube removal is usually performed 18–24 hours following successful tracheotomy tube occlusion.

ACKNOWLEDGMENTS

The authors wish to again thank Nelva Richardson (medical illustrator) for her time, energy, and artistic creativity.

REFERENCES

1. Goldman JL, Blaugrund SM, Friedman WH. Tracheostomy. In: English GM, ed. *Otolaryngology. Plastic and Reconstructive Surgery of the Head and Neck*, vol 4. Hagerstown, MD: Harper and Row, 1983.
2. Galloway TC. Tracheostomy in bulbar poliomyelitis. *JAMA* 1943; 128, 1096.
3. Head JM. Tracheostomy in the management of respiratory problems. *N Engl J Med* 1961;264:578–591.
4. Jackson C. High tracheotomy and other errors—the chief causes of chronic laryngeal stenosis. *Surg Gynecol Obstet* 1923;32:392.
5. Cole AG, Kerr JH. Paratracheal abscess after tracheostomy. *Intensive Care Med* 1983;9:345.
6. Snow N, Richardson JD, Flint LM. Management of necrotizing tracheostomy infections. *J Thorac Cardiovasc Surg* 1981;82:341.
7. Bonnano PC. Swallowing dysfunction after tracheostomy. *Ann Surg* 1971;174:29–33.
8. Sasaki CT, Susuki M, Horiuchi M, Kirshner JA. The effect of tracheotomy on the laryngeal closure reflex. *Laryngoscope* 1977;87:1428.
9. Andrews MJ, Pearson FG. Incidence and pathogenesis of tracheal injury following cuffed tube tracheostomy with assisted ventilation. *Ann Surg* 1971;173:249–262.
10. Grillo HC. The management of tracheal stenosis following assisted respiration. *J Thorac Cardiovasc Surg* 1969;57:52–71.
11. Biller HF, Lawson W, Weisberg V. Staged repair of extensive tracheal and laryngotracheal stenoses. *Ann Otol Rhinol Laryngol* 1986; 95:586–589.
12. Cotton RT, Myer CM. Contemporary surgical management of laryngeal stenosis. *Am J Otolaryngol* 1984;5:360–368.
13. Strong MS, Healy GB, Vaughn CW. Endoscopic management of Laryngeal Stenosis. *Otolaryngol Clin North Am* 12:797–806.

Airway Management, edited by
L.H. Hanowell, M.D. and R.J. Waldron, M.D.,
Lippincott-Raven Publishers, Philadelphia © 1996.

CHAPTER 27

Emergency Airway Management on the Ward

William C. Wilson

INTRODUCTION

Maintenance of adequate gas exchange is the fundamental responsibility of the anesthesiologist involved in cardiorespiratory arrest (code blue) situations on the ward, just as they are in the operating room. Failure to maintain a patent airway for more than a few minutes can lead to brain injury or death. Emergency airway management on the ward can be even more perilous than in the operating room because equipment and help may not be accessible, and the patents are frequently in well-established cardiopulmonary distress or failure.

Morbidity and mortality during emergency airway management on the ward can be decreased when certain guidelines are followed. These guidelines can be summarized as the *nine requirements for safe airway management* and the *four emergency airway complications to avoid*. The principles inherent in these guidelines are elucidated in the final section of this chapter by describing airway management recommendations for several specific *clinical scenarios*.

All recommendations and guidelines are intended for use by a fully trained anesthesiologist or nurse anesthetist, although they should also prove useful to medical students, residents, and nurses who help with airway care.

W. C. Wilson: Department of Critical Care Medicine and Cardiothoracic Anesthesiology, University of California, San Diego Medical Center, San Diego, California 92103.

NINE REQUIREMENTS FOR SAFE AIRWAY MANAGEMENT

Regardless of the code situation, the following requirements for safe intubation must always be present:

1. Oxygen.
2. Bag-mask ventilation capability and airway equipment.
3. Suction.
4. Functioning IV line.
5. Vasopressors.
6. Airway assessment.
7. Patient preparation and positioning.
8. An alternate plan.
9. Extra help.

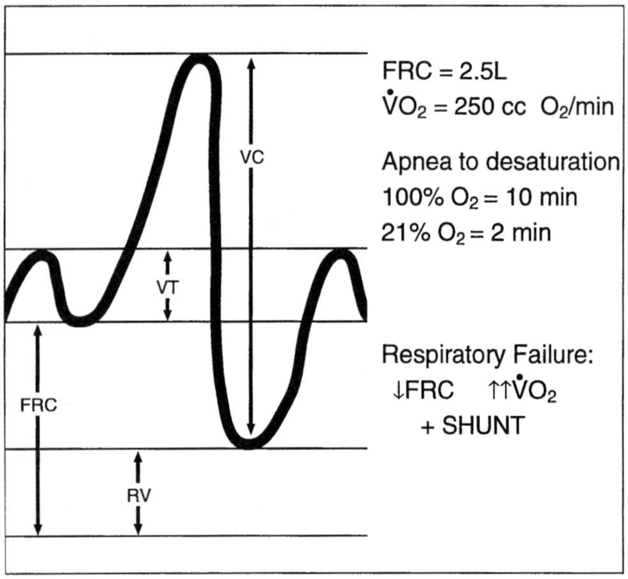

FIG. 1. FRC and relationship of oxygen reserve at various concentrations of inhaled oxygen consumption. FRC, functional residual capacity; RV, residual volume; V_T, tidal volume; VC, vital capacity; $\dot{V}O_2$, oxygen consumption.

Oxygen

Oxygen should always be applied during assessment of the patient and prior to intubation. The application of increased F_{IO_2} can be lifesaving because oxygen deficiency is frequently encountered in patients who are in respiratory failure on the ward.

Preoxygenation is an essential component of a "rapid sequence intubation" because it allows for a reserve of oxygen in the lungs during apnea (Fig. 1). Preoxygenation with 100% O_2 allows for up to 10 min of oxygen reserve following apnea (in a patient with healthy lungs). Patients in respiratory failure (as encountered during codes on the ward) will frequently desaturate sooner because these patients may have increased O_2 consumption, a decreased functional residual capacity (FRC), and an increased right-to-left transpulmonary shunt.

Bag-Mask Ventilation Capability

To ensure the ability to apply oxygen, positive pressure is used via a bag-mask device, along with oral and nasal airway adjuncts. Typically, the anesthesiologist brings these adjuncts to the code along with styletted endotracheal tubes, laryngoscopes, drugs, and adjunct equipment in a "code box."

Suction

Patients in respiratory failure on the ward may have thick secretions and/or may have regurgitated. In order to protect against aspiration and to better visualize the laryngeal anatomy, suctioning of the airway is frequently required during a code.

Functioning Intravenous Access

A functioning intravenous (IV) line is a very high priority and is mandatory when airway control is urgent but not emergent. The ability to administer fluids and cardiovascular support drugs is obviously essential. However, if confronted with a patient in "full arrest," the trachea must be intubated first and IV access secured secondarily. All Advanced Cardiac Life Support (ACLS) protocol drugs can be administered via the endotracheal tube (ETT) except for calcium and bicarbonate, which are not first-line drugs.

Vasopressors

Vasopressors must be available for immediate use because hypotension is a frequent side effect of tracheal intubation (reasons for hypotension are elaborated upon later in the section on hemodynamic compromise).

Airway Evaluation

Prior to attempting endotracheal intubation, the clinician should assess the patient's airway from a technical ease of ventilation/intubation vantage. Three easy-to-perform, no-risk, airway evaluation tests have emerged as highly predictive indicators of intubation difficulty: the relative tongue-to-pharyngeal size (Mallampati class) (1, 2), the space anterior to the larynx (also known as *hyomental* or *thyromental distance*) (3), and atlanto-occipital joint extension (4). When the results of these three tests are combined for the same patient, the predictive power becomes quite substantial. Since these tests are easy to perform and without risk to the patient, they should be done on all patients who require tracheal intubation (see Chapters 4 and 8).

Adequate Patient Preparation/Position

Regardless of whether an awake topicalized technique or a rapid sequence technique is chosen, proper patient positioning and preparation are important.

Awake Technique Preparation

If a blind nasal or fiberoptic intubation is planned, the patient should be psychologically prepared, and the clinician must be patient in ensuring that the nasopharynx and oropharynx are properly anesthetized with topically applied local anesthesia. Elevating the head of the bed by at least 45° will facilitate these techniques (see Chapter 16).

"Sniffing" Position: Preparation for Rapid Sequence Technique

The sniffing position is the optimal position for direct laryngoscopy and endotracheal intubation when using a rapid sequence technique. One of the most common reasons for difficulty with laryngoscopy and intubation is failure of the clinician to place the patient in the correct position. The sniffing position involves forward flexion of the neck on the chest and extension of the head at the neck. This aligns the oropharyngeal, laryngeal, and tracheal axes. The easiest way to accomplish this is to place at least two folded towels under the head of the supine patient. The first attempt at laryngoscopy should be a well-prepared attempt. Once the patient is placed in an adequate sniffing position, it is important to have a helper apply cricoid pressure to protect against regurgitation of gastric contents.

Alternate Plan

After assessment of the airway and evaluation of the patient's underlying pathologic condition, a plan for intubation must be devised. If there is any concern that the patient's airway will be difficult, an awake technique with spontaneous ventilation should be chosen. If the patient is in full arrest, rigid direct laryngoscopy should be performed immediately after administering 2–3 large breaths with a bag-mask device. For patients in respiratory failure on the ward, a blind nasal intubation should be considered a high option. However, there must always be a "plan B."

Extra Help

Whenever securing the airway, extra help is a must, as is communication with the patient and with helpers. Everyone must have the same game plan.

FOUR EMERGENCY AIRWAY COMPLICATIONS TO AVOID

There are four emergency airway complications to avoid when managing airways of patients on the ward:

1. Failure to intubate/ventilate.
2. Unrecognized esophageal intubation.
3. Aspiration of gastric contents.
4. Hemodynamic compromise.

We will examine each of these pitfalls in turn.

Failure To Intubate/Ventilate

It is now well recognized that failure to maintain a patent airway for more than a few minutes leads to brain damage or death and is the single most common cause of anesthesia-related morbidity and mortality (5). Patients in respiratory failure on the ward can be troublesome to intubate on the basis of a difficult airway, but also because they are sick (cardiopulmonary failure). Furthermore, difficulty can occur because proper equipment and help may be missing.

Difficult Airway

Several outstanding reviews of the anesthetic implications of the difficult airway exist (6,7). Benumof (8) has recently reviewed the difficult airway and the American Society of Anesthesiologists (ASA) difficult airway algorithm. The review by Benumof is recommended because it is current and has direct applicability to the intensive care unit (ICU) and to the patient in cardiorespiratory failure on the ward (see Chapter 8). The ASA difficult airway algorithm makes many specific management recommendations:

1. If concerned about losing the airway under general anesthesia, secure the airway awake.
2. Have plans B, C, and D physically and mentally ready to go—think ahead.
3. If trouble is encountered, stop (awaken or proceed to a surgical airway).
4. Decide on priorities (difficult airway versus risk of aspiration).
5. Do what you do best.
6. Extubation of the trachea of a patient with a known difficult airway should be over a jet stylet (preferably a fiberoptic bronchoscope), allowing for a controlled and reversible withdrawal from the airway (because ventilation and reintubation are possible at any time).

Three Emergency Airway Aids

When confronted with the cannot-ventilate–cannot-intubate patient, three alternative ventilation methods have recently been described: the laryngeal mask airway (LMA), the esophageal tracheal combitube (ETC), and transtracheal jet ventilation (TTJV). See Chapters 13–18 for more details on these advanced airway techniques. Once ventilation is established with one of these methods, other, more time-consuming techniques such as using a retrograde wire (9), or fiberoptic bronchoscopic-guided oral or nasotracheal intubation can be performed. However, if the reason for failure to ventilate is a laryngeal or sublaryngeal problem (i.e., laryngeal tumor), the LMA and ETC are contraindicated because they are both supralaryngeal airway solutions. Transtracheal jet ventilation is an effective means of providing adequate oxygenation for 30–40 min (10).

Unrecognized Esophageal Intubation

Esophageal intubation is more a problem of recognition, rather than of prevention. Indeed, unrecognized esophageal intubation has been identified as a significant contributor to cardiac arrests attributed solely to anesthesia (11). Esophageal intubations occur during code situations on the ward, as well. Because capnography is not available on the ward, other methods of detection must be employed.

Clinical Esophageal Intubation Detection Methods Are Error-Prone

Few esophageal intubation detection techniques are error-free. Indeed, Birmingham et al. (12) have elucidated sources of error with most clinical esophageal intubation detection maneuvers, including: chest movement, chest and epigastric auscultation, balloting the balloon in the suprasternal notch, tube condensation, reservoir bag compliance, etc.

Direct vision of the endotracheal tube passing through the cords is considered the "gold standard." The only foolproof techniques for confirming an endotracheal position are seeing the tube pass through the cords and looking through the endotracheal tube into the trachea with a fiberoptic bronchoscope.

Two Indirect Methods for Determining ETT Position

Two indirect methods of determining ETT position are useful for patients outside the operating room (end tidal CO_2 measurement and the esophageal detector device).

End Tidal CO_2 Measurement

The CO_2 detection devices are quite good. However, in code situations with little or no cardiac output, very little CO_2 will be detected. Conversely, patients with CO_2 in the stomach from $NaHCO_3$ or soft drinks can give a false positive test (13). Barring these two relatively rare events, end tidal CO_2 measurement is a reliable indication of endotracheal position. The CO_2 detection devices are now available in hand-size colorimetric versions that are accurate and can be used to detect esophageal intubation. Furthermore, these devices can be used to quantify the efficacy of cardiopulmonary resuscitation (CPR) (14). [See Chapter 21, Fig. 15.]

The Esophageal Detector Device

Recently, an esophageal detector (comprised of an Ellicks evacuator applied to the supposed "tracheal" tube) has proven to be highly sensitive and specific for esophageal detection (15). If the tube is in the esophagus, the deflated bulb fails to expand because suction applied to the esophageal wall causes the mucosa to obstruct the ETT; whereas, the tracheal-placed tube will allow air to flow out of the lungs and will reinflate the bulb because the tracheal rings keep the airway open. [See Chapter 21, Fig. 13.]

Delayed Desaturation May Indicate Esophageal Intubation

The problem of esophageal intubation is further compounded by the fact that, following adequate preoxygenation, the patient may not desaturate for as long as 10 min (Fig. 1). Thus, any cyanosis or desaturation that occurs in this time frame should be considered an esophageal intubation until proven otherwise and demands immediate reverification of endotracheal tube positioning.

Aspiration of Gastric Contents

The severity of gastric aspiration is a function of the volume, pH, and nature of material aspirated. Patients at high risk for aspiration should either receive a rapid sequence induction or have an awake topicalized intubation technique (16).

The purpose of the rapid sequence induction (with cricoid pressure) is to seal the airway with a cuffed endotracheal tube as soon as possible after the loss of airway reflexes. A rapid sequence induction is used when contraindications to a blind nasal intubation are present and when the risk of aspiration of gastric contents is high (trauma, acute abdomen, obesity, hiatal hernia).

In preparation for rapid sequence intubation, the patient is preoxygenated (where possible) for 3 min or for 4 vital capacity breaths prior to rendering the patient apneic (17). Anesthesia is induced, followed immediately with administration of a neuromuscular blocking drug, such as succinylcholine, or a rapid-onset, nondepolarizing neuromuscular blocking drug, such as rocuronium (18). Vecuronium can also be used, providing that 3–4 times the estimated dose to produce 95% depression of neuromuscular function (ED_{95}) is administered or a priming dose is used. Vecuronium causes somewhat less vagolysis than does rocuronium (19).

Hemodynamic Compromise

Hemodynamic compromise almost always occurs following a rapid sequence induction and sometimes following a topicalized awake technique during airway manipulations on the ward. Hypotension occurs secondary to lysis of catecholamine output and due to decreased venous return with positive pressure ventilation (especially in hypovolemic patients).

Four Factors Increase Catecholamines Preinduction

Prior to intubation/induction, four factors help sustain the patient's blood pressure through increased endogenous catecholamine elaboration:

1. Stress (fear of dying and dyspnea)
2. Pain (trauma)
3. Elevated $PaCO_2$ (ventilatory failure)
4. Hypovolemia.

Elevated catecholamines preinduction/preintubation sustain blood pressure, but can also lead to myocardial irritability.

Four Factors Cause the Blood Pressure to Plummet Following Induction

Following induction/intubation, the blood pressure frequently falls in patients with respiratory failure on the ward (especially following a rapid sequence induction). The hypotensive response can be attributed to four factors: loss of consciousness, drug effects, positive pressure ventilation, and decreased $PaCO_2$.

Loss of Consciousness

Intravenous drugs such as etomidate, ketamine (Ketaject, Ketaset, Ketalar), propofol, and thiopental sodium (Pentothal) lead to a loss of stress and pain perception (both involving the autonomic nervous system), therefore abolishing one important source of catecholamine production.

Direct Myocardial Depression and Vasodilation

Some IV drugs cause direct myocardial depression (thiopental, propofol, ketamine) and decreased systemic vascular resistance (SVR). There is very little myocardial depression with etomidate. Ketamine causes some myocardial depression but also has a sympathomimetic effect that can buoy the blood pressure (providing the patient is not already secreting the maximal amount of endogenous catecholamines) (20).

Decreased Right Ventricular Preload and Increased Right Ventricular Afterload

Positive pressure ventilation will decrease venous return to the right heart and thus decrease preload and increase afterload to the right heart (when alveolar pressure is greater than pulmonary capillary pressure). These changes, in turn, decrease filling of the left heart, tending to decrease stroke volume. These effects are especially pronounced when the patient is intravascularly volume-depleted (21).

Decreased $PaCO_2$

Hyperventilation will blow off the previously elevated $PaCO_2$, resulting in further decreasing the stimulus for catecholamine release. The combination of a patient who may be hypovolemic, with now-decreased endogenous catecholamine elaboration, and mechanical factors that inhibit cardiac output (positive pressure ventilation) can lead to catastrophic hypotension.

Techniques to Limit Hypotension Following Intubation

1. Use small doses of induction drugs (repeated as necessary).
2. Pretreat with a fluid load (if no congestive heart failure).
3. Have vasopressors drawn up and available for administration.
4. Do not overventilate following intubation.
5. Avoid general anesthesia if it is not necessary.

CLINICAL SCENARIOS

When called to the bedside of a patient for a code blue, the clinician must first determine whether the patient is truly a full arrest or whether the patient is in cardiopulmonary distress with impending arrest, the so-called pseudo code. In the case of the pseudo code, several specific recommendations apply.

True Code (Full Arrest)

In the case of a full arrest, no drugs are necessary; however, oxygen, suction, proper preparation, and patient positioning are important. Management begins with implementation of the ABCs (airway, breathing, circulation): application of cricoid pressure, opening of the airway, mask ventilation, and use of a direct laryngoscopic technique to intubate the trachea with a styletted endotracheal tube. Following intubation, endotracheal position must be verified, using clinical signs (symmetrical chest movement, equal bilateral breath sounds, fogging of the endotracheal tube) as well as the more reliable esophageal intubation detection devices [end tidal CO_2 (Nellcor®, Easy Cap™)] or infrared end tidal CO_2 measuring devices available in the operating room, such as the capnograph. It is important to attach the endotracheal tube securely to the patient's maxilla following intubation and to be cautious when manipulating the patient's head or body. This is the time when people "let down their guard" (since the airway is secured), and someone may inadvertently pull the endotracheal tube out of the trachea while reaching over to move the patient in performing some other manipulation. Finally, chest x-rays should be ordered and reviewed to verify the level of the endotracheal tube and to help establish the etiology of the cardiopulmonary failure.

Pseudo Code (Cardiopulmonary Arrest Imminent)

The pseudo code is characterized by the clinician being called "stat" for a code blue to the ward and, upon arrival, the patient is still ventilating and has a pulse and measurable blood pressure. The patient may or may not be in need of urgent airway management. The clinician must first decide if intubation is, indeed, necessary. If so, how urgently must intubation be performed and is the patient in the optimal setting? While these questions are being answered, the clinician should apply oxygen to the patient, listen to the patient's chest with a stethoscope, and (if necessary) assist ventilations with a bag-mask device. Next, the clinician should learn from members of the patient's primary team what history has led up to this event. The patient should also be interviewed regarding significant past medical problems, drug allergies, and current medications, including monoamine oxidase inhibitors (MAOs) and cardiac, pulmonary, or diuretic medications.

Specific Clinical Scenarios

There are several frequently encountered clinical scenarios that occur on the ward, in the emergency room, and in the ICU. Each has several specific management points. While the scenarios presented below represent patients who are in cardiopulmonary failure but have not yet arrested, improper or delayed therapy can lead to full arrest.

Respiratory Failure Due to Airway Compromise

Always be prepared to use TTJV or to perform a cricothyroidotomy when confronted with the patient who has a compromised airway. Clinical signs of airway compromise include stridor, chest retractions, CO_2 retention, and, ultimately, hypoxia. Airway compromise can occur secondary to tumor, foreign body, trauma, epiglottitis, or postoperative complications. Frequent postoperative causes of stridor include bleeding into a fresh surgical wound following carotid endarterectomy, thyroid, or parathyroid surgery, soft tissue swelling following anterior cervical discectomy, as well as edema in massively transfused or burned patients.

When confronted with the stridulous patient with impending airway obstruction, it is vital not to transform a partial airway obstruction into a complete airway obstruction. Therefore, a controlled, topicalized, awake technique is the recommended approach. However, when possible, airway management should be performed in the presence of another physician (preferably a surgeon) with particular expertise in gaining a surgical airway. These problems are quite well suited to treatment with a fiberoptic bronchoscopic technique following proper patient preparation and positioning.

In the case of the massively burned patient, it is frequently prudent to intubate electively early, even if there is no direct airway injury. Indeed, the first couple of hours following resuscitation can be associated with so much interstitial edema (from inflammatory mediators triggered by the massive burn, as well as the requisite fluid resuscitation) that airway swelling occurs, leading to a compromised airway and, occasionally, a difficult intubation.

In the case of hemorrhage into the closed surgical wound, the pressure from the bleeding vessels can be high enough to cause compression of the trachea. In this case, emergent opening of the wound can be lifesaving.

Respiratory Failure Due to Gas Exchange Problems (Shunt)

Primary pulmonary parenchymal problems (such as aspiration pneumonia, Pneumocystis pneumonia, respiratory distress syndromes, and sepsis) cause a large and variable right-to-left transpulmonary shunt. These patients typically have a high minute ventilation and are ideally managed via a blind nasal intubation technique. These patients may not require quite as much topicalization and analgesia as does a patient who presents for an elective operation. However, when time allows, proper topicalization and preparation is humane and can be the critical difference leading to success when securing the airway in this population.

Congestive Heart Failure

The patient who presents with respiratory insufficiency due to congestive heart failure must be considered to have poor myocardial function and be at a high resting catecholamine state. The high sympathetic output serves to maintain what little cardiac reserve and vascular tone the patient has. The clinician can occasionally temporize with high-flow oxygen and medical therapy. However, if the patient requires intubation, only very small doses of sedative/hypnotics should be administered (25–50 mg thiopental may be a suitable dose). Alternatively, a blind nasal intubation with careful topicalization is a very acceptable technique in this type of patient. However, it is essential that time is taken to carefully topicalize and prepare the patient to prevent patient distress and/or further increase in catecholamine output, leading to ventricular arrhythmias.

If the congestive heart failure is secondary to renal failure, caution should be taken concerning qualitative platelet defects and nasal bleeding. Renal failure is not a contraindication to a nasal technique, providing that careful and complete topicalization of the airway is performed.

The Asthmatic Patient

The asthmatic patient presents several difficult problems simultaneously. The patient may be very distressed and agitated, may be moving very little air, and may have wide swings in blood pressure due to the transmitted pleural and interior abdominal pressures and their effects on the cardiovascular system. Furthermore, a very significant problem for the anesthesiologist is the specter of unrecognized esophageal intubation resulting from difficulty hearing breath sounds in a patient during a severe asthmatic attack. Therefore, in the asthmatic patient, a rigid direct laryngoscopic technique to ensure visualization of the cords is superior to a blind technique, not only because it is difficult to hear breath sounds, but also because the chest wall excursions may be so minimal as to limit sounds of flow in and out of the endotracheal tube until positive pressure is applied. If a rigid, direct laryngoscopic technique is selected, ketamine is the ideal induction drug because ketamine provides hemodynamic stability and, most importantly, bronchial dilation.

Ventilatory Failure Due to Pain, Splinting, and Atelectasis

In some cases of ventilatory failure, analgesia is the only treatment necessary. For example, the patient who presents following trauma to the chest with multiple rib fractures or following a thoracotomy may be significantly improved following the administration of adequate analgesia. These patients are splinting, and because of this, their lungs become atelectatic and they may progress to respiratory failure, especially if the baseline pulmonary status is marginal. For these patients, an epidural (especially thoracic) mode of analgesia may be all that is necessary for the patient to then cough, deep breathe, and reexpand the atelectatic lung segments.

Pneumothorax

In the case of a pneumothorax, which may occur in patients with chronic obstructive pulmonary disease or following trauma, patients can be treated solely with a chest tube. Therefore, given the proper history and physical findings on presentation of the patient (decreased breath sounds on one side, deviation of the trachea away from the side of the pneumothorax), consideration should be given to placing a large-bore angiocath into the second interspace on the expected side of the pneumothorax. Preferably, if time allows, first obtain a chest x-ray to confirm a pneumothorax. The treatment would then be a chest tube.

The Comatose Patient (Medical Etiologies)

The comatose patient cannot protect the airway and may have regurgitated prior to arrival. Thus, blind manipulation of the airway should be avoided. These patients cannot protect the airway and will need intubation for this reason. Additionally, if the etiology of coma is thought to be a mass in the brain, there may be a requirement for hyperventilation, as well. For medical causes of coma, such as drug overdose, a postictal state or liver failure, a rigid, direct laryngoscopic technique is recommended. A blind nasal technique may lead to gagging, retching, vomiting, and aspiration.

Coma Following Head Injury or Intracerebral Hemorrhage

If the etiology of coma is thought to be due to a space-occupying lesion within the calvarium, it must be remembered that hyperventilation is an urgent requirement to decrease intracranial pressure (ICP). Another important factor to keep in mind is that cerebral perfusion pressure (CPP) must be kept up in patients with mass-occupying lesions.

$$\text{CPP} = \text{mean arterial pressure (MAP)} - \text{ICP}$$

Care must be taken not to overshoot blood pressure as this can increase bleeding into the brain or subdural–epidural space. At the same time, any drug administration or maneuvers used to secure the airways should be sure not to cause hypotension. In this scenario, etomidate is frequently the best choice, although thiopental titrated in small doses is also acceptable.

Etomidate increases cerebral perfusion pressure with an induction dose of 0.3 mg/kg; neural protection is provided and cardiac stability is maintained. The neural protective effect results from a decrease in ICP and a reduction in $CMRO_2$ of approximately 45%, with a concomitant decrease in cerebral blood flow of around 34%. All of this occurs with very little change in MAP, wedge pressure stroke volume, cardiac index, or SVR.

The Acutely Traumatized Patient

Four specific considerations that universally apply to trauma patients must be considered and can be summarized as the four cardinal rules for airway management in

TABLE 1. *Four rules for trauma airway management*

The cervical spine is always unstable.
The stomach is always full.
The patient is always dry.
Avoid maneuvers that will convert a partial airway obstruction into a complete airway obstruction (i.e., laryngeal fracture).

the trauma patient (Table 1). As we consider manipulations to maintain airway patency or place an endotracheal tube, we must always consider the trauma patient to have an unstable cervical spine [until proven otherwise], a full stomach, and to be intravascularly hypovolemic. We must also avoid airway manipulations that might convert a partial airway disruption into a complete airway loss.

C-Spine Issues

Head and neck should remain immobilized with in-line stabilization. It is recommended that radiographic C-spine clearance be achieved first (when practical). Nasal intubation is acceptable unless the patient is apneic or has major facial/nasal trauma or obvious basal skull fracture. Awake oral or nasal techniques versus anesthetized oral or nasal techniques are equal in terms of causing further neurologic injury, providing the neck is not moved (do what you do best).

Full Stomach Issues

Trauma, pain, and apprehension are all associated with an increased volume and decreased pH of gastric contents (22), thus increasing the risk that aspiration of passively regurgitated vomitus would progress to aspiration syndrome. Therefore, all trauma patients are considered to have full stomachs, and a rapid sequence induction with endotracheal intubation to protect the airway is indicated unless superseded by other issues (i.e., difficult airway). If a difficult airway is anticipated, intubate the trachea using an awake technique (16).

Hypovolemia Considerations

Trauma patients should always be considered hemodynamically unstable (due to intravascular volume depletion) until proven otherwise. Airway management decisions (and, indeed, anesthetic drug administration) must involve consideration that the patient has lost blood.

In the case of hypotension due to exsanguinating hemorrhage, if the patient is in a state of full arrest, the trachea is intubated without any drug administration. However, if the patient is agitated, combative, hypotensive, and requiring airway intubation, then very small doses of sedative or hypnotics should be given. These patients should have the trachea intubated with succinylcholine after a small dose of thiopental, ketamine, or etomidate (versus none at all). Once the patient's blood volume has been repleted and the hemodynamic status stabilized, the patient may receive further anesthetic drugs.

Above All, Do Not Lose the Airway

If the patient is maintaining spontaneous ventilation but needs emergent definitive airway management, techniques should be utilized that are best suited to preserving a patent airway throughout the airway manipulation.

Problems of recall in trauma patients are significant, as Bogetz and Katz have shown (23). Approximately 40% of the patients initially treated without sedative/hypnotics will have some recall of the event. However, having recall of the event is superior to not being around to tell the story. Other specific requirements for the traumatized airway are discussed in Chapter 23. It must be remembered that hemodynamic stability is always a problem in trauma and that the patient may have as much as a 30% blood loss with only a baseline tachycardia and a modest decrease in blood pressure.

SUMMARY

Emergency airway management on the ward is fraught with danger for the patient because, on average, these patients tend to be sicker than patients presenting for elective operating room care, and because equipment and help may be difficult to obtain in a timely manner.

The morbidity and mortality of emergency airway manipulation on the ward can be decreased by careful preparation of the clinician and of the patient for the planned manipulation, as well as preparation of alternate plans. Thinking ahead helps avoid the four major complications of emergency airway management: failed intubation/lost airway, unrecognized esophageal intubation, aspiration of gastric contents, and hemodynamic compromise.

REFERENCES

1. Mallampati SR, Gatt SP, Gugino LD, et al. A clinical sign to predict difficult tracheal intubation: a prospective study. *Can J Anaesth* 1985; 32:429.
2. Lewis M, Keramati S, Benumof JL, et al. What is the best way to determine oropharyngeal calssification and mandibular space length to predict difficult laryngoscopy? *Anesthesiology* 1994;81:69.
3. Finucane BT, Santora AH. Evaluation of the airway prior to intubation. In: *Principles of Airway Management*. Philadelphia: FA Norris Co., 1988;69.
4. Bellhouse CP, Dore C. Criteria for estimating likelihood of difficult intubation with the Macintosh laryngoscope. *Anesth Intensive Care* 1988;16:329.

5. Caplan RA, Posner KL, Ward RJ, et al. Adverse respiratory events in anesthesia: a closed claims analysis. *Anesthesiology* 1990;72:828–833.
6. Cormack RS, Lehane J. Difficult tracheal intubation in obstetrics. *Anaesthesia* 1984;39:1105.
7. McIntyre JRW. The difficult intubation. *Can J Anaesth* 1987;34:204.
8. Benumof JL. Management of the difficult airway. *Anesthesiology* 1991;75:1087.
9. Dhara SS. Retrograde intubation—a facilitated approach. *Br J Anaesth* 1992;69:631.
10. Benumof JL, Scheller, MS. The importance of transtracheal jet ventilation in the management of the difficult airway. *Anesthesiology* 1989;71:769.
11. Keenan RL, Boyan CP. Cardiac arrest due to anesthesia: a study of incidence and causes. *JAMA* 1985;253:2373.
12. Birmingham PK, Cheney FW, Ward RJ. Esophageal intubation. *Anesth Analg* 1986;65:886.
13. Sum Ping ST, Mehta MP, Symreng T. Reliability of capnography in identifying esophageal intubation with carbonated beverage or antacid in the stomach. *Anesth Analg* 1992;74:333.
14. Ornato JP, Shipley JB, Racht EM, et al. Multicenter study of a portable hand held colorometeric end-tidal carbon dioxide detection device. *Ann Emerg Med* 1992;21:518.
15. Williams KN, Nunn JF. The esophageal detector device. *Anaesthesia* 1989;44:412.
16. Ovassapian A, Krejcie TC, Yelich SJ, et al. Awake fiberoptic intubation in the patient at high risk of aspiration. *Br J Anaesth* 1989;62:13.
17. Gambee AM, Hertzka RE, Fisher DM. Preoxygenation techniques: comparison of three minutes and four breaths. *Anesth Analg* 1987;66:468.
18. Magorian T, Flannery KB, Miller RD. Comparison of rocuronium, succinylcholine, and vecuronium for rapid-sequence induction of anesthesia in adults patients. *Anesthesiology* 1993;79:913.
19. McCoy EP, Maddineni VR, Elliott P, et al. Haemodynamic effects of rocuronium during fentanyl anesthesia: comparison with vecuronium. *Can J Anaesth* 1993;40:703.
20. Kakayama DK, Waggoner T, Venkataraman ST, et al. The use of drugs in emergency airway management in pediatric trauma. *Ann Surg* 1992;216:205.
21. Perel A, Reuven P, Cotev S. Systolic blood pressure variation is a sensitive indicator of hypovolemia in ventilated dogs subjected to graded hemorrhage. *Anesthesiology* 1987;67:498.
22. Miller, RD, ed. *Anesthesia*, 3rd ed. New York: Churchill Livingstone, 1990.
23. Bogetz MS, Katz JA. Recall of surgery for major trauma. *Anesthesiology* 1984;61:6–9.

Airway Management, edited by
L.H. Hanowell, M.D. and R.J. Waldron, M.D.,
Lippincott-Raven Publishers, Philadelphia © 1996.

CHAPTER 28

Essential Aspects of Transport Ventilators

Russell T. Reid, Charles P. Kingsley, and Leland H. Hanowell

HISTORICAL PERSPECTIVE OF PATIENT TRANSPORT AND MECHANICAL VENTILATION

Every conceivable mode of transportation has been used over the centuries to transport the critically injured. For example, wounded soldiers were evacuated during the Battle of Blenheim in the 18th century by horse-drawn wagons by order of the Duke of Marlborough (1). Transport was by hot-air balloon during the Franco-Prussian War in 1870 (2), and public transportation was utilized in 19th century England (3). In the modern era of transport, the systematic use of helicopters during the conflict in Vietnam resulted in a 97.5% survival rate for all personnel reaching a U.S. field hospital (4).

Current management of the critically ill involves myriad settings, ranging from simple interhospital transport to disaster care in remote or austere environments (Table 1). Such transport may involve evacuation from the scene of motor vehicle or industrial accidents, the increasingly common rescue after injuries related to interpersonal violence, transport for performance of special procedures (MRI, radiation therapy, other), interhospital transport, or long-range transport (interstate or intercontinental) for definitive care (trauma care, organ transplant).

Like the modes of transport, airway management and ventilation of the lungs have undergone a marked transition. Paracelsus, who attempted ventilation with a fireplace bellows attached to a tube placed in a patient's mouth (5), was probably the first to conceive of a manual resuscitator. We now perform similar techniques with modern methods of intubation and mechanical ventilation, by either a manual resuscitator bag or portable transport ventilator.

PHYSIOLOGIC CHANGES ASSOCIATED WITH MECHANICAL VENTILATION DURING TRANSPORT

Waddell (6) found that 20% of critically ill patients developed clinically significant hypotension and arrhythmias during intrahospital transport. No specifics regard-

R. T. Reid: Department of Respiratory Care, University of California, Davis Medical Center, Sacramento, California 95817.
C. P. Kingsley: Department of Anesthesiology, The Pennsylvania State University School of Medicine, Hershey, Pennsylvania 17033.
L. H. Hanowell: Department of Anesthesiology, University of California, Davis School of Medicine and Medical Center, Sacramento, California 95817.

TABLE 1. *Settings for critical care transport*

Evacuation of injured from accidents
Interpersonal violence
Military conflict
Transport for special procedures
Interhospital transport

ing ventilatory parameters of the patients studied were defined; however, some patients required mechanical ventilation. Braman et al. (7) prospectively evaluated 36 intrahospital transports during critical illness to determine the ventilatory changes associated with manual resuscitator bags vs. portable mechanical ventilators. Fourteen of 20 patients ventilated by a manual resuscitator bag had alterations in $PaCO_2$ greater than 10 mm Hg or in pH greater than 0.05 units. These physiologic changes were significantly correlated with hemodynamic disturbances (hypotension and cardiac arrhythmias). Only 6 of 16 patients managed with portable transport ventilators had alterations in $PaCO_2$ and pH, and these changes were significantly less in magnitude than those in the manually ventilated group.

Gervais et al. (8) conducted a prospective analysis of 30 ventilator patients by randomizing patients to one of three groups ventilated by either 1) manual resuscitator bag, 2) manual resuscitator with volume measurements, or 3) portable transport ventilator. The groups that were ventilated by manual resuscitator without volume measurement and the group ventilated by portable transport ventilator demonstrated significant reduction in $PaCO_2$ and central venous PO_2, with a concomitant increase in arterial pH. These physiologic changes were smaller in the portable ventilator group. The portable transport ventilator exceeded its preset minute ventilation by 2.35 L/min; however, it is not clear whether the excess minute ventilation was caused by patient demand (additional patient-triggered breaths). The group that was manually ventilated with volume measurement experienced no significant changes in $PaCO_2$, central venous PO_2, or arterial pH. These investigators concluded that minute ventilation should be monitored during transport.

Finally, a study by Hurst and colleagues (9) clearly demonstrated the complication of acute respiratory alkalosis induced by manual ventilation during transport of the critically ill as evidenced by significant reduction of $PaCO_2$ and elevation of pH. The mean pretransport values were a pH of 7.39 and $PaCO_2$ of 39, compared with a mean pH of 7.51 and $PaCO_2$ of 30 during transport.

Respiratory alkalosis has been associated with reduced myocardial and cerebral blood flows with a simultaneous shift of the oxyhemoglobin dissociation curve to the left, resulting in decreased delivery of oxygen to the tissues. Hyperventilation can lead to coronary artery vasospasm and subsequent myocardial ischemia (10,11). Additionally, in neurosurgical patients who are being hyperventilated to prevent cerebral edema, cerebral blood flow may be reduced precipitously by any additional fall in $PaCO_2$ associated with inadvertently excessive hyperventilation (12).

It is clear from these studies that patients transported while being ventilated with a manual resuscitator suffer from inconsistent ventilation and clinically significant upward swings in pH. Patients in these studies were critically ill; such patients may be unable to tolerate the inconsistent ventilatory parameters that have been documented during manual ventilation and result in respiratory alkalosis.

Manual ventilation is associated with other potential problems during patient transport: 1) difficulty in the consistent delivery and monitoring of exhaled volumes and inspiratory pressures; 2) difficulty in manually ventilating the patient while rounding corners, entering an elevator, and negotiating other obstacles that may be encountered; and 3) inability to detect rapidly any inadvertent disconnections of the oxygen source in some of the manual resuscitator designs currently on the market. The use of a portable transport ventilator may eliminate many of these problems and, therefore, would appear to be the optimal method of transporting a ventilator-dependent and critically ill patient.

Potential problems do exist with the use of portable transport ventilators, such as inaccurate volume delivery, loss of power supply, mechanical failure, and inappropriate alarm settings. Any of these may lead to difficulty in detecting variable delivery of ventilation. On balance, however, it would appear that the use of portable transport ventilators should be recommended in the transport of critically ill patients.

VENTILATOR SELECTION

The selection of a transport ventilator depends on a multitude of factors, including performance characteristics, patient population served, size and weight of the device, cost, durability, complexity, and operational environment (Table 2). All these factors should be consid-

TABLE 2. *Selection of transport ventilators: factors involved*

Performance, durability
Patient population to be treated
Size, weight
Cost
Complexity
Operational environment

TABLE 3. *Selection of transport ventilators: pertinent features*

Range of
Respiratory rates, tidal volumes
Inspiratory times
PEEP
Accuracy of delivered volumes
Modes of ventilation

PEEP, positive end expiratory pressure.

ered prior to the selection of a portable transport ventilator. The discussion that follows focuses on the evaluation of the most important of these factors.

Consideration of the above-mentioned factors allows the selection process to proceed in a logical manner, with elimination of several potential transport ventilators. Are the majority of transports in adult, pediatric, or neonatal patients? It is extremely difficult, if not impossible, for one transport ventilator to serve all patients safely and effectively.

The pertinent characteristics that should be considered when selecting a transport ventilator for any patient population are the range of tidal volumes, accuracy of delivered tidal and minute volumes, work of breathing (i.e., continuous vs. demand flow, sensitivity, pneumatic valve design, surface area of exhalation valve), availability of various sizes of ventilator circuits, range of respiratory rates, range of inspiratory times, range of positive end expiratory pressure (PEEP), minimal and maximal flow capabilities, type of cycling mechanisms (time vs. pressure vs. volume), and available modes of ventilation (Table 3).

The makeup of the transport team is an important consideration when selecting a transport ventilator, as it relates to the complexity of the ventilator. It may be difficult for an individual without a background in respiratory care or expertise in the function of ventilators to operate and detect malfunctions in some transport ventilators. Conversely, an individual with specialized training in the function of mechanical ventilators should be capable of operating the most sophisticated transport ventilator if the requirements of the transport population being served, the physical requirements (size, weight), and/or the environment so dictate.

The operating environment may require specifically designed portable ventilators, as for example during helicopter transport, when barometric pressure may significantly affect ventilator performance. Similarly, MRI requires specialized ventilator construction with nonferrous components; otherwise, shielding of the ventilator from the magnetic field is necessary (13). The transport of patients receiving advanced ventilatory modalities, such as high-frequency jet ventilation, may require even further specialized equipment and personnel (14).

Gas Consumption and Oxygen Supply

Gas consumption (oxygen) by the transport ventilator may be a critical factor. Supply of medical gas is limited in certain environments, such as aircraft, and this may be a factor that eliminates some portable transport ventilators from further consideration. An aircraft with four E-cylinders on board has a total gas capacity of 2488 L. Each E-cylinder contains 622 L of gas when full (15). In contrast, an ambulance that carries one (full) H-cylinder has a total oxygen gas capacity of 6900 L (15).

Standard formulas for estimating the duration of cylinder gas supply (assuming a 500-lb safety factor) illustrate time differences in depletion of compressed gas reservoirs as a function of the transport ventilator selected (16). Transporting a patient who is administered a ventilation of 15 L/min using a Bio-Med IC-2A ventilator, with a *system* gas consumption of 12 L/min, requires a total gas consumption of 27 L/min. At this rate of oxygen consumption (minute ventilation plus system gas requirement), each E-cylinder provides only 15.5 minutes of ventilation before depletion, requiring four E-cylinders for each hour of transport ventilation. By comparison, the one H-cylinder would last for 2.9 hours. Weight limitations, of course, in most (short-range, civilian) air transports preclude the feasibility of H-cylinders for oxygen supply. Once the factors of transport population, physical requirements (size, weight), and operational environment have been reviewed and several potential portable transport ventilators eliminated, the individual performance characteristics for the remaining portable transport ventilators can be evaluated.

Essential Performance Characteristics of Mechanical Ventilators

Performance characteristics that should be considered include the following: 1) ventilator classification, 2) available modes of ventilation, 3) tidal volume ranges, 4) respiratory rate ranges, 5) PEEP range, 6) minimal and maximal flow capabilities, 7) duration and type of power source, 8) inspiratory-to-expiratory (I:E) ratio options, 9) F_{IO_2} range, 10) pneumatic valve design, 11) alarm features and ranges, 12) monitoring capabilities, and 13) availability of accessory equipment. Table 4 lists the performance characteristics of 11 transport ventilators currently available.

Characteristics of the Ideal Transport Ventilator

A survey conducted by Branson et al. in 1986 (17) identified the following characteristics of the ideal transport ventilator as identified by air medical programs: 1) provides intermittent mechanical ventilation, 2) has variable tidal volume, 3) has variable respiratory rate (2 to 30

TABLE 4. *Performance characteristics of commercially available transport ventilators*

Ventilator feature	Hamilton MAX	PneuPAC	Autovent 3000	Bird Mini TXP	Bio-Med IC-2A	Newport E100i	Logic 07a	Bird Avian	P-B 2801	Uni-Vent 750	Omni-Vent
Modes	IMV	CMV	IMV, CMV	CMV	CMV, SIMV, CPAP	CMV, AMV, SIMV, CPAP	CMV	CMV, AMV, SIMV, CPAP, Sigh	CMV, AMV, SIMV, Sigh	CMV, AMV, SIMV, Sigh	CMV, IMV
Rate (breaths/min)	2–30	11–14, 16,19, 21	Ped 9–27, Adult 8–20	4–15	1–66	1–120	10–40	0–150	1–69	1–150	
Tidal volume (mL)	50–1500	340–1450	Ped 200–600, Adult 400–1200	50–2500	0–3000	100–3600	100–2000	50–2000	50–2800	10–3000	30–3000
Max. pressure (cm H_2O)	60	55	45	Variable	≤ 100	≤ 100	70	100	100	100	NS
Peak flow (L/min)	90	40	48	120	75	80	65	100	120	100	45
FiO_2	1.0	.45 or 1.0	1.0	.45–.60	1.0	.12–1.0	.5 or 1.0	1.0	.21–1.0	1.0	1.0
PEEP (cm H_2O)	No	No	No	No	No	0–25	No	0–25 (external valve)	No	No	No
Alarms	Low battery, audible high pressure	Audible high pressure	Audible high pressure	None	None	Audible/visual high & low pressure, inverse I:E, low battery, apnea, visual external power failure	Audible high pressure	Audible/visual high & low pressure, inverse I:E, external power failure, apnea, disconnect, PEEP not set, battery low	Audible/visual high & low pressure, inverse I:E, apnea, low battery, ventilator malfunction, power failure	Audible/visual high & low pressure, disconnect, inverse I:E, low battery, apnea, PEEP not set, power failure	None
Monitoring	Airway pressures	None	None	None	Airway pressures	Airway pressures, battery charge, power source	Airway pressures	Airway pressures, respiratory rate, I. time, flow	Airway pressures, sensitivity, flow, volume, voltage	Airway pressures	Airway pressures
Gas consumption (L/min)	0	.5	.5	0	12	9	2	0	0	0	0
Weight (kg/lb)	5.0/11.0	1.3/2.9	0.68/1.5	1.2/2.6	3.85/8.5	5.4/11.9	5.0/11.0	5.0/11.0	17.6/35.5	2.9/6.4	2.0/4/5
Dimensions (cm)	30×8×16.5	18×9×6	NS	7×6×8.5	8.6×15.6 ×26	24×18×15	18×13×15	25.4×30.5 ×13	32.4×27 ×33.7	22×29×11	10×13×15

IMV, intermittent mandatory ventilation; CMV, controlled mechanical ventilation; SIMV, synchronized intermittent mandatory ventilation; CPAP, continuous positive airway pressure; AMV, assisted mechanical ventilation; NS, not specified; I:E, inspiratory-to-expiratory ratio; PEEP, positive end expiratory pressure; I. time, inspiratory time.

breaths per minute), 4) provides a minute ventilation of 4 to 20 L/min, 5) has low- and high-pressure alarms, 6) provides PEEP (0 to 20 cm H_2O), 7) has a pneumatic demand valve, and 8) monitors airway pressure.

MECHANICAL VENTILATION MODES DURING TRANSPORT VENTILATION

A variety of ventilator modes are available for use with the current generation of portable transport ventilators; these include 1) controlled mechanical ventilation (CMV), 2) assisted mechanical ventilation (AMV), 3) intermittent mandatory ventilation (IMV), 4) synchronized intermittent mandatory ventilation (SIMV), 5) continuous positive airway pressure (CPAP), and 6) a modified form of pressure-controlled ventilation (PCV).

A complete discussion of the use of various modes of ventilation is beyond the scope of this chapter (18–23). However, a few precautions are noteworthy. The risk for hyperventilation and subsequent acute respiratory alkalosis exists in patients with intact respiratory drive who become agitated during transport and ventilation in the assist/control mode. On the other hand, care must also be taken to ensure that patients in spontaneous modes of ventilation (such as CPAP) are not subjected to depression of their respiratory drive by narcotic or other sedative administration (benzodiazepines) during diagnostic procedures at the transport destination.

Performance of Mechanical Ventilators: Compliance and Airway Resistance

It has been recommended that tidal volume delivery in transport ventilators should vary no more than 10% from the set tidal volume (13). McGough and co-workers (24) examined the variations in the delivered tidal volume of eight transport ventilators, utilizing a mechanical lung model, under conditions of changing airway resistance and lung compliance. This study demonstrates that fluctuations in delivered tidal volumes occur as compliance decreases or airway resistance increases independently of one another or in tandem. Under the most rigorous conditions (compliance of 0.02 L/cm H_2O and airway resistance of 20 cm H_2O/L/s), the portable ventilators delivered tidal volumes that varied from 20 to 590 mL below the set volume. The manufacturer's use of preset, internal pop-off valves limited the delivered volumes in several of these ventilators, while the use of a Venturi mechanism to generate flow was responsible for the decreased tidal volume in at least one of the machines.

Power Sources for Transport Ventilators

The power source used in transport ventilators is another critical issue that should be taken into consideration when selecting a transport ventilator. There are two types of power sources commonly available: 1) electric and 2) pneumatic (Table 5). The type of battery (lead-acid, gel cell, rechargeable alkaline) utilized in the electrically powered device affects total ventilator weight, duration of power supply, and battery recharge time. In general, electrically powered devices consume less gas than pneumatically powered transport ventilators. Some electrically powered portable transport ventilators utilizing blenders may, however, have significant "bleed" flows that allow gas to leak at a controlled rate from the blender. This factor must be taken into consideration when calculating estimated gas usage (25), particularly when the compressed gas reservoir is limited by the transport mode for which the ventilator is to be utilized.

TABLE 5. *Power sources for transport ventilators*

Electric
Battery type affects
Weight
Duration of power supply
Recharge time
Pneumatic
Light and compact
Greater gas consumption
Barometric pressure changes cause variable
Inspiratory time
Ventilation frequency
Positive inspiratory pressure
Tidal volume

Pneumatically powered fluidic logic transport ventilators have the advantage of lighter weight and more compact dimensions. However, in addition to generally higher gas consumption, these ventilators have the disadvantage of significant variances in the operator-set parameters of respiratory rate, inspiratory time, peak inspiratory pressure and tidal volume when barometric pressure changes (26,27). Large barometric pressure changes could occur in environments such as an unpressurized rotary (or fixed) wing aircraft cabin or a hyperbaric chamber. For this reason, it is imperative that respiratory rate, exhaled tidal volume, inspiratory time, and peak inspiratory pressure be continuously monitored when this type of transport ventilator is used.

Alarm Features of Transport Ventilators

Alarm features should be considered when selecting a transport ventilator; they should give the clinician both audible and visual feedback. The ventilator should minimally be equipped with a high- and low-pressure alarm. The high-pressure alarm is adequate to warn of high-pressure conditions that occur secondary to patient coughing, obstruction of the endotracheal tube, displacement of the endotracheal tube, pneumothorax, airway

TABLE 6. *Specifications for transport ventilators: alarms*

Audible and visual feedback
High- and low-pressure alarms
Electrically powered ventilators
"Low battery" prior to loss of function
Display of battery charge/voltage
Apnea alarm
Note: Alarms DO NOT replace clinical observation.

TABLE 7. *Specifications for transport ventilators: control panel and indicators*

Airway pressure manometer
Indicators for breath type
Battery-in-use indicator (if applicable)
Plainly labeled, calibrated control knobs
Circuit connections plainly labeled
Fittings of different sizes
Visual indicators in helicopter/ambulance

obstruction, bronchospasm, and other events leading to an increase in peak airway pressures.

The high-pressure alarm should ideally be an integral part of the ventilator, capable of terminating the breath on detection of the high-pressure situation (Table 6). A mechanical pressure-limiting device completely independent of the electronically based high-pressure alarm should be incorporated into the ventilator circuit. The mechanical pressure pop-off serves as a secondary pressure-relief mechanism when the electronic pressure pop-off is functioning properly and becomes the primary pop-off valve in the event of electric failure or if an electronic high-pressure alarm is not an integral part of the transport ventilator.

The low-pressure alarm is used to detect any events leading to inadequate ventilation of the patient, such as disconnection of the ventilator circuit, ventilator circuit leaks, loss of power source, or mechanical failure. However, the low-pressure alarm by itself is inadequate if the ventilator is being used as a pressure-limited, time-cycled ventilator. Anything leading to airway obstruction in this mode will allow the ventilator to pressurize the ventilator circuit, effectively defeating the low-pressure alarm, even though the patient is in fact being hypoventilated. If the ventilator is used routinely as a pressure-limited, time-cycled ventilator, then an accessory alarm that displays exhaled tidal volume and has user-definable high and low minute ventilation alarms should be employed.

Any electrically powered transport ventilator should also incorporate an alarm indicating low battery voltage prior to actual loss of battery function and, ideally, an independent analog meter or digital display indicating the state of battery charge or absolute battery voltage.

An apnea alarm is recommended in any transport ventilator utilizing a completely spontaneous mode of ventilation such as CPAP. The alarm trigger mechanism typically is referenced to decreases in airway pressure. This alerts the operator to apnea or to respiratory efforts that are insufficient to reset the alarm.

It may be difficult to find a transport ventilator that incorporates all the alarm features that have been previously discussed. There are, however, many ventilator manufacturers and third-party vendors that offer accessory alarm packages that can be easily retrofitted to existing transport ventilators. It is important to determine the level of alarm protection that is necessary prior to purchase of a transport ventilator, since accessory alarms are expensive. Finally, there is no level of alarm protection that can replace observation of the patient by a skilled clinician.

Control Panel and Indicator Specifications

A number of visual indicators should be present on transport ventilators to enable the operator to monitor the patient visually and ensure safe operation of the ventilator (Table 7). These include an airway pressure manometer, indicators for breath type (i.e., assisted mechanical, mechanical, or spontaneous), and battery-in-use indicator (if applicable). Calibrated controls with plainly labeled knobs, easily readable from a distance of several feet, are ideal. All circuit connections should be plainly labeled and have fittings of different sizes to minimize the risk of inappropriate assembly. For example, if fittings are not diameter-indexed, conduits for the external exhalation valve and proximal airway pressure can inadvertently be transposed when being reconnected during unfavorable environmental conditions (poor ambient light, situations of high anxiety, rapid movement). Visual indicators are particularly important in a helicopter or ambulance, where noise levels have been shown to exceed 100 dB (28,29).

VENTILATORS FOR TRANSPORT: AUSTERE CONDITIONS AND MILITARY IMPLICATIONS

Ventilators for the care and transport of patients under nontraditional circumstances have been given a great deal of attention by military planners. The respiratory system requires either supportive care or therapeutic intervention in many wounded. Although spontaneous ventilation is possible with inhalation-based techniques, or with intravenous agents such ketamine or newer agents such as propofol, midazolam, and alfentanil, most general anesthetics require ventilatory support. Injuries to the chest and abdomen from shrapnel or conventional high-velocity military weapons are frequently fatal, although the advent and widespread use of body armor has increased the survival rates. However, these victims frequently have significant blunt trauma to the chest and may develop respiratory failure, requiring ventilatory support. The heavy reliance on mechanized armor in modern military operations increases the risk for thermal injury and associated inhalation injury. Fire-suppression systems may enhance the survival of occupants of armored vehicles and of personnel involved in naval and air operations, who are at significant risk for thermal injury. Many individuals injured under these circumstances are in closed spaces and sustain pulmonary injury resulting from the inhalation of steam or toxic by-products of combustion, in addition to burns and other injuries. Lastly, the respiratory system serves both as a portal of entry and as an organ system that is affected by chemical and biologic agents. Chemical agents can cause both respiratory paralysis and chemical pneumonitis leading to respiratory failure. Infectious agents are spread by aerosolization and enter through the respiratory tract, with the respiratory system being one of multiple end-organ systems targeted by these agents. While many of these injuries can be survived, they require sophisticated medical and supportive care.

Such care is technically demanding in regard to equipment, personnel, and supplies. Unlike treatment of other conventional wounds, which may consist of initial stabilization and repeated dressing changes and debridements, respiratory care is a continually demanding process that may be required for a protracted period of time and throughout all echelons of the medical-evacuation chain. In fact, in contrast to treatment of other types of injuries, for which simple life-saving care allows survival and evacuation to higher levels for more sophisticated care, respiratory support of high quality must be available at all levels of care, from the initial point of entry throughout the evacuation chain, if such patients are to survive their injuries.

The need for sophisticated respiratory care has posed a significant problem for military medical planners. The concept of the ideal ventilator has long been discussed. Many efforts have been made to adapt current ventilator technology to these conditions. However, with conventional ventilators for hospital use, there has been no need for constraints on size or weight. Gas supplies of air and oxygen have been readily available from piped-in supplies or from large cylinders and air compressors. Engineering and research have been devoted to understanding and better approximating normal respiratory mechanics to avoid barotrauma.

In addition, blood gas analysis has been readily available and has become the mainstay of the ventilator management of these patients. Physicians using these tools have made dramatic strides in the treatment of the adult respiratory distress syndrome that was initially described in soldiers wounded in Vietnam. Military planners and developers have been tasked with the nearly impossible job of bringing the ventilator technology currently available to the field setting, without sacrificing any therapeutic modalities or versatility. In addition, they must develop a group of technicians capable of operating and repairing sophisticated equipment and provide both a supply system and a laboratory system to support care.

TABLE 8. *Specifications for transport ventilators: military applications*

Lightweight, portable, durable
Economical use of compressed gas
Able to function in extreme climates and at high altitudes
Able to interface with protective filters
Able to withstand decontamination
Chemical, biologic, and nuclear
Aeromedical: meet RFI standards

RFI, radio-frequency interference.

Ideally, a single ventilator would be able to function at all levels of the field medical care system and evacuation chain (Table 8). The equipment should be lightweight and portable. It should be economical in the use of compressed gases. It must meet military specifications for durability and be able to function under extreme climatic conditions and at high altitudes without significant changes in function. If gas-operated, gas consumption requirements for power should be minimal. If electrically operated, it should function off multiple voltages and the software should be tolerant of variations in voltage and current. An integrated battery system is essential and should be capable of being charged while the ventilator is in operation. The equipment should tolerate storage for long periods of time with minimal maintenance. Alarms should be both visual and audible and operator-controlled, as this equipment may be used under conditions in which noise and light discipline are necessary. If this equipment is to be used throughout the evacuation chain, it must be simple to operate (as relatively untrained personnel may be called on to use it) and yet offer a wide range of ventilatory parameters. Circuitry should include an anti-asphyxiation valve to protect the patient from circuit obstruction during spontaneous or assisted ventilation. This circuitry should be simple to disassemble and clean, and additional circuits must be readily available. The entire ventilator must be capable of being integrated with a protective filter system and withstand decontamination procedures for use in an environment of chemical, biologic, or nuclear contamination. If the ventilator is to accompany the patient throughout the evacuation chain, then it must meet radio-frequency-interference (RFI) standards for aeromedical evacuation.

While it is attractive for this ventilator also to be suitable for use during the anesthetic management of these patients, current anesthesia delivery systems do not work with the types of ventilators that are currently available. The Ohmeda model 885-A field anesthesia machine (Ohmeda, Madison, Wisconsin) requires a bellows system in conjunction with the circle system; the bellows serves as a reservoir for respiratory gases between ventilatory cycles. The Ohmeda model 7000 ventilator is used with this anesthesia machine. The Ohmeda PAC drawover anesthesia system is a drawover delivery system that has an open circuit. This requires a reservoir from which respiratory gas is drawn through the vaporizer and subsequently forced into the patient. Pressurization of the vaporizer by a ventilator to force gas through the vaporizer to the patient results in altered anesthetic concentrations. No ventilator is available in the inventory for use with this system. The growing interest and development of total intravenous anesthesia delivery systems with computer-controlled infusion technology and modern short-acting narcotics (and other narcotics), hypnotics, and muscle relaxants make this an attractive alternative to the more traditional inhalational anesthetic techniques. Total intravenous anesthesia (TIVA) techniques would allow for the use of field ventilators and obviate the need for separate ventilators for anesthesia care.

The requirements for ventilators under field conditions are similar but more rigorous than the requirements for other circumstances. Transport ventilators such as those listed in Table 4 meet many if not all of the criteria and are either currently under evaluation or are included in the military inventory for respiratory care in the field.

Optimal Mechanical Ventilation for Transport and/or Care in Austere Conditions or Extreme Circumstances

Even standard anesthesia ventilators may not adequately ventilate those with chest, abdominal, or other trauma when adult respiratory distress syndrome (ARDS) or other disease produces gross abnormalities in lung or chest wall compliance. Ventilators of the type used in intensive care units are required under these circumstances (30). Those involved in the transport of seriously injured patients or patients with abnormal pulmonary compliance or excessive frictional airway resistance must make careful transport ventilator selections to assure sufficient ventilation under these circumstances. Pressure-controlled ventilation and inverse-ratio ventilation are used for victims of thoraco-abdominal trauma with noncompliant lungs and poor oxygenation when high concentrations of inspired oxygen and optimal PEEP are not sufficient. These modalities of ventilation are occasionally required during transport of the critically ill. The challenge in development and even selection of optimal transport ventilation systems for the ill and injured is a formidable one (Table 9). New developments that permit ventilation 1) with a variety of standard and enhanced ventilation modalities, 2) in a compact and durable device with flexible requirements in respect to power, and 3) with limited fresh gas flow requirements are vital to the effort of providing optimal care to those undergoing transport and/or treatment in austere or extreme environments.

TABLE 9. *Specifications for transport ventilators: summary of requirements*

Provide standard and enhanced ventilation modes
Perform reliably and effectively in
Critical care transport
Austere/remote environments
Be appropriately selected for
Specific patient population
Environment

CONCLUSION

In conclusion, the use of a portable transport ventilator leads to more consistent and safe ventilation and oxygenation of the patient requiring ventilatory support. The appropriate selection of a portable transport ventilator is based on a host of factors but primarily the patient transport population, specialized environmental considerations, and cost.

REFERENCES

1. Britten AG, Rogers MC. Transportation of critically ill children. In: Rogers MC, ed. *Textbook of Pediatric Intensive Care*. Baltimore: Williams & Wilkins; 1987:1385–1400.
2. Dobrin RS, Block B, Gilman JL, Massero TA. The development of a pediatric emergency transport system. *Pediatr Clin North Am* 1980; 27:633–646.
3. Hart HW. The conveyance of patients to and from hospitals, 1720–1850. *Med Hist* 1978;22:397–407.
4. Boyd DR. Comprehensive regional trauma and emergency medical service delivery systems: a goal of the 1980's. *Crit Care Q* 1982; 5:1–21.
5. On tubes, techniques and procedures. In: Burton GG, Gee GN, Hodgkin JE, eds. *Respiratory Care: a Guide to Clinical Practice*, 1st ed. Philadelphia: JB Lippincott; 1977:501–538.
6. Waddell G. Movement of critically ill patients within hospital. *Br Med J* 1975;2:417–419.
7. Braman SS, Dunn SM, Amico CA, Millman RP. Complications of intrahospital transport in critically ill patients. *Ann Intern Med* 1987; 107:469–473.
8. Gervais HW, Eberle B, Konietzke D, Hennes HJ, Dick W. Comparison of blood gases of ventilated patients during transport. *Crit Care Med* 1987;8:761–763.
9. Hurst JM, Davis K, Branson RD. Comparison of blood gases during transport using two methods of ventilatory support. *J Trauma* 1989; 29:1637–1640.
10. Girotti LA, Crosatto JR, Messutti H, et al. Hyperventilation test as a method for developing successful therapy in Prinzmetal's angina. *Am J Cardiol* 1982;49:834.
11. Freeman LJ, Nixon PGF. Are coronary artery spasm and progressive damage to the heart associated with the hyperventilation syndrome? *Br Med J* 1985;291:851.
12. Wollman H, Alexander SC, Cohen PJ, et al. Cerebral circulation during general anesthesia and hyperventilation in man. *Anesthesiology* 1965;26:329
13. Branson RD. Intrahospital transport of critically ill, mechanically ventilated patients. *Respir Care* 1992;37:775–795.
14. Scuderi J, Elton CB, Elton DR. A cart to provide high frequency jet ventilation during transport of neonates. *Respir Care* 1992;37:129–136.

15. McPherson SP. Primary systems: cylinders and piping systems. *Respiratory Therapy Equipment*. St. Louis: CV Mosby; 1977:36.
16. Oakes D. Equations. *Clinical Practitioner's Pocket Guide to Respiratory Care*. Old Town, Maine: Health Educator Publications; 1988: 180–199.
17. Branson RD, Hurst JM, Adams KS, Kessinger CK. Utilization of mechanical ventilators in hospital based air ambulance programs. *Hosp Aviation* 1986;5(Suppl 1):6–7.
18. Sassoon CSH, Mahutte CK, Light RW. Ventilator modes: old and new. *Crit Care Clin* 1990;6:605–634.
19. Marini JJ. Strategies to minimize breathing effort during mechanical ventilation. *Crit Care Clin* 1990;6:635–661.
20. Hinson JR, Marini JJ. Principles of mechanical ventilator use in respiratory failure. *Annu Rev Med* 1992;341–361.
21. Downs JB, Klein EF, Desautels D, et al. Intermittent mandatory ventilation: a new approach to weaning patients from mechanical ventilators. *Chest* 1973;64:331–335.
22. MacIntyre NR. New forms of mechanical ventilation in the adult. *Clin Chest Med* 1988;9:47–54.
23. Hubmayr RD, Martin DA, Rehder K. Physiologic approach to mechanical ventilation. *Crit Care Med* 1990;18:103–113.
24. McGough EK, Banner MJ, Melker RJ. Variations in tidal volumes with portable transport ventilators. *Respir Care* 1992;37:233–239.
25. Newport Medical Instruments, Inc. *Newport Ventilator E100i Operating Manual*. Rev. 1/89, Second Release:55.
26. Eyler R, Reid R. Effects of altitude on the Bio-Med MVP-10 transport ventilator. *Air Med J* 1993;9:341(abst).
27. Blanch PB, Desautels DA, Gallagher TJ. Deviations in function of mechanical ventilators during hyperbaric compression. *Respir Care* 1992;36:803–814.
28. Ridenour J, Schreiber V, Kelin K, Heller M, Menegazzi J. Noise exposure to flight crew from the MBB BO-105 and MBBK-117 helicopter. *J Air Med Transport* 1990;9:76(abst).
29. Campbell AN, Lightstone AD, Smith JM, Kirpalani H, Peralman M. Mechanical vibration and sound levels experienced in neonatal transport. *Am J Dis Child* 1984;138:967–970.
30. Marks JD, Schapera A, Kraemer RW, Katz J. Pressure and flow limitations of anesthesia ventilators. *Anesthesiology* 1989;71:403–408.

VI

Appendix

Appendix A

PATIENTS WHO MAY CAUSE DIFFICULTIES AT INTUBATION

This is a partial list. In patients with these conditions, it is advisable to consider alternatives or extra help as conventional intubation techniques may be inadequate.

Problems with the upper airway:

- Congenital deformities, e.g., Pierre-Robin, Treacher-Collins, cleft palate, microstomia
- Trismus (traumatic, infectious)
- Facial injuries (fractures of mandible or middle third face)
- Pregnancy (preeclampsia)
- Oral infections (especially submandibular and peritonsillar abscesses/ Ludwig's angina)
- Epistaxis and nasopharyngeal bleeding
- Burns (contractures and edema)
- Epiglottitis/ croup

Positioning problems:

- Cervical spine fracture or instability, e.g, rheumatoid arthritis/Down syndrome
- Cervical spine ankylosis or fusion (including kyphosis)
- Obesity, Cushing syndrome, pregnancy

Problems with the trachea:

- Foreign body
- Tracheal stenosis or compression (thyroid, tumor)
- Bacterial tracheitis/croup
- Tracheomalacia
- Traumatic tracheobronchial disruption/bronchopleural fistulae

Problems with response to intubation:

- Head injuries, cerebral aneurysms, cerebral arteriovenous malformations
- Penetrating eye injuries
- Cardiovascular disease (hypertension, ischemic heart disease, ruptured abdominal aortic aneurysms)

Problems concerning drug administration:

- Allergy
- Shock, hypovolemia
- Compromised myocardium
- Idiosyncratic (succinylcholine apnea, malignant hyperthermia)
- Myopathies and muscular dystrophies
- Burns (contractures, hyperkalemia with succinylcholine)
- Altered drug handling, e.g., renal/liver failure, neonates, elderly

Appendix B

INDICATIONS FOR INTUBATION

Remember: there are absolute and relative indications. The list below covers the most common indications for intubation.

1. Resuscitation
   a) cardiac or respiratory failure /arrest
      e.g., cardiac arrest, chest trauma, flail chest, pneumothorax, pulmonary embolus, obstructed airway (epiglottitis, croup, bilateral recurrent laryngeal nerve palsy)
   b) control of carbon dioxide
      e.g., head injuries, raised intracranial pressure
2. Protection of the Airway
   a) unconscious patient
      e.g, stroke, drug overdose, diabetic coma, other causes of coma
   b) full stomach, bleeding in the airway
      e.g ,general anesthesia for caesarian section, inadequate fasting, faciomaxillary trauma, epistaxis
   c) paralysis (chemical or traumatic)
3. Surgical access to site of operation
   a) faciomaxillary surgery/remote diagnostic procedures
      e.g., MRI, CT scan
   b) shared airway procedures
      e.g., microlaryngoscopy, rigid esophagoscopy, tonsillectomy
   c) patient positioning, i.e., prone, lateral
   d) prolonged surgery

Endotracheal Absorption of Drugs

The following drugs may be given via an endotracheal tube in emergency situations where intravenous access has not been secured. Note that consideration should be given to absorption via the lungs.

Lidocaine
Atropine
Epinephrine
Isoproterenol
Naloxone

Indications for Nasotracheal Intubation

Certain intraoral and plastic operations on the head
Repair of fractured mandible
Ankylosis of the temporomandibular joint
Conditions that make laryngoscopy and oral intubations difficult
Some intubations in the intensive care setting

Contraindications for Nasotracheal Intubation

Choanal atresia
Coagulopathy
Fractured base of skull (otorrhea, bleeding from ear after trauma)
Presence of cerebrospinal fluid rhinorrhea (anterior cranial fossa fracture)
Severe intranasal pathology
Fractured middle third of face (Le Forte)

Appendix C

SELECTION OF ENDOTRACHEAL TUBES

Age	Size (mm ID)
Premature	
Under 1500 gm	2.5
1500–5000 gm	3.0
Infant 3–6 months	3.0–3.5
6–12 months	3.5–4.0
1–6 years	[Age (years) /3]+3.75
Over 6 years	[Age (years) /4]+4.5

AVERAGE DIMENSIONS AND INSERTION DISTANCE OF ENDOTRACHEAL TUBES

Age	Internal diameter	External diameter	Insertion distance at teeth (at nose)
Adult (≥ 14 yrs)	8.0–9.0 mm	10.8–12.1 mm	20–21 (24–25) cm
10 years	6.5 mm	8.9 mm	17 (21) cm
6 years	5.5 mm	7.5 mm	15 (19) cm
4 years	5.0 mm	6.9 mm	14 (17) cm
1 year	4.0 mm	5.6 mm	11 (14) cm
3 months	3.5 mm	4.9 mm	10 (12) cm
Newborn (≤ 3 kg)	3.0 mm	4.9 mm	6 (7.5) cm

Appendix D

INSERTION OF OTHER AIRWAY DEVICES

Laryngeal Mask Airways

Range of LMAs

LMA size	1	2	2.5	3	4	5
rLMA size		2	2.5	3	4	
Patient weight (kg)	0–6.5	6.5–20	20–30	30–70	70–90	>90
Cuff Volume (ml)	2–5	7–10	12–15	15–20	25–30	35–40

LMA, laryngeal mask airway; rLMA, reinforced laryngeal mask airway

Size of ETTs througlh the LMA

LMA size	1	2	2.5	3	4	5
Length (cm)	10	11.5	12.5	19	19	20
ID/OD	5.25/8.0	7.0/11.0	8.4/13.0	10/15.0	10/15.0	11.5/16.5
ETT size (uncuffed)	3.5	4.5	5.0	6.5	6.5	8.0
ETT size (cuffed)	-	-	-	6.0	6.0	7.5
FFB size (outer diameter)	2.7	3.5	4.0	5.0	5.0	6.5

ID, Internal diameter; OD, Outer diameter; FFB, flexible fiberoptic bronchoscope

Combitubes

Insertion:
Head in neutral position
Chin lift
If necessary, use laryngoscope to lift tongue AWAY (do NOT attempt to visualize vocal cords)
Apply gentle pressure and insert so that the 2 black lines are at the level of the upper teeth.
Patient must be flaccid
Cuff Inflation:
Use entire 100 cc for oropharyngeal (#l) balloon first and then 15 cc for the esophageal (#2) balloon
ETC should "pop out" 1 cm with inflation of cuffs
Ventilation:
Ventilate # 1 (Blue) lumen first
94%–98% chance esophageal placement
DO NOT manipulate ETC/head when changing ventilation from lumen #1 to lumen #2
Contraindications:
1. Patients under 5 feet tall
2. Patients with intact gag reflex
3. Patients with known esophageal disease
4. Patients who have ingested caustic substances
5. Upper airway (supralaryngeal) obstruction

Appendix E

COMMONLY USED DRUGS FOR THE CONTROL OF AIRWAYS

Below is a list of commonly used anesthetic drugs and suggested drug dosages. There are many side effects and precautions for all these agents–refer to more detailed texts.

Intravenous Induction Agents

Many of these drugs may be used as sedatives in appropriate dosages. The suggested dosages given here are for induction of anesthesia *only* in normal, fit, healthy adults. Please note there are many patients who require far less than these dosages, e.g., shock/hypovolemia, neonates, elderly, concurrent administration of other sedatives/opiates/local anesthetic agents.

Drug	Typical Concentration	Induction Dosage
Thiopental	2.5% (25 mg/ml)	3–5 mg/kg
Propofol	1% (10 mg/ml)	2–2.5 mg/kg
Etomidate	0.2% (2 mg/ml)	0.25 mg/kg
Ketamine	50 mg/ml or 100 mg/ml	2–3 mg/kg
Midazolam	0.1% (1 mg/ml)	0.15–0.30 mg/kg

Neuromuscular Blockers

These drugs should only be given to patients who are already or about to be ventilated. They have no sedative, analgesic, or anesthetic action other than paralyzing patients. Intubation dosages are given here. Subsequent doses for patients already intubated and paralyzed are generally one-quarter the intubation dose. Succinylcholine is an exception.

Drug	Dosage	Clinical Duration
Succinycholine	1.5–2 mg/kg	5–10 minutes
Mivacurium	0.2–0.25 mg/kg	10–15 minutes
Rocuronium[a]	0.6–0.8 mg/kg	20–30 minutes
Vecuronium[a]	0.08–0.1 mg/kg	20–30 minutes
Atracurium	0.4–0.5 mg/kg	20–30 minutes
Pancuronium	0.8–1.0 mg/kg	45–60 minutes

[a]Drug is suitable in a higher dose for rapid sequence induction of anesthesia.

Subject Index

ISBN 0-397-51520-0

9 780397 515202